INSURANCE HANDBOOK
FOR THE MEDICAL OFFICE

14TH EDITION

INSURANCE HANDBOOK
FOR THE MEDICAL OFFICE

MARILYN TAKAHASHI FORDNEY, CMA-AC (AAMA)

Formerly Instructor of Medical Insurance,
Medical Terminology, Medical Machine
Transcription, and Medical Office Procedures
Ventura College
Ventura, California

ELSEVIER

ELSEVIER

3251 Riverport Lane
St. Louis, Missouri 63043

INSURANCE HANDBOOK FOR THE MEDICAL OFFICE   ISBN: 978-0-323-31625-5
FOURTEENTH EDITION

Notices

Knowledge and best practice in this field are constantly changing. As new research and experience broaden our understanding, changes in research methods, professional practices, or medical treatment may become necessary.

Practitioners and researchers must always rely on their own experience and knowledge in evaluating and using any information, methods, compounds, or experiments described herein. In using such information or methods they should be mindful of their own safety and the safety of others, including parties for whom they have a professional responsibility.

With respect to any drug or pharmaceutical products identified, readers are advised to check the most current information provided (i) on procedures featured or (ii) by the manufacturer of each product to be administered, to verify the recommended dose or formula, the method and duration of administration, and contraindications. It is the responsibility of practitioners, relying on their own experience and knowledge of their patients, to make diagnoses, to determine dosages and the best treatment for each individual patient, and to take all appropriate safety precautions.

To the fullest extent of the law, neither the Publisher nor the authors, contributors, or editors, assume any liability for any injury and/or damage to persons or property as a matter of products liability, negligence or otherwise, or from any use or operation of any methods, products, instructions, or ideas contained in the material herein.

Previous editions copyrighted 2014, 2012, 2010, 2008, 2006, 2004, 2002, 1999, 1997, 1995, 1989, 1981, and 1977.

Library of Congress Cataloging-in-Publication Data

Fordney, Marilyn Takahashi, author.
  Insurance handbook for the medical office / Marilyn Takahashi Fordney. -- 14th edition.
     p. ; cm.
  Includes bibliographical references and index.
  ISBN 978-0-323-31625-5 (pbk. : alk. paper)
  I. Title.
  [DNLM: 1. Insurance, Health--United States--Handbooks. 2. Clinical Coding--United States--Handbooks. 3. Insurance Claim Reporting--United States--Handbooks. 4. Insurance, Liability--United States--Handbooks. 5. Office Management--United States--Handbooks. W 49]
  HG9396
  368.38'2002461--dc23
                                                                                          2015027189

Executive Content Strategist: Jennifer Janson
Content Development Manager: Ellen Wurm-Cutter
Senior Content Development Specialist: Rebecca Leenhouts
Publishing Services Manager: Jeff Patterson
Book Production Specialist: Bill Drone
Book Designer: Paula Catalano

 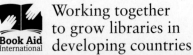
Printed in China.

Last digit is the print number: 9 8 7 6 5 4 3 2 1

I dedicate the fourteenth edition:

To the memory of my parents, Margaret O'Brien Uchiyamada
and Toshio James Takahashi, who gave me positive reinforcement
throughout their lives.

To my husband, Sándor Havasi, who has helped to guide and nurture
the Havasi Wilderness Foundation and Fordney Foundation that were
created as a result of the success of this publication.

To my youngest sister, Esme Takahashi, who offered encouragement
throughout my years of writing. And to her daughter, Gemma Hiranuma.

To all of the Elsevier Science/Saunders, Health Career editors
and production department teams, who always managed to meet target
dates for 40 years.

To the reviewers, who have helped to make this a better publication through
their suggestions and comments.

To the contributors, who have implemented new ideas and updated many
chapters to keep the material current.

To the thousands of students who used this textbook in the past and
to those who will use it in the future to obtain a better job.

Share peace and love.

Marilyn Takahashi Fordney

About the Author

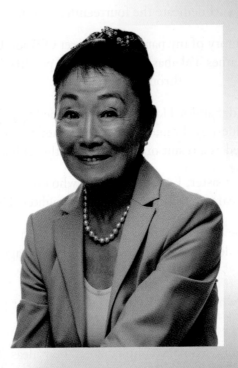

A dedicated professional, Marilyn Takahashi Fordney worked as a medical assistant for 14 years in various settings. During her 19-year teaching career, she taught courses in administrative medical assisting, medical insurance, and medical terminology at many community colleges and in adult education schools. Fordney is a Certified Medical Assistant. In 1977, she was named "Woman of the Year" by the Business and Professional Women's Club of Oxnard, California. In June 2005, Fordney was inducted into the Council of Fellows by the Text and Academic Authors Association in Las Vegas, Nevada.

Fordney's books have won national awards. This textbook, *Insurance Handbook for the Medical Office*, won the William Holmes McGuffey Award in Life Sciences for its excellence and longevity in the field. *Medical Insurance Billing and Coding: An Essentials Worktext*, a spin-off of the *Handbook*, won the Texty Excellence Award in its first edition.

The success of Fordney's books has allowed her to establish two foundations. The Fordney Foundation for DanceSport (www.fordneyfoundation.org) is a nonprofit foundation for amateur ballroom dancers aged 6 to 25 years. The foundation's objective is to help children and young adults to realize their dreams of artistic expression through ballroom dancing. The Havasi Wilderness Foundation (www.havasiwf.org) is a nonprofit foundation to assist in the preservation and protection of the earth's most precious places for future generations. It gives funds to schools for field trips so that students can learn about the wilderness in state and national or private parks. The foundation provides educational in-classroom interactive PowerPoint presentations to elementary school children.

Welcome to the Fourteenth Edition

When this textbook was first published in 1977, few people were aware of how important the subject of health insurance would become. *Insurance Handbook for the Medical Office* now celebrates its fortieth year. I have told others around me, "I don't think I ever dreamed I would be writing this long," and sometimes I pinch myself to see if it is really true. Through the years, this textbook has become the leader in its field because of its interactive learning system. The *Handbook* has gained wide acceptance across the nation among educators and working insurance billing specialists and coders.

Because of the many federal and state legislative mandates and technologic advances that have occurred since the previous edition, putting the fourteenth edition together has been challenging and exciting. Because changes occur daily in the insurance industry, *Insurance Handbook for the Medical Office* is revised every 2 years to keep the information current.

PURPOSE

The goals of this textbook are to prepare students to excel as insurance billing specialists and to increase efficiency and streamline administrative procedures for one of the most complex tasks of the physician's business: insurance coding and billing.

Why Is This Book Important to the Profession?

In the past two decades, health care professionals and the community have witnessed the emergence of an administrative medical specialty known variously as insurance billing specialist, medical biller, or reimbursement specialist. Several national organizations offer certification in the field, which has quickly achieved recognition and professionalism. Thus, the *Handbook* has been written to address this specialty as another branch of the administrative medical assistant profession. Health care reform has led to an explosion of jobs in the medical field, especially for those trained in coding and processing insurance claims both electronically and manually. Training in this area is necessary because, as a result of a lack of knowledge among office personnel, it is common to find medical practices either undercharging or not charging for billable services.

Insurance claims are being submitted for patients on the recommendation of management consultants to control cash flow, obtain correct reimbursement amounts, honor insurance contracts, compete with other medical practices, and maintain a good relationship with patients. Even offices that do not routinely complete insurance claims for patients make exceptions for elderly patients or patients with mental incompetence, illiteracy, diminished eyesight, or a poor command of the English language. When the amount of the bill is hundreds or thousands of dollars or when a surgical report is required, the physician's office should submit the bill to obtain maximum reimbursement. Individuals who administer the federal government's Medicare program increasingly promote electronic transmission of insurance claims for medium-sized and large medical practices. Because of these factors, as well as federal mandates to document care electronically, the amount of knowledge and skills that one must have has substantially increased. This textbook addresses all clerical functions of the insurance billing specialist, and illustrations throughout the text feature generic forms created to help simplify billing procedures.

Who Will Benefit From This Book?

Numerous schools and colleges have established 1-year certificate programs for those interested in a career as an insurance billing specialist, and many programs offer medical insurance as a full-semester, 18-week course on campus or as a hybrid course (mix of online and face-to-face classroom instruction). Community college extension divisions also offer community service classes and short courses in this subject. Some schools include it as part of a medical assisting program's curriculum, so the individual has knowledge in all administrative functions of a physician's office. The textbook may be used as a learning tool and resource guide in all of those programs as well as in vocational or commercial training institutes and welfare-work programs. *Insurance Handbook for the Medical Office* also serves as a text for in-service training in the private medical office. The *Handbook* may be used for independent home study, if no formal classes are available in the community. The layperson who is not pursuing a career in the medical field will find the textbook useful when working with a claims assistance professional or for billing his or her insurance plans. Insurance companies and their agents have found the *Handbook* to be a valuable reference tool when answering clients' questions.

The textbook is designed primarily for students who plan to seek employment in an outpatient setting (e.g., physician's office or clinic) or who wish to establish an independent billing business and need a thorough understanding of the reimbursement process. Many types of insurance coverage are available in the United States. The types most commonly encountered in physicians' offices and clinics have been emphasized in this textbook in simple, nontechnical explanations and tables. Electronic documentation in the medical record is the key to substantiating procedure and diagnostic code selections for proper reimbursement. Thus, in this edition, Chapter 4, *Medical Documentation and the Electronic Health Record*, has been further updated and enhanced. In recent years, the federal government targeted this issue with the introduction of Medicare compliance policies related to documentation and confidentiality; such issues are therefore covered to help physicians comply with possible reviews or audits of their billing practices. Because of the implementation by October 2015 of the *International Classification of Diseases*, Tenth Revision, Clinical Modification (ICD-10-CM), this diagnostic code system information has been greatly expanded throughout the textbook and workbook. It will help to ease the transition to this larger and more specific code system. Since health care reform affects federal programs, employers, and health insurance companies, information about the legislation and when it phases in is explained throughout various chapters. Finally, the textbook may be used as a stand-alone reference source or as an educational tool to increase the knowledge of someone currently working as an insurance billing specialist in a private medical office.

CONTENT

General Features

Each chapter has been updated to reflect current policies and procedures.

- All chapters have been completely restructured for better organization and flow of content, with legal information included where applicable to insurance billing and coding. The information presented is not a substitute for legal advice, and the physician and his or her insurance billing specialist should always seek legal counsel about specific questions of law as they relate to medical practice.

- "Service to Patients" color-screened boxes at the beginning of each chapter highlight patient service with regard to the topic being discussed.
- HIPAA Compliance Alerts are interspersed throughout all chapters for emphasis.

- Objectives are provided at the beginning of each chapter, sequenced to match the technical content, and help to guide instructors in preparing lecture material and inform readers about what material is presented.
- By reviewing the key terms that introduce each chapter, students are alerted to important words for the topic. Key abbreviations follow the key terms; spellouts of the abbreviations are provided in a section that follows the Glossary near the back of the textbook.
- Boxed examples are provided throughout each chapter.
- Key points are presented at the end of each chapter, summarizing and emphasizing the most important technical information in the chapter.

Many experts in the field reviewed the chapters in the thirteenth edition and several key chapters for this fourteenth edition so that improvements in content, clarity of topics, and deletions could be considered. The unique color-coded icons have been visually updated and are featured throughout the textbook to denote and clarify information specific to each type of payer. This system makes the learning process more effective by helping students to identify each insurance payer with a specific color and graphic. These icons follow:

 Property and Casualty Claims: All payer guidelines, including all private insurance companies and all federal and state programs.

 Medicaid: State Medicaid programs.

 Medicare: Federal Medicare programs, Medicare/Medicaid, Medicare/Medigap, and Medicare Secondary Payer (MSP).

 TRICARE: TRICARE Standard (formerly CHAMPUS), TRICARE Prime, and TRICARE Extra.

CHAMPVA: Civilian Health and Medical Program of the Department of Veterans Affairs.

Workers' Compensation: State workers' compensation programs.

Managed Care: All managed care organizations.

Maternal and Child Health Program: State and federal program for children under 21 years of age and with special health needs.

Disability Income Insurance: Insurance programs that replace income lost due to illness, injury, or disease.

Consumer-Directed Health Plans: Self-directed health plans that often pair a high-deductible preferred provider organization (PPO) plan with a tax-advantaged account.

Indemnity Health Insurance: Traditional or fee-for-service health plans.

ORGANIZATION

- Chapters 1 through 6 show basic health insurance information and coding examples for persons who are studying for a certification examination. Special emphasis is placed on correct and incorrect procedural codes and appropriate documentation—the keys to obtaining maximum reimbursement.
- Chapter 2, *Compliance, Privacy, Fraud, and Abuse in Insurance Billing*, focuses on the Health Insurance Portability and Accountability Act (HIPAA). The chapter explains HIPAA's effect on insurance reform and administrative simplification, along with other topics related to privacy, fraud, and abuse.
- Chapter 7, *The Paper Claim: CMS-1500 (02-12)*, uses a unique block-by-block approach specific to each different payer that denotes and clarifies information about the recently revised CMS-1500 (02-12) insurance claim form. The icons and graphics system is used to help students retain information. Templates

illustrate placement of information on the form consistent with the National Uniform Claim Committee's guidelines.

- Chapter 8, *The Electronic Claim*, has been updated. It contains additional HIPAA information on requirements for electronic transmission of insurance claims and explains the security rules.
- Chapters 9 through 16 provide many specific quick-action solutions for insurance problems and information about tracing delinquent claims and appealing denied claims. Thorough up-to-date information is presented for Medicare, Medicaid, TRICARE, private plans, workers' compensation, managed care plans, disability income insurance, and disability benefit programs. Helpful billing tips and guidelines for submitting insurance claims are given for each type of insurance program covered.
- Chapter 17, *Hospital Billing*, is intended especially for those students interested in pursuing a career in the hospital setting. Information about the *International Classification of Diseases*, Tenth Revision, Procedure Classification System (ICD-10-PCS) is presented. Additionally, step-by-step procedures are stated for processing a new patient for admission and to verify insurance benefits.
- Chapter 18, *Seeking a Job and Attaining Professional Advancement*, provides information pertinent to seeking a position as an insurance billing specialist, a self-employed claims assistance professional, or an electronic claims processor using high-tech procedures. The chapter explains the effect of HIPAA compliance policies on a business associate when hired by a medical practice to do insurance claim submission.
- The appendix aids the insurance billing specialist in locating audiotapes, books, newsletters, periodicals, software, and videotapes from various resources. It lists names, addresses, toll-free telephone numbers, and websites.
- An extensive glossary of basic medical and insurance terms and a comprehensive list of all technical abbreviations within each chapter, along with their spellouts, is included.

ANCILLARIES

Workbook

Users of the *Workbook* that accompanies this edition of the textbook will find the following features:

- Competency-based education is discussed. A point system has been applied to code and claims completion for *Workbook* assignments for instructors who need to document and gather statistics for competency-based education. The worksheets for each assignment are available on the Evolve website. *Handbook* learning objectives, *Workbook* performance objectives for all assignments, use of the tutorial software with reinforcement by *Workbook* assignments, the test section at the end of the *Workbook*, the quizzes of key terms featured on the website, and incorporation of classroom activities and suggestions from the *TEACH Instructor's Resource Manual* (available on the companion Evolve website) provide a complete competency-based educational program.

- Expanded Self-Assessment Quizzes for each chapter are available on the Evolve website for student use.
- Patient records and ledgers have been updated and reworded to correspond with the 2015 procedural codes and ICD-10-CM diagnostic code books.
- All chapters have fill-in-the-blank, multiple-choice, mix-and-match, and true/false review questions. Answers have been put into the *TEACH Instructor's Resource Manual* (available on the companion Evolve website).

General Features

For students, the *Workbook* that accompanies the textbook is a practical approach to learning insurance billing. It progresses from easy to more complex issues within each chapter and advances as new skills are learned and integrated. Chapter outlines serve as a lecture guide. Each chapter has performance objectives for assignments that indicate to students what will be accomplished. Key terms are repeated for quick reference when studying. Key abbreviations followed by blank lines are listed alphabetically so that students can assemble their own reference list for each chapter, thus reinforcing the abbreviations' spellouts. Patients' medical records, financial accounting statements, and encounter forms are presented as they might appear in the physician's files, so that students may learn how to abstract information to complete claim forms properly and accurately. Patient records and ledgers have been completely updated for technical clinical content and reworded to correspond with the 2015 procedural and ICD-10-CM diagnostic code books. Easily removable forms and other sample documents are included in the *Workbook* for completion and to enhance keying skills. Insurance claim forms and letterheads are available on the Evolve website. Some assignments give students hands-on experience in keying insurance claims on the CMS-1500 (02-12) claim forms using standardized guidelines developed by the National Uniform Claim Committee. Current procedural and diagnostic code exercises are used throughout the *Workbook* to facilitate and enhance coding skills for submitting a claim or posting to a patient's financial account statement. Critical thinking problems are presented in each chapter. Special appendixes are included at the end of the *Workbook*. These include a simulated practice, the College Clinic,

with a group of physicians who employ the student; a mock fee schedule with codes and fees (including Medicare); and an abbreviated Medicare Level II Healthcare Common Procedure Coding System (HCPCS) alphanumeric code list. The appendixes may be used as reference tools to complete the procedural code problems. These appendixes include the following:

- Appendix A details information for a simulated practice called *College Clinic*. Information is provided about the group of physicians and a mock fee schedule is included with codes and fees (including Medicare).
- Appendix B provides an abbreviated Medicare Level II HCPCS alphanumeric code list with a list of modifiers.
- Appendixes C and D contain reference tables from ICD-10-PCS for characters in codes created for medical/surgical procedures.

Student Software Challenge (Located on Evolve)

The Student Software Challenge located on Evolve is user-friendly software that provides students with another opportunity for hands-on learning. This software simulates a realistic experience by having students gather necessary documents and extract specific information to complete the CMS-1500 (02-12) insurance claim form. All source documents appear on screen and may be viewed simultaneously in a separate window. The Student Software Challenge also allows users to print the claim form for evaluation and edit it to correct errors.

The main objective is to complete CMS-1500 (02-12) forms for each case and insert accurate data, including diagnostic and procedural code numbers. Instructors may want their students to work through the first case or basic cases (1 through 4) strictly for learning and to use Case 5 for testing and grading. Cases 6 through 10, which are advanced and insurance-specific (e.g., Medicare, TRICARE), may be used for practice or testing. This simulated learning methodology makes possible an easier transition from classroom to workplace.

Additional features of the Student Software Challenge for the fourteenth edition of this textbook include the following:

- Blank interactive forms that can be typed into and printed or saved to be turned in to the instructor. This creates clean claims that are easier to read and grade.
- Complete fee schedule to simplify the insertion of fees on the CMS-1500 (02-12) claim form or financial accounting record.

TEACH Instructor's Resource Manual (Located on Evolve)

The *TEACH Instructor's Resource Manual* is available on the Evolve site; it contains lesson plans, *Workbook* answer keys, a test bank, and PowerPoint slides. This resource allows instructors the flexibility to quickly adapt the textbook for their individual classroom needs and to gauge students' understanding. The *TEACH Instructor's Resource Manual* features the following:

- Guidelines for establishing a medical insurance course
- Answer keys to the *Workbook* and Student Software Challenge assignments and tests with rationales, optional codes, and further explanations for most of the code problems
- Lesson plans for each chapter
- Suggested classroom activities and games
- Ideas on how to use the text as an adjunct to an administrative medical assisting or medical office procedures course
- Pretests for each chapter

Evolve Companion Website

Evolve is an interactive learning environment that works in coordination with the textbook. It provides internet-based course management tools that instructors can use to reinforce and expand on the concepts delivered in class. It can be used for the following:

- To publish the class syllabus, outline, and lecture notes
- To set up "virtual office hours" and e-mail communication
- To share important dates and information through the online class calendar
- To encourage student participation through chat rooms and discussion boards

Evolve also provides online access to free Learning Resources designed specifically to give students the information they need to quickly and successfully learn the topics covered in this textbook. These Learning Resources include the following:

- Self-assessment quizzes to evaluate students' mastery through multiple-choice, true/false, fill-in-the-blank, and matching questions. Instant scoring and feedback are available at the click of a button.
- Technical updates to keep up with changes in government regulations and codes as well as other industry changes.

- SimChart for the Medical Office application cases focused on the Billing and Coding module. SCMO customers can utilize this resource to reinforce practice management and EHR skills.
- Performance Evaluation Checklists.

Elsevier Adaptive Learning (Additional Purchase Required)

Elsevier Adaptive Learning is a uniquely personalized and interactive tool that enables students to learn faster and remember longer. It's fun; it's engaging; and it's constantly tracking student performance and adapting to deliver content precisely when it's needed to ensure information is transformed into lasting knowledge.

- Greater student performance
- Long-term knowledge storage
- Individualized learning
- Cognitive skills training
- Time management Dashboards and reporting
- Mobile app

SUMMARY

The *Handbook* and its ancillaries provide a complete competency-based educational program. *Handbook* learning objectives, *Workbook* performance objectives, assignments, tests, Student Software Challenge, and incorporation of lesson plans and suggested classroom activities from the *TEACH Instructor's Resource Manual* ensure that students know everything they need to succeed in the workforce. Escalating costs of medical care, the effect of technology, and the rapid increase of managed care plans have affected insurance billing procedures and claims processing and have necessitated new legislation for government and state programs. Therefore it is essential that all medical personnel who handle claims continually update their knowledge. This may be accomplished by reading bulletins from state agencies and regional insurance carriers, speaking with insurance representatives, or attending insurance workshops offered at local colleges or local chapters of professional associations, such as those mentioned in Chapters 1 and 18. It is hoped that this textbook will resolve any unclear issues pertaining to current methods and become the framework on which the insurance billing specialist builds new knowledge as understanding and appreciation of the profession are attained.

Marilyn Takahashi Fordney, CMA-AC (AAMA)
Agoura Hills, California

Acknowledgments

First, a special thank you to my husband, Sándor Havasi, who has encouraged and motivated me with his support to continue writing in this challenging and ever-changing career field.

Three contributors have assisted in updating and lending their expertise to eight of the chapters. I wish to thank Linda M. Smith, Karen M. Levein, and Payel Bhattacharya Madero for their diligence in meeting deadlines and doing an excellent job.

During my 14 years as a medical assistant, 19 years of teaching, and more than 40 years of writing, hundreds of students, physicians, friends, colleagues, and instructors have contributed valuable suggestions and interesting material for this textbook. I thank all of them, especially the following individuals:

- Lois C. Oliver, retired professor, Pierce College, Woodland Hills, California, helped me to organize my first medical insurance class in 1969 and offered assistance and encouragement throughout the preparation of the first edition of the *Handbook*.
- Marcia O. "Marcy" Diehl, CMA-A (AAMA), CMT, a former co-author and retired instructor, Grossmont Community College, El Cajon, California, generously shared her knowledge, ideas, and class materials. Marcy motivated me to submit my first manuscript to several publishers, and without her urging I probably would not have taken action in that direction.
- Members of the California Association of Medical Assistant Instructors (CAMAI) contributed suggestions for improving the textbook and gave me motivation to continue the project.
- Mary E. Kinn, CPS, CMA-A (AAMA), author and retired assistant professor, Long Beach City College, Long Beach, California, provided a perspective review of my syllabus. Without her positive endorsement, the first edition of this book might not have been published.
- The students of Linda French's former classes at Simi Valley Adult School and Career Institute in Simi Valley, California, who contributed their criticisms, shared technical subject matter, offered suggestions, and through voluntary participation, helped to enhance and create *Workbook* assignments for one of the previous editions.
- Karen Levein, CPC, CPC-I, Instructor at Burbank Adult School and The Coding Source, who offered clarification suggestions for the *Handbook*, gave technical assistance for the *Workbook* assignments, and updated many codes in the *TEACH Instructor's Resource Manual* answer keys. Her input is due to current classroom experiences with students.

I gratefully acknowledge the work of Paula Catalano, Art and Design, Elsevier, for the design of this edition. Sun West Studio of Ventura, California, took the photograph for "About the Author." I acknowledge and thank them both.

I also thank the print shop staff, Publications Department, Ventura College, Ventura, California, who printed the first California syllabus of this text.

I am indebted to many individuals on the staff at Elsevier for encouragement and guidance. I express special appreciation to Jennifer Janson, Executive Content Strategist; Rebecca Leenhouts, Senior Content Development Specialist; William Drone, Book Production Specialist; and Jeff Patterson, Publishing Services Manager, for coordination of the entire project.

Numerous supply companies were kind enough to cooperate by providing forms and descriptive literature of their products and their names are found throughout the textbook and *Workbook* figures.

However, colleagues, production staff, and editors working as a team do not quite make a book; there are others to whom I must express overwhelming debt and enduring gratitude, and these are the consultants who reviewed some of the chapters or who provided vital information about private, state, and federal insurance programs. Without the knowledge of these advisers, the massive task of compiling an insurance textbook that is truly national in scope might never have been completed. Although the names of all of those who graciously assisted me are too numerous to mention, I take great pride in listing my principal consultants for this fourteenth edition.

Marilyn Takahashi Fordney, CMA-AC (AAMA)
Agoura Hills, California

Contributors and Reviewers

CONTRIBUTORS

Karen Levein, CPC, CPC-I
Medical Professions Instructor
Burbank Adult School
Burbank, California

Payel Bhattacharya Madero, RHIT, MBA
AHIMA Approved ICD-10 Trainer
COO, PPJ Enterprises
Upland, California

Linda Smith, CPC, CPC-I, CEMC, PCS, CMBS
Consultant/Educator
MedOffice Resources
Greene, New York

EDITORIAL REVIEW BOARD

Sandra Alexander, MPA, BAS, CMA (AAMA)
Program Director/Coordinator
El Centro College
Dallas, Texas

Deborah A. Balentine, MEd, RHIA, CCS-P, CHTS-TR
Adjunct Instructor
Truman College, City College of Chicago
Chicago, Illinois

Kimberly Head, DC
Director of Healthcare Programs
Continuing Education Health Sciences
Collin College
Plano, Texas

Geri Kale-Smith, MS, CMA
Coordinator, Medical Office Programs
Associate Professor, Health Careers Division
Harper College
Palatine, Illinois

Colleen O. Kim, BS
Certified SHIP Counselor, Senior Management Fraud
    Counselor, Adjunct Professor
Manchester Community College
Manchester, Connecticut

Jennifer K. Lester, RBA, CMAA, CBCS
Certified Allied Health Instructor, Adjunct Instructor
Charleston Jobs Corps Center, Kanawha Valley
    Community & Technical College
Charleston, West Virginia

Michelle C. Maus, MBA
Program Chair/Assistant Professor of Healthcare
    Administration
Tiffin University
Tiffin, Ohio

PREVIOUS EDITION REVIEWERS

Pamela Audette, MBA, MT(ASCP), RMA
Assistant Professor and Program Director, Finlandia
    University, Hancock, Michigan

Megan Baez, CPC, CMA (AAMA)
Medical Coding & Billing Instructor, Everest University,
    Lakeland, Florida

Kelly Berge, MSHA, CPC, CBCS
Assistant Dean, Online, Berkeley College, Clifton,
    New Jersey

Ruth Berger, MS, RHIA
Instructor, Health Information Technology, Chippewa
    Valley Technical College, Eau Claire, Wisconsin

Peggy Black, RN, CCS, AHIMA-Approved ICD-10-CM/PCS Trainer
Medical Coding and Billing Instructor, Winter Park Tech,
    Winter Park, Florida

Carrie Cosson, CMA (NCCT), RMA (AMT)
Medical Assisting Instructor, Everest University, Lakeland,
    Florida

Gerard Cronin, DC, CCA
Assistant Professor, Salem Community College, Carneys
    Point, New Jersey

Brian Edward Dickens, MBA, RMA, CHI
Program Director–MA, Southeastern College, Greenacres,
    Florida

Jennifer Flippin, CPC
Medical Billing and Coding Program Coordinator, Pinnacle Career Institute, Kansas City, Missouri

Carol Hendrickson, MS Ed, CCS-P
Medical Coding & Health Information Management Instructor, Pasco Hernanado Community College, New Port Richey, Florida

Mary A. Johnson, BA, CPC
Program Manager, Medical Record Coding, Central Carolina Technical College, Sumter, South Carolina

Judith Leonhart, MBA
Instructor, Adult Education, OCM BOCES, Liverpool, New York

Angela MacLeod, MS, RHIA
Medical Coding & Billing Instructor, Certified Medical Assistant Program Director, Gogebic Community College, Ironwood, Michigan

Cassondra Major, MBA
Academic Program Director, Medical, Everest College, Henderson, Nevada

JanMarie C. Malik, MBA, RHIA, CCS-P
Coding, Billing, Reimbursement, and Office Procedures Instructor, Shasta Community College; National University, Redding, California

Laura Melendez, BS, RMA, RT BMO
Allied Health Instructor, Medical Assisting, Southeastern College, Greenacres, Florida

Deborah Newton, MA, PhD
Program Director, Medical Billing/Coding, Great Falls College Montana State University, Great Falls, Montana

Bhamini Patel, BSHIM, CPC, CPC-H
Medical Coding and Billing Instructor, Everest University, Lakeland, Florida

Jeanice Porta, BSEd, CPC, CPC-I
Medical Coding/Billing Instructor, Lee County High Tech Center North, Cape Coral, Florida

Susan Shear, MHA, CPC
Assistant Professor, Medical Information Technology, Bluegrass Community and Technical College, Danville, Kentucky

Tara Shepherd, CMA (AAMA)
Allied Health Director, Apollo Career Center, Lima, Ohio

Phaedra Spartan, RMA, CMAS, BS, MSHA
Healthcare Programs, Director, Medical, Vatterott College, Springfield, Missouri

Mia K. Thompson, MIBC, MAA
Program Director, Everest Institute, Marietta, Georgia

Deanne Ulrich, CPC-A
Instructor, Business, Hawkeye Community College, Waterloo, Iowa

Chris Welch, MBA, CPC, CMC, CEC, CMPE
Medical Insurance Billing and Coding, Program Director, Everest University, Orange Park, Florida

Nancy C. Withee, CPC, CPMA
Program Coordinator, Medical Office Administration and Health Information Technology, Great Bay Community College, Portsmouth, New Hampshire

Contents

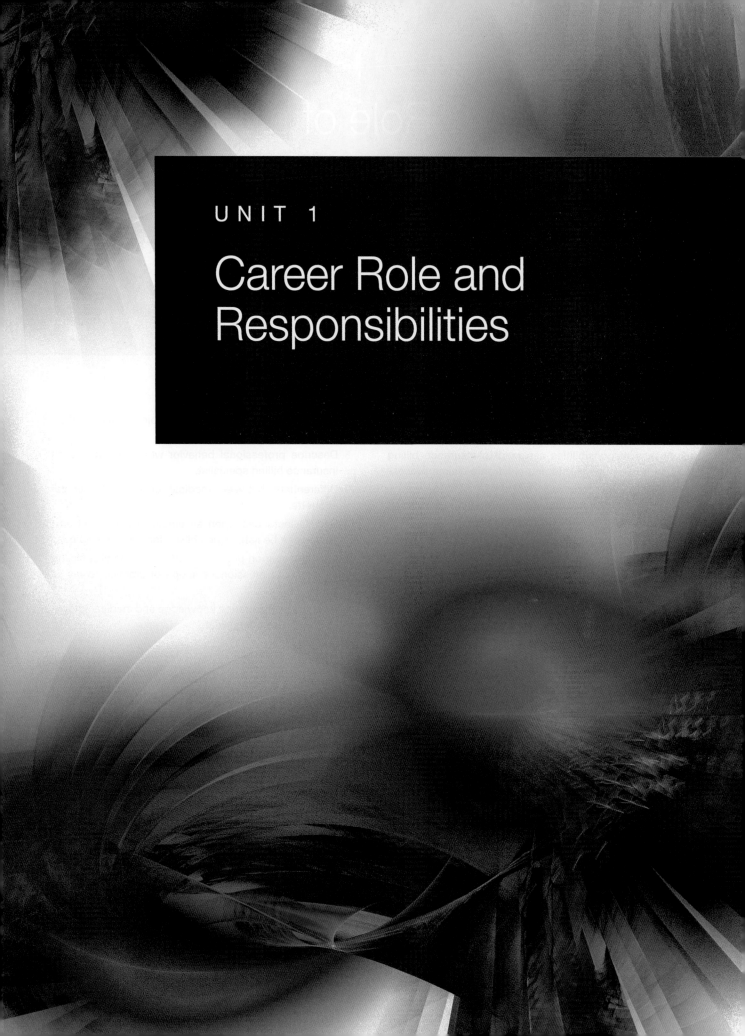

UNIT 1

Career Role and Responsibilities

CHAPTER

1

Role of an Insurance Billing Specialist

Marilyn Takahashi Fordney

OBJECTIVES

After reading this chapter, you should be able to:

1. Identify the background and importance of accurate insurance claims submission, coding, and billing.
2. Assess responsibilities assigned to insurance billing and coding specialists and electronic claims processors.
3. Name and discuss the office procedures performed during a workday that may affect billing.
4. Specify the educational requirements for a job as an insurance billing specialist and a coder.
5. Describe the variety of career advantages and areas of specialization open to those trained as insurance billing specialists.
6. List qualifications, attributes, and skills necessary to be an insurance billing specialist.

7. State the personal image to be projected as an insurance billing specialist.
8. Describe professional behavior when working as an insurance billing specialist.
9. Differentiate between medical ethics and medical etiquette.
10. Specify instances when an employer and/or an employee can be liable when billing for medical services.
11. Identify common practices and limitations of a claims assistance professional's scope of practice to his or her clients.
12. Explain how insurance knowledge and medical knowledge can be kept current.

KEY TERMS

American Health Information
   Management Association
American Medical Association
cash flow
claims assistance professional
electronic mail

ethics
etiquette
facility billing
insurance billing specialist
list service
medical billing representative

multiskilled health practitioner
professional billing
reimbursement specialist
respondeat superior
senior billing representative

KEY ABBREVIATIONS

AAMA	ASHD	GED	MSHP
ACA	CAP	HIPAA	MSO
AHIMA	e-mail	listserv	NPP
AMA			

Service to Patients

When choosing a profession as an insurance billing specialist, it is critical to match your talents to the career selected. An attitude directed at serving the patient's needs should be your priority as a medical insurance billing specialist. Be alert to discover ways in which you can best serve the patient while carrying out your job duties. A medical insurance billing specialist's primary goal is to assist in the revenue cycle, both helping the patient to obtain maximum insurance plan benefits and ensuring a cash flow to the health care provider. Revenue is the total income produced by a medical practice and the cycle is the regularly repeating set of events for producing it. The insurance billing specialist's responsibility is to conduct business in an ethical manner. Service to patients provides the opportunity to show high values, principles, and moral character, which will be appreciated and noticed.

BACKGROUND OF INSURANCE CLAIMS, CODING, AND BILLING

Welcome to the world of insurance billing, an exciting, ever-changing, and fast-growing career field. To help you focus on important terms and definitions, some of the basic words in this and subsequent chapters appear in **bold** or *italic* type. See the Glossary at the end of this text for a comprehensive list of key abbreviations and key terms with detailed definitions to broaden your knowledge.

A physician may have many problems that can affect obtaining maximum payment for services. He or she relies on professionals to handle billing, electronic transmission, and follow-up of claims. The health care industry is one of the most heavily regulated industries in the United States.

A number of billing and payment mechanisms are associated with third-party health insurance payers. A number of health insurance policy issues pertaining to compliance are connected with each payer. An insurance billing specialist must be aware of the health care system and all of the components, interrelationships, and interdependencies, such as hospitals, outpatient laboratories, insurance companies, federal government, patients, patient families, other physicians, and co-workers.

Two billing components exist: facility billing and professional billing. **Facility billing** is charging for services done in hospitals, acute care hospitals, skilled nursing or long-term care facilities, rehabilitation centers, or ambulatory surgical centers. **Professional billing** is charging for services performed by physicians or *non-physician practitioners (NPPs)*. An NPP is an individual, such as a physician assistant, nurse practitioner, advanced registered nurse practitioner, certified nurse anesthetist, physical therapist, speech therapist, licensed clinical social worker, or certified registered nurse practitioner, who has not

obtained a medical degree but is allowed to see patients and prescribe medications. These people are sometimes referred to as *physician extenders*. An **insurance billing specialist** must realize that NPPs should have a provider number and are permitted to submit claims to third-party payers. There may be occasions when the patient does not see a physician but is directed to the NPP. Proper authorization and documentation is required and then a financial record source document called an *encounter form* is generated for the NPP. Hence, this course is designed for professional billing.

Payment schedules for payment of professional services are based on the payer type (for example, managed care, workers' compensation, or Medicare). Under Medicare, physicians are paid according to relative value units, which are based on three things: (1) the cost (overhead) of delivering care, (2) malpractice insurance, and (3) the physician's work. A fee schedule is published by the Centers for Medicare and Medicaid Services (CMS), a federal organization that sets the mandates for financing and delivery of care to Medicare and Medicaid beneficiaries in the United States. Managed care organizations establish their own physician fee schedules. Their rates are close to what Medicare pays.

Whether you are employed to perform hospital or professional billing functions, the basic setup of a business office encompasses the following units or combined departments: reception of the patient, rendering of medical services, documentation of the services, and financial accounting. You must understand their functions in relation to the business office and the practice as a whole and how they affect payment for services. The flow of information is one of the most vital components of an organization. Knowing the job duties within the organization can assist in the effective flow of information, such as by written documents, telephone calls, oral communication among co-workers, or electronic mail (e-mail).

Office procedures performed throughout a workday include the following:

- *Scheduling appointments* involves assigning time slots for patients' visits. Canceling and rescheduling may also be involved. If the time is not properly assigned, there may be an influx or low volume of patients at a given time. Paperwork required for the visit must also be produced. It is important to record why the patient requires a visit.
- *Registering patients* may involve preregistration for visits by using a questionnaire referred to as a *patient registration form*. Financial and personal data are collected and accurately recorded (input) in a timely manner. Incorrect information affects the back office procedures and submission and payment of claims.

- *Documenting* pertinent clinical notes and assigning a diagnosis and service code to the patient's condition and visit is done by the provider of service. The notes in the patient's medical record include the reason for the visit, history, physical examination, diagnostic tests, results, diagnosis, and plan of treatment. The insurance billing specialist may be required to contact the insurance company to obtain authorization for treatment by secondary providers. He or she must also ensure that forms are properly completed and data are input into the system. Both proper documentation and assignment of the correct code for service affect reimbursement.
- Posting (inputting) a *charge entry* for patient care service rendered into the system by the charge entry staff member. The insurance biller must make certain that the insurance is correctly sequenced in the system (for example, primary versus secondary health insurance, workers' compensation, or automobile insurance versus primary health insurance). This person must ensure that the diagnosis coincides with the service rendered. For example, an obstetrics/gynecology visit should not have a diagnosis related to ophthalmology. Many times, individuals have the same names, so billing service dates and the name of the patient seen must be accurate. The charge entry staff member must ensure that the correct charge is assigned to the correct patient. Proper charge entry ensures timely billing and reimbursement.
- *Bookkeeping and accounting* is the posting of payments received (cash, checks, electronic funds transfer, or debit and credit cards) to patients' financial accounts. The bookkeeper or accountant must pay special attention to adjustments, denials, and write-offs. These entries may require investigation for validation. He or she may also receive insurance third-party payer remittance advices and may be assigned to follow up on denials.

ROLE OF THE INSURANCE BILLING SPECIALIST

In the past, administrative front office staff working in a physician's office performed both administrative and clinical duties. As decades passed, staff members' duties entailed either one or the other. Currently, because of changes in government regulations and standards for the insurance industry, specific medical assisting job tasks have become specialized. In a medical practice, it is commonplace to find administrative duties shared by a number of employees (for example, administrative medical assistant, bookkeeper, file clerk, insurance billing specialist, office manager, or receptionist). Several job title names are associated with medical billing personnel. The professional title used may depend on the region within the United States. Some of the most popular titles include insurance billing specialist, electronic claims processor,

medical biller, **reimbursement specialist, medical billing representative,** and **senior billing representative.** Hence, the title suggests that the employee is proficient in all aspects of medical billing. In this handbook, the title *insurance billing specialist* is used throughout. In clinics and large practices, it is common to find a billing department made up of many people; within the department, each position is specialized, such as Medicare billing specialist, Medicaid billing specialist, coding specialist, insurance counselor, collection manager, and medical and financial records manager.

Some medical practices and clinics contract with management services organizations (MSOs), which perform a variety of business functions, such as accounting, billing, coding, collections, computer support, legal advice, marketing, payroll, and management expertise. An insurance billing specialist may find a job working for an MSO as a part of this team.

Cost pressures on health care providers are forcing employers to be more efficient, and hiring **multiskilled health practitioners (MSHPs)** may achieve this. An MSHP is a person cross-trained to provide more than one function, often in more than one discipline. Knowledge of insurance claims completion and coding enhances skills so that he or she can offer more flexibility to someone hired in a medical setting.

Individuals called **claims assistance professionals (CAPs)** work for the consumer. They help patients organize, file, and negotiate health insurance claims of all types; assist the consumer in obtaining maximum benefits; and tell the patient how much to pay the providers to make sure there is no overpayment. It is possible for someone who has taken a course on insurance billing to function in this role.

Job Responsibilities

Whether employed by the medical practice of an academic medical center or hospital or by a self-employed biller, you should be able to perform any and all duties assigned pertaining to the business office. Front and back office personnel work together to ensure a strong billing cycle and enhanced reimbursement. Examples of generic job descriptions are shown in Figures 1-1 and 1-2 to illustrate the job duties, skills, and requirements that might be encountered for various insurance billing and coding positions. Job descriptions are used as tools by assisting managers, supervisors, and employers in recruiting, supervising, and evaluating individuals in these positions for salary increases. Companies have had to modify their job descriptions to address individuals with physical impairments who may be affected by the Americans with Disabilities Act.

GENERIC JOB DESCRIPTION FOR ENTRY LEVEL INSURANCE BILLING SPECIALIST

Knowledge, skills, and abilities:
1. Minimum education level consists of certificate from one-year insurance billing course, associate degree, or equivalent in work experience and continuing education.
2. Knowledge of basic medical terminology, anatomy and physiology, diseases, surgeries, medical specialties, and insurance terminology.
3. Ability to operate computer, printer, photocopy, and calculator equipment.
4. Written and oral communication skills including grammar, punctuation, and style.
5. Ability and knowledge to use procedure code books.
6. Ability and knowledge to use diagnostic code books.
7. Knowledge and skill of data entry.
8. Ability to work independently.
9. Certified Procedural Coder (CPC) or Certified Coding Specialist (CCS) status preferred.

Working conditions:
Medical office setting. Sufficient lighting.

Physical demands:
Prolonged sitting, standing and walking. Use of word processor or computer equipment. Some stooping, reaching, climbing, and bending. Occasional lifting of _____ lbs to a height of 5 feet. Hearing and speech capabilities necessary to communicate with patients and staff in person and on telephone. Vision capable of viewing computer monitors, calculators, charts, forms, text, and numbers for prolonged periods.

Salary:
Employer would list range of remuneration for the position.

Job responsibilities:	**Performance standards:**
1. Abstracts health information from patient records.	1.1 Uses knowledge of medical terminology, anatomy and physiology, diseases, surgeries, and medical specialties.
	1.2 Consults reference materials to clarify meanings of words.
	1.3 Meets accuracy and production requirements adopted by employer.
	1.4 Verifies with physician any vague information for accuracy.
2. Exhibits an understanding of ethical and medicolegal responsibilities related to insurance billing programs.	2.1 Observes policies and procedures related to federal privacy regulations, health records, release of information, retention of records, and statute of limitations for claim submission.
	2.2 Meets standards of professional etiquette and ethical conduct.
	2.3 Recognizes and reports problems involving fraud, abuse, embezzlement, and forgery to appropriate individuals.

FIGURE 1-1 Generic job description for an insurance billing specialist.

Continued.

3. Operates computer
to transmit insurance claims.

3.1 Operates equipment skillfully
and efficiently.
3.2 Evaluates condition of equipment and
reports need for repair or replacement.

4. Follows employer's policies
and procedures.

4.1 Punctual work attendance and is dependable.
4.2 Answers routine inquiries related to
account balances and dates insurance
forms submitted.

5. Transmits insurance
claims accurately.

5.1 Updates insurance registration and
account information.
5.2 Processes payments and posts to
accounts accurately.
5.3 Handles correspondence related to
insurance claims.
5.4 Reviews encounter forms for accuracy
before submission to data entry.
5.5 Inserts data for generating insurance claims
accurately.
5.6 Codes procedures and diagnoses
accurately.
5.7 Telephones third-party payers with
regard to delinquent claims.
5.8 Traces insurance claims.
5.9 Files appeals for denied claims.
5.10 Documents registration data from patients
accurately.
5.11 Maintains separate insurance files.

6. Enhances knowledge and
skills to keep up to date.

6.1 Attends continuing education activities.
6.2 Obtains current knowledge applicable to
state and federal programs as they relate
to insurance claim submission.
6.3 Keeps abreast and maintains files of current
changes in coding requirements from Medicare,
Medicaid, and other third-party payers.
6.4 Assists with updating fee schedules and
encounter forms with current codes.
6.5 Assists in the research of proper coding
techniques to maximize reimbursement.

7. Employs interpersonal
expertise to provide good
working relationships with
patients, employer, employees,
and third-party payers.

7.1 Works with employer and employees
cooperatively as a team.
7.2 Communicates effectively with patients
and third-party payers regarding
payment policies and financial obligations.
7.3 Executes job assignments with diligence
and skill.
7.4 Assists staff with coding and reimbursement problems.
7.5 Assists other employees when needed.
7.6 Assists with giving fee estimates to
patients when necessary.

FIGURE 1-1, cont'd

GENERIC JOB DESCRIPTION FOR AN ELECTRONIC CLAIMS PROCESSOR

Knowledge, skills, and abilities:
1. Minimum education level consists of certificate from one-year insurance billing course, associate degree, or equivalent in work experience and continuing education.
2. Knowledge of basic medical terminology, anatomy and physiology, diseases, surgeries, medical specialties, and insurance terminology.
3. Ability to operate computer and printer, as well as photocopy and calculator equipment.
4. Written and oral communication skills including grammar, punctuation, and style.
5. Ability and knowledge to use procedure code books.
6. Ability and knowledge to use diagnostic code books.
7. Knowledge and skill of data entry.
8. Ability to work independently.
9. Certified Electronic Claims Processor (CECP) status preferred.

Working conditions:
Medical office setting. Sufficient lighting.

Physical demands:
Prolonged sitting, standing and walking. Use of computer equipment. Some stooping, reaching, climbing, and bending. Occasional lifting of _____ lbs to a height of 5 feet. Hearing and speech capabilities necessary to communicate with patients and staff in person and on telephone. Vision capabilities necessary to view computer monitors, calculators, charts, forms, text, and numbers for prolonged periods.

Salary:
Employer would list range of remuneration for the position.

Job responsibilities:	Performance standards:
1. Acts as a link between the medical provider or facility and third-party payers.	1.1 Uses knowledge of medical terminology, anatomy and physiology, diseases, surgeries, and medical specialties.
	1.2 Understands computer applications and equipment required to convert and transmit patient billing data electronically.
	1.3 Consults reference materials to clarify meanings of words.
	1.4 Meets accuracy and production requirements adopted by employer.
	1.5 Verifies with physician any vague information for accuracy.
	1.6 Reduces volume of paperwork and variety of claim forms providers need to submit claims for payment.
2. Converts patient billing data into electronically readable formats.	2.1 Inputs data and transmits insurance claims accurately, either directly or through a clearinghouse.
	2.2 Answers routine inquiries related to account balances and dates insurance data transmitted to third-party payers.

FIGURE 1-2 Generic job description for an electronic claims processor.

Continued.

3. Uses software that eliminates common claim filing errors, provides clean claims to third-party payers, expedites payments to providers or facilities, and follows up on delinquent or denied claims.

2.3 Updates and maintains software applications with requirements of clearinghouses and third-party payers.

3.1 Codes procedures and diagnoses accurately.
3.2 Telephones third-party payers about delinquent claims.
3.3 Traces insurance claims.
3.4 Files appeals for denied claims.

4. Exhibits an understanding of ethical and medicolegal responsibilities related to insurance billing programs and plans.

4.1 Observes policies and procedures related to federal privacy regulations, health records, release of information, retention of records, and statute of limitations for claim submission.
4.2 Meets standards of professional etiquette and ethical conduct.
4.3 Recognizes and reports problems involving fraud, abuse, embezzlement, and forgery to appropriate individuals.

5. Operates computer equipment to complete insurance claims.

5.1 Operates equipment skillfully and efficiently.
5.2 Evaluates condition of equipment and reports need for repair or replacement.

6. Follows employer's policies and procedures.

6.1 Must have punctual work attendance and be dependable.

7. Enhances knowledge and skills to keep up to date.

7.1 Attends continuing education skills activities.
7.2 Obtains current knowledge applicable to state and federal programs as they relate to transmission of insurance claims.
7.3 Keeps abreast and maintains files of current changes in coding requirements from Medicare, Medicaid, and other third-party payers. Assists in the research of proper coding techniques to maximum reimbursement.

8. Employs interpersonal expertise to provide good working relationships with patients, employer, employees, and third-party payers.

8.1 Works with employer and employees cooperatively as a team.
8.2 Communicates effectively with patients and third-party payers regarding payment policies and financial obligations.
8.3 Executes job assignments with diligence and skill.
8.4 Assists staff with coding and reimbursement problems.
8.5 Assists other employees when needed.
8.6 Assists with giving fee estimates to patients when necessary.

FIGURE 1-2, cont'd

Administrative front office duties have gained in importance for the following reasons. Documentation is vital to good patient care. It must be done comprehensively for proper reimbursement to ensure continued existence of the medical office practice. Diagnostic and procedural coding must be reviewed for its correctness and completeness. Insurance claims must be promptly submitted, ideally within 1 to 5 business days, to ensure continuous cash flow. **Cash flow** is the amount of actual money generated and available for use by the medical practice within a given period of time. Without money coming in, overhead expenses cannot be met and a practice will face financial difficulties. Data required for billing must be collected from all health care providers, as well as from hospitals, outpatient clinics, and laboratories involved in a case.

An insurance billing specialist in a large medical practice may act as an insurance counselor, taking the patient to a private area of the office to discuss the practice's financial policies and the patient's insurance coverage, as well as to negotiate a reasonable payment plan. The insurance billing specialist discusses claims processing with contracted and noncontracted third-party payers, the billing of secondary insurance payers and patients once the third-party payer pays its portion, self-pay billing, and time payment plans. Federal and state programs require the provider to submit claims for the patient. In other plans, it is the patient's obligation, rather than the provider's, to send the claim to the third-party payer. However, most providers submit claims for patients as a courtesy. Any copayments or deductible amounts should be collected from the patient at each visit. Also, self-pay patients should be reminded that payment is due at the time of service. This is done to ensure that the physician will be paid for services rendered and to develop good communication lines. Patients who are informed are patients who pay their bills. The counselor learns the deductible amount and verifies with the insurance company whether any preauthorization, precertification, or second-opinion requirements exist. Credit counseling helps obtain payment in full when expensive procedures are necessary. In some offices, the insurance biller may act as a collection manager who answers routine inquiries related to account balances and insurance submission dates; assists patients in setting up a payment schedule that is within their budget; follows up on delinquent accounts; and traces denied, "adjusted," or unpaid claims (Figure 1-3).

Having large accounts receivables (total amount of money owed for professional services rendered) in a health care practice is often a direct result of failure to verify insurance plan benefits, obtain authorization or precertification, or collect copayments and deductibles or inadequate claims filing. The rush to get a claim

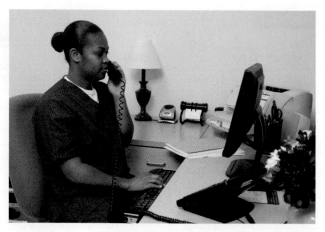

FIGURE 1-3 Insurance biller talking to a patient on the telephone about copayment required for an office visit under the patient's insurance plan.

"out the door" cannot be justified when a practice has thousands or millions of dollars in unpaid or denied claims. Accounts receivables will be low and revenue high if a practice takes the extra time to ensure that the claim is 100% accurate, complete, and verified.

In 1997 the American Association of Medical Assistants (AAMA) developed a role delineation study analyzing the many job functions of the medical assistant; it was updated in 2002 and 2007 and renamed and published in 2008. Table 1-1 shows the 2007–2008 Advanced Practice of Medical Assisting Skills, with arrows indicating material covered in this text. The Occupational Analysis of the CMA (AAMA) was updated and the 2012–2013 version is available for download on the AAMA's website (www.aama-ntl.org). The topics shown in Table 1-1 must be studied to pass the certification examination offered by the AAMA. Further information about many types of certification and registration is provided in Chapter 18.

Educational and Training Requirements

Generally, a high school diploma or general equivalency diploma (GED) is required for entry into an insurance billing or coding specialist accredited program. The accredited program usually offers additional education in medical terminology, insurance claims completion, procedural and diagnostic coding, anatomy and physiology, computer skills, **ethics** and medicolegal knowledge, and general office skills. Completion of an accredited program for coding certification or an accredited health information technology program is necessary for a job as a coder.

Experience in coding and insurance claim processing or management, completion of a 1-year insurance

Table 1-1   **General, Clinical, and Administrative Skills* of the CMA (AAMA)**

General Skills

COMMUNICATION	LEGAL CONCEPTS	INSTRUCTION	OPERATIONAL FUNCTIONS
• Recognize and respect cultural diversity. • Adapt communications to individual's understanding. • Use professional telephone and interpersonal techniques. • Recognize and respond effectively to verbal, nonverbal, and written communications. • Use and apply medical terminology appropriately. ➔• Receive, organize, prioritize, store, and maintain transmittable information using electronic technology. • Serve as "communication liaison" between the physician and patient. ➔• Serve as patient advocate professional and health coach in a team approach in health care. • Identify basics of office emergency preparedness.	➔• Perform within legal (including federal and state statutes, regulations, opinions, and rulings) and ethical boundaries. • Document patient communication and clinical treatments accurately and appropriately. • Maintain medical records. ➔• Follow employer's established policies dealing with the health care contract. • Comply with established risk management and safety procedures. • Recognize professional credentialing criteria. ➔• Identify and respond to issues of confidentiality.	• Function as a health care advocate to meet individual's needs. • Educate individuals in office policies and procedures. • Educate the patient within the scope of practice and as directed by supervising physician in health maintenance, disease prevention, and compliance with patient's treatment plan. • Identify community resources for health maintenance and disease prevention to meet individual patient needs. • Maintain current list of community resources, including those for emergency preparedness and other patient care needs. • Collaborate with local community resources for emergency preparedness. ➔• Educate patients in their responsibilities relating to third-party reimbursements.	• Perform inventory of supplies and equipment. • Perform routine maintenance of administrative and clinical equipment. ➔• Apply computer and other electronic equipment techniques to support office operations. • Perform methods of quality control. • Receive, organize, prioritize, store, and maintain transmittable information using electronic technology. • Serve as patient advocate professional and health coach in a team approach in health care.

Clinical Skills

FUNDAMENTAL PRINCIPLES	DIAGNOSTIC PROCEDURES	PATIENT CARE
• Identify the roles and responsibilities of the medical assistant in the clinical setting. • Identify the roles and responsibilities of other team members in the medical office. • Apply principles of aseptic technique and infection control. • Practice standard precautions, including handwashing and disposal of biohazardous materials. • Perform sterilization techniques. • Comply with quality assurance practices.	• Collect and process specimens. • Perform CLIA-waived tests. • Perform electrocardiography and respiratory testing. • Perform phlebotomy, including venipuncture and capillary puncture. • Use knowledge of principles of radiology.	• Perform initial-response screening following protocols approved by supervising physician. • Obtain, evaluate, and record patient history using critical thinking skills. • Obtain vital signs. • Prepare and maintain examination and treatment areas. • Prepare patient for examinations, procedures, and treatments. • Assist with examinations, procedures, and treatments. • Maintain examination/treatment rooms, including inventory of supplies and equipment. • Prepare and administer oral and parenteral (excluding IV) medications and immunizations (*as directed by supervising physician and as permitted by state law*). • Use knowledge of principles of IV therapy. • Maintain medication and immunization records. • Screen and follow up on test results. • Recognize and respond to emergencies.

Table 1-1	General, Clinical, and Administrative Skills* of the CMA (AAMA)—cont'd
Administrative Skills	
ADMINISTRATIVE PROCEDURES	**PRACTICE FINANCES**
• Schedule, coordinate, and monitor appointments. • Schedule inpatient/outpatient admissions and procedures. ➔• Apply third-party and managed care policies, procedures, and guidelines. • Establish, organize, and maintain patient medical records. • File medical records appropriately.	➔• Perform procedural and diagnostic coding for reimbursement. ➔• Perform billing and collection procedures. ➔• Perform administrative functions, including bookkeeping and financial procedures. ➔• Prepare submittable ("clean") insurance forms.

AAMA, American Association of Medical Assistants; *CLIA*, Clinical Laboratory Improvement Amendments; *CMA*, certified medical assistant; *IV*, intravenous.
*All skills require decision making based on critical thinking concepts.

MEDICAL INSURANCE SPECIALIST CERTIFICATE PROGRAM

PROGRAM DESCRIPTION: The Medical Insurance program prepares you for employment in the area of medical insurance and health care claims processing. This program also serves the needs of health care personnel interested in upgrading their professional skills. Training in computerized medical billing, CPT-4 and ICD-10-CM coding, and processing medical insurance claims are included in the curriculum. Students may be enrolled on a full-time or part-time basis, and may complete the program by attending either day or evening classes. Accelerated or fast track courses are also available for those wishing to complete this program within a short time period. The program graduates students with marketable skills that are in demand. They are employed in hospitals, insurance companies, private medical laboratories, billing bureaus, and doctors' offices. Graduates may apply credits toward other certificate or associate degree programs.

The following courses are included in this program:

First Semester

Medical Terminology	3 Credits
Administrative Medical Office Management	4 Credits
Biology	3 Credits
Keyboarding	3 Credits
Computer I	2 Credits
	TOTAL 15 Credits

Second Semester

Principles and Applications of Medical Insurance	3 Credits
Current Issues of Medical Insurance	3 Credits
Medical Financial Management	3 Credits
Word Processing	3 Credits
Basic Principles of Composition	3 Credits
	TOTAL 15 Credits

FIGURE 1-4 Example of a 1-year medical insurance specialist certificate program offered at a community college. Basic coding is taught as a part of the course in Administrative Medical Office Management and advanced coding is covered in Principles and Applications of Medical Insurance. Biology may be titled Anatomy and Physiology in some colleges. *(Reprinted with permission from Community College of Allegheny County, Pittsburgh, Pa.)*

specialist certificate program at a community college, or both are usually required for a job as an insurance billing specialist. The curriculum that might be offered in a 1-year certificate program is shown in Figure 1-4. You might find that the courses in your locale are labeled with different titles and time frames; the information in Figure 1-4 is specifically from a community college in Pennsylvania. Courses should cover medical terminology, anatomy and physiology, introduction to computer technology, procedural and diagnostic coding, and comprehensive medical insurance billing. A 2-year educational course can result in obtaining an associate's degree. Training prepares an individual for a wide range of employment opportunities. Knowledge of computer hardware and software, electronic data transmission requirements, and health care claim reimbursement is recommended for people planning to become electronic claims processors. Many accredited programs include an externship (on-the-job) period of training that may be paid or unpaid.

The **American Health Information Management Association (AHIMA)** has published diagnostic and procedure coding competencies for outpatient services and diagnostic coding and reporting requirements for physician billing. Refer to these competencies for a more inclusive list of educational and training requirements by visiting the AHIMA website (www.ahima.org).

A moderate to high degree of knowledge of the health insurance business is necessary if your goal is to become a self-employed insurance billing specialist or CAP. In addition to insurance terminology, claims procedures, and coding, you must know commercial third-party payers' requirements as well as Medicare and state Medicaid policies and regulations. You also need human relations skills and proficiency in running a business, including marketing and sales expertise.

To reach a professional level, certification is available from many national associations, depending on the type of certification desired. Refer to Chapter 18 for more information on this topic.

Career Advantages

Jobs are available in every state, ranging from nonmanagement to management positions. Insurance billing specialists can receive a salary of $8000 part-time to $50,000 full-time or more per year, depending on knowledge, experience, duties, responsibilities, locale, and size of the employing institution. Jobs are available in consulting firms, insurance and managed care companies, medical clearinghouses, ambulatory surgical centers, clinics, hospitals, multispecialty medical groups, and private physicians' practices. You can also be an instructor, a lecturer, or a consumer advocate. You can be your own boss by either setting up an in-home billing service or establishing an office service for billing.

Self-Employment or Independent Contracting

After gaining some experience, many people establish independently owned and self-operated businesses within their communities as medical insurance billing specialists, coders, claim assistance professionals, or collectors. However, the responsibilities are greater in this area because such work demands a full-time commitment, a lot of hard work, long hours to obtain clients, and the need to advertise and market the business. This means you are responsible for everything: advertising, billing, bookkeeping, and so on. Some billers work from their homes and others rent or lease an office. If you eventually plan on self-employment and you are weak in an area, such as accounting, then take a bookkeeping course. Chapter 18 discusses setting up your own business.

Flexible Hours

Another advantage of this career field is the opportunity to have flexible hours. Most other employees in the physician's office must adhere to the physician's schedule. However, the medical insurance billing specialist may want to come in early to transmit electronic claims during off-peak hours or stay late to make collection calls. It may be advantageous to both the physician and insurance specialist to vary his or her schedule according to the needs of the practice. In-home or office billing services save a medical practice valuable time, money, and overhead costs because the physician does not have to cover benefits or equipment.

Disabled Workers

A career as an insurance billing specialist or a collector of delinquent accounts can be rewarding for persons with disabilities. These jobs are for individuals who have current knowledge of health care insurance billing as well as state and federal collection laws. Interacting well with people both in person and by telephone is essential in these roles. The financial management responsibilities and other jobs involving telephone communications are an opportunity for someone who is visually impaired because he or she is usually a good listener when properly and specifically trained. Special equipment, such as a Braille keyboard, magnified computer screen, audible scanner, or digital audio recorder, may be necessary to enhance job performance.

Working independently from a home office may appeal to a physically disabled person when there is no need to commute to a physician's office on a daily basis. Accessing information remotely via the computer and fax machine is a manageable method for success. However, it is important first to gain experience before trying to establish a home office business.

The government amended the Rehabilitation Act in 1998 to "require Federal agencies to make their electronic and information technology accessible to people with disabilities" because inaccessible technology obviously may interfere with one's ability to obtain and use information quickly and easily. Section 508 was enacted to diminish barriers in information technology. This makes new opportunities available for people with disabilities.

Inquire at your local vocational rehabilitation center for training disabled individuals. Specific to being a delinquent account collector, you may contact ACA International (formerly known as the American Collectors Association [ACA]) in Minneapolis (the website is www.acainternational.org), which has developed a collections training program for the visually impaired. Chapter 10 is devoted to the topic of collections.

Qualifications and Attributes

An individual must have a variety of characteristics or qualities to function well as an insurance billing specialist. Strong critical thinking and reading skills with good comprehension are a must. Being a logical and practical thinker, as well as a creative problem solver, is important. Being meticulous and neat makes it easier to get the job done at the workstation. A person with good organizational skills who is conscientious and loyal is always an asset to the employer. Because a large amount of specific data must be obtained, this work requires an individual who is detail oriented. A person with a curious nature will dig deeper into an issue and not be satisfied with an answer unless the "whys" and "whats" are defined. This also helps one to grow while on the job and not become stagnant. Equally important are time management and social skills. This list is by no means complete; perhaps you can think of additional attributes that might lead to a more successful career.

Skills

A person who completes insurance claims must have many skills. One needs the following skills to be proficient:

- Solid foundation and working knowledge of medical terminology, including anatomy, physiology, disease, and treatment terms, as well as the meanings of abbreviations.
  Application: Interpretation of patient's chart notes and code manuals.
  Incorrect: Final diagnosis: ASHD.
  Correct: Final diagnosis: Arteriosclerotic heart disease.
  Locating the diagnostic code using an abbreviation is difficult; therefore you must be able to translate it.
- Expert use of procedural and diagnostic code books and other related resources.
  Application: Code manuals and other reference books are used to assign accurate codes for each case billed.
- Precise reading skills.
  Application: Differentiate between the technical descriptions of two different but similar procedures.

Procedure (CPT) Code No. 43352 Esophagostomy (fistulization of esophagus, external; cervical approach).
Procedure (CPT) Code No. 43020 Esophagotomy (cervical approach, with removal of foreign body).
Note that the additional letter "s" to the surgical procedure in the first part of the example changes the entire procedure.
- Basic mathematics.
  Application: Calculate fees and adjustments on the insurance claim forms and enter them into the patient accounts. It is essential that these figures be accurate.
- Knowledge of medicolegal rules and regulations of various insurance programs.
  Application: Avoid filing of claims considered fraudulent or abusive because of code selection and program policies.
- Knowledge of compliance issues.
  Application: Federal Privacy, Security, Transaction rules in addition to Fraud, Waste, and Abuse. For further information, see Chapter 2.
- Basic keyboarding and computer skills.
  Application: Good keyboarding and data entry skills and knowledge of computer programs are essential because the industry increasingly involves practice management software and electronic claims submission; handwritten claims are a format of the past.
- Proficiency in accessing information through the internet.
  Application: Obtain federal, state, and commercial insurance regulations and current information as needed through the internet. Sign on as a member of a **list service (listserv)**, which is a service run from a website where questions may be posted. Find one composed of working coders to obtain answers on how to code complex, rare, or difficult medical cases.
- Knowledge of billing and collection techniques.
  Application: Use latest billing and collection ideas to keep cash flow constant and avoid delinquent accounts.
- Expertise in the legalities of collection on accounts.
  Application: Avoid lawsuits by knowing state and federal collection laws as they apply to medical collection of accounts receivable.
- Generate insurance claims with speed and accuracy.
  Application: If you develop your own business as a medical claims and billing specialist, you may be paid according to the amount of paid claims the health care practice is reimbursed. Because you will rely on volume for an income, the more expeditious you become, the more money you earn. Therefore accuracy in selecting the correct codes and data entry and motivation in completing claims also become marketable skills. Measure your

correct claim productivity for precision and time when you complete the insurance claim forms for this course, and see how many accurate claims you can generate.

Personal Image

To project a professional image, be attentive to apparel and grooming (Figure 1-5). If a person works at home, the tendency is to dress casually (for example, blue jeans, sneakers, shorts, and tank tops). In a work setting, however, a uniform may be required, or you might be expected to wear business attire that is conservative and stylish but not trendy. For women, this includes a business suit, dress, or skirt of appropriate length; slacks; sweaters; blouses; and dress shoes. For men, a business suit or dress slacks and jacket, shirt, tie (optional), and dress shoes are appropriate.

When hired, it is important to discuss appropriate dress code with the supervisor. Keep in mind that fragrances can be offensive or cause allergies to some clients and patients; therefore use good judgment. Fingernails should be carefully manicured and appropriate to the dress code. For women, subdued eye makeup is appropriate for day use. Consult the employer for the office policy regarding body piercings and tattoos.

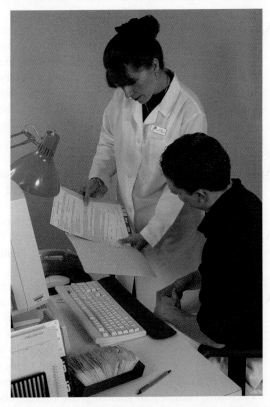

FIGURE 1-5 Male and female medical personnel who project a clean, fresh, and professional image.

Remember that you are in a professional environment and must present yourself in such a way.

Behavior

Many aspects make an individual a true professional: getting along with people rates high on the list, as does maintaining confidentiality of patients' medical histories and ongoing medical treatment. An insurance billing specialist depends on many co-workers for information needed to bill claims (for example, the receptionist who collects the patient information). Therefore it is necessary to be a team player and treat patients and co-workers with courtesy and respect. Consider all co-workers' duties as important because they are part of the team helping you reach the goal of processing the billing and obtaining maximum reimbursement for the patient and physician. Communicate effectively. Be honest, dependable, and on time. Never take part in office gossip or politics. Be willing to do the job and be efficient in how you carry it out.

MEDICAL ETIQUETTE

Before beginning work as an insurance billing specialist, it is wise to have a basic knowledge of medical **etiquette** as it pertains to the medical profession, the insurance industry, and the medical coder. Medical etiquette has to do with how medical professionals conduct themselves. Customs, courtesy, and manners of the medical profession can be expressed in three simple words: *consideration for others.*

In every business that interacts with customers or clients, the focus begins with good customer service. The Service to Patients box in this chapter emphasizes this point; if you did not read it, go back and do so now. If you work in an office in which patients go by your desk, acknowledge them with a smile, a nod, or a greeting. Patients may arrive for their appointments ill or injured and suffering from a lot of negativity. If a mistake is made, there is power in an apology given at the first sign of trouble. Attentiveness and a helpful, friendly atmosphere can smooth out the kinks and wrinkles of stressful and negative situations. All people have the need to feel special and they gravitate toward individuals who make them feel that way. All of these personal skills mean good customer service and satisfaction and can lead to professional success for you and the medical practice.

Several points about medical etiquette bear mentioning, as follows:
1. Never keep another physician who wants to talk to your physician/employer about a medical case waiting longer than necessary in the reception room. Usher him or her into the physician's office as soon as it is unoccupied.

2. Always connect another physician who is calling on the telephone to your physician immediately, asking as few questions as possible. The only exception is if you know the physician calling is treating one of your patients and you wish to verify the name to pull the chart or other data for your physician.
3. Follow the basic rules of etiquette with co-workers while working in the office, such as acknowledging people who enter your office or come to your desk by saying, "I'll be with you in a moment."
4. Identify yourself to callers and people you call.
5. Do not use first names until you know it is appropriate to do so.
6. Maintain a professional demeanor and a certain amount of formality when interacting with others. Remember to be courteous and always project a professional image.
7. Observe rules of etiquette when sending e-mail messages and placing or receiving cellphone calls. These rules fall under the Health Insurance Portability and Accountability Act (HIPAA) and are stated in detail in Chapters 1 and 4.

Electronic Mail Etiquette

Electronic mail (e-mail) is the transmitting, receiving, storing, and forwarding of text, voice messages, attachments, or images by computer from one person to another. Every computer user subscribing to an online service may establish an e-mail address. See Example 1-1.

Example 1-1 Electronic Mail Address
Electronic mail (e-mail) address mason@aol.com means:

Mason individual user (Mason)
@   at
aol   site (America Online, an online service provider)
com   type of site (commercial business)

Because this is a more cost-effective and efficient method of sending a message to someone and obtaining a quicker response, you may be composing, forwarding, and responding via e-mail with staff in other locations, with patients, and with insurance billers (Figure 1-6). It is important to set some standards to follow when communicating via e-mail. The messages you send are a reflection of your professional image.

1. Identify yourself and the reason for the message.
2. Compose the message in a clear and concise manner using good grammar and proper spelling. Make sure it cannot be misconstrued.
3. Include a descriptive subject line. If a reply changes the topic, then change the subject line.
4. Do not put confidential information in an e-mail message (e.g., patient-identifiable information).
5. Encrypt (code) all files about patients and e-mail attachments and limit the size of attachments. Some users pay a per-minute connect time and will be downloading the attachment.

Address →	To: apcmonitor@shore.net
Subject Line →	Subj: **anesthesia modifiers**
Date →	Date: Thursday, April 7, 2016
Sender Address →	From: brownm@aol.com
Salutation →	Dear Madam or Sir:
Left →	Question: Is conscious sedation considered anesthesia in
Justified	relationship to modifier -73 and -74? A speaker at a recent
Brief Message	conference said "yes" but another said it had not yet been
With Proper	clarified by CMS. Our fiscal intermediary manual has an
Grammar	example that said modifier -52 would be used in conjunction
	with a colonoscopy with conscious sedation. What is correct?
Complimentary	
Closing →	Sincerely,
Signature Line →	Mary Brown
Title →	Insurance Billing Specialist
Location →	Smith Medical Center
E-mail address →	brownm@aol.com
Confidentiality	IMPORTANT WARNING: This e-mail (and any attachments) is
Statement →	only intended for the use of the person or entity to which it is
	addressed, and may contain information that is privileged and
	confidential. You, the recipient, are obligated to maintain it in a
	safe, secure and confidential manner. Unauthorized re-
	disclosure or failure to maintain confidentiality may subject you
	to federal and state penalties. If you are not the intended
	recipient, please immediately notify us by return e-mail, and
	delete this message from your computer.

FIGURE 1-6 Electronic mail message sent to *APC's Weekly Monitor* asking a question about the use of modifiers.

6. Recognize that all e-mail is discoverable in legal proceedings, so be careful with content and choice of words.
7. Do not use all capital letters for more than one word.
8. Insert a blank line between paragraphs.
9. Surround URLs (long web addresses) with angle brackets [ ] to avoid problems occurring at the end of a line due to the word wrap feature.
10. Do not use variable text styles (bold or italic) or text colors.
11. Quote sparingly when automatically quoting the original message in replies. Some programs allow you to select some text in the original message by pressing a keyboard shortcut, and only that text will be quoted in the reply. Quotation marks should be inserted to differentiate original and new text.
12. Avoid sending or forwarding junk messages (e.g., welcome messages, congratulation messages, jokes, chain messages).
13. Avoid "emoticons," a short sequence of keyboard letters and symbols used to convey emotion, gestures, or expressions (e.g., "smiley" (; :-)).
14. Do not respond immediately if a person's e-mail makes you angry or emotional. Put the message aside until the next day and then answer it diplomatically.
15. Do not write anything that is racially or sexually offensive.
16. Insert a short signature at the end of the message that includes your name, affiliation, and e-mail and/or URL address.

MEDICAL ETHICS

Medical **ethics** are not laws but standards of conduct generally accepted as moral guides for behavior by which an insurance billing or coding specialist may determine the propriety of his or her conduct in a relationship with patients, the physician, co-workers, the government, and insurance companies. You are entrusted with holding patients' medical information in confidence, collecting money for your physician, and being a reliable resource for your co-workers. To act with ethical behavior means carrying out responsibilities with integrity, decency, honesty, competence, consideration, respect, fairness, trust, and courage.

The earliest written code of ethical principles and conduct for the medical profession originated in Babylonia about 2500 B.C. and is called the *Code of Hammurabi*. Then, about the fifth century B.C., Hippocrates, a Greek physician who is known as the "Father of Medicine," conceived the Oath of Hippocrates.

In 1980 the **American Medical Association (AMA)** adopted a modern code of ethics, called the *Principles of Medical Ethics*, for the benefit of the health professional

---

> **Box 1-1   Principles of Medical Ethics of the American Medical Association**
>
> **Preamble**
>
> The medical profession has long subscribed to a body of ethical statements developed primarily for the benefit of the patient.
>
> As a member of the profession, a physician must recognize responsibility not only to patients, but also to society, to other health professionals, and to self. The following principles adopted by the AMA are not laws but standards of conduct that define the essentials of honorable behavior for the physician.
>
> I. A physician shall be dedicated to providing competent medical service with compassion and respect for human dignity.
>
> II. A physician shall deal honestly with patients and colleagues, and strive to expose those physicians deficient in character or competence, or who engage in fraud or deception.
>
> III. A physician shall respect the law and also recognize a responsibility to seek changes in those requirements that are contrary to the best interests of the patient.
>
> IV. A physician shall respect the rights of patients, of colleagues, and of other health professionals, and shall safeguard patient confidences within the constraints of the law.
>
> V. A physician shall continue to study, apply, and advance scientific knowledge; make relevant information available to patients, colleagues, and the public; obtain consultation; and use the talents of other health professionals when indicated.
>
> VI. A physician shall, in the provision of appropriate patient care, except in emergencies, be free to choose whom to serve, with whom to associate, and the environment in which to provide medical services.
>
> VII. A physician shall recognize a responsibility to participate in activities contributing to an improved community.

---

and to meet the needs of changing times. The Principles of Medical Ethics of the AMA (Box 1-1) guide physicians' standards of conduct for honorable behavior in the practice of medicine.

It is the coder's responsibility to inform administration or his or her immediate supervisor if unethical or possibly illegal coding practices are taking place. Illegal activities are subject to penalties, fines, and/or imprisonment and can result in loss of morale, reputation, and the goodwill of the community. Standards of ethical coding developed by AHIMA are available at its website (www.ahima.org).

The following are principles of ethics for the insurance billing specialist:
● Never make critical remarks about a physician to a patient or anyone else. Maintain dignity; never belittle patients.
● In certain circumstances, it may be unethical for two physicians to treat the same patient for the same condition. Always notify your physician if you discover

that a patient in your practice may have questionable issues of care, conduct, or treatment with your office or another physician's practice.
● Maintain a dignified, courteous relationship with all persons in the office—patients, staff, and the physician—as well as with insurance adjusters, pharmaceutical representatives, and others who come into or telephone the office.
● Do not make critical statements about the treatment given a patient by another physician.

Anyone who uses the internet for health-related reasons has a right to expect that organizations that provide health products, services, or information online will uphold ethical principles. The Internet Healthcare Coalition has developed an eHealth Code of Ethics, which is available at its website (www.ihealthcoalition.org).

It is *illegal* to report incorrect information to government-funded programs, such as Medicare, Medicaid, and TRICARE. Federal legislation has been passed on fraud and abuse issues that relate to federal health care programs. Chapter 2 explains in detail the Criminal False Claims Act and HIPAA mandates. However, private third-party payers operate under different laws and it is *unethical but may not be illegal, depending on state laws,* to report incorrect information to private third-party payers. Incorrect information may damage the individual and the integrity of the database, allow reimbursement for services that should be paid by the patient, or deny payment that should be made by the insurance company.

Examples of illegal and unethical coding follow.
1. Violating guidelines by using code numbers or modifiers to increase payment when the case documentation does not warrant it.
2. Coding services or procedures that were not performed for payment.
3. Unbundling services provided into separate codes when one code is available and includes all of the services provided.
4. Failing to code a relevant condition or complication when it is documented in the health record or, vice versa, assigning a code without documentation from the provider.
5. Coding a service in such a way that it is paid when usually it is not covered.
6. Coding another condition as the principal or primary diagnosis when most of the patient's treatment is for a preexisting condition.

AHIMA has established a code of ethics. This code is appropriate for persons handling health information, whether they are health information specialists, insurance billing specialists, or coders (Figure 1-7).

In the final analysis, most ethical issues can be reduced to right and wrong with the main focus being the moral dictum to do no harm.

EMPLOYER LIABILITY

As mentioned, insurance billing specialists can be either self-employed or employed by physicians, clinics, or hospitals. Physicians are legally responsible for their own conduct and any actions of their employees performed within the context of their employment. This is referred to as *vicarious liability,* also known as **respondeat superior,** which literally means "let the master answer." However, this does not mean that an employee cannot be sued or brought to trial. Actions of the insurance biller may have a definite legal ramification on the employer, depending on the situation. For example, if an employee knowingly submits a fraudulent Medicare or Medicaid claim at the direction of the employer and subsequently the business is audited, both the employer and employee can be brought into litigation by the state or federal government. An insurance biller always should check with his or her physician-employer to determine whether he or she is included in the medical professional liability insurance policy, otherwise known as *malpractice insurance.* If not included, he or she could be sued as an individual. It is the physician's responsibility to make certain all staff members are protected.

> **HIPAA Compliance Alert** **CONFIDENTIALITY**
>
> An insurance billing specialist must be held responsible for maintaining confidentiality when working with patients and their records. The next chapter presents information related to the privacy issues of the Health Insurance Portability and Accountability Act (HIPAA).

EMPLOYEE LIABILITY

Billers and coders can be held personally responsible under the law for billing errors and have been listed as defendants in billing-fraud lawsuits. If you knowingly submit a false claim or allow such a claim to be submitted, you can be liable for a civil violation. If you conceal information or fail to disclose it to obtain payment, you can be held liable. If you are not the person preparing a false claim but you mail or electronically file it, you can be implicated in mail or wire fraud.

Errors and omissions insurance is protection against loss of money caused by failure through error or unintentional omission on the part of the individual or service submitting the insurance claim. Some physicians may contract with a billing service to handle claims submission, and some agreements contain a clause stating that the physician will hold the company harmless from "liability resulting from

STANDARDS OF ETHICAL CODING

Coding professionals should:

1. Apply accurate, complete, and consistent coding practices for the production of high-quality healthcare data.

2. Report all healthcare data elements (e.g. diagnosis and procedure codes, present on admission indicator, discharge status) required for external reporting purposes (e.g. reimbursement and other administrative uses, population health, quality and patient safety measurement, and research) completely and accurately, in accordance with regulatory and documentation standards and requirements and applicable official coding conventions, rules, and guidelines.

3. Assign and report only the codes and data that are clearly and consistently supported by health record documentation in accordance with applicable code set and abstraction conventions, rules, and guidelines.

4. Query provider (physician or other qualified healthcare practitioner) for clarification and additional documentation prior to code assignment when there is conflicting, incomplete, or ambiguous information in the health record regarding a significant reportable condition or procedure or other reportable data element dependent on health record documentation (e.g. present on admission indicator).

5. Refuse to change reported codes or the narratives of codes so that meanings are misrepresented.

6. Refuse to participate in or support coding or documentation practices intended to inappropriately increase payment, qualify for insurance policy coverage, or skew data by means that do not comply with federal and state statutes, regulations and official rules and guidelines.

7. Facilitate interdisciplinary collaboration in situations supporting proper coding practices.

8. Advance coding knowledge and practice through continuing education.

9. Refuse to participate in or conceal unethical coding or abstraction practices or procedures.

10. Protect the confidentiality of the health record at all times and refuse to access protected health information not required for coding-related activities (examples of coding-related activities include completion of code assignment, other health record data abstraction, coding audits, and educational purposes).

11. Demonstrate behavior that reflects integrity, shows a commitment to ethical and legal coding practices, and fosters trust in professional activities.

FIGURE 1-7 AHIMA Codes of Ethics, revised and adopted by AHIMA House of Delegates, 2008. *(Copyright © 2008 American Health Information Management Association. All rights reserved.)*

claims submitted by the service for any account." This means the physician is responsible for mistakes made by the billing service. Thus errors and omissions insurance would not be necessary in this instance. If a physician asks you as the insurance biller to do something that is the least bit questionable, such as writing off patient balances for certain patients automatically, make sure you have a legal document or signed waiver of liability relieving you of the responsibility for such actions. If you notice a problem, it is your responsibility to correct it and to document your actions in writing.

SCOPE OF PRACTICE

An individual who works as a CAP acts as an informal representative of patients (policyholders and Medicare beneficiaries), helping them to obtain insurance reimbursement. A CAP reviews and analyzes existing or potential policies, renders advice, and offers counseling, recommendations, and information. A CAP may not interpret insurance policies or act as an attorney. The legal ability of a CAP to represent a policyholder is limited. When a claim cannot be resolved after a denied claim has been appealed to the insurance company, the CAP must be careful in rendering a personal opinion or advising clients that they have a right to pursue legal action. Always check in your state to see whether there is a scope of practice. In some states, a CAP could be acting outside the scope of the law by giving advice to clients on legal issues, even if licensed as an attorney but not practicing law full-time. If the client wishes to take legal action, it is his or her responsibility to find a competent attorney specializing in contract law and insurance. In some states, giving an insured client advice on purchase or discontinuance of insurance policies is construed as being an insurance agent.

A number of states require CAPs to be licensed, depending on the services rendered to clients. CAPs who perform only the clerical function of filing health insurance claims do not have to be licensed. Check with your state's department of insurance and insurance commissioner (see Chapter 9) to determine whether you should be licensed.

If working as a CAP who does not handle checks or cash, inquire about an errors and omissions insurance policy by contacting the Alliance of Claims Assistance Professionals (ACAP).*

FUTURE CHALLENGES

As you begin your study to become an insurance billing specialist, remember that you are expected to profitably manage a medical practice's financial affairs or patient accounts; otherwise, you will not be considered qualified for this position. In subsequent chapters, you will learn the important information and skills necessary to help you achieve this goal. You will be expected to do the following:

- Know billing regulations for each insurance program and managed care plan in which the practice is a participant.
- Know the aspects of compliance rules and regulations.
- State various insurance rules about treatment and referral of patients.
- Become proficient in computer skills and use of various medical software packages.
- Learn electronic billing software and the variances of each payer.
- Develop diagnostic and procedural coding expertise.
- Know how to interpret third-party remittance advice summary reports, explanation of benefit documents, or both.
- Attain bookkeeping skills necessary to post, interpret, and manage patient accounts.
- Keep current and stay up to date by reading the latest health care industry association publications, participating in e-mail listserv discussions, joining a professional organization for networking, and attending seminars on billing and coding. Train so that you become familiar with other aspects of the medical practice.
- Strive toward becoming certified as an insurance billing specialist and/or coder and, once certified, seek continuing education credits to become recertified. Chapter 18 has more information about the professional organizations that offer certification.

*ACAP, 25500 Hawthorne Blvd., Suite 1158, Torrance, CA 90505.

KEY POINTS

This is a brief chapter review, or summary, of the key issues presented. To further enhance your knowledge of the technical subject matter, review the key terms and key abbreviations for this chapter by locating the meaning for each in the Glossary at the end of this text, which appears in a section before the index.

1. The person who does billing for physicians has become a proficient specialist known by a number of job titles, such as insurance billing specialist or reimbursement specialist.

2. Individuals who help patients organize and file claims are called *claims assistance professionals (CAPs)*.

3. Insurance claims must be promptly submitted to ensure continuous cash flow for a medical practice. If not, overhead expenses cannot be met and a practice will face financial difficulties.

4. Because of the increased technical knowledge that a biller must have, education and training must be more comprehensive and skills must be developed in coding and claims completion. When proficiency is reached, a person can work for a medical practice or may possibly set up his or her own billing service. In this career, jobs can be rewarding for persons with disabilities.

5. Individuals who do billing and complete insurance claims must have many skills, such as knowledge of medical terminology and abbreviations, expert use of procedural and diagnostic code books, precise reading skills, ability to perform basic mathematic calculations, knowledge of medicolegal rules and regulations of various insurance programs, ability to understand and apply compliance issues, basic computer skills (keyboarding and software applications), proficiency in accessing information via the internet, ability to carry out billing and collection techniques, expertise in the legalities of collection on accounts, and ability to generate insurance claims expediently and accurately.

6. Becoming a professional is a gradual process and one must project an appropriate image and develop as a courteous and respectful team player.

7. Etiquette in a medical setting must be adhered to routinely and one must behave ethically at all times.

8. A physician who employs an insurance billing specialist is legally responsible for any actions his or her employees perform within the context of their employment. This is referred to as vicarious liability, also known as *respondeat superior*.

9. Remember, ignorance of the law is not a protection for anyone working in the medical office, so one must stay up to date and well informed on state and federal statutes.

💻 STUDENT ASSIGNMENT

Read the Introduction in the *Workbook*, which explains how you will be working as an insurance billing specialist during this course.

✔ Study Chapter 1.
✔ Answer the fill-in-the-blank, multiple-choice, and true/false questions in the *Workbook* to reinforce the theory learned in this chapter and help prepare for a future test.

✔ Complete the assignments in the *Workbook* to help develop critical thinking and writing skills. As you proceed through the assignments in the *Workbook*, you will broaden your knowledge of medical terminology and gain an entry-level skill in diagnostic and procedural coding and insurance claim completion.

✔ Turn to the Glossary at the end of this text for a further understanding of the key terms and key abbreviations used in this chapter.

CHAPTER 2

Compliance, Privacy, Fraud, and Abuse in Insurance Billing

Linda Smith

OBJECTIVES

After reading this chapter, you should be able to:

1. Define compliance.
2. Name the two provisions of the Health Insurance Portability and Accountability Act (HIPAA) that relate most to health care.
3. Explain the difference between *Title I: Health Insurance Reform* and *Title II: Administrative Simplification*.
4. Define and discuss HIPAA roles, relationships, and key terms, including HIPAA in the practice setting.
5. Describe the Privacy Rule under HIPAA.
6. Define and discuss protected health information (PHI).
7. Identify the difference between disclosure and use of PHI and discuss exceptions to HIPAA.
8. Illustrate the difference between privileged and non-privileged information.
9. Explain patient rights under HIPAA.
10. Explain responsibilities of the health care organization to protect patient rights under HIPAA.
11. State the guidelines for HIPAA privacy compliance.
12. List the three major categories of security safeguards under HIPAA.
13. Discuss the Security Rule and how it relates to coding and billing.
14. Define the provisions of the HITECH Act.
15. Explain the purpose of the HIPAA Omnibus Rule.
16. List consequences of noncompliance with HIPAA and the HITECH Act.
17. Discuss how HIPAA affects all areas of the health care office, including the organization and staff responsibilities in protecting patient rights.
18. Identify the difference between fraud and abuse.
19. Identify the federal and state laws that regulate health care fraud and abuse.
20. List the various fraud and abuse audit programs.
21. Describe the basic components of an effective compliance program.
22. Discuss what to expect from your health care practice when it comes to various HIPAA policies and procedures.

KEY TERMS

abuse
American Recovery and
   Reinvestment Act
authorization
authorization form
breach of confidential
   communication
business associate
Civil Monetary Penalty

clearinghouse
clustering
compliance
compliance plan
Comprehensive Error Rate Testing
confidential communication
confidentiality
consent
covered entity

disclosure
electronic media
embezzlement
fraud
Health Care Fraud Prevention
   and Enforcement
   Action Team
health care provider
HIPAA Omnibus Rule

individually identifiable health
 information
mitigation
nonprivileged information
Notice of Privacy Practices
phantom bills
privacy

privacy officer, privacy official
privileged information
protected health information
psychotherapy notes
qui tam
Recovery Audit Contractor
security officer

Security Rule
Self-Disclosure Protocol
state preemption
transaction
use
Zone Program Integrity
 Contractor

KEY ABBREVIATIONS

ARRA	ePHI	HIPAA	OSHA
CD	FBI	HITECH	P&P
CERT	FCA	IIHI	PHI
CLIA	FDIC	MIP	PO
CMP	FERA	NPP	RAC
CMS	FTP	OCR	SDP
DHHS	HCFAC	OIG	TPO
DOJ	HEAT	ORT	ZPIC

Service to Patients

The insurance billing specialist has many opportunities to serve patients' needs. Although you may be delegated the task of obtaining required paperwork, keep in mind that many patients are experiencing pain, anxiety, and concern when entering the doctor's office. When presenting the Notice of Privacy, greet the patient with a smile and have a helpful and caring attitude. Be ready to answer questions regarding the notice. Have the notice available in those languages spoken by a significant portion of the medical practice's patient population. Serve patients by respecting their privacy and keeping their health information confidential, disclosing it only according to the medical practice's correct policies and procedures that comply with federal regulations. Communicate your physician's commitment to improve quality of care and to ensure patient safety by avoiding errors.

Use of electronic formats in the health care industry is a driving force behind electronic communications that will make a full circle to complete the patient care process. It is your duty to understand how health information and electronic technologies tie together. As an educated and informed employee, you can better serve the patients who visit your office.

COMPLIANCE DEFINED

Compliance in the health care industry is the process of meeting regulations, recommendations, and expectations of federal and state agencies that pay for health care services and regulate the industry. Health care compliance encompasses the claims reimbursement processes, managed care procedures, protection of patients' privacy, Occupational Safety and Health Administration (OSHA) guidelines, Clinical Laboratory Improvement Amendments (CLIA) provisions, licensure, and due diligence in obeying the law.

Health care is one of the most highly regulated industries, holding the health care worker to the highest levels of scrutiny. Any individual working in health care and any business that is involved with the health care industry must conform to the principles and practices identified by state and federal agencies. A compliance strategy provides a standardized process for handling business functions, much like a "user's manual." This will enable consistent and effective management and staff performance.

The first step toward achieving compliance is identifying the laws that regulate the industry, which are outlined further in this chapter. It is crucial to understand and follow the laws; failure to comply with the associated mandates can lead to criminal penalties and/or civil fines.

Government agencies, including the Department of Justice (DOJ), the Department of Health and Human Services (DHHS or HHS), Office for Civil Rights (OCR), Office of the Inspector General (OIG), and the Centers for Medicare and Medicaid Services (CMS), are charged with enforcing these laws.

HEALTH INSURANCE PORTABILITY AND ACCOUNTABILITY ACT

One of the most significant pieces of legislation to have an impact on **health care providers,** health care workers, and individuals receiving health care services is the Health Insurance Portability and Accountability Act (HIPAA) of 1996, Public Law 104-191. The Act is made up of five titles. Among these five titles, there are two provisions of HIPAA that relate most to health care, *Title I: Health Insurance Reform* and *Title II: Administrative Simplification*. The HIPAA legislation projected long-term benefits that include lowered administrative costs, increased accuracy of data, increased patient and customer satisfaction, and reduced revenue cycle time, ultimately improving financial management.

Title I: Health Insurance Reform

The primary purpose of HIPAA *Title I: Health Insurance Reform* is to provide continuous insurance coverage for workers and their insured dependents when they change or lose jobs. This aspect of HIPAA affects individuals as consumers, not particularly as patients. Previously, when an employee left or lost a job and changed insurance coverage, a "preexisting" clause prevented or limited coverage for certain medical conditions. HIPAA now limits the use of preexisting condition exclusions, prohibits discrimination for past or present poor health, and guarantees certain employers and individuals the right to purchase new health insurance coverage after losing a job. Additionally, HIPAA allows renewal of health insurance coverage regardless of an individual's health condition that is covered under the particular policy.

Title II: Administrative Simplification

The goals of HIPAA *Title II: Administrative Simplification* focus on the health care practice setting and aim to reduce administrative costs and burdens. Standardizing electronic transmissions of administrative and financial information reduces the number of forms and methods used in the claims processing cycle and reduces the nonproductive effort that results from processing paper or nonstandard electronic claims. Additional provisions are meant to ensure the privacy and security of an individual's health data.

Two parts of the Administrative Simplification provisions are as follows.
1. Development and implementation of standardized electronic transactions using common sets of descriptors (that is, standard code sets) to represent health care concepts and procedures when performing health-related financial and administrative activities electronically (Box 2-1). HIPAA has been part of a great shift in processing electronic data. Transaction

standards apply to the following, which are called *covered entities* under HIPAA: health care third-party payers, health care providers, and health care clearinghouses. A health care **clearinghouse** is an organization that acts as an intermediary between a medical provider and the entity to which health care information is transmitted. It is an independent organization that receives insurance claims from the physician's office, performs software edits, and redistributes the claims electronically to various third-party payers.
2. Implementation of privacy and security procedures to prevent the misuse of health information by ensuring the following:
   ● Privacy and confidentiality
   ● Security of health information

Administrative simplification has created uniform sets of standards that protect and place limits on how confidential health information can be used. For years, health care providers have locked medical records in file cabinets and refused to share patient health information. Patients now have specific rights regarding how their health information is used and disclosed because federal and state laws regulate the protection of an individual's privacy. Knowledge of and attention to the rights of patients are important to the compliance endeavor in a health care practice. Providers are entrusted with health information and are expected to recognize when certain health information can be used or disclosed.

Patients have the legal right to request (1) access and amendments to their health records, (2) an accounting of those who have received their health information, and (3) restrictions on who can access their health records. Understanding the parameters concerning these rights is crucial to complying with HIPAA.

Health care providers and their employees can be held accountable for using or disclosing patient health information inappropriately. HIPAA regulations will be enforced, as clearly stated by the US government.

Defining HIPAA Roles, Relationships, and Key Terms
Department of Health and Human Services

The Department of Health and Human Services (DHHS or HHS) is the United States government's principal agency for protecting the health of all Americans and providing essential human services. HIPAA legislation required the DHHS to establish national standards and identifiers for electronic transactions as well as to implement privacy and security standards. In regard to HIPAA, *Secretary* refers to the DHHS Secretary or any officer or employee of DHHS to whom the authority involved has been delegated.

Box 2-1	Examples of Administrative and Financial Data

Administrative Data	Financial Data
● Referral certification and authorization for services	● Health care claim submission for services
● Enrollment or disenrollment of individual in or from health plan	● Process health plan premium payment
● Health plan eligibility	● Check status of a previously submitted claim
	● Health care payment and remittance advice
	● Coordination of benefits

Office of E-Health Standards and Services

The Office of E-Health Standards and Services within the Centers for Medicare and Medicaid Services (CMS) enforces the insurance portability and transaction and code set requirements of HIPAA for Medicare and Medicaid programs.

The Office for Civil Rights

The Office for Civil Rights (OCR) enforces privacy and security rules.

Key HIPAA Terms

Electronic media refers to the mode of electronic transmission, including the following:

- Internet (online mode—wide open)
- Extranet or private network using internet technology to link business parties
- Leased telephone or dial-up telephone lines, including fax modems (speaking over the telephone is not considered an electronic transmission)
- Transmissions that are physically moved from one location to another using removable or transportable digital memory medium such as magnetic tape or disk, optical disk, or digital memory card.

A **transaction** refers to the transmission of information between two parties to carry out financial or administrative activities related to health care. These data transmissions include information that completes the health care insurance claim process and are discussed further in Chapter 8.

Refer to Box 2-2 for titles of additional entities that oversee HIPAA-related functions.

HIPAA in the Practice Setting

Under HIPAA, the term **covered entity** applies to any health care provider who transmits any health information in electronic form. HIPAA does not affect only medical physicians; HIPAA's definition of a health care provider extends to anyone who provides health care services to a patient. In addition to physicians, this includes clinics, physician's assistants, nurse practitioners, social workers, chiropractors, dentists, nursing homes, pharmacies, and others.

It is important to remember that health care providers who transmit any health information in electronic form in connection with a HIPAA transaction are covered entities. Electronic form or media can include optical disk (compact disk [CD] or DVD), USB flash drive, or file transfer protocol (FTP) over the internet.

Box 2-2 Overseers of HIPAA Functions

A covered entity transmits health information in electronic form in connection with a *transaction* covered by HIPAA. The covered entity may be (1) a health care coverage carrier, such as Blue Cross/Blue Shield; (2) a health care clearinghouse through which claims are submitted; or (3) a health care provider, such as the primary care physician.

A business associate is a person who, on behalf of the covered entity, performs or assists in the performance of a function or activity involving the use or disclosure of individually identifiable health information, including claims processing or administration, data analysis, processing or administration, utilization review, quality assurance, billing, benefit management, practice management, and repricing. For example, if a provider's practice contracts with an outside billing company to manage its claims and accounts receivable, the billing company would be a business associate of the provider (the covered entity).

A health care provider is a person trained and licensed to provide care to a patient and also a place that is licensed to give health care, such as a hospital, skilled nursing facility, inpatient/outpatient rehabilitation facility, home health agency, hospice program, physician, diagnostic department, outpatient physical or occupational therapy, rural clinic, or home dialysis supplier.

Privacy and security officers oversee the HIPAA-related functions. These individuals may or may not be employees of a particular health care practice. A privacy officer or privacy official (PO) is designated to help the provider remain in compliance by setting policies and procedures (P&P) and by training and managing the staff regarding HIPAA and patient rights. The PO is usually the contact person for questions and complaints.

A **security officer** protects the computer and networking systems within the practice and implements protocols such as password assignment, backup procedures, firewalls, virus protection, and contingency planning for emergencies.

Voice-over-modem faxes, meaning a telephone line, are not considered electronic media, although a fax from a computer (for example, using the WinFax program) is considered an electronic medium.

HIPAA requires the designation of a **privacy officer** or **privacy official (PO)** to develop and implement the organization's policies and procedures (P&P). The organization's PO may hold another position within the practice or may not be an employee of the practice at all. Often the PO is a contracted professional who is available to the practice through established means of contact.

A **business associate** is a person or entity that performs certain functions or activities using health care information on behalf of a covered entity. It is considered an extension of the provider practice and is held to the same standards under HIPAA. For example, if the office's medical transcription is performed by an outside service, the transcription service is a business associate of the covered entity (the health care provider or practice). See Boxes 2-2 and 2-3.

HIPAA privacy regulations as a federal mandate apply unless the state laws are contrary or more stringent regarding privacy. A state law is contrary if it is impossible to comply with the state law while complying with federal requirements or if the state law stands as an obstacle to the purposes of the federal law. **State preemption,** a complex technical issue not within the scope of the health care provider's role, refers to instances when state law takes precedence over federal law. The PO determines when the need for preemption arises.

THE PRIVACY RULE: CONFIDENTIALITY AND PROTECTED HEALTH INFORMATION

What I may see or hear in the course of the treatment or even outside of the treatment in regard to the life of men, which on no account one must spread abroad, I will keep to myself holding such things shameful to be spoken about.

Hippocrates, 400 B.C.

The Hippocratic Oath, federal and state regulations, professional standards, and ethics all address patient privacy. Because current technology allows easy access to health care information, HIPAA imposes new requirements on health care providers. Since computers have become indispensable in the health care office, confidential health data have been sent across networks, e-mailed over the internet, and even exposed by hackers, with few safeguards taken to protect data and prevent information from being intercepted or lost. With the implementation of standardizing electronic transactions of health care information, the use of technologies poses new risks for privacy and security. These concerns were addressed under HIPAA and regulations now closely govern how the industry handles its electronic activities.

Privacy is the condition of being secluded from the presence or view of others. **Confidentiality** is using discretion in keeping secret information. Integrity plays an important part in the health care setting. Staff of a health care organization need a good understanding of HIPAA's basic requirements and must be committed to protecting the privacy and rights of the practice's patients.

Health care organizations and staff members use and disclose health information on a regular basis. **Use** means the sharing, application, utilization, examination, or analysis of health information within the organization. When a patient's billing record is accessed to review the claim submission history, the individual's health information is in "use."

Disclosure means the release, transfer, provision of access to, or divulging in any other manner of information outside the entity holding the information. An example of a disclosure is giving information about a patient you are scheduling for a procedure to the hospital's outpatient surgery center.

Consent is the verbal or written agreement that gives approval to some action, situation, or statement. In health care, a consent is a general document that gives health care providers permission to routinely use or disclose protected health information (PHI) for treatment, payment, or health care operations (TPO). Although many practices obtain signed consents from their patients, the Privacy Rule does not require a covered entity to obtain patient consent for routine uses and disclosures.

Treatment includes coordination or management of health care between providers or referral of a patient to another provider. PHI can be disclosed to obtain reimbursement. Other health care operations include performance reviews, audits, training programs, and certain types of fundraising (Figures 2-1 to 2-4).

In contrast to a consent, the HIPAA Privacy Rule requires a signed **authorization** for any uses and disclosures that are not routine and are not otherwise allowed by the Rule. Authorization is an individual's formal, written permission to use or disclose his or her personally identifiable health information for purposes other than TPO. For some "extra" activities, including marketing, research, and **psychotherapy notes,** an **authorization form** is necessary for use and disclosure of PHI that is not included in any existing consent form agreements. **Individually identifiable health information (IIHI)** is any part of an individual's health information, including demographic information (for example, address or date of birth), collected from the individual that is created or received by a covered entity. This information relates to the individual's past, present, or future physical or mental health or condition; the provision of health care to the individual; or the past, present, or future payment for the provision of health care. IIHI data identify the individual or establish a reasonable basis to believe that the information can be used to identify the individual. For example, if you as a health care provider are talking to an insurance representative, you will likely give information such as the patient's date of birth and last name. These pieces of information would make it reasonably easy to identify the patient. If you are talking to a pharmaceutical representative about a drug assistance program that covers

**REQUIRED ELEMENTS
OF HIPAA AUTHORIZATION**

Identification of person (or class) authorized to request

Identification of person (or class) to whom covered entity is to use/disclose

Description of information to be released with specificity to allow entity to know which information the authorization references

Description of each purpose of the requested use or disclosure

Expiration date, time period, or event

Statement that is revocable by written request

Individual's (patient's) signature and date

Statement of representative's authority

Authorization for Release of Information

PATIENT NAME: ___Levy___ ___Chloe___ ___E.___ _____
LAST   FIRST   MI   MAIDEN OR OTHER NAME
DATE OF BIRTH: _02_-_12_-_1950_ SS# _320_-_21_-_3408_ MEDICAL RECORD #: ___3075___
MO DAY YR
ADDRESS: ___3298 East Main Street___ CITY: ___Woodland Hills___ STATE: _XY_ ZIP: _12345-0001_

DAY PHONE: ___013-340-9800___ EVENING PHONE: ___013-549-8708___

I hereby authorize ___Gerald Practon, MD___ (Print Name of Provider) to release information from my medical record as indicated below to:
NAME: ___Margaret L. Lee, MD___
ADDRESS: ___328 Seward Street___ CITY: ___Anytown___ STATE: _XY_ ZIP: _45601-0731_

PHONE: ___013-219-7698___ FAX: ___013-290-9877___

INFORMATION TO BE RELEASED:
DATES:
☒ History and physical exam ___6-8-20XX___
☐ Progress notes _____
☐ Lab reports _____
☐ X-ray reports _____
☐ Other: _____ _____

I specifically authorize the release of information relating to:
☐ Substance abuse (including alcohol/drug abuse)
☐ Mental health (including psychotherapy notes)
☐ HIV related information (AIDS related testing)
X _____
SIGNATURE OF PATIENT OR LEGAL GUARDIAN   DATE

PURPOSE OF DISCLOSURE: ☐ Changing physicians ☒ Consultation/second opinion ☐ Continuing care
☐ Legal   ☐ School   ☐ Insurance   ☐ Workers Compensation
☐ Other (please specify): _____

1. I understand that this authorization will expire on ___09/01/20XX___ (Print the Date this Form Expires) days after I have signed the form.

2. I understand that I may revoke this authorization at any time by notifying the providing organization in writing, and it will be effective on the date notified except to the extent action has already been taken in reliance upon it.

3. I understand that information used or disclosed pursuant to this authorization may be subject to redisclosure by the recipient and no longer be protected by Federal privacy regulations.

4. I understand that if I am being requested to release this information by ___Gerald Practon, MD___ (Print Name of Provider) for the purpose of: _____

   a. By authorizing this release of information, my health care and payment for my health care will not be affected if I do not sign this form.
   b. I understand I may see and copy the information described on this form if I ask for it, and that I will get a copy of this form after I sign it.
   c. I have been informed that ___Gerald Practon, MD___ (Print Name of Provider) will/will not receive financial or in-kind compensation in exchange for using or disclosing the health information described above.

5. I understand that in compliance with ___XY___ (Print the State Whose Laws Govern the Provider) statute, I will pay a fee of $ _5.00_ (Print the Fee Charged). There is no charge for medical records if copies are sent to facilities for ongoing care or follow up treatment.

___Chloe E. Levy___   ___6/1/XX___ OR _____
SIGNATURE OF PATIENT   DATE   PARENT/LEGAL GUARDIAN/AUTHORIZED PERSON   DATE

_____   _____   ☐ _____
RECORDS RECEIVED BY   DATE   RELATIONSHIP TO PATIENT

FOR OFFICE USE ONLY
DATE REQUEST FILLED _____   BY: _____
IDENTIFICATION PRESENTED _____   FEE COLLECTED $_____

FIGURE 2-1 Completed authorization for release of information form for a patient who is relocating to another city. The required elements for HIPAA authorization are indicated. Note: This form is used on a one-time basis for reasons other than treatment, payment, or health care operations (TPO). When the patient arrives at the new physician's office, a consent for TPO form will need to be signed. *(From* Federal Register *64[212]: Appendix to Subpart E of Part 164: Model Authorization Form, November 3, 1999.)*

RELEASE OF MEDICAL INFORMATION

PATIENT INFORMATION

Patient Name _____

Address _____ Social Security # _____

City _____ State _____ ZIP _____ Birth date ____/____/____

Phone (Home) _____ Work _____

RELEASE FROM:

Name _____

Address _____

City _____ State _____ ZIP_____

RELEASE TO:

Name _____

Address _____

City _____ State _____ ZIP_____

INFORMATION TO BE RELEASED:

1. GENERAL RELEASE:

____Entire Medical Record (excluding protected information)

____Hospital Records only (specify)_____

____Lab Results only (specify) _____

____X-ray Reports only (specify) _____

____Other Records (specify) _____

2. INFORMATION PROTECTED BY STATE/FEDERAL LAW:
If indicated below, I hereby authorize the disclosure and release of information regarding:

____Drug Abuse Diagnosis/Treatment

____Alcoholism Diagnosis/Treatment

____Mental Health Diagnosis/Treatment

____Sexually Transmitted Disease

PATIENT AUTHORIZATION TO RELEASE INFORMATION:

   Authorization is valid for 60 days only from the date of my signature. I reserve the right to revoke this authorization at any time prior to 60 days (except for action that has already been taken) by notifying the medical office in writing.

   I understand that my records are protected under HIPAA (Health Insurance Portability and Accountability Act) Standards for Privacy of Individually Identifiable Information (45 CFR Parts 160 and 164) unless otherwise permitted by federal law. Any information released or received shall not be further relayed to any other facility or person without my written authorization. I also understand that such information will not be given, sold, transferred, or in any way relayed to any other person or party not specified above without my further written authorization.

   I hereby grant authorization to release the information listed above. I certify that this request has been made voluntarily and that the information given above is accurate to the best of my knowledge.

_____   _____
Signature of Patient/Legally Responsible Party   Date

_____   _____
Witness Signature   Date

FIGURE 2-2 Consent for release of information form. *(Modified from Bonewit-West K, Hunt S, Applegate E:* Today's medical assistant: clinical & administrative procedures, *ed 2, St. Louis, 2013, Saunders.)*

a new pill for heartburn and you say that your practice has a patient living in your town who is indigent and has stomach problems, you are not divulging information that would identify the patient.

   Protected health information (PHI) is any information that identifies an individual and describes his or her health status, age, sex, ethnicity, or other demographic characteristics, whether that information is or is not stored or transmitted electronically. It refers to IIHI that is transmitted by electronic media, maintained in electronic form or transmitted, or maintained in any other form or medium. See Example 2-1. Traditionally, the focus was on protecting paper medical records and documentation that held patient's health information, such as laboratory results and radiology reports. HIPAA Privacy Rule expands these protections to apply to PHI. The individual's health information is protected regardless of the type of medium in which it is maintained. This includes paper, the health care provider's computerized practice management and billing system, spoken words, and x-ray films.

Example 2-1	Protected Health Information in a Medical Office
Intake forms	Encounter sheets
Laboratory work requests	Physician notes
Physician–patient conversations	Prescriptions
Conversations that refer to patients by name	Insurance claim forms
Physician dictation tapes	X-rays
Telephone conversations with patients	E-mail messages

   HIPAA imposes requirements to protect not only disclosure of PHI outside of the organization but also internal uses of health information. PHI may not be used or disclosed without permission of the patient or someone authorized to act on behalf of the patient, unless the use or disclosure is specifically required or permitted by the rule (for example, TPO). The two types of disclosure required by HIPAA Privacy Rule are to the individual

COLLEGE CLINIC
4567 Broad Avenue
Woodland Hills, XY 12345-0001
Phone: 555/486-9002
Fax: 555/487-8976

CONSENT TO THE USE AND DISCLOSURE OF HEALTH INFORMATION

I understand that this organization originates and maintains health records which describe my health history, symptoms, examination, test results, diagnoses, treatment, and any plans for future care or treatment. I understand that this information is used to:

- plan my care and treatment.
- communicate among health professionals who contribute to my care.
- apply my diagnosis and services, procedures, and surgical information to my bill.
- verify services billed by third-party payers.
- assess quality of care and review the competence of health care professionals in routine health care operations.

I further understand that:

- a complete description of information uses and disclosures is included in a *Notice of Information Practices* which has been provided to me.
- I have a right to review the notice prior to signing this consent.
- the organization reserves the right to change their notice and practices.
- any revised notice will be mailed to the address I have provided prior to implementation.
- I have the right to object to the use of my health information for directory purposes.
- I have the right to request restrictions as to how my health information may be used or disclosed to carry out treatment, payment, or health care operations.
- the organization is not required to agree to the restrictions requested.
- I may revoke this consent in writing, except to the extent that the organization has already taken action in reliance thereon.

☐ I request the following restrictions to the use or disclosure of my health information.

_____

_____   _____
Date   Notice Effective Date

_____   _____
Signature of Patient or Legal Representative   Witness

_____   _____
Signature   Title

Date _____   __ Accepted __ Rejected

FIGURE 2-3 An example of a consent form used to disclose and use health information for treatment, payment, or health care operations (TPO). This is not required under HIPAA, but you may find that some medical practices use it. *(From Fordney MT, French L: Medical insurance billing and coding: a worktext, Philadelphia, 2003, Elsevier.)*

who is the subject of the PHI and to the Secretary of DHHS to investigate compliance with the rule.

Confidential Information

The insurance billing specialist must be responsible for maintaining confidentiality of patients' health information when working with patients and their medical records. Example 2-1 lists some of the PHI that is typical in a medical office and that falls under HIPAA compliance regulations.

The patient record and any photographs obtained are confidential documents and require an authorization form that must be signed by the patient to release information (see Figures 2-1 to 2-4). If the form is a photocopy,

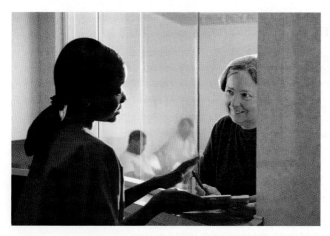

FIGURE 2-4 Patient signing a consent form.

it is necessary to state that the photocopy is approved by the patient or write to the patient and obtain an original signed document.

Exceptions to HIPAA

Unauthorized release of information is called **breach of confidential communication** and is considered a HIPAA violation, which may lead to fines.

Confidentiality between the physician and patient is automatically waived in the following situations:

1. When the patient is a member of a managed care organization (MCO) and the physician has signed a contract with the MCO that contains a clause that states "for quality care purposes, the MCO has a right to access the medical records of their patients, and for utilization management purposes," the MCO has a right to audit that patient's financial records. Other managed care providers need to know about the patients if they are involved in the care and treatment of members of the MCO.
2. When patients have certain communicable diseases that are highly contagious or infectious and state health agencies require providers to report, even if the patient does not want the information reported.
3. When a medical device breaks or malfunctions, the Food and Drug Administration (FDA) requires providers to report certain information that will allow it to be advised of the break or malfunction.
4. When a patient is suspect in a criminal investigation or to assist in locating a missing person, material witness, or suspect, police have the right to request certain information.
5. When the patient's records are subpoenaed or there is a search warrant. The courts have the right to order providers to release patient information.
6. When there is a suspicious death or suspected crime victim, providers must report cases to proper authorities (law enforcement).
7. When the physician examines a patient at the request of a third party who is paying the bill, as in workers' compensation cases.
8. When state law requires the release of information to police that is for the good of society, such as reporting cases of child abuse, elder abuse, domestic violence, or gunshot wounds.

For information on confidentiality as it relates to computer use, refer to Chapter 8.

The purpose of the Privacy Rule is to ensure that patients who receive medical treatment can control the manner in which specific information is used and to whom it is disclosed. **Confidential communication** is a privileged communication that may be disclosed only with the patient's permission. Everything you see, hear, or read about patients remains confidential and does not leave the office. Never talk about patients or data contained in medical records where others may overhear. Some employers require employees to sign a confidentiality agreement (Figure 2-5). Such agreements should be updated periodically to address issues raised by the use of new technologies.

Privileged Information

Privileged information is related to the treatment and progress of the patient. The patient must sign an authorization to release this information or selected facts from the medical record. Some states have passed laws allowing certain test results (for example, disclosure of the presence of the human immunodeficiency virus [HIV] or alcohol or substance abuse) and other information to be placed separate from the patient's medical record. A special authorization form is used to release this information.

Nonprivileged Information

Nonprivileged information consists of ordinary facts unrelated to treatment of the patient, including the patient's name, city of residence, and dates of admission or discharge. This information must be sensitized against unauthorized disclosure under the privacy section of HIPAA. The patient's authorization is not necessary for the purposes of treatment, payment, or health care operations, unless the record is in a specialty hospital (for example, for alcohol treatment) or a special service unit of a general hospital (for example, psychiatric unit). Professional judgment is required. The information is disclosed on a legitimate need-to-know basis, meaning that the medical data should be revealed to the attending physician because the information may have some effect on the treatment of the patient.

EMPLOYEE CONFIDENTIALITY STATEMENT

As an employee of _____ABC Clinic, Inc._____ (employer), having been trained as an insurance billing specialist with employee responsibilities and authorization to access personal medical and health information, and as a condition of my employment, I agree to the following:

A. I recognize that I am responsible for complying with the Health Insurance Portability and Accountability Act (HIPAA) of 1996 policies regarding confidentiality of patients' information, which, if I violate, may lead to immediate dismissal from employment and, depending on state laws, criminal prosecution.

B. I will treat all information received during the course of my employment, which relates to the patients, as confidential and privileged information.

C. I will not access patient information unless I must obtain the information to perform my job duties.

D. I will not disclose information regarding my employer's patients to any person or entity, other than that necessary to perform my job duties, and as permitted under the employer's HIPAA policies.

E. I will not access any of my employer's computer systems that currently exist or may exist in the future using a password other than my own.

F. I will safeguard my computer password and will not show it in public.

G. I will not allow anyone, including other employees, to use my password to access computer files.

H. I will log off of the computer immediately after I finish using it.

I. I will not use e-mail to transmit patient information unless instructed to do so by my employer's HIPAA privacy officer.

J. I will not take patient information from my employer's premises in hard copy or electronic form without permission from my employer's HIPAA privacy officer.

K. Upon termination of my employment, I agree to continue to maintain the confidentiality of any information learned while an employee and agree to relinquish office keys, access cards, or any other device that provides access to the provider or its information.

Mary Doe
_____
Signature

September 14, 20XX
_____
Date

Mary Doe
_____
Print name

Brenda Shield
_____
Witness

FIGURE 2-5 An example of an employee confidentiality agreement that may be used by an employer when hiring an insurance billing specialist.

Patients' Rights

Right to Privacy

All patients have a right to privacy. It is important never to discuss patient information other than with the physician, an insurance company, or an individual who has been authorized by the patient. If a telephone inquiry is made and you need to verify that callers are who they say they are, you should do the following:

● Ask for one or more of the following items: patient's full name, home address, date of birth, Social Security number, mother's maiden name, dates of service.
● Ask for a call-back number and compare it with the number on file.

● Ask the patient to fax a sheet with his or her signature on it so that you can compare it with the one on file.
● Some hospitals may assign a code word or number that may be a middle name or date that is easy for patients to remember. If a patient does not know the code word, then ask for personal identifying information as mentioned.

If a telephone inquiry is made about a patient, ask the caller to put the request in writing and include the patient's signed authorization. If the caller refuses, have the physician return the call. If a relative telephones asking about a patient, have the physician return the call.

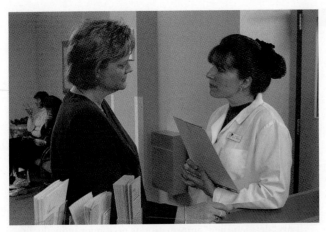

FIGURE 2-6 Insurance billing specialist consulting with the supervisor or office manager about office policies regarding release of a patient's medical record.

When you telephone a patient about an insurance matter and reach voice mail, use care in choosing your words when leaving a message in the event that the call is inadvertently received at the wrong number. Leave your name, the office name, and the return telephone number. Never attempt to interpret a report or provide information about the outcome of laboratory or other diagnostic tests to the patient. Let the physician do it (Figure 2-6).

Do's and Don'ts of Confidentiality

Don't: Discuss a patient with acquaintances, yours or the patient's.

Don't: Leave patients' records or appointment books exposed on your desk. If confidential documents are on your desk and patients can easily see them as they walk by, either turn the documents over or lock them in a secure drawer when you leave your desk, even if you are gone for only a few moments.

Don't: Leave a computer screen with patient information visible, even for a moment, if another patient may see the data. If patient information is on your computer, either turn the screen off or save it on disk, lock the disk in a secure place, and clear the information from the screen.

Do: Properly dispose of notes, papers, and memos by using a shredding device.

Do: Be careful when using the copying machine, because it is easy to forget to remove the original insurance claim or medical record from the document glass.

Do: Use common sense and follow the guidelines mentioned in this chapter to help you maintain your professional credibility and integrity.

Privacy Rules: Patient Rights Under HIPAA

Patients are granted the following six federal rights that allow them to be informed about PHI and to control how their PHI is used and disclosed:

1. *Right to **Notice of Privacy Practices (NPP)***, a document in plain language that is usually given to the patient at the first visit or at enrollment. The staff must make a reasonable "best effort" to obtain a signature from the patient acknowledging receipt, and this must be done once only. If the patient cannot or will not sign, this should be documented in the patient's health record. The NPP must be posted at every service delivery site and be available in paper form for those who request it. A provider's website must have the NPP placed on the site and must deliver a copy electronically on request.

2. *Right to request restrictions on certain uses and disclosures of PHI.* Patients have the right to ask for restrictions on how a medical office uses and discloses PHI for TPO (for example, a patient had a successfully treated sexually transmitted infection many years ago and requests that, whenever possible, this material not be disclosed). A provider is not required to agree to these requests but must have a process to review the requests, accept and review any appeal, and give a sound reason for not agreeing to a request. Restrictions must be documented and followed. See Box 2-4, which details the regulations for disclosing the minimum necessary PHI, de-identification of PHI, marketing related to the patient, and fundraising activities related to patients.

3. *Right to request confidential communications* by alternative means or at an alternative location (for example, calling at work rather than at the residence or test results sent in writing instead of communicated by telephone). The patient does not need to explain the reason for the request. The health care office must have a process in place both to evaluate requests and appeals and to respond to the patient. Patients may be required by the office to make their requests in writing. A written document protects the practice's compliance endeavors.

4. *Right to access (inspect and obtain a copy of) PHI.* Privacy regulations allow the provider to require that the patient make the request for access in writing. Generally, a request must be acted on within 30 days. A reasonable, cost-based fee for copies of PHI may include only the costs for supplies and labor for copying, postage when mailed, and preparing a summary of the PHI if the patient has agreed to this instead of complete access. If a digital office copier is used, ensure that precautions are taken to digitally shred information after every copy, print scan, or fax job so that information is kept secure. If a patient requests an electronic copy of his or her information

Box 2-4   HIPAA Help

These key terms are addressed in the Notice of Privacy Practices (NPP) that applies to the patient's right to request restrictions on certain uses and disclosures of protected health information (PHI).

- **Minimum Necessary.** Privacy regulations require that use or disclosure of only the minimum amount of information necessary to fulfill the intended purpose be permitted. There are some exceptions to this rule. You do not need to limit PHI for disclosures regarding health care providers for treatment, the patient, DHHS for investigations of compliance with HIPAA, or as required by law.

   Minimum Necessary determinations for *uses of PHI* must be made within each organization and reasonable efforts must be made to limit access to only the minimum amount of information needed by identified staff members. In smaller offices, employees may have multiple job functions. If a medical assistant helps with the patient examination, documents vital signs, and then collects the patient's copayment at the reception area, the assistant will likely access clinical and billing records. Simple procedure and policy (P&P) about appropriate access to PHI may be sufficient to satisfy the Minimum Necessary requirement. Larger organizations may have specific restrictions regarding who should have access to different types of PHI, because staff members tend to have more targeted job roles. Remain knowledgeable about your office's policy regarding Minimum Necessary. If you are strictly scheduling appointments, you may not need access to the clinical record. An x-ray technician likely will not need to access the patient billing records.

   Minimum Necessary determinations for *disclosures of PHI* are distinguished by two categories within the Privacy Rule:
   1. For disclosures made on a routine and recurring basis, you may implement policies and procedures, or standard protocols, for what will be disclosed. These disclosures would be common in your practice. Examples may include disclosures for workers' compensation claims or school physical forms.
   2. For other disclosures that would be considered nonroutine, criteria for determining the Minimum Necessary amount of PHI should be established and

each request for disclosure should be reviewed on an individual basis. A staff member (for example, privacy officer [PO], medical records supervisor) will likely be assigned to determine this situation when the need arises.
As a general rule, remember that you must limit your requests to access PHI to the Minimum Necessary to accomplish the task for which you will need the information.
- **De-identification of Confidential Information.** Other requirements relating to uses and disclosures of PHI include health information that does not identify an individual or leaves no reasonable basis to believe that the information can be used to identify an individual. This "de-identified" information is no longer individually identifiable health information (IIHI). Most providers will never need to de-identify patient information and the requirements for de-identifying PHI are lengthy. The regulations give specific directions on how to ensure that all pieces of necessary information are removed to fit the definition. De-identified information is not subject to the privacy regulations because it does not specifically identify an individual.
- **Marketing.** When communicating about a product or service, the goal is to encourage patients to purchase or use the product or service. For example, a dermatologist may advertise for a discount on facial cream when you schedule a dermabrasion treatment. You will not likely be involved in marketing but keep in mind the general rule that PHI (including names and addresses) cannot be used for marketing purposes without the specific authorization of the patient. Sending appointment reminders and general news updates about your organization and the services you provide is not considered marketing and does not require patient authorization.
- **Fundraising.** Again, you will likely not be involved in fundraising activities but HIPAA allows demographic information and dates of care to be used for fundraising purposes without patient authorization. The disclosure of any additional information requires patient authorization. Your organization's NPP will state that patients may receive fundraising materials and are given the opportunity to opt out of receiving future solicitations.

---

or requests that it be transmitted to another person, the covered entity generally must produce it in the form requested if readily producible. Under HIPAA Privacy Rule, patients do not have the right to access the following:
- Psychotherapy notes (Box 2-5)
- Information compiled in reasonable anticipation of, or for use in, legal proceedings
- Information exempted from disclosure under the CLIA

The office may deny patient access for the previously mentioned reasons without giving the patient the right to review the denial.

If the health care provider has determined that the patient would be endangered (or cause danger to

another person) as a result of accessing the confidential health information, access may be denied. In this case, the patient has the right to have the denial reviewed by another licensed professional who did not participate in the initial denial decision.

Regarding psychotherapy notes, HIPAA gives special protection to PHI. Disclosure of a patient's mental health records requires specific patient permission. This means that when an insurance payer requests the health records to review the claim, a patient authorization is required.

Certain clinical data are excluded from the definition of psychotherapy notes. In other words, when an individual is using the services of a mental health professional, not all information gathered and recorded in the health record of the mental health provider is

---

Box 2-5   HIPAA Help

According to the HIPAA Privacy Rule, the term *psychotherapy notes* means notes that are recorded (in any medium) by a health care provider who is a mental health professional documenting or analyzing the contents of conversation during a private counseling session or a group, joint, or family counseling session and that are separated from the rest of the individual's medical record.

Box 2-6   HIPAA Help

In summary, *patients have the right to* the following:
- Be informed of the organization's privacy practices by receiving a Notice of Privacy Practices (NPP)
- Have their information kept confidential and secure
- Obtain a copy of their health records
- Request to have their health records amended
- Request special considerations in communication
- Restrict unauthorized access to their confidential health information

Patients cannot prevent their confidential health information from being used for treatment, payment, or routine health care operations (TPO), nor may they force amendments to their health record. As you become acclimated to your organization's policies and procedures regarding the handling of protected health information (PHI), you will be better able to recognize that your position plays an important part in HIPAA compliance.

---

considered psychotherapy notes. The law lists the following specific items that are excluded from such notes:
- Medication prescription and monitoring
- Counseling session start and stop times
- Modalities and frequencies of treatment furnished
- Results of clinical tests
- Any summary of the following items: diagnosis, functional status, treatment plan, symptoms, prognosis, and progress to date

In general, the major difference between what are and are not considered psychotherapy notes is the information that is the *recorded (in any manner) documentation and/or analysis of conversation*. This information should be kept separate from the medical section of the patient health record to be distinguished as psychotherapy notes. For example, Jane Doe tells her psychologist the details of her childhood trauma. The documented conversation specific to her trauma (for example, what occurred and how she felt) is considered the psychotherapy notes and cannot be released without Jane Doe's specific permission.

It is also important to understand that patients do not have the right to obtain a copy of psychotherapy notes under HIPAA. However, the treating mental health provider can decide when a patient may obtain access to this health information.

State law must always be considered. Some states allow patients access to their psychotherapy notes; therefore state law would take precedence over HIPAA as a result of the state preemption allowance.

5. *Right to request an amendment of PHI.* Patients have the right to request that their PHI be amended. As with other requests, the provider may require the request to be in writing. The provider must have a process to accept and review both the request and any appeal in a timely fashion. The health care provider may deny this request in the following circumstances:
- The provider who is being requested to change the PHI is not the creator of the information (for example, office has records sent by a referring physician).
- The PHI is believed to be accurate and complete as it stands in the provider's records.
- The information is not required to be accessible to the patient (see item 4: *Right to access [inspect and obtain a copy of] PHI*).

Generally, the office must respond to a patient's request for amendment within 60 days. If a request is denied, the patient must be informed in writing of the reason for the denial. The patient must also be given the opportunity to file a statement of disagreement.

6. *Right to receive an accounting of disclosure of PHI.* Providers should maintain a log of all disclosures of PHI, either on paper or within the organization's computer system, other than those made for TPO, facility directories, and some national security and law enforcement agencies. The process for providing an accounting should be outlined in the practice's policy manual. Patients may request an accounting (or tracking) of disclosures of their confidential information and are granted the right to receive this accounting once a year without charge. Additional accountings may be assessed a cost-based fee. See Boxes 2-6 and 2-7.

These accountings started on April 14, 2003, when privacy regulations became enforceable. Items to be documented must include the following:
- Date of disclosure
- Name of the entity or person who received the PHI, including their address, if known
- Brief description of the PHI disclosed
- Brief statement of the purpose of the disclosure

Verification of Identity and Authority

Before any disclosure, you must verify the identity of persons requesting PHI if they are unknown to you. You may request identifying information, such as date of birth, Social Security number, or even a code word stored in your practice management system that is unique to each patient. Public officials may present badges, credentials, official letterheads, and other legal documents of authority for identification purposes.

Box 2-7   HIPAA Help

Health care providers and staff likely will not be reading the *Federal Register* and thus will want to familiarize themselves with the general forms used in their practice setting. They should be aware of the following:

- **Written acknowledgment.** After providing the patient with the Notice of Privacy Practices (NPP), a "good faith" effort must be made to obtain written acknowledgment from the patient receiving the document. If the patient refuses to sign or is unable to sign, this must be documented in the patient record.
- **Authorization forms.** Use and disclosure of protected health information (PHI) is permissible for treatment, payment, or routine health care operations (TPO) because the NPP describes how PHI is used for these purposes. The health care provider is required to obtain signed authorization to use or disclose health information for situations beyond TPO. This functions as protection for the practice. Providers must learn about the particular "authorization" forms used in their office. Psychotherapy notes are handled separately under HIPAA. Such notes have additional protection, specifically that an authorization for any use or disclosure of psychotherapy notes must be obtained.

Your organization will be expected to handle requests made by patients to exercise their rights. You must know your office's process for dealing with each specific request. With your understanding of HIPAA and your organization's policy manual, you will be guided in procedures specific to your health care practice.

Additionally, you must verify that the requestor has the right to have and the need for the PHI. Exercising professional judgment fulfills your verification requirements for most disclosures because you are acting on "good faith" in believing the identity of the individual requesting PHI. It is good practice when making any disclosure to note the "authority" of the person receiving the PHI and how this was determined. This evidence of due diligence on your part enforces a needed structure on your staff and dampens any complaints that might arise.

Validating Patient Permission

Before making any uses or disclosures of confidential health information other than for the purposes of TPO, your office must have appropriate patient permission. Always check for conflicts between various permissions your office may have on file for a given patient (Table 2-1). This information should be maintained either in your practice management system or in the medical chart, where it can be easily identified and retrieved.

For example, if a covered entity has agreed to a patient's request to limit how much of the PHI is sent to a consulting physician for treatment but then receives the patient's authorization to disclose the entire medical record to that physician, this would be a conflict. In general, the more restrictive permission would take precedence. Privacy regulations allow resolving conflicting permissions either by obtaining new permission from the patient or by communicating orally or in writing with the patient to determine the patient's preference. Be sure to document any form of communication in writing.

Obligations of the Health Care Provider
Training

Under HIPAA regulations, a covered entity must train all members of its workforce. This training must include the practice's P&P with respect to PHI as "necessary and appropriate for the members of the workforce to carry out their function within the covered entity." This training will address how your role relates to PHI in your office and you will be instructed on how to handle confidential information. The PO at your health care practice will likely be the instructor for this training. HIPAA training focuses on how to handle confidential information securely in the office, as discussed later in this chapter.

Safeguards: Ensuring that Confidential Information Is Secure

Every covered entity must have appropriate safeguards to ensure the protection of an individual's confidential health information. Such safeguards include administrative, technical, and physical measures that will "reasonably safeguard" PHI from any use or disclosure that violates HIPAA, whether intentional or unintentional (Box 2-8).

Complaints to Health Care Practice and Workforce Sanctions

Individuals, both patients and staff, must be provided with a process to make a complaint concerning the P&P of the covered entity. If a violation involves the misuse of PHI, this incident should be reported to the practice's PO. Should there be further cause, the OCR also may be contacted.

Workforce members are subject to appropriate sanctions for failure to comply with the P&P regarding PHI set forth in the office. The types of sanctions applied vary, depending on factors involved with the violation. Sanctions can range from a warning to suspension to termination. This information should be covered in the P&P manual. Written documentation of complaints and sanctions must be prepared with any disposition.

Mitigation

Mitigation means to "alleviate the severity" or "make mild." In reference to HIPAA, the covered entity has an

Table 2-1	Title II: Administrative Simplification: Uses and Disclosures of Protected Health Information
PERMITTED DISCLOSURES (NO AUTHORIZATION REQUIRED)	**WHAT IT MEANS FOR YOUR PRACTICE**
Disclose PHI to patient	You may discuss the patient's own medical condition with him or her. **Doing so does not require signed authorization from the patient.**
Disclose PHI for treatment	Treatment includes speaking with the patient, ordering tests, writing prescriptions, coordinating his or her care, and consulting with another health care provider about the patient. **"Treatment" does not require signed authorization from the patient.**
Disclose PHI for payment	Payment includes obtaining the patient's eligibility or benefits coverage information from the insurance payer, obtaining preapproval for treatment, and billing and managing the claims process. **"Payment" does not require signed authorization from the patient.**
Disclose PHI for health care operations	Do not confuse this with performing surgery. The term *health care operations* refers to the business activities in which your organization participates. Examples include case management, certification, accreditation, medical reviews, and audits to detect fraud and abuse. **"Operations" do not require signed authorization from the patient.**
Disclose PHI for public purposes	PHI may be disclosed for public health purposes, such as reporting a communicable disease, injury, child abuse, domestic violence, judicial and administrative proceedings, law enforcement, coroner or medical examiner, or research purposes, if PHI is "de-identified." This is not an all-inclusive list but **these examples do not require signed authorization from the patient.**
Disclose PHI for workers' compensation	You may disclose PHI as authorized by the laws relating to workers' compensation. Such disclosures to programs that provide benefits for work-related injuries or illness **do not require signed authorization from the patient.**
DISCLOSURES THAT REQUIRE PATIENT'S OPPORTUNITY TO AGREE OR OBJECT	**WHAT IT MEANS FOR YOUR PRACTICE**
Disclose PHI to persons involved with the patient	You must provide patients with an opportunity to object to sharing PHI with family, friends, or others involved with their care. The health care provider can use professional judgment when disclosing PHI to a person involved with the patient's care when the patient is not present. **This requires the patient to have the opportunity to agree or object.**
DISCLOSURES (AUTHORIZATION REQUIRED)	**WHAT IT MEANS FOR YOUR PRACTICE**
Disclose psychotherapy	Psychotherapy notes may not be disclosed without authorization except for use by the notes' originator (therapist) for treatment. **Signed authorization *is* required.**
Disclose PHI to a child's school for permission to participate in sports	You may not disclose a child's PHI to a school to permit the student's participation in a sports activity. **Signed authorization *is* required.**
Disclose PHI to employer	You may not disclose PHI to a patient's employer unless the information is necessary to comply with OSHA, MSHA, or other state laws. **With certain exceptions, signed authorization *is* required.**
Disclose PHI to insurer	You may not disclose PHI to an insurer for underwriting or eligibility without authorization from the patient (for example, if the patient is trying to obtain a life insurance policy). **Signed authorization *is* required.**
Disclose PHI for fundraising or marketing	If your health care practice does fundraising or marketing, you may not disclose PHI without prior authorization from the patient. **Signed authorization *is* required.**

MSHA, Mine Safety and Health Administration; *OSHA,* Occupational Safety and Health Administration; *PHI,* protected health information.

affirmative duty to take reasonable steps in response to breaches. If a breach is discovered, the health care provider is required to mitigate, to the extent possible, any harmful effects of the breach. For example, if you learn that you have erroneously sent medical records by fax to an incorrect party, steps should be taken to have the recipient destroy the PHI. Mitigation procedures also apply to activities of the practice's business associates. Being proactive and responsible by mitigating reduces the potential for a more disastrous outcome from the breach or violation.

Refraining from Intimidating or Retaliatory Acts

HIPAA privacy regulations prohibit a covered entity from intimidating, threatening, coercing, discriminating against, or otherwise taking retaliatory action against the following:

● Individuals, for exercising HIPAA privacy rights
● Individuals, for filing a complaint with DHHS; for testifying, assisting, or participating in an investigation about the covered entity's privacy practices; or for reasonably opposing any practice prohibited by the regulation

Box 2-8	Examples of Safeguards	
Administrative	**Technical**	**Physical**
Verifying the identity of an individual picking up health records	Create username and password required to access patient records from computer	Locked, fireproof filing cabinets for storing paper records
Apply sanctions against workforce members who fail to comply with security policies and procedures	Establish procedures to obtain necessary ePHI during an emergency	Establish procedures that allow facility access in support of restoration of lost data under the disaster recovery plan
Perform regular records review of information system activity, such as audit logs, access reports, and security incident tracking reports.	Implement procedures that terminate an electronic session after a predetermined time of inactivity	Implement physical safeguards for all workstations that access ePHI, to restrict access to authorized users
Identify a security official who will be responsible for the development of policies and procedures	Implement a mechanism to encrypt and decrypt ePHI	Implement policies and procedures to limit physical access to electronic information systems by identifying authorized individuals by title and/or job function

ePHI, Electronic protected health information.

Guidelines for HIPAA Privacy Compliance

As an insurance billing specialist, you will likely answer the telephone and speak during the course of your business, and there will be questions about what questions you can and cannot answer. Reasonable and appropriate safeguards must be taken to ensure that all confidential health information in your office is protected from unauthorized and inappropriate access, in both verbal and written forms.

Some of the following situations may be referred to as incidental disclosures. This topic is discussed in further detail with additional examples later in this chapter.

1. Consider that conversations occurring throughout the office may be overheard. The reception area and waiting room are often linked and it is easy to hear the scheduling of appointments and exchange of confidential information. It is necessary to observe work areas and maximize efforts to avoid unauthorized disclosures. Simple and affordable precautions include using privacy glass at the front desk and having conversations away from settings where other patients or visitors are present. Health care providers can move their dictation stations away from patient areas or wait until no patients are present before dictating. Telephone conversations made by providers in front of patients, even in emergency situations, should be avoided. Providers and staff must use their best professional judgment.

2. Be sure to check in both the patient's medical record and your computer system to determine whether there are any special instructions for contacting the patient regarding scheduling or reporting test results. Follow these requests as agreed by the office.

3. Patient sign-in sheets are permissible but limit the information you request when a patient signs in and change the sheet periodically during the day. A sign-in sheet must not contain information such as a reason for the visit or the patient's medical condition. Because some providers specialize in treating patients with sensitive issues, simply showing that a particular individual has an appointment with your practice may pose a breach of patient confidentiality.

4. Make sure to have patients sign a form acknowledging receipt of the NPP. The NPP allows you to release the patient's confidential information for billing and other purposes. If your practice has other confidentiality statements and policies besides HIPAA mandates, these must be reviewed to ensure that they meet HIPAA requirements.

5. Formal policies for transferring and accepting outside PHI must address how your office keeps this information confidential. When using courier services, billing services, transcription services, or e-mail, you must ensure that transferring PHI is done in a secure and compliant manner. Data that must be removed from e-mail before being sent are name of patient; address information other than city, state, and zip code; telephone and fax numbers; e-mail address; Social Security number; medical record number; health plan beneficiary number; account number; certificate/license numbers; vehicle identifier; device identifiers; device serial number; website address; biometric identifiers; full-face photograph; geographic subdivisions smaller than state; dates

(except for years) related to birth, death, admission, and discharge; and any other unique identifying number, code, or characteristic, unless otherwise permitted.

6. Computers are used for a variety of administrative functions, including scheduling, billing, and managing medical records. Computers are typically present at the reception area. Keep the computer screen turned so that viewing is restricted to authorized staff. Screen savers should be used to prevent unauthorized viewing or access. The computer should automatically log off the user after a period of being idle, requiring the staff member to reenter his or her password.

7. Keep your username and password confidential and change them often. Do not share this information. An authorized staff member, such as the PO, will have administrative access to reset your password if you lose it or if someone discovers it. Also, practice management software can track users and follow their activity. Do not set yourself up by giving out your password. Safeguards include password protection for electronic data and storing paper records securely.

8. Safeguard your work area; do not place notes with confidential information in areas that are easy to view by nonstaff. Cleaning services will access your building, usually after business hours; ensure that you safeguard PHI.

9. Place medical record charts face down at reception areas so that the patient's name is not exposed to other patients or visitors. When placing medical records on the door of an examination room, turn the chart so that identifying information faces the door. If you keep medical charts on countertops or in receptacles, it is your duty to ensure that nonstaff persons will not access the records. Handling and storing medical records will certainly change because of HIPAA guidelines.

10. Do not post the health care provider's schedule in areas viewable by nonstaff individuals. Schedules are often posted for the convenience of the professional staff but this may be a breach of patient confidentiality.

11. Fax machines should not be placed in patient examination rooms or in any reception area where nonstaff persons may view incoming or sent documents. Only staff members should have access to the faxes.

12. If you open office mail or take telephone calls pertaining to medical record requests, direct these requests to the appropriate staff member.

13. Send all privacy-related questions or concerns to the appropriate staff member.

14. Immediately report any suspected or known improper behavior to your supervisor or the PO so that the issue may be documented and investigated.

15. If you have questions, contact your supervisor or the PO.

THE SECURITY RULE: ADMINISTRATIVE, TECHNICAL, AND PHYSICAL SAFEGUARDS

The **Security Rule** comprises regulations related to the security of electronic protected health information (ePHI), which refers to any protected health information that is produced, saved, transferred, or received in an electronic form. The Security Rule provides regulations related to electronic transactions and code sets, privacy, and enforcement, which make up the administrative simplification provisions of HIPAA. Security measures encompass all administrative, physical, and technical safeguards in an information system. The Security Rule addresses only ePHI but the concept of preserving PHI that will become ePHI makes attention to security for the entire office important. The policies and procedures required by the Security Rule must be maintained for 6 years. The Security Rule is divided into three main sections: administrative safeguards, technical safeguards, and physical safeguards.

- *Administrative safeguards* prevent unauthorized use or disclosure of PHI through administrative actions and P&P to manage the selection, development, implementation, and maintenance of security measures to protect ePHI.
- *Technical safeguards* are technologic controls in place to protect and control access to information on computers in the health care organization.
- *Physical safeguards* also prevent unauthorized access to PHI. These physical measures and P&P protect a covered entity's electronic information systems and related buildings and equipment from natural and environmental hazards and unauthorized intrusion.

The Security Rule is discussed further in Chapter 8.

HEALTH INFORMATION TECHNOLOGY FOR ECONOMIC AND CLINICAL HEALTH ACT

The Health Information Technology for Economic and Clinical Health Act (HITECH Act) was a provision of the **American Recovery and Reinvestment Act (ARRA)** of 2009 signed into law by President Obama. ARRA contains provisions for incentives related to adapting health care information technology that are designed to speed up the adoption of electronic health record systems among health care providers. Because this legislation promotes a massive expansion in the exchange of ePHI, the purpose of the HITECH Act was to strengthen the HIPAA privacy protections and rights. The Act updates and enhances the privacy and security responsibilities of covered entities that were established under HIPAA. The HITECH Act brought significant compliance changes to three very specific areas: (1) business associates,

(2) notification of breach, and (3) civil penalties for non-compliance with the provisions of HIPAA.

Business Associates

Under HIPAA, the covered entity was responsible and liable for all activities related to their business associates. If a covered entity became aware of a breach involving a business associate, the covered entity was expected to terminate the contract if the breach was not corrected. The HITECH Act brought greater responsibility to the business associate. It required all business associates to comply with the HIPAA Security Rule by February 17, 2010, in the same manner that a covered entity would. Business associates are expected to implement physical and technical safeguards as outlined in the Security Rule. They are expected to conduct a risk analysis, to develop and implement related policies and procedures, and to comply with written documentation and workforce training requirements. The business associate is now subject to the application of civil and criminal penalties, just as a covered entity is.

Notification of Breach

The HITECH Act defines a breach as the unauthorized acquisition, access, use, or disclosure of PHI that compromises the security or privacy of such information, except where an unauthorized person to whom such information is disclosed would not reasonably have been able to retain such information. Breach does not include any unintentional acquisition or use of PHI or any inadvertent disclosure of PHI.

Under the HITECH Act, if a breach were to occur, the Act requires a covered entity to notify the affected party directly and individually without unreasonable delay and in no case later than 60 calendar days after the discovery of a breach by the covered entity. Enforcement of the notification of breach began on February 22, 2010.

Effective September 23, 2013, the standard for reporting breaches of unsecured health information was modified. Any breach is presumed reportable unless the covered entity or business associated can demonstrate that there is a low probability that the information has been compromised based on a risk assessment of certain factors or unless the breach fits within certain exceptions. Health care organizations must develop policies that apply to these standards.

HIPAA Compliance Audits

The HITECH Act further requires DHHS to provide periodic audits to ensure that covered entities and business associates are complying with HIPAA Privacy and Security Rules and Breach Notification standards. The OCR has developed an audit program that will be used to assess HIPAA privacy and security programs and compliance efforts. It will examine mechanisms for compliance, identify best practices, and discover risks and vulnerabilities that may not have been identified through its ongoing complaint investigations and compliance reviews. All covered entities, including health plans, health care clearinghouses, health care providers, and business associates, are eligible for an audit. The likely area of focus for OCR audits that began in 2014 will be whether organizations have conducted a timely and thorough HIPAA security risk assessment, because that was the common weak spot found in pilot audit programs and breach investigations.

Increased Penalties for Noncompliance with the Provisions of HIPAA

There are both civil and criminal penalties for failure to comply with HIPAA regulations. The HITECH Act significantly increased the penalty amounts that may be imposed for violations related to failure to comply with HIPAA rules.

- $100 to $50,000 if the covered entity did not know about the violaton
- $1000 to $50,000 if the violation was due to reasonable cause
- $10,000 to $50,000 if the violation was due to willful neglect and was corrected
- $50,000 or more if the violation was due to willful neglect and was not corrected

The HITECH Act set a maximum penalty of $1.5 million for all violations of an identical provision in a calendar year.

Individuals also can be held personally responsible for HIPAA violations, with criminal actions as follows:

- Knowing violations: up to $50,000 and/or 1 year in prison.
- Misrepresentation or offenses under false pretenses: up to $100,000 and/or 5 years in prison
- Intent to sell, distribute, etc.: up to $250,000 and/or 10 years in prison

HIPAA Omnibus Rule

The final **HIPAA Omnibus Rule** is an update to the existing HIPAA law and HITECH Act that modified both privacy and security rules for covered entities and their business associates. The new rules were effective March 26, 2013, but covered entities and their business associates had until September 23, 2013, to comply. The rule enhanced patients' privacy rights and protections and strengthened the ability to enforce the HIPAA privacy and security protections. Furthermore, the new rule expanded many of the requirements of business associates who receive PHI and clarified when breaches of unsecured health information must be reported to DHHS. The new rule required covered entities to update policies applicable to deceased persons, stating that a covered entity may disclose PHI to a coroner or medical examiner for the purpose of identifying a deceased person and determining the cause of death or other duties as authorized by law. The rule strengthened the need for timeliness in response to a patient's request for records. It also added a provision permitting providers to disclose proof of a child's immunization records to schools if the school is required by law to have such proof. The rule also makes it easier for parents and others to disclose the child's immunization records by giving them the ability to authorize the disclosure through oral consent.

Consequences of Noncompliance with HIPAA and the HITECH Act

The prosecution of HIPAA violations is handled by different governing bodies. DHHS handles issues regarding transaction code sets and security. Complaints can be filed against a covered entity for not complying with these rules. The OCR oversees privacy issues and complaints, referring criminal issues to the OIG. The OIG provides the workup for referral cases, which may involve the Federal Bureau of Investigation (FBI) and other agencies.

DHHS announced its first enforcement action resulting from a violation of the HITECH Act Breach Notification Rule in 2012, which placed a monetary settlement of $1.5 million per breach on the accused. This enforcement action clearly sends a message to the health care community that the OCR expects health care organizations to have a carefully designed and active HIPAA compliance plan in place.

APPLICATION TO PRACTICE SETTING

HIPAA affects all areas of the health care office, from the reception area to the provider. In addition to being educated and trained in job responsibilities, every staff member must be educated about HIPAA and trained in the P&P pertinent to the organization.

Reasonable safeguards are measurable solutions based on accepted standards that are implemented and periodically monitored to demonstrate that the office is in compliance. Reasonable efforts must be made to limit the use or disclosure of PHI. If you are the front desk receptionist and you close the privacy glass between your desk and the waiting area when making a call to a patient, this is a reasonable safeguard to prevent others in the waiting room from overhearing.

Incidental uses and disclosures are permissible under HIPAA only when reasonable safeguards or precautions have been implemented to prevent misuse or inappropriate disclosure of PHI. When incidental uses and disclosures result from failure to apply reasonable safeguards or adhere to the minimum necessary standard, the Privacy Rule has been violated. If you are in the reception area and you close the privacy glass before having a confidential conversation but are still overheard by an individual in the waiting room, this would be "incidental." You have applied a reasonable safeguard to prevent your conversation from being overheard. The OCR has addressed what is permissible regarding incidental disclosures. Examples follow.

1. Health care professionals may discuss a patient's condition in a treatment area or over the telephone with the patient, a provider, or a family member. However, when telephoning a patient about an insurance matter and reaching voice mail, care in choice of words must be used when leaving a message in case the call is inadvertently received at the wrong number. Leave your name, the office name, and a return telephone number. Never provide information about the results of diagnostic tests to the patient. Let the physician do it.
2. Health care professionals may discuss laboratory test results with a patient or other provider in a joint treatment area. A *health care professional* is an individual who has been trained in a health-related field, whether clinical or administrative. The professional may be licensed, certified, or registered by a state or government agency or professional organization.
3. A physician may discuss a patient's condition or treatment regimen in the patient's hospital room.
4. A pharmacist may discuss a prescription with a patient over the pharmacy counter or with a physician or the patient by telephone.
5. A physician may give instructions to a staff member to bill a patient for a certain procedure even if other individuals in the reception room can overhear the conversation.
6. A patient's name may be called out in the reception room; however, some offices prefer to use first names and not call out last names.

Organization and Staff Responsibilities in Protecting Patient Rights

The covered entity must implement written P&P that comply with HIPAA standards. P&P are tailored guidelines established to accommodate each health care practice and designed to address PHI. HIPAA requires each practice to implement P&P that comply with privacy and security rules. The office should have a P&P manual to train providers and staff and to serve as a resource for situations that need clarification. Revisions to P&P must be made as needed and appropriate to comply with laws as they change. Documentation must be maintained in written or electronic form and retained for 6 years after its creation or when it was last in effect, whichever is later.

Health care organizations face challenges in implementing the HIPAA requirements; do not let these overwhelm you. Your office is required to take reasonable steps to build protections specific to your health care organization. Compliance is an ongoing endeavor involving teamwork. Understand your office's established P&P. Monitor your own activities to ensure that you are following the required procedures. Do not take shortcuts when your actions involve patient privacy and security.

Be alert to other activities in your office. Help your co-workers change work habits that do not comply with HIPAA. Do not ignore unauthorized uses and disclosures of PHI and do not allow unauthorized persons to access data. You have an obligation to your employer and to the patients you serve.

FRAUD AND ABUSE LAWS

The CMS has stated that perpetrators of health care fraud steal billions of dollars each year from federal and state government programs, resulting in higher costs for everyone in the health care system. With many regulations and laws in place, there are very tight controls on medical billing by health care organizations, holding the insurance billing specialist to very high standards. In light of complex government regulations and constant scrutiny, it is important for those involved in the reimbursement process to clearly understand the agencies that oversee health care compliance and what exactly constitutes fraud and abuse.

Fraud can occur when deception is used in a claim submission to obtain payment from the payer. Individuals who knowingly, willfully, and intentionally submit false information to benefit themselves or others commit fraud. Fraud can also be interpreted from mistakes that result in excessive reimbursement. No proof of "specific intent to defraud" is required for fraud to be considered. Fraud usually involves careful planning. Examples are listed in Box 2-9.

Abuse means incidents or practices by physicians, not usually considered fraudulent, that are inconsistent with accepted sound medical business or fiscal practices. Examples are listed in Box 2-10.

Box 2-9	**Examples of Fraud**

- Bill for services or supplies not provided (**phantom bills** or invoice ghosts) or for an office visit if a patient fails to keep an appointment and is not notified ahead of time that this is office policy
- Alter fees on a claim form to obtain higher payment
- Forgive the deductible or copayment
- Alter medical records to generate fraudulent payments
- Leave relevant information off a claim (for example, failing to reveal whether a spouse has health insurance coverage through an employer)
- Upcode (for example, submit a code for a complex fracture when the patient had a simple fracture)
- Shorten (for example, dispense less medication than billed for)
- Split billing schemes (for example, bill procedures over a period of days when all treatment occurred during one visit)
- Use another person's insurance card to obtain medical care
- Change a date of service
- Post adjustments to generate fraudulent payments
- Solicit, offer, or receive a kickback, bribe, or rebate in return for referring a patient to a physician, physical therapist, or pharmacy or for referring a patient to obtain any item or service that may be paid for in full or in part by Medicare or Medicaid
- Restate the diagnosis to obtain insurance benefits or better payment
- Apply deliberately for duplicate payment (for example, bill Medicare twice, bill Medicare and the beneficiary for the same service, or bill Medicare and another insurer in an attempt to be paid twice)
- Unbundle or explode charges (for example, bill a multichannel laboratory test as if individual tests were performed)
- Collusion between a physician and an employee of a third-party payer when the claim is assigned (If the physician deliberately overbilled for services, overpayments could be generated with little awareness on the part of the Medicare beneficiary.)
- Bill based on gang visits (for example, a physician visits a nursing home and bills for 20 visits without furnishing any specific services to or on behalf of individual patients)
- Knowingly bill for the same item or service more than once or another party bills the federal health care program for an item or service also billed by the physician

---

Defining Fraud and Abuse Roles, Relationships, and Key Terms
Centers for Medicare and Medicaid Services

CMS is the federal agency that administers and oversees the Medicare program and monitors the Medicaid program run by each state. CMS is committed to providing health care services to Medicare and Medicaid beneficiaries while also partnering with various entities and law enforcement agencies to prevent and detect health care fraud and abuse.

Box 2-10   Examples of Medical Billing Abuse

- Refer excessively to other providers for unnecessary services
- Charge excessively for services or supplies
- Perform a battery of diagnostic tests when only a few tests are required for services
- Violate Medicare's physician participating agreement
- Call patients for repeated and unnecessary follow-up visits
- Bill Medicare beneficiaries at a higher rate than other patients
- Submit bills to Medicare and not to third-party payers (for example, claims for injury from an automobile accident, in a store, or at the workplace)
- Breach an assignment agreement
- Fail to make required refunds when services are not reasonable and necessary
- Require patients to contract to pay their physician's full charges, in excess of the Medicare charge limits
- Require a patient to waive rights to have the physician submit claims to Medicare and obligate a patient to pay privately for Medicare-covered services
- Require patients to pay for services not previously billed, including telephone calls with the physician, prescription refills, and medical conferences with other professionals
- Require patients to sign a global waiver agreeing to pay privately for all services that Medicare will not cover and using these waivers to obligate patients to pay separately for a service that Medicare covers as part of a package or related procedures

---

The Office of the Inspector General

Since its establishment in 1976, the OIG's mission has been to safeguard the health and welfare of the beneficiaries of DHHS programs and to protect the integrity of DHHS programs (Medicare and Medicaid). The OIG was established to identify and eliminate fraud, abuse, and waste and "to promote efficiency and economy in departmental operations." HIPAA legislation has radically changed the focus and mission within the OIG. HIPAA pushed the OIG into a new era, guaranteeing funds for the OIG programs and mandating initiatives to protect the integrity of all health care programs. The OIG undertakes nationwide audits as well as investigations and inspections to review the claim submission processes of providers and reimbursement patterns of the programs. Recommendations are made to the DHHS Secretary and the US Congress on correcting problematic areas addressed in the federal programs according to the OIG.

Health Care Fraud and Abuse Control Program

Efforts to combat fraud were consolidated and strengthened under Public Law 104-191, the Health Insurance Portability and Accountability Act (HIPAA) of 1996. The Act established a comprehensive program to combat fraud committed against all health plans, both public and private. The legislation required the establishment of a national Health Care Fraud and Abuse Control (HCFAC) Program, under the joint direction of the Attorney General and the Secretary of the DHHS acting through the department's Inspector General (DHHS/OIG). The HCFAC Program is designed to coordinate federal, state, and local law enforcement activities with respect to health care fraud and abuse. HIPAA requires DHHS and the DOJ to detail in an annual report the amounts deposited and appropriated to the Medicare Trust Fund as well as the source of such deposits. The Affordable Care Act of 2010 provides additional tools and resources to help fight fraud that will help to boost HCFAC Program activities. These resources include enhanced screenings and enrollment requirements, increased data sharing across government, expanded overpayment recovery efforts, and greater oversight of private insurance abuses.

The text that follows contains very important information from federal fraud and abuse laws that are crucial for anyone in the health care field to become familiar with and to follow to avoid violations that can result in criminal penalties and civil fines.

Criminal False Claims Act (18 US Code §287)

The criminal False Claims Act stated that anyone who knowingly makes or presents a false, fictitious, or fraudulent claim to any department or agency of the United States shall be imprisoned not more than 5 years and shall be subject to a fine. The law did not apply specifically to the health care industry; however, HIPAA amendments to the criminal code include the following:

- Theft or Embezzlement (18 US Code §669). This law brings fines and imprisonment against any individual who "knowingly and willfully embezzles, steals, or otherwise without authority converts to the use of any person other than the rightful owner, or intentionally misapplies any of the moneys, funds, securities, premiums, credits, property, or other assets of a health care benefit program." In addition to health care organizations that deal with the Medicare and Medicaid programs, this law applies to financial service industries, bookkeeping and accounting firms, and all business types and industries. **Embezzlement** means stealing money that has been entrusted to one's care. In cases of insurance claims embezzlement related to health care, the physician can be held as the guilty party and may have to pay huge sums to a third-party payer when false claims are submitted by an employee. If an undiscovered embezzler leaves the employer and you are hired to replace that person, you could be accused some months later of doing something you did not do. Take precautions as an employee to protect the medical practice. These precautions are discussed in Chapter 10.

- False Statement Relating to Health Care Matters (19 US Code §1035). Any individual who knowingly and willfully "falsifies, conceals, or covers up by any trick, scheme, or device, a material fact; or makes any materially false, fictitious, or fraudulent statements or representations, or makes or uses any materially false writing or document knowing the same to contain any materially false, fictitious, or fraudulent statement or entry, in connection with the delivery of or payment for health care benefits, items, or services" is subject to fines and imprisonment.
- Health Care Fraud (18 US Code §1347). Any individual who knowingly and willfully "executes, or attempts to execute, a scheme or artifice to defraud any health care benefit program; or to obtain, by means of false or fraudulent pretenses, representations, or promises, any of the money or property owned by, or under the custody or control of, any health care benefit program, in connection with the delivery or of payment for health care benefits, items, or services" is subject to fines and imprisonment. If serious bodily injury or death occurs, the person may face life imprisonment.
- Obstruction of Criminal Investigations of Health Care Offenses (18 US Code §1518). An individual is subject to fines and imprisonment when the person "willfully prevents, obstructs, misleads, delays or attempts to prevent, obstruct, mislead, or delay the communication of information or records relating to a violation of a federal health care offense to a criminal investigator."

Civil False Claims Act (31 US Code §3729-3733)

The federal civil False Claims Act authorizes the United States to recover monetary damages from parties who file fraudulent or false claims for payment by the federal government. "A false claim is a claim for payment for services or supplies that were not provided specifically as presented or for which the provider is otherwise not entitled to payment." Presenting a claim for an item or service based on a code known to result in greater payment or to submit a claim for services not medically necessary is also a violation of the False Claims Act (FCA). The government uses the FCA in conjunction with other fraud and abuse laws and as a primary enforcement tool.

Although no proof of specific intent to defraud is required, liability can occur when a person knowingly presents or causes to present such a claim or makes, uses, or causes a false record or statement to have a false or fraudulent claim paid or approved by the federal government.

A coder or biller who has knowledge of fraud or abuse should take the following measures:

- Notify the provider both personally and with a dated written memorandum.
- Document the false statement or representation of the material fact.
- Send a memorandum to the office manager or employer stating your concern if no change is made.
- Maintain a written audit trail with dated memoranda for your files.
- Do not discuss the problem with anyone who is not immediately involved.

Civil penalties for violations of the FCA can result in fines of up to three times the programs' loss plus $11,000 per claim filed. Criminal penalties for submitting false claims may include fines, imprisonment, or both.

The FCA was amended in 2009 and 2010 under the Fraud Enforcement and Recovery Act of 2009 (FERA) and the Patient Protection and Affordable Care Act (PPACA). One significant change to the FCA under PPACA was clarification that overpayments under Medicare and Medicaid must be reported and returned within 60 days of discovery. Failure to report and return an overpayment exposes a provider of health care services to liability under the FCA.

Qui Tam Provision

Qui tam (pronounced kwee tam) in the FCA provisions allows a private citizen to bring a civil action suit for a violation on behalf of the federal government (Example 2-2). This involves fraud by government contractors and other entities that receive or use government funds. The individual who files a qui tam suit is known as a "relator" and also referred to as a "whistleblower." The whistleblower shares in any money recovered from a successful qui tam action.

Example 2-2   Qui Tam Action
A qui tam relator alleged that a hospital violated the False Claims Act (FCA) by bundling tests when billing nursing homes and unbundling those charges when billing Medicare, double billing, and submitting multiple and excessive bills.

Exclusion Statute (42 US Code §1320a-7)

Individuals, health care providers, and health care organizations who have been convicted of a misdemeanor or criminal offense related to health care risk being excluded by the OIG from future participation in any federal health care programs.

According to OIG:

No program payment will be made for anything that an excluded person furnishes, orders, or prescribes. This payment prohibition applies to the excluded person, anyone who employs or contracts with the excluded person, any hospital or other provider where the excluded person provides services, and anyone else. The exclusion applies regardless of who submits the claims and applies to all administrative and management services furnished by the excluded person.

Employers of health care staff are required to screen all prospective employees and contractors against the OIG's List of Excluded Individuals and Entities prior to hire. Organizations that hire or contract with excluded individuals may be subject to civil monetary penalties. Be sure to check the updated exclusion listings at the OIG website (https://oig.hhs.gov).

Civil Monetary Penalties Law (41 US Code §1320a-7a)

A civil penalty is a fine assessed for violation of a law or regulation. The US Congress enacted the **Civil Monetary Penalty (CMP)** statute to provide administrative remediation to combat health care fraud and abuse. CMP imposes civil monetary penalties and assessments against a person or organization for making false or improper claims against any federal health care program. Penalties can range from $10,000 to $50,000 per violation and may also include an assessment of up to three times the amount claimed for each item or service.

Stark I and II Laws (42 US Code §1395nn)

The Stark Law is commonly referred to as the Physician Self-Referral Law. Stark II laws prohibit the submission of claims for "designated services" or referral of patients if the referring physician has a "financial relationship" with the entity that provides the services. Originally named "Stark I," this law pertained only to clinical laboratories that prohibited physicians from referring a patient to a clinical laboratory in which the doctor or a member of his or her family had a financial interest. Stark laws carry exceptions, so it is important to understand the referral processes and in-office ancillary services used by your health care organization. Penalties for violations of the Stark Law include fines and exclusion from participation in the federal health care programs.

Anti-Kickback Statute (42 US Code §1320a-7b[b])

In the federal health care program, paying for referrals is a crime. Accepting discounts, rebates, or other reductions in price may violate the Anti-Kickback Statute because such arrangements induce the purchase of items or services payable by Medicare or Medicaid. Penalties for paying or accepting kickbacks can include fines, jail terms, and exclusion from participating in federal health care programs. Penalties up to $50,000 per kickback plus three times the amount of the remuneration can be imposed. The PPACA strengthened this statute by clarifying that "a person need not have actual knowledge of this section or specific intent to commit a violation of this section."

Safe Harbors

Safe harbors specify various business and service arrangements that are protected from prosecution under the Anti-Kickback Statute. These include certain investments, care in underserved areas, and other arrangements.

Certain arrangements are not violations of the Anti-Kickback Statute and are clearly allowed if they fall within a "safe harbor." One safe harbor protects certain discounting practices. A "discount" is the reduction in the amount a seller charges a buyer for a good or service based on an "arm's-length" transaction. To be protected under the discount safe harbor, the discount must apply to the original item or service purchased or furnished. In 2013 a safe harbor that allows hospitals to provide physician practices with electronic health record systems and training to operate them was extended by CMS and the OIG through 2021. This safe harbor was extended to continue to facilitate the adoption of electronic health records technology throughout the health care community.

Operation Restore Trust

Launched in 1995, Operation Restore Trust (ORT) was designed to coordinate the activities of the OIG along with CMS and other DHHS entities in identifying and preventing fraud. An established hotline (1-800-HHS-TIPS) for the public allows individuals to report issues that might indicate fraud, abuse, or waste. ORT has been successful because of planning with the DOJ and other law enforcement agencies, training state and local organizations to detect fraud and abuse, and implementing statistical methods to identify providers for audits and investigations.

Additional Laws and Compliance

Other laws pertaining to fraud and abuse include the Federal Deposit Insurance Corporation (FDIC) mail and wire fraud provisions, as follows:
- §1341. Frauds and swindles. An individual is subject to both fines and imprisonment when having "devised or intending to devise any scheme or artifice to defraud, or for obtaining money or property by means of

false or fraudulent pretenses" by use of the US Postal Service, whether sent by or delivered to the Postal Service.

- §1343. Fraud by wire, radio, or television. An individual will be fined and/or imprisoned "for having devised or intending to devise any scheme or artifice to defraud, or for obtaining money or property by means of false or fraudulent pretenses, representations, or promises, transmits or causes to be transmitted by means of wire, radio, or television communication."

The US government is clearly committed to the investigation and prosecution of health care fraud. As with HIPAA policies and procedures, it is imperative that health care entities develop their own compliance program to identify and prevent fraud.

Increased Compliance Audits and Oversight

One of the greatest challenges for health care providers, workers, and organizations is the growing number of government and third-party fraud and abuse audit programs that scrutinize payment of health care services.

Recovery Audit Contractors

Recovery Audit Contractors (RACs) are companies that contract with Medicare to recoup money from inappropriately paid claims. They receive information from Medicare about paid claims and then data mine for potential claim payment errors using computer programs. RACs are paid a percentage of the money they recover and are highly motivated to find claim errors.

Medicare and Medicaid Integrity Programs

HIPAA includes a provision establishing the Medicare Integrity Program (MIP). That provision gives the CMS specific contracting authority, consistent with Federal Acquisition Regulations, to enter into contracts with entities to promote the integrity of the Medicare program.

The goals of the MIP are to identify and reduce Medicare overpayments through a series of audits and reviews of provider claims and cost report data. Initiatives of MIP include identifying plan beneficiaries with additional insurance and educating health care providers. Program integrity contractors help expand the scope of the MIP. This endeavor has recovered several billions of dollars in the fight against fraud, waste, and abuse in the Medicare program. Similar programs have recently extended into state Medicaid programs and are referred to as Medicaid Integrity Programs, which work to identify and recover inappropriate Medicaid payments.

Zone Program Integrity Contractors

Zone Program Integrity Contractors (ZPICs) have replaced the Medicare program safeguard contracts (PSCs) and Medicare drug integrity contractors (MEDICs). They focus on reviewing claims for providers who have suspicious billing patterns or submit more claims to Medicare than the majority of providers in the community. If fraud and abuse are detected, ZPICs report this to the OIG for further investigation.

Comprehensive Error Rate Testing

The CMS implemented the **Comprehensive Error Rate Testing (CERT)** program to measure accuracy of payments in the Medicare fee-for-service (FFS) program at both national and regional levels. Claims are randomly selected for CERT review. The provider of services receives a letter from CMS requesting medical documentation to substantiate services that have been paid. Instructions for returning the documentation is provided and all documentation related to the services in question must be sent to the CERT Documentation Contractor within 75 days of the request. Failure to submit documentation will result in a CERT denial and recoupment of Medicare payments. CERT error rates are calculated based on review of records and are then used to form OIG target issues. CERT errors are also used by CMS to measure performance of Medicare contractors.

Health Care Fraud Prevention and Enforcement Action Team

In 2009 the DOJ and DHHS established the **Health Care Fraud Prevention and Enforcement Action Team (HEAT)** to build and strengthen existing programs to combat Medicare and Medicaid fraud and to crack down on fraud perpetrators. HEAT efforts have included expansion of the DOJ-DHHS Medicare Fraud Strike Force that has been successful in fighting fraud. In 2011, HEAT coordinated the largest-ever federal health care fraud takedown, involving $530 million in fraudulent billing. It continues its efforts, which are outlined in annual reports issued by the DHHS Press Office.

Special Alerts, Bulletins, and Guidance Documents

The health insurance specialist should follow all *special fraud alerts* published by the OIG to alert the industry of specific patterns or trends related to fraudulent or abusive activities regarding the Medicare and Medicaid programs. *Special advisory bulletins* report industry practices and arrangements that may indicate fraud and abuse. Other guidance documents include updates, response letters, and alerts important to more specifically targeted matters. All notices are available at the OIG website and you can sign up for their mailing list.

A special alert was issued in 2009 when the DHHS and OIG sent an open letter to all health care providers in refining the OIG's **Self-Disclosure Protocol (SDP)** originally established in 2006. The SDP is a vehicle for providers and health care organizations to voluntarily disclose self-discovered evidence of potential fraud and work collaboratively with the OIG in resolving issues efficiently and fairly. The OIG updated the SDP again in 2013 in an effort to improve efficient resolution of SDP matters.

COMPLIANCE PROGRAM GUIDANCE FOR INDIVIDUAL AND SMALL GROUP PHYSICIAN PRACTICES

A compliance program is a comprehensive set of policies, procedures, and guidelines designed to ensure that an organization conducts its business in accordance with applicable laws and regulations. The OIG's *Compliance Program for Individual and Small Group Physician Practices* and the *Compliance Program Guidance for Third-Party Medical Billing Companies* are two publications in a series for the health care industry that provide guidance and acceptable principles for business operations.

The OIG published *Compliance Program for Individual and Small Group Physician Practices* in September 2000. At that time, the guidance recommended by the OIG was voluntary. It was provided as a means for health care organizations to effectively reduce the risk of legal action and create a "good faith" effort in combating fraud, waste, and abuse. Under federal legislation known as the Affordable Care Act of 2010, mandatory compliance program requirements were implemented and became effective January 1, 2011, for Medicare Advantage (MA) and Medicare Part D programs. Upon finalization of the Affordable Care Act provisions, the DHHS Secretary has the authority to define providers, suppliers, and physicians who must adopt a compliance plan. Thereafter, nursing homes were mandated to have an effective complaint program as of March 2013, with further expansion of mandated provider compliance programs expected.

A **compliance plan** requires that a health care practice review all billing processes through audits and establish controls that will correct weaknesses and prevent errors. The organization's governing authority should be knowledgeable about the contents of the plan and exercise reasonable oversight of its implementation and effectiveness, while high-level management should be assigned overall responsibility for the program.

A well-designed compliance program can (1) speed the claims processing cycle, (2) optimize proper payment or claims, (3) minimize billing mistakes, (4) reduce the likelihood of a government audit, (5) avoid conflict with Stark laws and the Anti-Kickback Statute, (6) show a "good faith" effort that claims will be submitted appropriately, and (7) relay to staff that there is a duty to report mistakes and suspected or known misconduct.

If you are a claims processing staff member, your organization's claims processing supervisor should research industry sector program guidance to help with specific concerns regarding the specialty or facility setting. Check the OIG website (https://oig.hhs.gov/) to view addenda, comments, and drafts of additional compliance guidance subjects.

Increased Productivity and Decreased Penalties with a Compliance Plan

The presence of an OIG compliance program can significantly mitigate imposed penalties in the event of an OIG audit or other discovery of fraudulent billing activities. These P&P can be found in the provider's P&P manual. For those not currently in the role of a privacy/security/compliance officer, knowledge of P&P as they pertain to both HIPAA and OIG is invaluable.

Because health care providers rely on the expertise of their billing and coding staff to process claims accurately and promptly, they also look to these staff members for advice and guidance. If you are directly involved in this area of your organization, you will likely be expected to understand the complexities of the various laws and regulations governing the medical claims process.

Compliance plans effectively become a "meeting of the minds" among the players; providers, claims processing staff, and payers all agree to process claims in accordance with shared values. Consider your organization's OIG compliance program as a way to integrate regulatory requirements directly into your claims processing procedures. OIG views the experienced claims processing staff as the critical screen for the health care provider's claims. The common denominators in the key benefits identified by OIG are efficiency, consistency, and integrity.

Seven Basic Components of a Compliance Plan

OIG outlines the following seven components of an effective program guidance plan specifically for individual and small group physician practices:
1. Conducting internal monitoring and auditing
2. Implementing compliance and practice standards
3. Designating a compliance officer or contact

4. Conducting appropriate training and education
5. Responding appropriately to detected offenses and developing corrective action
6. Developing open lines of communication
7. Enforcing disciplinary standards through well-publicized guidelines

Conducting Internal Monitoring and Auditing

A comprehensive auditing and monitoring program will not eliminate misconduct within an organization but will minimize the risk of fraud and abuse by identifying the risk areas. The compliance officer, with the committee's assistance, should identify problem areas and have established auditing priorities and procedures as part of the organization's compliance program.

Special attention should be paid to the risk areas associated with claims submission and processing. Also, a thorough review of the organization's standards and written P&P should be conducted to ensure proper guidelines for complying with state and federal laws and insurance payer requirements.

Implementing Compliance and Practice Standards

Written standards and procedures address risk areas that an office needs to monitor and follow. Specific risk areas* identified by OIG include the following:
- Billing for items or services not rendered or not provided as claimed
- Submitting claims for equipment, medical supplies, and services that are not reasonable and necessary
- Double billing resulting in duplicate payment
- Billing for noncovered services as though covered
- Known misuse of provider identification numbers, which results in improper billing
- Unbundling, or billing for each component of the service instead of billing or using an all-inclusive code
- Failure to use coding modifiers properly
- **Clustering;** reporting one level of service for all patient visits, regardless of the patient's presenting problem or the amount of work or time spent with the patient
- Upcoding the level of service provided; reporting a higher level of service for patient visits, regardless of the patient's presenting problem or the amount of work or time spent with the patient

In addition to these risk areas, policies should be developed that address the following:
- Definition of reasonable and necessary
- Proper medical documentation

*Data from *Federal Register* 65 (194): 59439, 2000.

- Federal sentencing guidelines
- Record retention

You should be able to access your organization's P&P manual to review the standards and protocol for these issues involving your practice.

Designating a Compliance Officer or Contact

As with the HIPAA PO, the compliance officer is the key individual who oversees your organization's compliance program monitoring with the support of the compliance committee. The number of members on your compliance committee is not important and prospective staff members from human resources, claims auditing, billing, legal, and medicine departments can ensure a comprehensive mix. You may currently participate on your office's compliance committee or may be asked to do so in the future. The compliance committee acts as a review board. Some committees consist of provider-client office staff and billing company staff. Some committees are simply the provider-client and the billing company staff or a combination of the provider-client, their practice manager, and the billing company staff. The committee, empowered by management, legitimizes the compliance strategy within your organization. In addition to possessing professional experience in claims processing and auditing, committee members are expected to use good judgment and high integrity to fulfill committee obligations.

Conducting Appropriate Training and Education

Because OIG compliance program guidelines are based on Federal Sentencing Guidelines, significant elements of an effective compliance program involve proper education and training of staff. Every employee and individual who interacts with your health care organization may be accountable for potential misconduct and should be considered in the organization's training sessions.

You should be required to attend training in a "general" compliance training session at least annually. For staff members involved in claims processing (coding and billing), a separate training session should be held to cover internal procedures, federal and state laws regarding fraud and abuse, and specific government and other payer reimbursement policies. Periodic professional courses in continuing education should be available. Coding and billing personnel should receive training at least annually to remain updated on diagnostic and procedural codes for each year. You will attend training on site, at a remote location, or both.

Effective training can reduce potential errors, penalties, and fines. An educated staff makes fewer errors, reduces your organization's risks, and requires less micromanagement.

Responding Appropriately to Detected Offenses and Developing Corrective Action

When faced with the discovery of an offense or an error, inaction may be interpreted as indifference. This could jeopardize the reputation of the health care provider's practice. Your office should have a process for investigating problems and taking necessary corrective action. Issues that raise concern include significant changes in claims that are rejected; software edits that show a pattern of misuse of codes or fees; an unusually high volume of charges, payments, or rejections; and notices from insurance payers regarding claims submitted by your office.

You and your fellow staff members should be encouraged to report concerns for any suspected or known misconduct, with an established chain of command in the reporting path. Some incidences of misconduct may violate criminal, civil, or administrative law. If the situation warrants it, the compliance officer should report the misconduct promptly to the appropriate government authority.

Fraud and abuse should be reported. Contact the DHHS OIG as follows:
- Telephone hotline: 1-800-HHS-TIPS (1-800-447-8477)
- TTY: 1-800-377-4950
- Fax: 1-800-223-8164
- E-mail: HHSTIPS@oig.hhs.gov
- Website: http://www.oig.hhs.gov/fraud/hotline

Developing Open Lines of Communication

Effective lines of communication provide a channel for employees to report suspected or known misconduct without immediately reporting to an external agency. In this way, your health care organization can resolve issues internally. "Open door" policies ensure an environment in which staff members feel secure to ask about the organization's existing P&P and to report questionable activities. Your role as a conscientious employee allows you to know the steps to take in reporting any suspicious business activity.

You will learn your office's procedure for reporting misconduct. It is important to follow these guidelines to protect your reputation and credibility within the workplace. Depending on the size of the practice, the methods for contacting managerial staff may include anonymous telephone calls through a "hotline" or written report forms.

Enforcing Disciplinary Standards Through Well-Publicized Guidelines

The unfortunate downside to compliance is that misconduct does occur. For this reason, health care organizations must have established disciplinary guidelines and must make these well known to employees and other agents who contract with the organization. We all want to know what will happen if we "make a mistake" and what progressive forms of discipline await situations involving misconduct. Disciplinary standards include the following:
- Verbal warning
- Written warning
- Written reprimand
- Suspension or probation
- Demotion
- Termination of employment
- Restitution of any damages
- Referral to federal agencies for criminal prosecution

Whether the misconduct was intentional or negligent, all levels of employees need to know what is expected of them. Your office must publish this information and disseminate it to all employees.

WHAT TO EXPECT FROM YOUR HEALTH CARE PRACTICE

Health care workers must be aware of the potential liabilities when submitting claims for payment that are deemed to be "fraudulent" or inappropriate by the government. The government may impose significant financial and administrative penalties when health care claims are not submitted appropriately, including criminal prosecution against the offending party. According to the OIG, fraud can result from deliberate unethical behavior or simply from mistakes and miscues that cause excessive reimbursement.

If you are involved in the claims processing procedures in your organization, note the importance and urgency in following the legal and ethical path when performing your duties. Your "honest mistake" could lead to a situation that puts the health care provider at risk for investigation of fraud, waste, or abuse if it continues and is not corrected.

Although every health care organization or practice has different policies and procedures, you now know what to expect in the workplace, as follows:
- Adherence to all laws and guidelines that regulate and pay for health care services
- Privacy/security/compliance officer (even if one person)
- P&P manual
- Employee training and education (at least annually and whenever there are changes in business operations that affect staff members directly)

KEY POINTS

This is a brief chapter review, or summary, of the key issues presented. To further enhance your knowledge of the technical subject matter, review the key terms and key abbreviations for this chapter by locating the meaning for each in the Glossary at the end of this text, which appears in a section before the Index.

1. The Health Insurance Portability and Accountability Act (HIPAA) has affected confidentiality and disclosure of protected health information (PHI), completion and electronic transmission of insurance claims, fraud and abuse in claims submission, and implementation of compliance and practice standards.

2. While employed by a medical practice, the insurance billing specialist's duty is to have complete knowledge and understanding of HIPAA mandates, carry out policies and procedures that comply with federal regulations, and keep up to date with these statutes. This will assist both the physician and the patients.

3. The primary purpose of HIPAA *Title I: Health Insurance Reform* is to provide continuous insurance coverage for workers and their insured dependents when they change or lose jobs. *Title II: Administrative Simplification* focuses on the health care practice setting and aims to reduce administrative costs and burdens.

4. Serious civil and criminal penalties, such as fines and imprisonment, apply for HIPAA noncompliance.

5. PHI refers to data that identify an individual and describe his or her health status, age, sex, ethnicity, or other demographic characteristics, whether that information is or is not stored or transmitted electronically.

6. Under HIPAA, PHI may not be used or disclosed without permission of the patient or someone authorized to act on behalf of the patient, unless the use or disclosure is specifically required or permitted by the regulation (for example, treatment, payment, or routine health care operations [TPO]). The two types of disclosure required by the HIPAA Privacy Rule are to the individual who is the subject of the PHI and to the Secretary of the DHHS to investigate compliance with the rule.

7. When comparing privileged and nonprivileged information, privileged information is related to the treatment and progress of the patient. The patient must sign an authorization to release this information or selected facts from the medical record. Non-privileged information consists of ordinary facts unrelated to treatment of the patient, including the patient's name, city of residence, and dates of admission or discharge.

8. Under HIPAA, a Notice of Privacy Practices (NPP) document must be given to the patient at the first visit or at enrollment, explaining the individual's rights and the physician's legal duties regarding PHI. Use and disclosure of PHI is permissible for TPO because the NPP describes how PHI is used for these purposes. Thus a consent form is not required. The health care provider is required to obtain a signed authorization form to use or disclose health information for situations beyond the TPO. This is a protection for the practice. Psychotherapy notes are handled separately under HIPAA. Such notes have additional protection, specifically that an authorization for any disclosure of psychotherapy notes must be obtained.

9. *Disclosure* means the release, transfer, provision of access to, or divulging in any other manner of information outside the entity holding the information. *Use* means the sharing, employment, application, utilization, examination, or analysis of IIHI within an organization that holds such information. When a patient's billing record is accessed to review the claim submission history, the individual's health information is in "use."

10. The three major categories of security safeguards are administrative, technical, and physical measures that will reasonably protect PHI from any use or disclosure that is in violation of HIPAA.

11. The difference between *fraud* and *abuse* is that fraud can occur when deception is used in a claim submission to obtain payment from the payer. Individuals who knowingly, willfully, and intentionally submit false information to benefit themselves or others commit *fraud. Abuse* means incidents or practices by physicians, not usually considered fraudulent, that are inconsistent with accepted sound medical business or fiscal practices.

You must strongly consider the lessons learned from the privacy, transaction, and security rules in conjunction with OIG compliance recommendations. The most important points are to read your organization's P&P manual and to ask questions about the general operations of your organization. Always use your ethical and "best practice" approach to be an informed and effective employee.

🖥 STUDENT ASSIGNMENT

✔ Study Chapter 2.

✔ Answer the fill-in-the-blank, multiple-choice, and true/false questions in the *Workbook* to reinforce the theory learned in this chapter and help prepare for a future test.

✔ Complete the assignments in the *Workbook* to give you experience in making decisions regarding situations of fraud, abuse, incidental disclosures, compliance violations, consents, or authorizations.

✔ Turn to the Glossary at the end of this text for a further understanding of the key terms and key abbreviations used in this chapter.

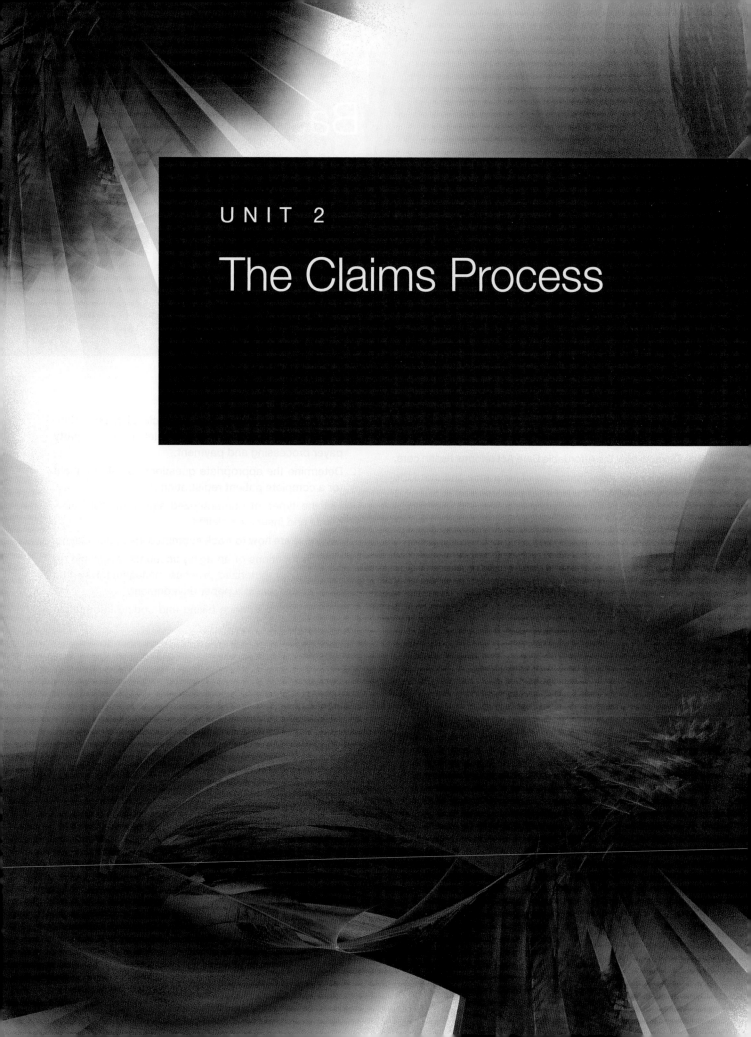

UNIT 2
The Claims Process

Basics of Health Insurance

Linda Smith

OBJECTIVES

After reading this chapter, you should be able to:

1. Describe the history of insurance in the United States.
2. Explain the reasons for the rising cost of health care.
3. Discuss how the Affordable Care Act reforms health care.
4. Discuss the legal principles of insurance and state the four concepts of a valid insurance contract.
5. Explain the difference between an implied and an expressed physician–patient contract and discuss different types of patients.
6. Discuss the intricacies of the insurance policy and define common insurance terms.
7. List and describe the choices a person has when it comes to choosing and obtaining health insurance.
8. State the types of health insurance coverage.
9. Describe in general terms the important federal, state, and private health insurance plans.
10. Relate the entire billing process to simple and complex medical cases.
11. Explain the administrative life cycle of a physician-based insurance claim from completion to third-party payer processing and payment.
12. Determine the appropriate questions to ask a patient for a complete patient registration form.
13. List the types of computerized signatures for documents and insurance claims.
14. Demonstrate how to track submitted insurance claims.
15. List the functions of an aging accounts receivable report in a computerized practice management system or a "tickler" file in a paper environment.
16. Explain how insurance billing and coding information can be kept up to date.
17. Describe the proper information to post to the patient's financial account after claims submission and payment received.

KEY TERMS

accounts receivable
   management
applicant
assignment
blanket contract
cancelable
claim
coinsurance
competitive medical plan
conditionally renewable
Consumer Directed Health Plan

contract
coordination of benefits
copayment (copay)
daysheet
deductible
disability income insurance
electronic signature
eligibility
emancipated minor
encounter form
Exchanges

exclusions
exclusive provider organization
expressed contract
extended
financial accounting record
foundation for medical care
guaranteed renewable
guarantor
health insurance
health maintenance organization
implied contract

indemnity
Indemnity Health Insurance
independent or individual
    practice association
insured
major medical
mandated benefits
Maternal and Child Health
    Program
Medicaid
medically necessary
Medicare
Medicare/Medicaid
member
noncancelable policy

nonparticipating physician
    or provider
optionally renewable
participating physician or
    provider
patient registration form
personal insurance
point-of-service plan
posted
preauthorization
precertification
predetermination
preexisting conditions
preferred provider organization
premium

running balance
State Children's Health
    Insurance Program
State Disability Insurance
subscriber
TRICARE
Unemployment Compensation
    Disability
Veterans Affairs Outpatient Clinic
Veterans Health Administration
    (CHAMPVA)
workers' compensation
    insurance

KEY ABBREVIATIONS

AAPC	EPO	MCHP	ROA
ACA	FMC	Medi-Medi	SCHIP
ADSM	FSA	MGMA	SDHP
AMBA	HBMA	MSA	SDI
A/R	HCERA	nonpar	SHOP
CDHP	HDHP	NPP	SOF
CHAMPVA	HFMA	PAHCOM	UCD
CMP	HMO	par	VA
COB	HRA	PMS	WC
COBRA	HSA	POS plan	
DoD	IPA	PPACA	
DOS	MAB	PPO	

Service to Patients

Good customer service is emphasized in most industries that serve the consumer; when processing insurance matters, it is equally important. Some suggestions are as follows:
- You must be friendly and courteous to each patient when handling insurance claims to maintain a harmonious physician–patient relationship. Collections often can be significantly improved and simplified if the patient feels free to discuss personal financial problems at any time and is educated regarding the physician's fees.
- Quickly obtain precertification, preauthorization, or predetermination so that the patient's treatment plan may be carried out without delay.
- Assist and instruct the patient in filling out a patient information form so that data are accurate and complete.
- Explain and answer the patient's questions about your office's Notice of Privacy Practices (NPP). Remember, it is important for you to understand what the NPP states.
- Promptly transmit accurate insurance claim data to the third-party payer so that reimbursement is received in a timely manner on behalf of the patient.

HISTORY OF HEALTH INSURANCE IN THE UNITED STATES

Health insurance is a contract between a policyholder and a third-party payer or government program to reimburse the policyholder for all or a portion of the cost of medical and/or preventive care on the basis of the contract purchased. Its main purpose is to help offset some of the high costs accrued during sickness or when an injury has occurred.

To understand our current health care system, you need to understand the history of health care in the United States and how it has evolved into what it currently is. The health care system we have now did not always exist.

Health care insurance originated in the mid-1800s in the United States when the Franklin Health Assurance Company of Massachusetts began offering insurance for nonfatal injury. About 10 years later, the Travelers Insurance Company of Hartford marketed a plan that is similar to today's health insurance. Other companies began writing health insurance policies and in 1911 Montgomery Ward and Company offered benefits to its ill or injured employees. This was the first group plan. These commercial plans paid only when an individual was sick or received an injury.

Only large employers offered health insurance to their employers prior to 1920; everyone else paid out of their own pockets. However, as doctors began learning more about diseases and effective treatments and as more people took advantage of the new medical technology and were treated in hospitals, the cost for health care increased. To help ease the burden of health care costs, Baylor Hospital in Dallas created a system that eventually became known as Blue Cross to help people pay their hospital bills. Its counterpart, Blue Shield started gaining interest in the late 1930s as a way for doctors to secure payment for health care services.

By the 1960s, the success of the Blue Cross and Blue Shield model encouraged other insurers to enter the health care market. The shortage of labor during World War II also had an impact on the health care market and employers began to offer health insurance as an added benefit to the employment package. Soon it was commonplace for employers to provide health insurance. Most private insurance companies sold policies that included hospital care, surgical fees, and physicians' services. In addition to those benefits, many plans began offering catastrophic health insurance coverage, preventive care, dental insurance, **disability income insurance,** and long-term care and home health care insurance for the chronically ill, disabled, and developmentally disabled.

In 1965, federal legislation was passed to assist the elderly and the poor with their health insurance expenses, which led to the Medicare and Medicaid programs. Although both programs started small, expenditures in Medicare and Medicaid grew dramatically and currently make up a large percentage of all health care expenses in the United States.

As additional benefits were offered by insurance carriers and there were increases in the use of health care, medical care costs escalated and **premium** rates increased. Developing technologies and an increase in the aging population with more advanced health care needs has pushed health care spending even higher.

To deal with the rising costs of health care, the federal government adopted cost-containment legislation for the **Medicare, Medicaid,** and **TRICARE** programs. The concept of managed care, which began in the 1930s

when Kaiser Industries developed a prepaid, integrated health care insurance model for their employees, started to be noticed by insurance carriers in the 1980s. Managed care principles, in which insurance carriers became more involved in decisions related to how much care a patient receives, what kind of care he or she receives, and who could provide it, were recognized as a method to help control rising health care expenditures. As a result, many new types of insurance plans arose across the nation to control the cost of medical care and help those who could not afford insurance.

HEALTH CARE REFORM

Over the past 75 years, leaders of the United States, from President Roosevelt to President Obama, have announced reforms of the health care system. A major restructuring of the United States health care system was necessary during the 1990s for the following reasons:

- A growing percentage of Americans were not covered by private or government insurance.
- Employers had to pay escalating health care premiums and did not want to cut wages to cover these costs.
- Government needed to reduce the deficit by controlling increases in the Medicare and Medicaid programs.
- Physicians and hospital costs soared, with no end in sight because of inflation, high-tech equipment, expensive medications, and so on.
- Patients spent more and more money for less and less care and coped with a system riddled with inefficiency and fraud.
- Services were overused by patients.

On March 23, 2010, the Patient Protection and Affordable Care Act (PPACA) was signed into law and the related Health Care and Education Reconciliation Act (HCERA), which modifies certain provisions of PPACA, was signed into law on March 30, 2010. These two laws together are commonly referred to as the *Affordable Care Act (ACA),* which put in place comprehensive health insurance reforms that hold insurance companies accountable, lower costs, guarantee choice, and enhance the quality of health care for all Americans. Implementation of the ACA began in 2010 and will continue through 2020 (Table 3-1).

The ACA helps to make health care available and affordable for the 32 million Americans who are without insurance coverage. Under the plan, it is expected that 94% of Americans will be insured. The ACA's goal is to make insurance more affordable by providing tax cuts for the middle class and by reducing premiums for families and small business owners who are unable to afford the premiums associated with health care. Essentially, the ACA is making sweeping changes in the existing laws

Table 3-1	Timeline for Implementation of the Affordable Care Act (ACA) from 2010 to 2020
YEAR	**TIMELINE**
2010	• Implementation of rules to prevent insurance companies from denying coverage to children with preexisting conditions. • Prohibits insurance companies from dropping coverage due to technical errors in insurance contracts when patients get sick. • Prohibits insurance companies from imposing lifetime dollar limits on essential benefits. • Regulates annual limits on insurance coverage. • Provides consumers with an easy way to appeal to their insurance company and to an outside board if the company denies coverage of a claim. • Creates an easy-to-use website where consumers can compare health insurance coverage options. • Tax credits to small businesses that provide insurance benefits to their workers. • Relief for seniors who hit the Medicare prescription drug "doughnut hole." • New insurance plans must cover certain preventive services without cost-sharing (that is, deductibles, copays, or coinsurance). • A prevention and public health fund to invest in proven prevention public health programs. • Further crack down on health care fraud through new resources and screening procedures for health care providers. • Access to insurance for uninsured Americans with preexisting conditions. • Extending coverage for young adults. • Coverage for early retirees. • Rebuilding the primary care workforce. • Holding insurance companies accountable for unreasonable rate hikes. • Allowing states to cover more people on Medicaid through additional federal funding. • Payments for rural health care providers.
2011	• Prescription drug discounts. • Free preventive care for seniors through annual wellness visits and personalized prevention plans. • Improving health care quality and efficiency. • Improving care for seniors after they leave the hospital. • New innovations to bring down costs. • Increased access to services at home and in the community. • Strengthen community health centers. • Bring down health care premiums. • Address overpayments to big insurance companies and strengthen Medicare Advantage (MA).
2012	• Link payment to quality outcomes. • Encourage integrated health systems through "Accountable Care Organizations." • Reduce paperwork and administrative costs by implementation of electronic health records. • Understand and fight health disparities through collection of racial, ethnic, and language data. • Provide new voluntary options for long-term care insurance.
2013	• Improve preventive health coverage through additional funding to state Medicaid programs. • Expanded authority to bundle payments and pay providers at a flat rate for an episode of care. • Increase Medicaid payments for primary care doctors. • Additional funding for the State Children's Health Insurance Program (SCHIP).
2014	• No discrimination due to preexisting conditions or gender. • Eliminate annual limits on insurance coverage. • Ensure coverage for individuals participating in clinical trials. • Make care more affordable. • Establish health insurance exchanges. • Small business tax credits. • Increase access to Medicaid. • Promote individual responsibility. • Ensure free choice through establishment of health insurance exchanges.
2015	• Pay physicians based on value, not volume. Physicians will receive higher payments based on the quality of care they provide. • Annual health insurance industry fees will be imposed on health insurance companies to fund some of the provisions of the ACA. The fees will continue to increase yearly until 2018.
2016	• States will be permitted to form health care choice compacts and allow insurers to sell policies in any state participating in the compact. • Reduce Medicare payments to certain hospitals for hospital-acquired conditions by 1%.
2018	• 40% excise tax will be imposed on high-cost group health plans.
2020	• Elimination of Medicare Part D (doughnut hole) coverage gap.

Data from www.whitehouse.gov/healthreform/timeline.

that govern employer-sponsored group plans, individual health coverage, and governmental health programs.

Individual Mandate

The ACA included an individual mandate, which required most Americans to have health insurance coverage or face a penalty. Because of the individual mandate, the constitutionality of the Act was challenged in March 2012. On June 28, 2012, the Supreme Court of the United States upheld the PPACA in its entirety.

Consequently, if an individual does not have health insurance, he or she will pay a tax penalty of $95 per individual or 1% of taxable income, whichever is greater, for 2014.

In 2015, the fine will be $325 per individual or 2% of taxable income. This will rise to $695 per individual or 2.5% of income in 2016. In each year after 2016 the government will refigure the fine based on a cost-of-living adjustment.

Health Benefit Exchanges

A primary issue in health care reform was to make health care more accessible and more affordable to the uninsured population. To facilitate accessibility and affordability, a key provision of the ACA insurance reform was the creation of **"Exchanges."** An Exchange is an organized marketplace where uninsured individuals and small-business owners can find health insurance coverage and select from all of the qualified private health plans available in their area. Exchanges are an effort to lower health care costs through the establishment of a new competitive private insurance market that will be regional and administered by a governmental agency or nonprofit organization. Small Business Health Options Program (SHOP) Exchanges will serve a similar function for small employers and the self-employed. The Act required that Exchanges be established and open on January 1, 2014.

The Exchanges are a central clearinghouse that offers a "one-stop shop" for researching, comparing, and purchasing health insurance coverage that makes the process of finding a health insurance policy easier and more efficient. Exchanges create larger individual and small employer insurance pools with many of the advantages that a larger pool enjoys. They provide individuals and very small employers with access to the ACA policies that were written using the uniform set of national rules, which are more consumer-friendly.

Those who buy insurance through the individual plan must purchase plans through the Exchange to take advantage of federal subsidies. Those who receive coverage through their employers will continue to select and purchase their plans via employers. Individuals and small businesses of up to 100 employees can purchase qualified coverage. States are permitted to allow businesses with more than 100 employees to purchase coverage in the SHOP Exchange beginning in 2017. Through establishment of Health Benefit Exchanges, millions of Americans and small businesses will have access to affordable coverage and the same choices of insurance that members of Congress will have. The ACA holds insurance companies accountable by keeping premiums down and preventing insurance industry abuses and denial of care, and it will end discrimination against Americans with preexisting conditions.

With the advent of health care reform in 2010, additional changes occurred that affect programs such as Medicare, Medicaid, and the Employee Retirement Income Security Act (ERISA). In this chapter and Chapters 11, 12, 13, and 15, this reform is explained in more detail.

LEGAL PRINCIPLES OF INSURANCE

The role of a medical insurance billing specialist is to complete the insurance **claim** accurately and assist claims submission so that optimal accurate reimbursement is received quickly. However, before developing the skill of coding and completing insurance claim forms, it is necessary to know frequently encountered legal problems and how to handle them. Legal situations occur daily in the performance of these job duties and involve confidentiality of medical records, accurate insurance claim transmission, fraud and abuse issues, credit and collection laws, and so on. An insurance billing specialist cannot escape liability by pleading ignorance. It cannot be overemphasized that keeping up to date on health care plan policies and procedures is essential. Most legal issues of private health insurance claims fall under civil law, while Medicare, Medicaid, and TRICARE programs fall under federal laws. Although the private health care insurance industry is regulated by state law and is not considered a federally regulated industry, the Health Insurance Portability and Accountability Act (HIPAA) and Office of the Inspector General (OIG) federal regulations help to govern the entire industry.

Insurance Contracts

The first legal item in the business of handling medical insurance is the insurance contract, also known as a *policy*. A **contract** is a legal and binding written document that exists between two or more parties. Essentially, any agreement between two or more persons that is enforceable by law is considered a contract. There is no standard health insurance contract. Individuals who take out a policy receive an original document composed by the insuring company.

The following four considerations are involved in drawing up a valid insurance contract:

1. The person must be a mentally competent adult and not under the influence of drugs or alcohol when signing the contract.
2. The insurance company must make an offer (the signed application) and the person must accept the offer (issuance of the policy), without concealment or misrepresentation of facts on the application.
3. An exchange of value (the first premium payment) submitted with the application, known as a *consideration*, must be present.
4. A legal purpose must exist, which is an insurable interest in the case of a health insurance policy. This means that the policyholder expects to continue in good health but the insurance policy will provide something of value if an accident or illness strikes.

A policy can be challenged and coverage may not be in effect when a fraudulent statement is made by the purchaser of the insurance policy or **subscriber.** After a policy has been in force for 2 years (3 years in some states), a policy becomes incontestable and may not be challenged. If the time limit has passed and a policy is **guaranteed renewable,** meaning that the insurer is obligated to continue coverage as long as premiums are paid, the policy becomes incontestable even if false statements were made on the application.

PHYSICIAN–PATIENT CONTRACTS AND FINANCIAL OBLIGATION

Implied or Expressed Contracts

A physician and his or her staff must be aware of the physician's obligations to each patient, as well as his or her liabilities in regard to service, and the patient's obligations to the physician. The physician–patient contract begins when the physician accepts the patient and agrees to treat him or her. This action can be either an implied or an **expressed contract.** An **implied contract** is defined as not manifested by direct words but implied or deduced from the circumstance, the general language, or the conduct of the patient. For example, if Mary Johnson goes to Dr. Doe's office and Dr. Doe gives Ms. Johnson professional services that she accepts, this is an implied contract. If the patient is unconscious when treatment is rendered, treatment is based on an implied-in-fact contract. An expressed contract can be verbal or written. However, most physician–patient contracts are implied.

Self-Pay Patients

For patients who do not have medical insurance, the contract for treatment is between the physician and the patient. The patient is liable for the entire bill and is considered a self-pay patient.

Guarantor

A **guarantor** is an individual who promises to pay the medical bill by signing a form agreeing to pay or who accepts treatment, which by this act constitutes an expressed promise. Usually a patient is the guarantor and must be of legal age (18 or 21 years, depending on state law). However, if the patient is a child of a divorced parent, the custodial parent bears the responsibility of the child's medical expenses unless the divorce decree states otherwise. An adoptive parent may be the custodial parent (guarantor) and therefore solely liable for the child's bill. A father is ordinarily responsible for his children's debts if they are minors and are not emancipated (Figure 3-1).

Emancipated Minor

An **emancipated minor** is a person younger than 18 years of age who lives independently, is totally self-supporting, is married or divorced, is a parent even if not married, or is in the military and possesses decision-making rights. College students living away from home, even when financially dependent on their parents, are considered emancipated. Parents are not liable for the medical expenses incurred by an emancipated minor. The patient record should contain the minor's signed statement that he or she is on his or her own.

Managed Care Patients

A physician under contract to a managed care plan may or may not periodically receive an updated list of current

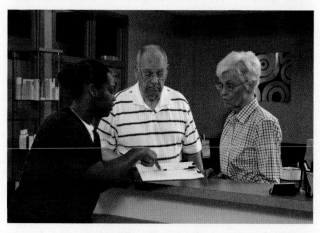

FIGURE 3-1 Receptionist explaining where a guarantor's signature goes on a patient registration form for the medical services rendered to a family member.

enrollees. The physician is obligated to see those individuals who are enrolled if one of them calls for an appointment. However, the contract for treatment occurs when the patient is first seen. If the primary care physician no longer wishes to treat a patient on a managed care plan, termination is handled according to the contract. Generally, approval must be obtained from the third-party administrator of the plan to have the patient reassigned.

An insurance billing specialist should be able to read and explain managed care plan contracts that the office participates with; however, if the specialist is unable to interpret these matters, professional assistance should be sought from the physician's attorney, the medical practice's accountant, or the managed care plan. The specialist should understand billing and collection requirements and track payments made by the managed care plan.

Employment and Disability Examinations

Courts in most jurisdictions have ruled that there is no physician–patient relationship in an employment or disability examination and that the doctor does not owe a duty of care to the person being examined. This is mainly because the insurance company is requesting the examination and the patient is not seeking the medical services of the physician.

Workers' Compensation Patients

Workers' compensation (WC) cases involve a person being injured on the job. These cases may be referred to as *industrial accidents* or *illnesses*. In these types of cases, the contract exists between the physician and the insurance company. When there is a dispute as to whether the injured party was hurt at work, a Patient Agreement form (see Figure 15-11) must be signed by the patient who agrees to pay the physician's fees if the case is declared to be non–work-related.

THE INSURANCE POLICY

Insurance policies are complex and contain a great deal of language that is difficult to understand. This can cause misunderstanding by patients or anyone trying to obtain information from the policy. Basic health insurance coverage includes benefits for hospital, surgical, and other medical expenses. **Major medical** or **extended** benefits contracts are designed to offset large medical expenses caused by prolonged illness or serious injury. Some of these policies include coverage for *extended care* or *skilled nursing facility* benefits. The **insured** is known as a *subscriber* or, in some insurance programs, a **member**, *policyholder*, or *recipient* and may not necessarily be

the patient seen for the medical service. The subscriber may or may not be the guarantor. The insured is the individual (enrollee) or organization protected in case of loss under the terms of an insurance policy. In group insurance, the employer is considered the insured and the employees are the risks. However, when completing an insurance claim form, the covered employee is listed as the insured. A policy might also include *dependents* of the insured. Generally, this term refers to the spouse and children of the insured but under some contracts, parents, other family members, and domestic partners may be covered as dependents. Under the health care reform legislation of 2010, health plans must allow employees to keep their children on their plans until the children are 26 years old.

Policy Application

Before a policy is issued, the insurance company decides whether it will enter into a contract with the **applicant** who is applying for the insurance coverage. Information is obtained about the applicant so that the company can decide whether to accept the risk. Generally, the application form has two sections: the first part contains basic information about the application and the second part concerns the health of the individual.

An insurance policy is a legally enforceable agreement, or contract. If a policy is issued, the applicant becomes part of the insurance contract or plan. The policy becomes effective only after the company offers the policy and the person accepts it and then pays the initial premium. If a premium is paid at the time the application is submitted, the insurance coverage can be put into force before the policy is delivered. Depending on the laws in some states, the applicant also can have temporary conditional insurance if the agent issues a specific type of receipt.

Policy Renewal Provisions

Health insurance policies may have renewal provisions written into the policy stating the circumstances under which the company may refuse to renew, may cancel coverage, or may increase the premium. It is important for the insurance billing specialist to understand that coverage may change from the last time the physician saw the patient for an appointment. It is always a good routine to verify insurance information each time the patient comes for an appointment. **Eligibility** verification means to check and confirm that the patient is a member of the insurance plan and that the member identification number is correct. This may seem redundant but it may avoid a lot of future confusion and delays in payment.

In private health insurance, there are five classifications: (1) cancelable, (2) optionally renewable, (3) conditionally renewable, (4) guaranteed renewable, and (5) noncancelable.

A renewable provision in a **cancelable** policy grants the insurer the right to cancel the policy at any time and for any reason. The company notifies the insured that the policy is canceled and refunds any advance premium the policyholder has paid. In some states, this type of policy is illegal.

In an **optionally renewable** policy, the insurer has the right to terminate coverage on the premium or anniversary date, as specified in the contract. The insurer may not cancel the policy at any time in between. **Conditionally renewable** policies grant the insurer a limited right to refuse to renew a health insurance policy at the end of a premium payment period. Reasons stated in the policy may relate to age, employment status, or both but may not relate to the insured's health status.

The guaranteed renewable classification is desirable because the insurer is required to renew the policy as long as premium payments are made. However, these policies may have age limits of 60, 65, or 70 years or they may be renewable for life.

In a **noncancelable policy,** the insurer cannot increase premium rates and must renew the policy until the insured reaches the age specified in the contract. Some disability income policies have noncancelable terms.

Policy Terms

To keep the insurance in force, a person must pay a monthly, quarterly, or annual fee called a *premium.* If the premium is not paid, a *grace period* of 10 to 30 days is usually given before insurance coverage ceases. In addition, usually a **deductible** (a specific amount of money) must be paid each year before the policy benefits begin. Generally, the higher the deductible is, the lower the cost of the policy is. Most policies, as well as Part B of the Medicare program, have a **coinsurance** or *cost-sharing* requirement, which means the insured will assume a percentage of the fee (for example, 20%) or pay a specific dollar amount (for example, $5 or $10) for covered services.

Managed care plans use the term **copayment (copay)** when referring to the amount the patient pays at the point of arriving in the office and before he or she sees the physician. It is not advisable to routinely waive copayments because the health care provider has agreed to accept a patient portion. Many insurance companies do not tolerate this practice. Not only

would it be a loss of income to the provider, but the federal government can assess penalties for not collecting coinsurance for patients seen under the Medicare program if the provider is audited. Generally, deductibles, coinsurance, and copayments should be collected at the time of service, with the exception of the Medicare program, which does not recommend collecting the deductible in advance from the beneficiary. In cases of financial hardship, a discount or waiver may be considered. Be sure to document this and obtain the patient's signature and any document that verifies the patient's financial status.

Health insurance policies consider an *accident* to be an unforeseen and unintended event. Some policies cover accidents that occur from the first day the policy is in force. Others may contain an *elimination period* or a *waiting period* before benefits for sickness or accident become payable.

Generally, it is the patient's responsibility to give a written notice of claim to the insurance company within a certain number of days, known as a *time limit.* However, some insurance carriers and Medicare guidelines require that the provider of service be obligated to submit the claim. Usually as a courtesy, the claim is filed for the patient by the provider of professional services. The insurance billing specialist must be able to abstract proper information from the patient record, which is used to code the diagnoses and services rendered, to complete an insurance claim form, to make entries (post) to a patient's **financial accounting record** (ledger), and to follow up on unpaid claims. If any one of these procedures is not done properly, correct reimbursement or payment (also called **indemnity**) from the third-party payer will not be generated.

Following up on unpaid claims is done by contacting the claims representative, called a *claims adjudicator* or an *adjuster.*

Coordination of Benefits

A **coordination of benefits (COB)** statement is included in most policies and contracts with providers.

When the patient has more than one insurance policy (dual coverage or duplication of coverage), this clause requires insurance companies to coordinate the reimbursement of benefits to determine which carrier is going to be primary and which carrier is going to be secondary, thus preventing the duplication or overlapping of payments for the same medical expense. The combination of payments from the primary and secondary carriers cannot be more than the amount of the provider's charges (Example 3-1).

Example 3-1	Coordination of Benefits for Dual Coverage Case

Mr. Smith has Insurance A and Insurance B. The claim is for $100. The claim is sent to Insurance A. Insurance A allows $80 for the procedure and pays $80. The claim is then sent to Insurance B. Insurance B also allows $80 for the procedure. The claim that was sent to Insurance B was not for $100 but for the remaining $20. The $20 is within the amount allowed by Insurance B; therefore Insurance B pays the $20. Some carriers try to play by their own rules by stating that because Insurance A paid $80 and the $80 equals the amount Insurance B pays, Insurance B will pay no more for the claim. These rules were established by the National Association of Insurance Commissioners and approved by every State Insurance Commissioner. Therefore be observant of insurance claims like this.

Birthday Rule

The birthday rule is an informal procedure that the health insurance industry has widely adopted for the coordination of benefits when children are listed as dependents on two parents' group health plans. Under the birthday rule, the health plan of the parent whose birthday comes first in the calendar year (month and day, *not* year) is designated as the primary plan. If both mother and father have the same birthday, the plan of the person who has had coverage longer is the primary payer. According to the National Association of Insurance Commissioners, the birthday rule is not insurance law. Some insurance plans do not follow these customs and it may be necessary to contact the plan for confirmation.

In cases of divorce, consider that you are not an enforcer of court laws and that the divorce decree is between the parents of the child. Have the parent accompanying the child pay the bill at the time of service. He or she can be reimbursed by the responsible party. If a copy of the court decision is presented, bill the insurance of the parent deemed responsible.

Finally, a carrier may pend or delay a claim, stating that the carrier is attempting to coordinate benefits with the other carrier. This process can be time consuming and may take 90 days or more to resolve. As an insurance billing specialist, you should be diligent in following up on this situation so that the stalled cash flow issue can be resolved. In some situations, the patient ultimately may be responsible for the bill; if you help the patient to understand that, this will bring payment and resolve the account balance quicker.

General Policy Limitations

Health insurance policies may contain **exclusions** or limitations of the policy. Exclusions are services that are never covered by the health insurance policy. These exclusions are typically outlined in the insurance policy and may include items such as acupuncture, eyeglasses, contact lenses, dental treatment or surgery, services related to sex transformations, and cosmetic and aesthetic treatments. Most insurance policies also have limitations for covered services that are not deemed medically necessary. **Medically necessary** refers to a decision by your health plan that your treatment, test, or procedure is necessary for your health or to treat a diagnosed medical problem. For example, a patient may request to have an electrocardiogram (ECG) performed because he or she has a family history of heart disease; however, the insurance may not pay for the service unless the patient presents with shortness of breath, chest pain, or other signs or symptoms that may indicate medical necessity for the procedure to be performed. In the past, insurance companies may have issued policies that did not provide benefits for conditions that existed and were treated before the policy was issued; these are called **preexisting conditions.** Under the health care reform legislation of 2010, insurance companies cannot deny coverage to children with preexisting medical problems. In 2014 the ACA prohibited insurers from denying coverage to *any* American with preexisting conditions or charging them more or from charging more for women.

Mandated benefits are state and/or federal laws that require coverage for treatment of specific health conditions by certain types of health care providers for some categories of dependents, such as children placed for adoption. Health care benefits may be mandated by state law, federal law, or in some cases both. For example, under the Newborns' and Mothers' Health Protection Act of 1996, health plans may not limit benefits for any hospital length of stay related to childbirth for the mother or newborn child. Additionally, there is a federal mandate that requires health plans to provide someone who is receiving benefits related to a mastectomy with coverage for reconstruction of the breast. The Americans with Disabilities Act (ADA) requires insurance companies to provide the same benefits to disabled and nondisabled individuals with regard to premiums, deductibles, and limits on coverage.

Case Management Requirements
Preapproval

Many private third-party payers and prepaid health plans have certain requirements that must be met before they approve hospital admissions, inpatient or outpatient surgeries, and elective procedures. First, eligibility requirements must be obtained. These are conditions or qualifying factors that must be met before the patient receives benefits (medical services) under a specified insurance plan, government program, or managed care plan.

COLLEGE CLINIC
4567 Broad Avenue
Woodland Hills, XY 12345-0000

Phone: 555/486-9002   Fax: 555/590-2189

Insurance Precertification Form

Date: _5/4/XX_

To: Insurance Carrier ___Cal-Net Care___   From: ___Janet___ Office Mgr.
    Address _____9900 Baker Street_____
            ___Los Angeles, CA 90067___

Check those that apply: Admission certification ✓   Outpatient ___ Inpatient ✓
                           Surgery certification ✓   Emergency situation ✓

Patient's name ___Ronald Stranton___   Date of Birth: _4-14-49_
Patient's address ___639 Cedar Street___   Sex: Male ✓ Female ___
                  ___Woodland Hills, XY 12345___   Social Security No. _527-XX-7250_
Insured's Name ___Same___   Policy Group ID No. _A59_
Insured's Address _____   Employer: _Aerostar Aviation_

Treating physician ___Clarence Cutler, M.D.___   NPI #: _430 500 47XX_
Primary Care Physician _Gerald Practon, M.D._   NPI #: _462 7889 7XX_

Name of Hospital ___College Hospital___   Admission Date: _5/4/XX_
                                                  Estimated Length of Stay: _3-5 d_
Admitting Diagnosis _Volvulus_   Diagnosis Code: _560.2_
Complicating conditions to substantiate need for inpatient hospitalization _____
                   ___Complete bowel obstruction___
Date current illness or injury began _5/2/XX_
Procedure/surgery to be done _Reduction of Volvulus_   Procedure code _44050_

Second opinion needed   Yes ___ No ✓ Date performed _____

Telephone precertification: ____Emergency Cert. 5/4/XX____
Name of representative certifying___McKenzie Kwan___
Direct-dial telephone number of representative ___1-800-463-9000 ext. 227___

Reason(s) for denial _____
Certification approved   Yes ✓ No ___ Certification approval No. _69874_
Authorization for services Yes ✓ No ___ Authorization No. _69874E_

Note: The information contained in this facsimile message is confidential and privileged information intended only for the use of the individual or entity named above. If the reader of this message is not the intended recipient, you are hereby notified that any dissemination, distribution, or copying of this communication is strictly prohibited. If you have received this communication in error, please immediately notify me by telephone and return the original facsimile to me via the U.S. Postal Service. Thank you.

FIGURE 3-2 Insurance precertification form. This form can be faxed to the insurance company or used when telephoning to obtain approval for hospitalization under a patient's insurance policy or managed care plan.

The carrier can refuse to pay part of or the entire fee if these requirements are not met. **Precertification** refers to discovering whether a treatment (surgery, hospitalization, tests) is covered under a patient's contract. **Preauthorization** relates not only to whether a service or procedure is covered, but also to finding out whether it is medically necessary. **Predetermination** means discovering the maximum dollar amount that the carrier will pay for surgery, consulting services, radiology procedures, and so on.

Obtain precertification or predetermination when a procedure is tentatively scheduled. The information that may be required to obtain precertification approval by fax or telephone is shown in Figure 3-2. Use the form shown in Figure 3-3 to obtain predetermination by mail. Figure 11-3 is an example of a preauthorization form. This form also can be used to document the information received when verifying the patient's insurance coverage by telephone. It should become part of the patient's record

COLLEGE CLINIC
4567 Broad Avenue
Woodland Hills, XY 12345-0001

Phone: 555/486-9002   Fax: 555/487-8976

INSURANCE PREDETERMINATION FORM

Perry Cardi, MD
Physician

Patient: __Leslee Austin__   Telephone # __(555) 486-8452__
Address: __209 Refugio Road__   Date of Birth __04-07-44__
City __Woodland Hills__ — State __XY__   ZIP __12345-0001__
Social Security # __629-XX-9260__   Accident Yes _____ No __X__
Insurance Company __American Insurance__   Member # __Am 45692__
Insurance Co. Address __4040 Broadway Ave__   Group # __123P__
__Valley Vista, XY 12345__   Telephone # __(555) 238-5000__
Policy holder __Leslee Austin__
Relationship to insured: Self __X__ Spouse_____ Child ____ Other____
Type of coverage: HMO __X__ PPO ____ 80/20 ____ 70/30 ____ Other____
Procedure/Service __Cardioversion (CPT 92960)__
Diagnosis __Atrial fibrillation (ICD–9–CM 427.31)__

- -

BENEFITS:
Coverage effective date: From __02/01/XX__ To __01/31/XX__   Maximum benefit or benefit limitation: __$1,000,000 lifetime__
Preexisting exclusions: __Lupus erythematosus__   Second opinion requirements: Yes _____ No __X__
Major medical   Yes __X__ No ____   Precertification/Preauthorization Yes __X__ No ____
Deductible   Yes _____ No __X__ Amount $_____   Reference # __432786__
  Per family: Yes _____ No __X__ Amount $_____   Authorized by: __Lucille Vasquez__
  Deductible paid to date: Amount $_____
Out of pocket expense limit: Amount $_____
                                        Per: _____

- -

COVERAGE: COVERAGE DETAILS AND LIMITS
  Procedures/Services
    Office visits   YES __X__   NO _____   Physical exam; one per year
    Consultations   YES __X__   NO _____   _____
    ER visits   YES __X__   NO _____   _____
    X-ray   YES __X__   NO _____   _____
    Laboratory   YES __X__   NO _____   Need authorization
    Office surgery   YES __X__   NO _____   Need authorization
    Hospital surgery   YES __X__   NO _____   _____
    Anesthesia   YES __X__   NO _____   Need authorization
    DME   YES __X__   NO _____   _____
  Physician payment schedule: RVS_____ RBRVS_____ UCR_____ Other __X__

- -

    Payment sent to: Provider __X__ Patient _____ Time limit after submission? __30 days__
    Verification by: __Karen Reynolds__   Date: __07-14-XX__

FIGURE 3-3 Insurance predetermination form. This form can be sent to the insurance company to find out the maximum dollar amount that will be paid for primary surgery, consulting services, postoperative care, and so on.

and be used for reference when billing future insurance claims.

After the information is received from the third-party payer, give the patient an estimate of fees for the proposed surgery, state how much the insurance payer is expected to pay, and make the patient aware of any balance amounts that may be due by him or her. It is further recommended that the patient sign a statement that he or she is aware of the patient responsibility

and agrees to pay it on receipt of a patient statement. An example of suggested wording for a letter is given in Figure 3-4. This written estimate makes collection quicker and easier.

CHOICE OF HEALTH INSURANCE

A person can obtain health insurance by taking out insurance through a group plan (contract or policy) or by paying the premium on an individual contract.

COLLEGE CLINIC
4567 Broad Avenue
Woodland Hills, XY 12345-0000

Phone: 555/486-9002   **Fax: 555/487-8976**

Current date

Patient's name
Address
City, State, ZIP code

Dear

This letter gives you an estimate of the fees for your proposed surgery. Verification of coverage and benefit information has been obtained from your insurance company. Listed are your benefits for the proposed surgical expenses and the estimated balance after your insurance carrier pays.

Surgical procedure	Craniotomy		
Date of surgery	February 21, 20XX		
Name of hospital	College Hospital		
Hospital address	4500 Broad Ave., Woodland Hills, XY 12345		

		Insurance pays	Estimated balance
Surgeon's fee	2548.09	1344.24	1203.85
Preoperative visit			
Preoperative tests			

You have a policy deductible of $1000   which ___ has ✓ has not been met.

The surgery requires the use of an anesthesiologist, assistant surgeon, and a pathologist. These physicians will bill you separately for their services. The hospital will also bill you separately.

This office will file your insurance claim for the surgical procedure, so the insurance payment should come directly to us. If the insurance carrier sends you the payment, then you are responsible to get the payment to this office within five days. Your balance after surgery should be approximately $1203.85. You are responsible for any remaining balance after our office receives the insurance payment.

This notice gives our estimation of the balance for which you will be responsible. Please sign below to indicate you have received and understand this notification.

_____   _____

Signature   Date

Thank you for choosing our medical practice. If you have any questions, please call me.

Sincerely,

Karen Martinez, CMA
Administrative Medical Assistant

FIGURE 3-4 Sample letter to a patient supplying an estimate of the fees for proposed surgery.

Individual Contract

Any insurance plan issued directly to an individual (and dependents) is called an *individual contract.* Usually this type of policy has a higher premium and often the benefits are less than those obtainable under a group health insurance plan. Sometimes this is called **personal insurance.**

Group Contract

A *group contract* is any insurance plan by which a group of employees (and their eligible dependents) or other homogeneous group is insured under a single policy issued to their employer or leader, with individual certificates given to each insured individual or family unit. A group policy usually provides better benefits and offers lower premiums. However, the coverage for each person in the group is the same. If a new employee declines enrollment, he or she must sign a waiver stating this fact. Under the health care reform legislation of 2010, employers may change the kind of medical benefits they offer their employees (for example, increase copayments and deductibles or reduce what the plans cover).

Conversion Privilege

Some individuals can obtain comprehensive group coverage through plans sponsored by the professional organizations to which they belong. Sometimes this is called a **blanket contract.** If the person leaves the employer or organization or the group contract is terminated, the insured may continue the same or lesser coverage under an individual policy if the group contract has a *conversion privilege.* Usually, conversion from a group policy to an individual policy increases the premium and could reduce the benefits.

Income Continuation Benefits

According to the Consolidated Omnibus Budget Reconciliation Act (COBRA) of 1985, when an employee is laid off from a company with 20 or more workers, federal law requires that the group health insurance coverage be extended to the employee and his or her dependents at group rates for up to 18 months. This also applies to those workers who lose coverage because of reduced work hours. In the case of death of a covered employee, divorced or widowed spouse, or employee entitled to Medicare, the extension of coverage may be for 36 months. However, the employee must pay for the group policy; this is known as *income continuation benefits.* See the section on COBRA in Chapter 12 for additional information on this topic.

Medical Savings Accounts

A *medical savings account (MSA)* is a type of tax-free savings account that allows individuals and their employers to set aside money to pay for health care expenses. An employer can set up an MSA for his or her employees and make an annual contribution to the MSA, which is tax-deductible for both employer and employee. MSA balances can be carried over from year to year tax-free. MSAs are portable, allowing individuals to take their MSA with them when they retire, change jobs, or relocate. When health care services are provided, the patient files a claim to receive reimbursement from these funds and uses the explanation of benefits (EOB) from the insurance company as documentation. Processing of the EOB for insurance claims with large deductibles (for example, more than $1000), even though you know the insurance company will not

be paying for the services, is necessary so that the patient/employee may submit documentation and recoup funds from the MSA. It also may be necessary to provide EOB documents from the insurance company to patients who do not receive them for this same purpose. Medicare beneficiaries are eligible to enroll in a similar tax-advantaged savings account, which may be referred to as a *Medicare medical savings account.*

Health Savings Accounts

The Medicare reform act was signed into law in December 2003, giving Americans a tool for defraying medical costs called *health savings accounts (HSAs).* HSAs are open to anyone younger than 65 years of age who enrolls in a high-deductible health plan (HDHP) (for example, more than $1250 per individual or $2500 per family in 2014). Annual out-of-pocket expenses (deductibles and copayments) apply and may not exceed $6350 for self-only coverage ($12,700 for family coverage) in 2014. Employers pay the monthly premiums. Employees pay the deductibles when they receive health care treatment and may share some of the costs of the plan via payroll deductions. These accounts are a tax-favored savings plan in which a working person can deposit money in an HSA and deduct the amount of the deposits from taxable income. Withdrawals from HSAs are tax-free when used for qualifying medical expenses. Money left unspent in an HSA may be rolled over year after year.

Health Reimbursement Arrangements

An alternative plan is a *health reimbursement account (HRA),* which has a high deductible and may be better than an HSA for a chronically ill person (for example, a person with diabetes). HRAs are typically offered in tandem with high-deductible plans. The employer owns the account and *only* the employer is eligible to make contributions. The employer is allowed to determine contribution limits and define covered expenses and can determine whether the balance can be rolled over from one year to the next. Employers may keep the money if a worker quits.

Flexible Spending Accounts

Another option is a health care flexible spending account (FSA). FSAs are employer sponsored, allow a specific amount of wages to be put aside for qualified medical expenses, and care for dependents who live with someone while that person is at work. Under the health care reform of 2010, over-the-counter medications, such as antihistamines and pain relievers, were added to the list of qualified medical expenses that are allowed using the FSA but a written prescription is required. An individual can put up to $2500 in an FSA each year, with the cap increasing by the annual inflation rate in subsequent years. Money deducted from an employee's pay into an FSA is not subject to payroll taxes, resulting in substantial payroll tax savings. Before the Affordable Care Act, one disadvantage of using an FSA was that funds not used by the end of the plan year were lost to the employee, known as the "use it or lose it" rule. Under the terms of the ACA and effective in 2013 plan years, the employee is allowed to carry over up to $500 per year to the following year without losing the funds.

High-Deductible Health Plans

HDHPs, also known as *consumer-directed health plans,* are combined with an HSA or HRA and give insurance coverage that has tax advantages to assist in saving for future medical expenses. They have annual out-of-pocket limits and a higher annual deductible than traditional health insurance plans.

TYPES OF HEALTH INSURANCE COVERAGE

Many forms of health insurance coverage are currently in effect in the United States. These are referred to as third-party payers (private insurance, government plans, managed care contracts, and workers' compensation). A brief explanation of the programs discussed in this text is given here, but for an in-depth study, refer to the appropriate chapters that follow.

 Competitive Medical Plan: A competitive medical plan (CMP) is a type of managed care organization created by the Tax Equity and Fiscal Responsibility Act of 1982 (TEFRA). This federal legislation allows for enrollment of Medicare beneficiaries in managed care plans (see Chapter 12).

 Consumer Directed Health Plans: These plans are a rapidly emerging approach to health care services that are also referred to as *Self-Directed Health Plans (SDHPs).* Consumer Directed Health Plans (CDHPs) allow the consumer to design and customize his or her own health plan, based on his or her specific needs and circumstances. Typically, the CDHP involves the pairing of a high-deductible preferred provider organization (PPO) plan with a tax-advantaged account, such as an HSA (see Chapter 11).

 Disability Income Insurance: Disability income insurance is a form of insurance that provides periodic payments to replace income when the insured is unable to work as a result of illness, injury, or disease (see Chapter 16). This type of insurance should not be confused with workers' compensation, because those injuries must be work-related.

 Exclusive Provider Organization: An exclusive provider organization (EPO) is a type of managed health care plan in which subscriber members are eligible for benefits only when they use the services of a limited network of providers. EPOs combine features of both health maintenance organizations (HMOs) and PPOs. Employers agree not to enter into an agreement with any other plan for coverage of eligible employees. EPOs are regulated under state health insurance laws (see Chapter 11).

 Foundation for Medical Care: A foundation for medical care (FMC) is an organization of physicians, sponsored by a state or local medical association, concerned with the development and delivery of medical services and the cost of health care (see Chapter 11).

 Health Maintenance Organization: A health maintenance organization (HMO) is an organization that provides a wide range of comprehensive health care services for a specified group at a fixed periodic payment. The emphasis is on preventive care. Physicians are reimbursed by capitation. An HMO can be sponsored by the government, medical schools, hospitals, employers, labor unions, consumer groups, insurance companies, or hospital medical plans (see Chapter 11).

Indemnity Health Insurance: Indemnity Health Insurance plans are referred to as *traditional* or *fee-for-service health plans.* They are designed to allow patients maximum flexibility and choice when it comes to providers. Subscribers pay a fixed monthly premium and services are paid at a percentage of covered benefits after an annual deductible is met. Providers are paid each time a service is rendered on a fee-for-service basis (see Chapter 11).

Independent or Individual Practice Association: An independent or individual practice association (IPA) is a type of managed care plan in which a program administrator contracts with a number of physicians who agree to provide treatment to subscribers in their own offices or clinics for a fixed capitation payment per month. Subscribers to IPA plans have limited or no choice of physician. IPA physicians continue to see their fee-for-service patients (see Chapter 11).

Maternal and Child Health Program: A Maternal and Child Health Program (MCHP) is a state and federal program for children who are younger than 21 years of age and have special health care needs. It assists parents with financial planning and may assume part or all of the costs of treatment, depending on the child's condition and the family's resources (see Chapter 13).

Medicaid: Medicaid is a program sponsored jointly by federal, state, and local governments to provide health care benefits to medically indigent persons on welfare (public assistance), aged individuals who meet certain financial requirements, and the disabled. Some states have expanded coverage for other medically needy individuals who meet special state-determined criteria. Coverage and benefits vary widely from state to state (see Chapter 13).

Medicare: Medicare is a national four-part program. It consists of a hospital insurance system (Part A), supplementary medical insurance (Part B), Medicare Plus Choice Program (Part C), and the Medicare Prescription Drug benefits (Part D). It is for individuals who are at least 65 years of age. It was created by the 1965 Amendments to the Social Security Act and is operated under the provisions of the Act. Benefits are also extended to certain disabled people (for example, those who are totally disabled or blind) and coverage and payment are provided for those who require kidney dialysis and kidney transplant services (see Chapters 12 and 13).

Medicare/Medicaid: Medicare/Medicaid is a program that covers those persons eligible for both Medicare and Medicaid (see Chapters 12 and 13). In some areas of the country, dual coverage in both programs may be referred to as Medi-Medi.

Point-of-Service Plan: A point-of-service (POS) plan is a managed care plan consisting of a network of physicians and hospitals that provides an insurance company or employer with discounts on its services. Patients can refer themselves to a specialist or see a nonprogram provider for a higher copayment (see Chapter 11).

Preferred Provider Organization: A variation of a managed care plan is a preferred provider organization (PPO). This is a form of contract medicine by which a large employer (for example, hospitals or physicians) or any organization that can produce a large number of patients (for example, union trusts or insurance companies) contracts with a hospital or a group of physicians to offer medical care at a reduced rate (see Chapter 11).

State Children's Health Insurance Program (SCHIP): The State Children's Health Insurance Program (SCHIP) is a state-sponsored program that provides free or low-cost health coverage for low-income children (see Chapter 13).

 TRICARE: A government-sponsored program called TRICARE provides military and nonmilitary hospital and medical services for spouses of active service personnel, dependents of active service personnel, retired service personnel and their dependents, and dependents of members who died on active duty. Active duty service members (ADSMs) are not eligible for TRICARE but have benefits like TRICARE Prime, in which the Department of Defense (DoD) covers all allowable charges for medically necessary care (see Chapter 14).

 Unemployment Compensation Disability: Unemployment Compensation Disability (UCD) or **State Disability Insurance** (SDI) is insurance that covers off-the-job injury or sickness and is paid for by deductions from a person's paycheck. This program is administered by a state agency in only six states (see Chapter 16).

 Veterans Affairs Outpatient Clinic: A Veterans Affairs Outpatient Clinic renders medical and dental services to a veteran who has a service-related disability (see Chapter 14).

 Veterans Health Administration (CHAMPVA): The Veterans Health Administration (or Civilian Health and Medical Program of the Department of Veterans Affairs [CHAMPVA]) is administered by the Department of Veterans Affairs (VA). This federal program shares the medical bills of spouses and children of veterans with total, permanent, service-connected disabilities or of the surviving spouses and children of veterans who died as a result of service-connected disabilities (see Chapter 14).

 Workers' Compensation Insurance: Workers' compensation insurance is a contract that insures a person against on-the-job injury or illness. The employer pays the premium for his or her employees (see Chapter 15).

Examples of Insurance Billing

Sometimes it is difficult to comprehend the full scale of insurance billing. As an example of total medical billing, six cases are presented to help you understand the entire billing picture from simple to complex.

CASE 1: A new patient comes in with complaints of a sore throat and an infected nail.
   The physician's office bills for:
   Office visit, penicillin injection
   Office surgery for infected nail
   Sterile surgical tray (may or may not be billed, depending on third-party payer)

CASE 2: A patient comes in because of an accident and has complaints that require evaluation and management services, x-ray films, and laboratory studies (urinalysis) performed in the physician's office.

The physician's office bills for:
Office visit x-ray studies (including interpretation) and laboratory tests (urinalysis, including interpretation)

CASE 3: A patient is seen by the family physician after office hours in the hospital emergency department.
   The physician's office bills for the visit to the hospital emergency department.
   The hospital bills for hospital (outpatient) emergency department services (use and supplies).

CASE 4: A physician sends a patient's Papanicolaou (Pap) test to a private clinical laboratory.
   The physician's office bills for:
   Office visit
   Handling of specimen
   The laboratory bills for the Pap test

CASE 5: A patient is sent to a local hospital for an upper gastrointestinal radiographic series. An x-ray technician obtains the films in the hospital and a privately owned radiologic group does the interpretation.

   The hospital bills for the technical component of the upper gastrointestinal x-ray series (use of equipment).

   The radiologic group bills for the professional component of the upper gastrointestinal x-ray series (the interpretation).

CASE 6: A patient is seen in the office and is immediately hospitalized for surgery.

   The physician's office bills for initial hospital admission and surgical procedure (for example, hysterectomy). (The physician is a surgeon.)

   The assistant surgeon bills for assisting the surgeon during hysterectomy. (Some third-party payers do not allow payment.)

   The anesthesiologist bills for anesthesia administered during hysterectomy.

   The hospital (inpatient) bills for hospital room, operating room, anesthesia supplies, medications, x-ray films, laboratory tests, and medical and surgical supplies (dressings, intravenous lines). The hospital (inpatient) might also bill for blood for transfusions, electrocardiogram, radiation therapy, and respiratory therapy.

An insurance billing specialist in the offices of the attending physician, assistant surgeon, anesthesiologist, radiologic group, and private clinical laboratory submits an itemized statement and/or insurance claim form for reimbursement to the insurance payer or gives the patient the necessary information to submit his or her own claim to the insurance company.

EXCEPTION

MEDICARE PATIENTS BY FEDERAL LAW MAY NOT SUBMIT THEIR OWN CLAIMS FOR PHYSICIAN OR HOSPITAL SERVICES. EXCEPTIONS ARE MENTIONED IN CHAPTER 12.

In the hospital and hospital emergency department, a member of the hospital staff inputs services into a central computer system that produces an itemized statement and completed insurance claim form via computer to be submitted to the third-party payer. Hospital billing is explained in Chapter 17.

HANDLING AND PROCESSING INSURANCE CLAIMS

Most offices today are computerized and use practice management software (PMS) for scheduling, **accounts receivable management** (coding and billing) and patient statements, electronic health records, and other administrative functions, such as generating patient reminders and letters. However, some smaller offices thrive in the paper environment and will continue to do so.

A computerized office may still generate paper insurance claim forms and send them to the insurance payer; however, this chapter differentiates health care practices that have computerized operations from those that are simply using paper ledgers and generating paper-only claims and do not use the computer for any administrative practice management functions.

To help you better understand the differences in methodologies used by paper-based offices versus the computerized office, use the icons as a guide.

Different methods exist for processing insurance claims for the health care practice. The most common ones follow.

1.   Posting charges and submitting to the insurance payer on the legacy paper CMS 1500 (02-12) claim form. This form has been used in the industry since 1975. The CMS 1500 (02-12) can be prepared manually by completing the claim information with a pen or electronically and transmitting it via computer.

2.   Contracting with an outside billing service company to prepare and electronically transmit claims on behalf of the health care provider's office.

3.   Direct data entry (DDE) in the payer's system. The billing specialist logs into the insurance company's system and keys in the data required to process the claim.

Keep in mind that HIPAA regulations will determine whether a health care provider is a covered entity and whether it is required to submit claims electronically.

Life Cycle of an Insurance Claim

When using any of these methods for processing of insurance claims, the administrative life cycle of an insurance claim showing the basic steps (Figure 3-5) in handling and processing insurance claims in a physician's office, to the insurance carrier, and after payment is received is as follows.

1.   **Preregistration—Patient Registration Information Form:** Some medical practices preregister a new patient during the initial telephone call, have a designated staff member contact the patient before the appointment time, or send a letter confirming the appointment with an informative

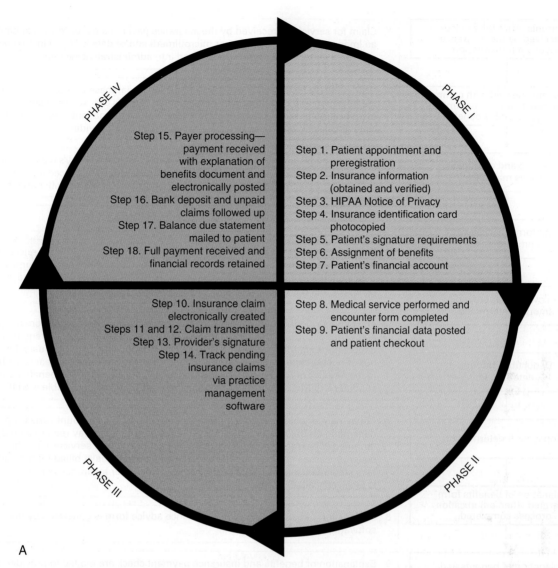

Continued

FIGURE 3-5 A, Revenue cycle overview showing the basic steps in processing an insurance claim in a physician's office, to the third-party payer, and after payment is received.

brochure about the medical practice and a **patient registration form.** This form may be printed off the practice's website, completed online, or completed when the patient arrives for his or her appointment. It is a good idea to give directions and/or a map of how to get to the office and to ask the patient to arrive early. An average window of time is 15 to 20 minutes before the scheduled appointment. This allows time to collect vital statistics and insurance information and to discuss the patient's responsibility with respect to payment policies. A patient registration form also may be called a *patient information form* or *intake sheet* (Figures 3-6 and 3-7). If the patient has a medical problem that makes it difficult to complete the form (such as rheumatoid arthritis of the hands or limited vision), then the insurance billing specialist should interview the patient and fill in the necessary data.

Instruct the patient to fill in all spaces and indicate not applicable (N/A) if an item does not apply. Read the form carefully after completion to ensure that *complete* and *accurate* personal and financial information have been obtained from the patient. The patient registration form should contain the following facts:

- Name: First, middle initial, and last. The name must match that shown on the insurance identification card. (Some pediatric patients do not have the same last name as their parents or stepparents.) Insurance payments show the policyholder's name and it is time consuming to find and give credit to the patient's account without this information

- Practice management systems allow a cross-reference of the patient, subscriber, and guarantor's names, as well as Social

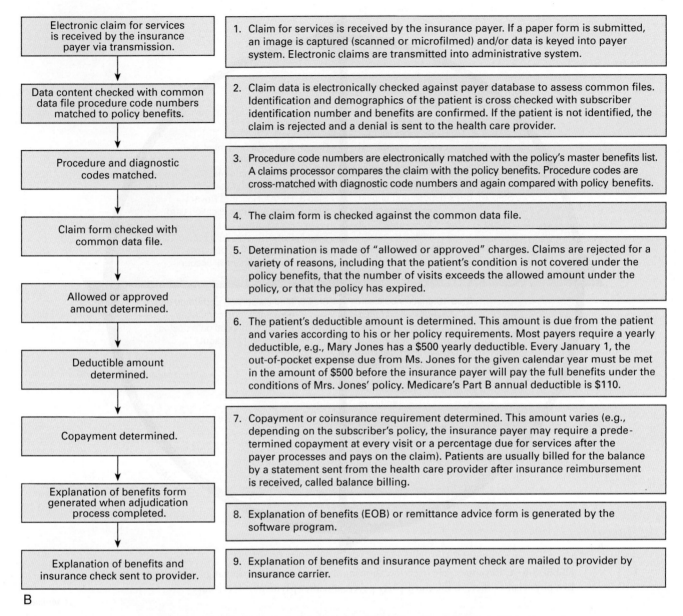

Electronic claim for services is received by the insurance payer via transmission.	1. Claim for services is received by the insurance payer. If a paper form is submitted, an image is captured (scanned or microfilmed) and/or data is keyed into payer system. Electronic claims are transmitted into administrative system.
Data content checked with common data file procedure code numbers matched to policy benefits.	2. Claim data is electronically checked against payer database to assess common files. Identification and demographics of the patient is cross checked with subscriber identification number and benefits are confirmed. If the patient is not identified, the claim is rejected and a denial is sent to the health care provider.
Procedure and diagnostic codes matched.	3. Procedure code numbers are electronically matched with the policy's master benefits list. A claims processor compares the claim with the policy benefits. Procedure codes are cross-matched with diagnostic code numbers and again compared with policy benefits.
Claim form checked with common data file.	4. The claim form is checked against the common data file.
Allowed or approved amount determined.	5. Determination is made of "allowed or approved" charges. Claims are rejected for a variety of reasons, including that the patient's condition is not covered under the policy benefits, that the number of visits exceeds the allowed amount under the policy, or that the policy has expired.
Deductible amount determined.	6. The patient's deductible amount is determined. This amount is due from the patient and varies according to his or her policy requirements. Most payers require a yearly deductible, e.g., Mary Jones has a $500 yearly deductible. Every January 1, the out-of-pocket expense due from Ms. Jones for the given calendar year must be met in the amount of $500 before the insurance payer will pay the full benefits under the conditions of Mrs. Jones' policy. Medicare's Part B annual deductible is $110.
Copayment determined.	7. Copayment or coinsurance requirement determined. This amount varies (e.g., depending on the subscriber's policy, the insurance payer may require a predetermined copayment at every visit or a percentage due for services after the payer processes and pays on the claim). Patients are usually billed for the balance by a statement sent from the health care provider after insurance reimbursement is received, called balance billing.
Explanation of benefits form generated when adjudication process completed.	8. Explanation of benefits (EOB) or remittance advice form is generated by the software program.
Explanation of benefits and insurance check sent to provider.	9. Explanation of benefits and insurance payment check are mailed to provider by insurance carrier.

B

FIGURE 3-5, cont'd B, Adjudication: Insurance payer life cycle of an insurance claim shows the basic steps of a third-party payer to pay an insurance claim and the documents generated.

Security number, so that when you recall the policyholder's name, the patient's name also appears.

- Street address, including apartment number, zip code, and telephone numbers with area code (cell and landline)
- Business address, telephone number with extension, and occupation
- E-mail address
- Date of birth (HIPAA requires eight digits [year/month/day] to be submitted to payers; for example, the eight-digit format of January 2, 1936, is 19360102). Your practice management system may collect these data in a different format but transmit in the required eight-digit format.

- Person responsible for account (guarantor) or insured's name
- Social Security number
- Spouse's name and occupation
- Referring physician's name or other referral source
- Driver's license number
- Emergency contact (close relative or friend with name, address, and telephone number)
- Insurance billing information: all insurance company names, addresses, policy numbers, and group numbers. This is important because of the COB clause written into some health insurance policies. Medicare and Medicaid patients are given the option of joining managed care programs and

Patient Registration

I was referred to this office by: __Margaret Taylor__   City: __Oxnard__   Date: __01/20/13__

PATIENT INFORMATION	PRIMARY INSURED INFORMATION

PATIENT INFORMATION

Name (Last)	(First)	(Middle)
Fuhr	Linda	L

Name you like to be called
Linda

Address
3070 Tipper street

City	State	Zip
Oxnard	CA	93030

Patient's birthdate	Sex	Home phone number
11-05-65	☐ M ☒ F	555-276-1101

SSN	Work phone number
550-XX-5172	555-372-1151

Email address	Cell phone number
LFUHR65@AOL.COM	555-243-1777

Employer or school name	Title
Macys	Sales associate

Patient status   ☒ Employed   ☐ Full time student

☐ Single   ☒ Married   ☐ Other

Ethnicity   ☐ Hispanic   ☐ Non-Hispanic   ☒ Not specified

Race   ☐ African American   ☐ Asian American
☒ Caucasian or European American
☐ Native American   ☐ Pacific Islander

Preferred language
English

PRIMARY INSURED INFORMATION

Name of insured (Last)	(First)	(Middle)
Fuhr	Gerald	T

Address (If different)

City	State	Zip

Policyholder's birthdate	Sex	Home phone number
06-15-64	☒ M ☐ F	555-276-1101

SSN	Work phone number
545-XX-2771	555-921-0075

Email address	Cell phone number
GFUHR64@AOL.COM	555-243-2736

Insurance name
ABC Insurance Company

Insurance address
P.O. Box 12340, Fresno, CA 93765

ID number	Group number
H-550-XX-5172-02	17098

Primary insured's relationship to patient
Spouse

Employer
Electronic Data Systems

Employer address
2700 West 5th Street
Oxnard, CA 93030

Comments
None

EMERGENCY CONTACT INFORMATION	SECONDARY INSURANCE INFORMATION

EMERGENCY CONTACT INFORMATION

Name	Relationship
Hannah Gildea	Aunt

Address
4621 Lucretia St. , Oxnard, CA 93030

Home phone number	Cell phone number
555-274-0132	555-243-1388

Email address
GILDEAH@YAHOO.COM

Does your emergency contact have power of attorney? ☐ Yes ☒ No   Advance health directive? ☒ Yes ☐ No

SECONDARY INSURANCE INFORMATION

Name of insured (Last)	(First)	(Middle)

Policy holder's birthdate	Sex
	☐ M ☐ F

Insurance name
None

Insurance address

ID number	Group number

FOR WORK-RELATED PROBLEMS, PLEASE FILL OUT BELOW

Workers' comp insurance	Policy number	Address	City	State	Zip

Claim number	Date of injury	Employer at time of injury

Has this injury been reported to the employer? ☐ Yes ☐ No	Employer address

INSURANCE SIGNATURE AUTHORIZATION

I authorize any holder of medical or other information about me to release to the insurance company any information needed for this or a related claim. I permit a copy of this authorization to be used in place of the original, and newest payment of medical insurance benefits to, (PHYSICIAN NAME OR PRACTICE NAME): _____

X *Linda Fuhr*   Jan. 20, 20XX

FIGURE 3-6 Patient registration information form showing a comprehensive listing of personal and financial information obtained from the patient on his or her first visit to the office. *(Courtesy Bibbero Systems, Inc., Petaluma, Calif. Telephone: 800-242-2376; fax: 800-242-9330; website: www.bibbero.com.)*

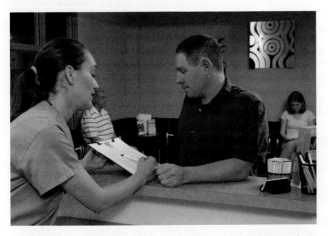

FIGURE 3-7 Receptionist giving instructions to a patient on how to complete the patient registration form.

are allowed to switch every 30 days. Always ask each older patient whether he or she is covered by traditional Medicare or a Medicare HMO. A good patient information sheet has space where this information can be written in by the patient.

2. **Verification of Insurance:** Verify insurance and all other information that may have changed since the last visit because patients may transfer from one insurance plan to another, move, or change jobs. This may be done by giving the patient a copy of the previously completed patient registration form and asking him or her to correct any incorrect data in red. Established patients may have changed employers or may have married or divorced.

3. **Notice of Privacy Practices:** Each patient is given a Notice of Privacy Practices (NPP) that explains how his or her health information is used. Obtain patient's acknowledgment of receipt of the NPP. If the patient refuses or is unable to sign, document this in his or her health record. An NPP is mandatory under federal law through HIPAA.

4. **Insurance Identification Card:** Photocopy front and back sides of all of the patient's insurance identification cards (Figure 3-8). A copy produces error-free insurance data and can be used in lieu of completing the insurance section of the patient registration form. Ask for photo identification, such as a driver's license, to verify that the person has not used someone else's card. If the insurance plan requires referral or precertification for any services, call the insurance company to verify coverage and applicable deductible or copayment. On a return visit, ask to see the card and check it with the data on file (Figure 3-9). If it differs, photocopy both sides and write the date on the copy, using this as the base for revising data on file.

RELEASE OF INFORMATION

If the physician is submitting an insurance claim for the patient, the patient is not required to sign a release of information form before information can be given to an insurance company for obtaining payment for professional services. However, some medical practices prefer to operate at a higher level of privacy and continue to obtain patients' signatures on release of information forms.

5. **Patient's Signature Requirements:** Under HIPAA regulations, a patient's signed authorization is not required for treatment, payment, or routine health care operations (TPO). However, many practices continue to have patient's sign an authorization allowing the release of any medical or other information necessary to process the claim. If the patient is physically or mentally unable to sign, the person representing the patient may sign for the patient.

 Electronic environment: Electronic billers are permitted to obtain a lifetime authorization from the beneficiary to release medical or other information necessary to process a claim. The signature should be retained in a file for future use on all electronic claims. This authorization allows the office to submit assigned and unassigned claims on the beneficiary's behalf. To use this procedure, the patient should sign a brief statement that reads as follows:

(Name of Beneficiary) (Health Insurance Claim Number)

"I request that payment of authorized benefits be made either to me or on my behalf to (name of physician or supplier) for any services furnished me by physician or supplier. I authorize any holder of medical information about me to release to my insurance carrier and its agents any information needed to determine these benefits or the benefits payable for related services."

Patient signature source codes are used on electronic claims to indicate the type of signatures on file for the patient. Under HIPAA Version 5010, adopted in 2013, they are no longer required, with the exception of a "P," which is reported if the signature was generated by the provider because the patient was not physically present for the service. If any other value is present on the electronic claim, it will be rejected.

Most patient registration forms include a statement to sign regarding these two authorizations (see bottom of Figure 3-6).

Paper Environment: Since the enforcement of HIPAA regulations, a patient's signature for the release of information in Block 12 is no longer required. If a signature is

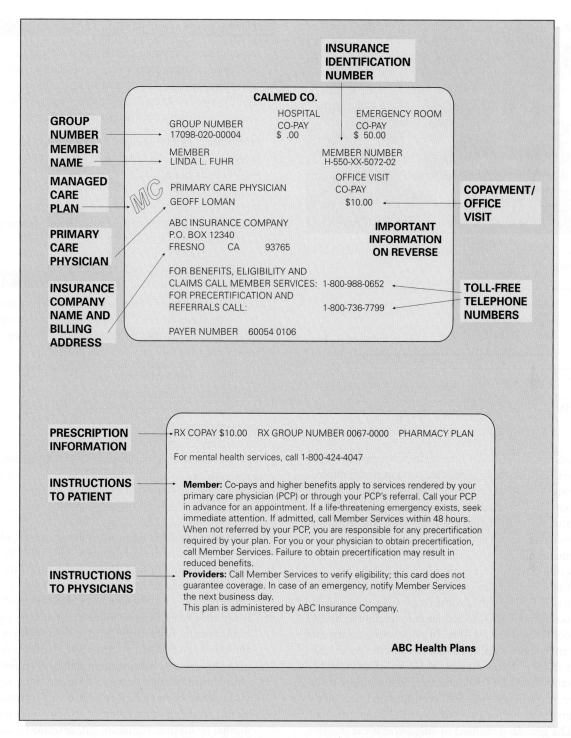

FIGURE 3-8 Front *(top)* and back *(bottom)* sides of an insurance card.

obtained on a separate form, it may be filed in the patient's health record and the abbreviation "SOF" or the preferred spelled-out notation "signature on file" may be used on the insurance claim form.

6. **Assignment of Benefits:** The signature requirement for the **assignment** of benefits is included in Block 13 of the CMS-1500 (02-12) insurance claim form (Figure 3-10). For the health care provider to receive

reimbursement directly from the insurance payer, the patient must sign an assignment of benefits statement for each insurance company. However, before explaining an assignment, it is important to define the difference between **participating (par)** and **nonparticipating (nonpar)** physicians or providers. A par provider has a contractual agreement with an insurance plan to render care to eligible beneficiaries

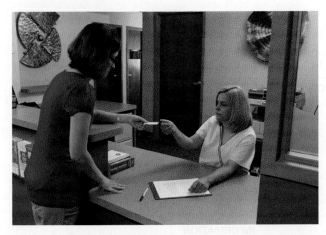

FIGURE 3-9 Patient presenting an insurance identification card to the receptionist for photocopying.

> 13. INSURED'S OR AUTHORIZED PERSON'S SIGNATURE I authorize payment of medical benefits to the undersigned physician or supplier for services described below.
>
> SIGNED _____

FIGURE 3-10 Section 13 from the health insurance claim form CMS-1500 (02-12), illustrating authorization for assignment of benefits.

and bills the third-party payer directly (Example 3-2). The third-party payer pays its portion of the allowed amount and the provider bills the patient for the balance not paid by the insurer after the disallowed portion is adjusted off of the account. Managed care plans also refer to par providers as *member physicians*. If the amount of the patient's responsibility can be determined, collect it at the time of the visit.

A nonpar provider is a physician without a contractual agreement with an insurance plan to accept an allowed amount and to render care to eligible beneficiaries (Example 3-3). The provider may or may not file an insurance claim as a courtesy to the patient and may obtain full payment at the time of service. The patient should be made aware that his or her insurance plan will cover a considerable amount less on the claim when receiving services from a nonpar provider.

The general definition of *assignment* is the transfer, after an event insured against, of an individual's legal right to collect an amount payable under an insurance

---

Example 3-2   Participating Provider

Dr. Gomez accepts assignment and is a par provider for the Liberty Health Insurance Plan. Pedro Nunez, a new patient, is seen in the office with complaints of a sore throat and infected nail, for which a $150 fee is charged for the office visit, office surgery, and penicillin injection. The patient has met his deductible for the year.

Provider fee (total billed amount)	$150
Provider contracted rate (allowable charge)	$140
Patient coinsurance or copayment amount	$10
Insurance claims payment	$130
Provider's adjusted (write-off) amount	$10

Dr. Gomez collects $10 from the patient and is paid a total of $140.

Example 3-3   Nonparticipating Provider

Dr. Warner does not accept assignment and is a nonpar provider for the XYZ Health Insurance Plan. Estelle Cutter, an established patient, is seen in the office complaining that her ears are full of earwax that needs to be removed. A $60 fee is charged.

Provider fee (total billed amount)	$60
Usual, customary, and reasonable (UCR)	$55
Patient coinsurance or copayment amount	$10
Insurance claims payment	$44
Provider may bill patient over UCR	$6

Dr. Warner collects $16 from the patient and is paid a total of $60 because he can collect the difference between his fee and the patient's copayment plus the insurance payment.

---

contract. Most of the time an agreement is obtained by having the patient sign an assignment of insurance benefits document that directs payment to the physician. However, the paper CMS-1500 (02-12) claim form contains a provision that, when signed by the insured, directs the insurance company to pay benefits directly to the provider of care on whose charge the claim is based. An assignment of benefits becomes a legally enforceable document but must refer to specific hospitalization, course of treatment, or office visits. Each course of treatment needs to have an assignment document executed by the patient unless an annual or lifetime signature authorization is accepted and in the patient's financial file, except when automobile or homeowners liability insurance is involved.

Private Carriers: For private insurance companies with whom the provider does not have a contractual agreement, accepting assignment means that the insurance check will be directed to the provider's office instead of to the patient. Because there is no signed agreement with the carrier, the difference between the billed amount and the carrier's allowed amount is not written off but collected from the patient as is any copayment or deductible. In private third-party liability cases, the physician needs to negotiate with the insurance company to make sure benefits are paid to him or her directly.

Managed Care: In managed care plans, a par provider (also called a *preferred provider*) is a physician who has contracted with a plan to provide medical services to plan members. A nonpar provider refers to a physician who has not contracted with a managed care plan to provide medical services to plan members. The assignment is automatic for individuals who have signed with managed care contracts.

Medicaid: For Medicaid cases, there is no assignment unless the patient has other insurance in addition to Medicaid. The Medicaid fiscal intermediary pays all providers directly.

Medicare: The words *participating*, *nonparticipating*, and *assignment* have slightly different meanings in the Medicare program. A physician who accepts assignment on Medicare claims is called a *participating (par) physician* and may not bill or accept payment for the amount of the difference between the submitted charge and the Medicare allowed amount. However, an attempt must be made to collect 20% of the allowed charge (coinsurance) and any amount applied to the deductible. A physician who does not participate is called a *nonparticipating (nonpar) physician* and has an option regarding assignment. The physician either may not accept assignment for all services or may exercise the option of accepting assignment for some services and collecting from the patient for other services performed at the same time and place. The physician collects the fee from the patient but may bill no more than the Medicare-limiting charge. The check is sent to the patient. When treating federal or state government employees or a Medicare recipient, the physician may lose the fee if government guidelines are not followed.

TRICARE: A provider who accepts TRICARE standard assignment (participates) agrees to accept the allowable charge as the full fee and cannot charge the patient the difference between the provider's charge and the allowable charge. The exception to this is when the provider does not accept assignment on the claim. A provider that participates or does not participate with TRICARE can submit a claim and not accept assignment on a claim-by-claim basis. In the event the provider does not accept assignment, TRICARE sends the sponsor all payments. TRICARE does not communicate with the provider if the provider has questions about the claim. It is up to the provider to bill the sponsor for payment. The provider can collect 115% of the TRICARE allowable from the patient when a CMS-1500 (02-12) claim form is marked "no" in the accepting assignment block.

Workers' Compensation: There is no assignment for industrial cases. The workers' compensation carrier pays the fee for services rendered according to its fee schedule, and the check automatically goes to the physician. The patient is not responsible for payment of services for any work-related injury or illness.

7. **Patient's Financial Account:** Patient information is entered into the practice management software program. Accuracy is crucial because the data will be used to construct the claim for transmission to the insurance company. If the medical practice is not computerized, a manual system includes paper day-sheets and patient ledger cards.

8a. **Encounter Form:** An **encounter form** (also called a *charge slip, multipurpose billing form, patient service slip, routing form, superbill,* or *transaction slip*) is attached to the patient's health record during the visit (Figure 3-11). This contains the patient's name, the date, and in some instances the previous balance due. It also contains the procedural and diagnostic codes and the date the patient should return for an appointment. This two- or three-part form is a combination bill, insurance form, and routing document used in both computer- and paper-based systems. This also can be a computerized multipurpose billing form that may be scanned to input charges and diagnoses into the patient's computerized account. Time is saved and fewer errors occur because no keystrokes are involved. Medical practices use the encounter form as a communications tool (routing sheet) and as an invoice to the patient. When used as a routing sheet, it becomes a source document for insurance claim data. The encounter form is completed by the provider. Both a procedural code for services performed and a diagnostic code are chosen by the provider of services. In some situations, a certified coder may review the patient's health record to assign

STATE LIC.# C1503X
SOC. SEC. # 000-11-0000
PIN # _____

College Clinic
4567 Broad Avenue
Woodland Hills, XY 12345-4700

Phone: 555-486-9002

☐ Private ☒ Bluecross ☐ Ind. ☐ Medicare ☐ Medi-cal ☐ Hmo ☐ Ppo

Patient's last name	First	Account #:	Birthdate	Sex ☐ Male	Today's date
Smith	Lydia	13845	09 / 13 / 92	☒ Female	09 / 17 / 20XX

Insurance company	Subscriber	Plan #	Sub. #	Group
Blue Shield of CA	Lydia Smith	0473	186-72-10XX	849-37000

ASSIGNMENT: I hereby assign my insurance benefits to be paid directly to the undersigned physician, I am financially responsible for non-covered services.
SIGNED: Patient, or parent, if minor *Lydia Smith*   Today's date 09 / 17 / 20XX

RELEASE: I hereby authorize the physician to release to my insurance carriers any information require to process this claim.
SIGNED: Patient, or parent, if minor *Lydia Smith*   Today's date 09 / 17 / 20XX

✓	DESCRIPTION	NEW	EST.	FEE	✓	DESCRIPTION	CODE	FEE	✓	DESCRIPTION	CODE	FEE
	OFFICE VISITS	NEW	EST.			Venipuncture	36415			OFFICE PROCEDURES		
	Blood pressure check		99211			TB skin test	86580			Anoscopy	46600	
	Level II	99202	99212			Hematocrit	85013			Ear lavage	69210	
	Level III	99203	99213			Glucose finger stick	82948			Spirometry	94010	
X	Level IV	99204	99214	70.92		IMMUNIZATIONS				Nebulizer Rx	94664	
	Level V	99205	99215			Allergy inj. X1	95115			EKG	93000	
	PREVENTIVE EXAMS	NEW	EST.			Allergy inj. X2	95117			SURGERY		
	Age 65 and older	99387	99397			Trigger pt. inj.	20552			Mole removal (1st)	17110	
	Age 40 - 64	99386	99396			Therapeutic inj.	96372			(2nd to 14th)	17003	
	Age 18 - 39	99385	99395			VACCINATION PRODUCTS				Flat warts (1st - 14th)	07110	
	Age 12 - 17	99384	99394			DPT	90701			15 or more	17111	
	Age 5 - 11	99383	99393			DT	90702			Biopsy, 1 lesion	11100	
	Age 1 - 4	99382	99392			Tetanus	90703			Addt'l. lesions	11101	
	Infant	99381	99391			MMR	90707			Endometrial Bx	58100	
	Newborn ofc		99432			OPV	90712			Skin tags to 15	11200	
	OB/NEWBORN CARE					Polio inj.	90713			Each addt'l. 10	11201	
	OB package		59400			Flu	90662			I & D abscess	10060	
	Post-partum visit N/C					Hemophilus B	90645			SUPPLIES/MISCELLANEOUS		
	LAB PROCEDURES					Hepatitis B vac.	90746			Surgical tray	99070	
	Urine dip		81000			Pneumovax	90670			Handling charge	99000	
	UA qualitative		81005			VACCINE ADMINISTRATION				Special report	99080	
X	Pregnancey urine		81025	20.00		Age: Through 18 yrs. (1st inj.)	90460			DOCTOR'S NOTES:		
	Wet mount		87210			Age: Through 18 yrs. (ea. addt'l. inj.)	90461					
	kOH prip		87220			Adult (1st inj.)	90471					
	Occult blood		82270			Adult (ea. addt'l. inj.)	90472					

DIAGNOSES   ICD-10-CM

Abdominal pain/unspec. . . R10.9	Colitis/unspec. K51.90	FUO R50.9	Osteoarthritis (site). . . . . . M19._
Absess . . . . L02._	Confusion R41.0	Gastritis K29.70	Otitis media . . . . H66.9_
Allergic reaction . . . . . . T78.40_	CHF I50.9	Gastroenteritis (colitis) . . K52.9	Parkinson's disease G20
Alzheimer's disease G30	Constipation K59.00	G.I. bleed K92.2	Pharyngitis, acute. J02.9
Anemia/unspec. D64.9	COPD J44.9	Gout/unspec. M10.9	Pleurisy R09.1
Angina/unspec. I20.9	Cough R05	Headache R51	Pneumonia. J18.9
Anorexia R63.0	Crohn's disease/unspec. . . K50.90	Health exam . . . . 200._	Pneumonia, viral J12.9
Anxiety/unspec. F41.9	CVA I63.9	Hematuria/unspec. R31.9	Prostatitis/unspec. N41.9
Apnea, sleep G47.30	Decubitus ulcer. . . . . . . L89._	Herpes simplex. B00.9	PVD I73.9
Arrhythmia, cardiac I49.9	Dehydration. E86.0	Herpes zoster. B02.9	Radiculopathy . . . . M54.1_
Arthritis, rheumatoid M06.9	Dementia/unspec. F03	Hiatal hernia K44.9	Rectal bleeding K62.5
Asthma/unspec. J45.909	Depression, major/unsp. . F32.9	HTN (HBP) I10	Renal failure. N19
Atrial fibrillation. I48.0	Diab I, no complications . . E10.0	Hyperlipidemia/unspec. . . E78.5	Sciatica. . . . . M54.3_
B-12 deficiency. E53.8	Diab II, no complications . . E11.9	Hypothyroidism/unspec. . E03.9	Shortness of breath R03.02
Back pain, low M54.5	w/kidney complic. . . . . . E11.2_	Impotentce . . . . N52._	Sinusitis, chr./unspec. . . . J32.9
BPH N40	w/ophthalmic compl. . . . E11.3_	Influenza, respiratory . . . J10.1	Syncope R55
Bradycardia/unspec. R00.1	w/neurolog.compl. . . . . . E11.4_	Insomnia G47.0	Tachycardia/unspec. R00.0
Broncitis, acute. . . . . J20._	w/circulatory cmpl. . . . . E11.5_	IBS, diarrhea . . . . K58.	Tachy., supraventric I47.1
Bronchitis, chronic. J42	Insulin use. Z79.4	Lupus, systemic erythim. . M32.9	Tendinitis/unspec. M77.9
Bursitis/unspec. M71.9	Diarrhea/unspec. R19.7	MI, acute . . . . I21._	TIA G45.9
CA, breast . . . . C50._	Diverticulitix. K57.92	MI, old I25.2	Ulcer, duodenal/unspec. . . K26.9
CA, lung . . . . C34._	Diverticulosis. K57.90	Migraine G43.9	Ulcer, gastric/unspec. . . . K25.9
CA, prostate C61	Dizziness. R42	Myalgia M79.1	Ulcer, peptic/unspec. K27.9
Cellulitis . . . . L03._	Dysuria R30.0	Neck pain M54.2	URI/unspec. J06.9
Chest pain/unspec. R07.9	Edema/unspec. R60.9	Neuropathy G62.9	UTI N39.0
Cirrhosis, liver/unspec. . . . K74.60	Endocarditis I38	Nausea R11.1	Vertigo R42
Cold, common J00	Esophageal reflux K21.0	X Nausea/vomiting R11.0	Weight gain R63.5
	Fatigue (lethargy) R53.83	Obesity/unspec. E66.9	Weight loss R63.4

Diagnosis/additional description:	Doctor's signature/date	
Pregnancy	*Dr. B. Caesar*	09-17-20XX

Return appointment information:	-with whom	(Self) other	Rec'd. by:	Total today's fee	90.92
Days ___ Wks. ___ (Mos.) 1 month			☐ Cash		
			☐ Check # ___	Amount rec'd. today	

PLEASE RMEMBER THAT PAYMENT IS YOUR OBLIGATION, REGARDLESS OF INSURANCE OR OTHER THIRD PARTY INVOLVEMENT.

INSUR-A-BILL ® BIBBERO SYSTEMS, INC. • PETULUMA, CA • © 7/90 (BM1092)   (REV. 7/11)

FIGURE 3-11 Encounter form: Procedural codes for professional services are taken from the Current Procedural Terminology (CPT) book and diagnostic codes are taken from the *International Classification of Diseases, Tenth Revision, Clinical Modification (ICD-10-CM)* book. (*Courtesy Bibbero Systems, Inc., Petaluma, Calif. Telephone: 800-242-2376; fax: 800-242-9330; website: www.bibbero.com.*)

a proper code on the basis of the documentation. The encounter form's procedure and diagnostic code sections should be updated and reprinted biannually with correct descriptions because changes, additions, and deletions occur that may affect the practice. Remove all codes not used or seldom used and revise and add current, valid, commonly used codes for the practice. Because there is no grace period, update encounter forms twice a year: by October 1 for changes in diagnostic codes and by January 1 for changes in procedural codes. Some practices develop encounter forms for different services (for example, surgical services, office services [within the facility], and out-of-office services [hospital visits, emergency, outpatient facility, nursing home, or house calls]). Examples of encounter forms are shown in Figures 8-3 and 10-9

8b. **Physician's Signature:** After examination and treatment, the physician or health care provider rendering services completes the encounter form by checking off the procedure (services and treatments) codes and diagnostic codes (Figure 3-12). The physician signs the encounter form and indicates whether the patient needs another appointment.

8c. **Determine Fees:** Some medical practices may have patients carry the encounter form to the reception desk, where fees are determined and input for billing (Figure 3-13). The patient is given the opportunity to pay and make a future appointment.

9. **Bookkeeping—Financial Accounting Record and Accounts Receivable Management:** The value of maintaining careful records of all insurance matters cannot be overemphasized. Accounts receivable (A/R) management breathes life into the practice's cash flow. Encompassed in A/R management is establishing the patient financial accounting record and carrying out the claims process. For compilation of claim data, services are entered into the computer by either front desk personnel or the in-office billing department. If the practice outsources this function, an off-site billing company retrieves the data and processes the claims. All charges and patient payments are **posted** to their respective accounts.

Electronic Environment: A financial account is set up in the practice management system. Data obtained from the patient registration process are keyed into the program and a patient account is established. Usually an account number is automatically assigned by the program and used for tracking and reporting. All items posted to each patient account are housed in the computer database for accurate and easy retrieval.

Paper Environment: In the paper environment, a ledger card is maintained for each patient who receives professional services (Figure 3-14). An established private patient who is injured on the job requires two ledgers, one for private care and one for posting workers' compensation insurance.

Using the encounter form, daily transactions are posted (recorded) by the billing staff. Professional fees (charges), payments (cash, check, or credit card), adjustments, and balance due are also posted in the practice management software program. Accuracy is especially important when keying data into the

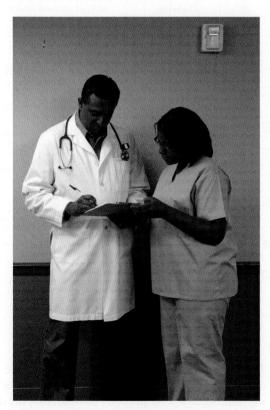

FIGURE 3-12 Physician checking off procedures on the encounter form at the conclusion of a patient's office visit.

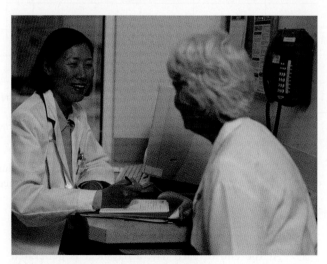

FIGURE 3-13 Insurance billing specialist discussing the encounter form with the patient at the medical office's checkout station.

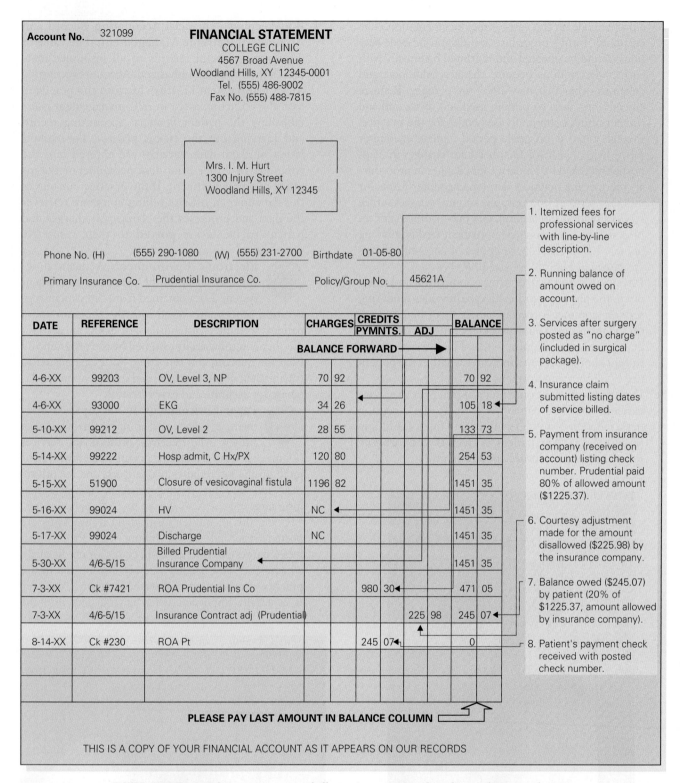

Account No. 321099

FINANCIAL STATEMENT
COLLEGE CLINIC
4567 Broad Avenue
Woodland Hills, XY 12345-0001
Tel. (555) 486-9002
Fax No. (555) 488-7815

Mrs. I. M. Hurt
1300 Injury Street
Woodland Hills, XY 12345

Phone No. (H) _____ (555) 290-1080 ___ (W) _(555) 231-2700_ Birthdate _01-05-80_

Primary Insurance Co. _Prudential Insurance Co._   Policy/Group No. ___45621A___

DATE	REFERENCE	DESCRIPTION	CHARGES	CREDITS PYMNTS.	ADJ	BALANCE
		BALANCE FORWARD →				
4-6-XX	99203	OV, Level 3, NP	70 92			70 92
4-6-XX	93000	EKG	34 26			105 18
5-10-XX	99212	OV, Level 2	28 55			133 73
5-14-XX	99222	Hosp admit, C Hx/PX	120 80			254 53
5-15-XX	51900	Closure of vesicovaginal fistula	1196 82			1451 35
5-16-XX	99024	HV	NC			1451 35
5-17-XX	99024	Discharge	NC			1451 35
5-30-XX	4/6-5/15	Billed Prudential Insurance Company				1451 35
7-3-XX	Ck #7421	ROA Prudential Ins Co		980 30		471 05
7-3-XX	4/6-5/15	Insurance Contract adj (Prudential)			225 98	245 07
8-14-XX	Ck #230	ROA Pt		245 07		0

PLEASE PAY LAST AMOUNT IN BALANCE COLUMN

THIS IS A COPY OF YOUR FINANCIAL ACCOUNT AS IT APPEARS ON OUR RECORDS

1. Itemized fees for professional services with line-by-line description.

2. Running balance of amount owed on account.

3. Services after surgery posted as "no charge" (included in surgical package).

4. Insurance claim submitted listing dates of service billed.

5. Payment from insurance company (received on account) listing check number. Prudential paid 80% of allowed amount ($1225.37).

6. Courtesy adjustment made for the amount disallowed ($225.98) by the insurance company.

7. Balance owed ($245.07) by patient (20% of $1225.37, amount allowed by insurance company).

8. Patient's payment check received with posted check number.

FIGURE 3-14 Financial accounting record illustrating posting of professional service descriptions, fees, payments, adjustments, and balance due.

computer because this is where the movable data start to build an insurance claim.

At the end of each day, a daysheet is generated and printed. A **daysheet,** or daily record sheet, is a register for recording daily business transactions.

The totals from this can be compared with the encounter forms to ensure that all charges, payments, and adjustments were properly posted. Also, the daysheet is a useful tool for "checks and balances" when assessing the bank deposit slip for accuracy.

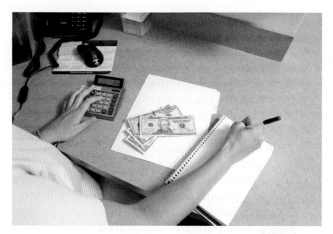

FIGURE 3-15 Medical office employee posting to a patient's financial accounting record or daysheet.

Paper Environment: The paper environment allows transactions to be recorded on the patient ledger cards. All patients seen on one day have their charges (debits) recorded on the daysheet, along with all payments and adjustments (credits). Each day the totals are carried forward and a new daysheet is set up to receive posting for that day (Figure 3-15). The ledger card should show an entry of the date an insurance claim is sent, including the date of services that were billed. Each service must be posted on a single line, and a **running balance** is calculated in the right column. When the ledger is completely filled, the account balance is brought forward (also known as *extended*) to a new card.

Step-by-step instructions for completing a ledger card are given at the end of this chapter in Procedure 3-1.

10. **Insurance Claim:** Under HIPAA guidelines, providers who are not small providers (institutional organizations with fewer than 25 full-time employees or physicians with fewer than 10 full-time employees) must send all claims electronically in the approved format.

Generally, the insurance billing specialist in the physician's office completes the claim information for the following cases: (1) all hospitalized (both surgical and medical) patients, (2) all claims in which the benefits are assigned to the physician, and (3) special procedures (minor surgery or extensive testing). In these cases, the insurance billing specialist generates an accurate claim to be submitted by using exact procedural and diagnostic codes, including the use of any appropriate documents (operative report or invoice), and mails it to the correct third-party payer when circumstances call for it to be sent in hard copy.

The minimum information required by third-party payers is as follows:

- What was done? (services and procedures, using procedure codes and appropriate modifiers discussed in Chapter 6)

- Why was it done? (diagnoses, using diagnostic codes discussed in Chapter 5)
- When was it performed? (date of service [DOS])
- Where was it received? (place of service [POS])
- Who did it? (provider name and identifying number)

A helpful hint is to group together, or batch, all outstanding charges to the same type of insurance at one time. This cuts down on errors, allows easier trackability, and in the paper environment makes manual completion of the forms less tedious.

It is preferable to electronically transmit claims as soon as possible after professional services are rendered. Time limits range from 30 days to 1½ years for filing an insurance claim from the DOS. This can vary depending on the commercial carrier, federal or state program, or whether the claim is for an illness or accident. Claims filed after the time limit will be denied and a detailed appeal process may be required to have the claim reconsidered. See further discussion in the chapters on Medicare (Chapter 12), Medicaid (Chapter 13), TRICARE (Chapter 14), and workers' compensation (Chapter 15).

Financial losses from delay can occur in the following instances. If a patient has had a long-term illness, insurance benefits can expire before a claim is processed. If several physicians treat the same patient, some insurance companies pay only one of the physicians. (Typically, whoever files the claim first is paid first.) In this scenario, the other physicians may have to wait for disbursement by the physician who received the check. Submit hospitalized patients' insurance claim forms promptly on discharge or on a regular schedule (weekly or twice a month depending on the office protocol), regardless of the discharge date for long-term inpatients.

Patients who pay at time of service and who wish to submit their own insurance claims are given two copies of the encounter form. The patient retains one copy for personal records and attaches the second copy to the insurance claim form and forwards it to the insurance company.

11. **Submitting the Paper Claim:** If a paper claim is submitted, a copy of the CMS-1500 (02-12) form is placed in the office's pending file or the patient's health record chart, depending on office protocol. The date the claim is mailed is noted on the patient's ledger card and recorded on the insurance claims register.

Mail claims in batches to each carrier to save on postage.

12. **Transmitting the Electronic Claim:** When filing claims electronically (details discussed in Chapter 8), a batch is created and a digital file is stored in a predetermined directory. These files are either transmitted directly to the

insurance payer or transmitted to a clearinghouse over a dial-up modem, digital subscriber line (DSL) modem, or via the internet.

Claims are transmitted electronically as required by HIPAA or in cases of exemption or waiver on a paper CMS-1500 (02-12) form. When sending paper claims, make a copy for office records and create an insurance claims register or spreadsheet to track and follow up claims.

Refer to Figure 3-5, *B*, for the phases of adjudication (claim settlement) by the third-party payer for payment, partial payment, denial, or rejection.

13. **Provider's Signature:** Providers rarely sign the CMS-1500 (02-12) insurance claim form. However, when a signature is required, it can be accepted in several formats—handwritten, facsimile stamp, or **electronic signature.** State and government programs require a signature. In the Medicare program, certificates of medical necessity require an original signature.

Physician's Representative: Sometimes a physician gives signature authorization to one person on the staff to sign insurance claims; that person then becomes known as the *physician's representative*, referred to in Figure 3-16 as the *attorney-in-fact*. For an authorization of this type, a document should be typed and signed before a notary public. This means that whoever signs the form is attesting to it because it is a legal document. If the medical practice is ever audited and fraud or embezzlement is discovered, the person who had signature authorization, as well as the physician, can be brought into the case. The federal government will prosecute if this involves a Medicare patient; the state government will prosecute if a Medicaid patient is involved.

Computerized Signatures: There are three levels of computerized or electronic signatures, listed in order of their strength. Level 1—digitized signature; Level 2—button, PIN, biometric, or token; and Level 3—digital signature. An electronic signature looks like the signer's handwritten signature (Example 3-4). The signer authenticates the document by key entry or with a pen pad using a stylus to capture the live signature.

PROVIDER'S NOTARIZED SIGNATURE AUTHORIZATION

State of ___Iowa___)
)ss
County of ___Des Moines___)

Know all persons by these presents:

That I ___John Doe, MD___ have made, constituted, and appointed and by these presents do make, constitute and appoint ___Mary Coleman___ my true and lawful attorney-in-fact for me and in my name place and stead to sign my name on claims, for payment for services provided by me submitted to the ___Blue Cross and Blue Shield of Iowa___, My signature by my said attorney-in-fact includes my agreement to abide by the full payment concept and the remainder of the certification appearing on all ___CMS-1500___ claim forms. I hereby ratify and confirm all that my said attorney-in-fact shall lawfully do or cause to be done by virtue of the power generated herein.

In witness whereof I have hereunto set my hand this ___20th___ day of ___January___ 20 __XX__.

___John Doe, MD___
(Signature)

Subscribed and sworn to before me this _20th_ day of January __20 XX__

_____
Notary Public

My commission expires _____ .

FIGURE 3-16 Example of a provider's signature authorization form that can be completed, notarized, and sent to the third-party payer after a copy is retained for the physician's records.

| Example 3-4 | Electronic Signature |

David Smith, MD

| Example 3-5 | Digital Signature |

Electronically signed:
David Smith, MD
07/12/2008 10:30:08

PROVIDER'S NOTARIZED FACSIMILE SIGNATURE AUTHORIZATION

State of ___Florida___)

County of ___Jacksonville___)ss)

___John Doe, MD___ being first duty sworn, deposes and says:

I hereby authorize the ___Blue Cross of Florida___
(Name of Fiscal Administrator)
to accept my facsimile signature shown below

___John Doe, MD___
(Facsimile or Stamp Signature)

as my true signature for all purposes under the ___Medicare___
(Name of Insurance Program)
in the same manner as if it were my actual signature, including my agreeing to abide by the full payment concept and the remainder of the certification normally signed by the source of care as it appears on all ___CMS-1500___ claim forms.

___John Doe, MD___
(Signature)

Subscribed and sworn to before me this _3rd_ day of ___January___ 20XX.

_____
Notary Public in and for
_____ County, State of_____
(SEAL)
My commission expires _____.

FIGURE 3-17 Example of a provider's facsimile authorization form that can be completed, notarized, and sent to the third-party payer after a copy is retained for the physician's records.

It also can be defined as an individualized computer access and identification system (for example, a unique personal identification number [PIN], series of letters, electronic writing, voice, computer key, token, or fingerprint transmission [biometric system]).

A *digital signature* may be lines of text or a text box stating the signer's name, date, and time and a statement indicating that a signature has been attached from within the software application (Example 3-5). Level 3 is the strongest signature because it protects the signature by a type of tamper-proof seal that breaks if the message content is altered. Refer to Chapter 8 for additional information on computerized signatures.

Signature Stamp—Paper Environment: In the past, some medical practices have used a signature stamp so that the staff can process insurance forms and other paperwork without interrupting the physician and waiting for her or his signature. For an authorization of this type, a document is typed and signed before a notary (Figure 3-17).

Use of a signature stamp is not recommended and most insurance carriers have updated signature policies advising providers that stamp signatures are no longer acceptable due to misuse or abuse.

State laws may require that insurance claims or other related documents have an original signature or otherwise bars the use of signature stamps. You must follow those rules regardless of any carrier manual regulations. For information on state laws, contact your state legislature at your state capitol. For data about signatures on hospital medical records, see Chapter 17.

14. **Track Pending Insurance Claims:** In the computerized practice management system, a date is noted each time a claim is generated for submission, whether it is sent electronically or is printed on a paper claim form from the computer. An aging A/R report to determine outstanding balances can be generated using the date the claim was filed as a point to assess how many days old the claim is. The *aging report* is used to obtain the total A/R amount, which shows a snapshot of how much money is due to the practice from each patient account.

Paper Environment: When submitting paper claims, keep a duplicate of the claim in the office pending file or in the computer system files in the event payment is not received within a predetermined amount of time and the claim must be followed up. This file also may be referred to as a suspense, follow-up, or "tickler" file. The term *tickler* came into existence because it tickles or jogs the memory at certain dates in the future. You may be accustomed to hearing the term *aging report* as discussed earlier.

If a computerized system is not being used, establish an insurance claims register (tracing file) to keep track of the status of each case that has been billed. Record to whom the claim was sent and the submission date on the insurance claims register and the patient's ledger card. The insurance billing specialist handling the insurance forms can see at a glance which claims are becoming delinquent and the amounts owed to the physician. This is an efficient method used for 30- to 60-day follow-up. Figure 3-18 shows a document generated by a practice management system to assist in following up on electronically transmitted claims.

Outstanding Claims
Primary Insurance
August 10, 20XX

Billing No.	Patient Name	Primary Insurance	Claim Sent	Bill Balance
1002	Simpson, Teri E	United Western Benefit		47.50
1003	Lee, Michael	United Western Benefit		83.55
1005	Bortolussi, Jabe	ABC Insurance Company	05/25/2007	465.00
1006	Blackwood, Crystal L	TRICARE	05/25/2007	16.07
1007	Helms, Clinton A	Medicare Health Systems Corporation	05/25/2007	33.25
1008	Jameson, Richard D	Royal Pacific Insurance Company	05/25/2007	41.07
1010	Kelsey, Ron	XYZ Insurance	06/09/2007	66.23
1011	Simpson, Teri E	United Western Benefit		16.07
1012	Simpson, Teri E	United Western Benefit		40.20
1013	Simpson, Teri E	United Western Benefit		16.07
1014	Simpson, Teri E	United Western Benefit		8.00
1015	Lee, Michael	United Western Benefit		16.07
1016	Lee, Michael	United Western Benefit		28.55
1017	Lee, Michael	United Western Benefit		40.20
1018	Martin, John R	Medicare Health Systems Corporation		149.86
1019	Jameson, Richard D	Royal Pacific Insurance Company		86.42
1020	Nunez, Margaret A	Aetna Health Plan		18.25
	Report Count: 17			1172.36

FIGURE 3-18 Practice management software screen showing outstanding claims, patients' balances due, and names of insurance companies to follow up on claims.

Keep two copies of each claim for the physician's records, one to be filed by patient name and the other by carrier name. Or, simply record the name of the insurance company on each patient's ledger card and keep a file for each carrier by date of service. Filing by carrier allows all inquiries to be included in a single letter to the insurance company to eliminate having to write to the same company three or four times.

Whether you are billing claims electronically or in paper format, you should check with the insurance carrier to determine if their company features an on-line claim-tracking service on its website. This will allow you to follow up on unpaid claims and to check the status of a claim quickly using the insurance company's website.

15. **Insurance Payments:** After the claim is processed by the insurance payer, an explanation of benefits (EOB) or remittance advice (RA) is generated and either sent on paper or transmitted electronically to the health care provider. Record of payment or denial of the claim is posted to the patient's financial account.

Paper Environment: The payment is posted (credited) to the patient's account (ledge card) and current daysheet indicating the date posted, name of insurance company, check or voucher number, amount received, contracted adjustment, and outstanding balance.

In both the electronic and payer environment, there may be claims that are not processed in a timely manner by the insurance payer. To follow up on these, a monthly review of outstanding claims, also known as an *unpaid claims report* or *aged receivables*, should be generated to determine further collection activity needed.

For further information on improper payments received and tracing delinquent claims, see Chapter 9.

16. **Bank Deposit:** The health care provider of services should receive a payment (check) from the third-party payer within 2 to 8 weeks from claim submission. The payment should accompany the remittance advice (described above) sent by the insurance payer. Electronic funds transfer (EFT) may be used in place of a mailed paper check. EFT allows the automatic deposit of funds from the payer to the provider's bank account, just as you may have set up with your own paycheck. In either electronic or paper office environments, all checks and cash are entered on the bank deposit slip and deposited at the bank.

17. **Monthly Statement:** The claim transaction is completed when the claim generated for each date of service has been processed by all responsible parties and the patient's financial account is at zero. For the patient who has insurance, a monthly statement for any outstanding balance should be sent indicating that insurance has been billed and the amount due is the patient's responsibility. The patient statement should always reflect the same fee as that submitted to the insurance company minus the amount paid by the patient copayment and/or the insurance

amount reimbursed. Patients who do not have insurance should receive a monthly statement indicating all outstanding balances due minus any payments or adjustments applied since the last billing statement.

Some companies offer services to enable patients to pay their bills online securely through the medical practice's website. They also have electronic or eStatements that reduce processing and mailing costs by delivering patient statements securely or leave balance due reminders. Online bill payment may be set up to automatically draft patients' debit/credit cards; this eliminates checks and postage and speeds payments.

18. **Financial Records Retained:** Whether your office is computerized or still operates in a paper-based environment, you will not escape the volumes of paperwork that business produces. Financial records must be retained and may include the following (not an all-inclusive list):

- Copy of the completed patient information form, patient authorization or signature-on-file for assignment of benefits form, copies of insurance identification cards, responsible-party authorization, and insurance correspondence
- Explanation of benefits or remittance advice documents sent from insurance payers
- Logs of all telephone conversations and actions taken regarding insurance disputes or collection activities. If you do not store these notes in the corresponding patient health record, you will likely have a master file set up where all logs are kept.
- Encounter forms and referral and authorization slips
- Daysheets and deposit slips

KEEPING UP TO DATE

- Make a folder or binder of pertinent insurance information. Obtain information booklets and policy manuals from the local offices of the various insurance companies. Obtain sample copies of all forms required for the insurance plans used most in your physician's office. Keep samples of completed claim forms.
- Changes occur daily and monthly, so keep well informed by reading your Medicaid, Medicare, TRICARE, and local medical society bulletins. Maintain a chronologic file on each of these bulletins for easy reference, always keeping the latest bulletin on top.
- Attend any workshops on insurance in the medical practice offered in your area. Network with other insurance specialists to compare policies and discuss common problems. The American Association of Medical Assistants (AAMA) has chapters in many states that feature educational workshops and lectures.
- Become a member of the American Academy of Professional Coders (AAPC), American Medical Billing Association (AMBA), Medical Association of Billers (MAB), Medical Group Management Association (MGMA), Healthcare Financial Management Association (HFMA), Healthcare Billing and Management Association (HBMA), Professional Association of Health Care Office Management (PAHCOM), and/or American Health Information Management Association (AHIMA). Each of these associations distributes journals or newsletters on a monthly basis featuring current information.
- Make good use of the internet.
- For addresses of the professional associations mentioned in this chapter, refer to Table 18-2.

PROCEDURE 3-1

Prepare and Post to a Patient's Financial Accounting Report

OBJECTIVES: To prepare; insert descriptions; and post fees, payments, credit adjustments, and balances due to a patient's ledger card

EQUIPMENT/SUPPLIES: Typewriter or computer, patient accounts or ledger cards, and calculator

DIRECTIONS: Follow these steps to post charges, payments, adjustments, and balances to a patient's ledger/account (see Figure 3-14) and practice this skill by completing the assignments in the *Workbook*.

Personal data: Insert the patient's name and address to prepare the ledger card. Some ledgers may require additional information (attending physician's name; type of insurance; insurance company's name with policy and group numbers; patient's home and work telephone numbers; birth date; Social Security number; driver's license number; spouse's and/or dependents' names; and name, address, and telephone number of nearest relative), depending on the style of card chosen for a medical practice.

Date: Post the date of service (DOS) in the date column, description of the services in the professional service description column, and charge amount in the charge column. The posting date is the actual date the transaction is recorded. If the DOS differs from the posting date, reference the DOS in the description column. This date column should never be left blank.

Reference: List a Current Procedural Terminology (CPT) procedure code number in the reference column.

Description: Write a brief description of the transaction that is being posted, such as OV for office visit or HV for hospital visit. Indicate the evaluation and management (E/M) service levels (1 through 5) using the last digit of the E/M code (for example, 99205 = Level **5**). List the name of other services or surgical procedures (for example, ECG, vaccination, tonsillectomy).

Charges: Add the charge to the running current balance and enter the current balance in the right column.

Payments: Post the date the payment is received and indicate received on account (ROA) and who made the payment (for example, patient [pt] or name of insurance company) in the description column. List the type of payment (cash, check, debit card, money order, or credit card) and voucher or check number (for example, ck #430) in the reference column.

Adjustments: Post the date the adjustment is being made and indicate the type of adjustment (for example, insurance plan adj., contract adj., courtesy adj.).

Billing comments: Indicate when the insurance company was billed by posting the current date and name of the insurance company. Include the dates of service being billed in the reference column (for example, 4/20/XX through 5/1/XX). Indicate when the patient statement was sent and amount due if different from the current balance (for example, patient billed $45.00 balance after insurance payment).

Other comments: Indicate other comments that pertain directly to the account (for example, account sent to ABC Collection Agency, account scheduled for small claims court).

Charges: Refer to the fee schedule and post each fee (charge) on a separate line in the "Charge" column. Charges are debited (subtracted) from the account balance.

Payments: Enter the amount paid in the "Payment" column, credit (subtract) the payment received from the amount in the running current balance column, and enter the current balance.

Adjustments: Post the contracted insurance plan discount in the "Adjustment" column by referencing the DOS, insurance company name, and type of contract discount (for example, HealthNet PPO discount or Medicare courtesy adjustment). Adjustments are credited to the account balance.

Current balance: Line by line, credit and debit by adding and subtracting postings to the running balance to determine the amount for the current balance column as shown in Figure 3-14. If a line is used to indicate a date an action was taken (for example, insurance company or patient billed, account sent to collection), bring down the running balance from the previous line. This column must always contain an amount and should never be left blank. *Optional:* Post the adjustment on the same line as the payment.

Submit an itemized billing statement to the patient for the balance due.

Date	Description	Charge	Payment	Adjustment	Balance
					1346.17
7-3-XX	ROA Prudential Ins #7421		980.30	120.80	245.07

KEY POINTS

This is a brief chapter review, or summary, of the key issues presented. To further enhance your knowledge of the technical subject matter, review the key terms and key abbreviations for this chapter by locating the meaning for each in the Glossary at the end of this text, which appears in a section before the Index.

1. An insurance contract (policy or agreement) is a legal document in which the insured (policyholder or subscriber) receives coverage that helps to offset costs when medical services are necessary. The four concepts of a valid insurance contract follow: (1) The person must be a mentally competent adult and not under the influence of drugs or alcohol when signing the contract. (2) The insurance company must make an offer (the signed application) and the person must accept the offer (issuance of the policy) without concealment or misrepresentation of facts on the application. (3) An exchange of value (the first premium payment) submitted with the application, known as a *consideration*, must be present. (4) A legal purpose must exist, which is an insurable interest in the case of a health insurance policy. This means that the policyholder expects to continue in good health but the insurance policy will provide something of value if an accident or illness strikes.

2. The insurance biller must understand insurance terminology and policy provisions as they relate to billing and claims submission. An implied contract is defined as not manifested by direct words but implied or deduced from the circumstance, the general language, or the conduct of the patient. On the other hand, an expressed contract can be verbal or written. However, most physician–patient contracts are implied.

3. There are many types of private and federal insurance programs, such as managed care, workers' compensation, Medicare, Medicaid, and TRICARE.

4. Establish an insurance claims register or log (tracing file) to keep track of the status of each case that has been billed. Record to whom the claim was sent and the submission date on the insurance claims register and the patient's ledger card.

5. The patient registration form must be reviewed for accuracy and completeness of the content. This information becomes critical when completing and following up on claims.

6. Verifying an insured's eligibility to receive benefits and obtaining prior approval from the insurance company to give a specific treatment are vital issues for collecting payment when medical services are provided.

7. An aging accounts receivable report to determine outstanding balances can be generated using the date that the claim was filed as a point to assess how many days old the claim is. This report is used to understand how much money is due to the practice from each patient account.

8. Each type of insurance has different time limits for claims submission; if electronically transmitted after the designated time, claims will be denied.

9. After insurance payments are received, they must be posted to each patient's account and any necessary adjustments made with the outstanding balance billed to the patient.

10. Because federal program regulations have ongoing changes and new diagnostic and procedural codes are adopted annually, it is imperative that the insurance biller keep up to date on technical information and have access to current reference books.

11. With the advent of health care reform in 2010, health benefit exchanges were created and changes occurred that affect the uninsured; preexisting conditions; prescription drugs; employers' responsibilities; and programs such as Medicare, Medicaid, and ERISA.

💻 STUDENT ASSIGNMENT

✔ Study Chapter 3.

✔ Answer the fill-in-the-blank, multiple-choice, and true/false questions in the *Workbook* to reinforce the theory learned in this chapter and to help prepare for a future test.

✔ Complete the assignments in the *Workbook* to help reinforce the basic steps in submitting an insurance claim form.

✔ Turn to the Glossary at the end of this text for a further understanding of the key terms and key abbreviations used in this chapter.

CHAPTER 4

Medical Documentation and the Electronic Health Record

Linda Smith

OBJECTIVES

After reading this chapter, you should be able to:

1. Identify the most common documents found in the medical record.
2. Discuss health record systems and list the advantages and disadvantages of an electronic health record system.
3. Describe the incentive programs established through federal legislation for adoption of electronic health records in physician offices and hospitals.
4. Define *meaningful use* and describe the implementation stages.
5. Define the various titles of physicians as they relate to health record documentation.
6. Explain the reasons that legible documentation is required.
7. Describe common billing errors found in medical records and define medical necessity.
8. Discuss various billing patterns that could cause possible audit.
9. Define common terminology related to medical, diagnostic, and surgical services.
10. Abstract information from the medical record to complete a life or health insurance application.
11. Describe the difference between prospective and retrospective review of records.
12. Respond appropriately to the subpoena of a witness and records.
13. Identify principles for retention of health records.
14. Formulate a procedure for termination of a case.
15. Discuss in-depth documentation requirements for evaluation and management services, including documentation guidelines for medical services, as well as the documentation of history, examinations, and medical decision making.

KEY TERMS

acute	critical care	high complexity
attending physician	degaussing	history of present illness
chief complaint	detailed	internal review
chronic	documentation	legible
cloned note	electronic health record	low complexity
comorbidity	emergency care	meaningful use
comprehensive	eponym	medical decision making
concurrent care	established patient	medical necessity
consultation	expanded problem focused	medical report
consulting physician	external audit	moderate complexity
continuity of care	family history	new patient
counseling	health record/medical record	non-physician practitioner

KEY TERMS

ordering physician	referral	subpoena
past history	referring physician	*subpoena duces tecum*
physical examination	resident physician	teaching physician
prepayment audit	retrospective review	treating, or performing,
primary care physician	review of systems	physician
problem focused	social history	zeroization
prospective review	straightforward	

KEY ABBREVIATIONS

ARRA	EPF level of history or	MC medical decision	POMR system
C level of history or	examination	making	RCU
examination	FH	MDM	RLQ
CC	HC medical decision	MU	R/O
CCU	making	NP	ROS
D level of history or	HIM	NPP	RUQ
examination	HIV	PCP	SF medical decision
dx or Dx	HPI	PE or PX	making
ED or ER	ICU	PF level of history or	SH
EHR	LC medical decision	examination	SOAP style
E/M service	making	PFSH	SOR system
EMR	LLQ	PH	WNL
	LUQ	PO	

Service to Patients

It is essential that all medical staff who work with health records serve patients by doing the following:

- Keeping their personal health information private and confidential.
- Following federal Health Insurance Portability and Accountability Act (HIPAA) guidelines for consent and disclosure of information to keep a medical practice compliant and patients confident that their medical records will be secure and safe.
- Helping patients manage their online electronic personal records by keeping them informed of the provider's role in access, update, and exchange of data.

THE DOCUMENTATION PROCESS

Health Record

The connection between insurance billing and the **health record,** also known for decades as the *medical record,* should be explained to better understand its importance as the foremost tool of clinical care and communication. A health record can be defined as written or graphic information documenting facts and events during the rendering of patient care. It may be kept in either a paper or an electronic format.

Contents of a health record vary from case to case but some of the most common medical office documents are as follows:

- Patient registration (demographic information)
- Medication record
- History and **physical examination** notes or report
- Progress or chart notes
- **Consultation** reports
- Imaging and x-ray reports
- Laboratory reports
- Immunization records
- Consent and authorization forms
- Operative reports
- Pathology reports

In a hospital setting, in addition to the aforementioned documents, there are **attending physician**'s orders, dates of admission, hospital stay dates, discharge dates, and discharge summaries. The key to substantiating procedure and diagnostic code selections for claim submission and to ensure appropriate reimbursement is supporting **documentation** in the health record. Proper documentation can prevent penalties and refund requests in the event that the physician's practice is reviewed or audited. Some states or facilities use different terminology, such as medical information, medical record, progress or chart note, hospital record, or health care record, when referring to the health record.

Health Record Systems

Any one of several record systems can be used in a medical practice. They are the problem-oriented medical record (POMR) system, the source-oriented record (SOR) system, and the integrated record system. An **electronic health record (EHR)** system can be kept as a POMR or SOR system.

The POMR system is designed to organize patient information by the presenting problem, allowing the provider to obtain a quick and structured overview of the patient's history when he or she presents. The record consists of flow sheets, charts, or graphs that allow a physician to quickly locate information and compare evaluations. These data sheets are commonly used to record blood sugar levels for diabetic patients, blood pressure readings for hypertensive patients, weight for obese patients, immunizations, medication refills, and so on. Using this type of system assists the provider in focusing on the patient's problems, their evolution, and the relationship between clinical events.

In the SOR system, documents are arranged according to sections (for example, history and physical section, progress notes, laboratory tests, radiology reports, or surgical operations). The integrated record system files all documents in reverse chronologic order; thus it may be more difficult to locate data because they are scattered throughout the record.

Electronic Health Records

Paper-based offices are fading into the past and the electronic format is gradually becoming the norm as the ability to share patient health records among other professionals who constitute the patient's health care team has become increasingly important.

In an EHR system, networked computers use practice management software and patient medical information software that interface. The medical information software uses either free-text or built-in templates to help structure documentation through a process of answering a series of questions and entering data. Thus an EHR is a collection of medical information about the past, present, and future of a patient that resides in a centralized electronic system. This system receives, stores, transmits, retrieves, and links data for giving health care services from many information systems, such as laboratory test results, radiology reports and

x-ray images, pathology reports, and financial documents. However, the difference between an EHR and an *electronic medical record (EMR)* is that an EMR is an individual physician's EMR for the patient, including medical history, allergies, and appointment information. In comparison, the EHR is all patient medical information from many information systems, including all components of the EMR.

Electronic Health Records in the Billing Process

Many EHR programs allow the insurance billing specialist to perform insurance verification automatically during the preregistration process. The electronic **medical report** is part of the health record and is a permanent legal document that formally states the outcomes of the patient's examination or treatment in letter or report form. It is this record that provides the information needed to complete the insurance claim form. Selection of procedure and diagnostic codes by the provider may be computer assisted prior to final review by a medical coder. The procedure and diagnostic codes are used for interpretation by the insurance company when processing a claim. When billing the insurance company, the date of service (DOS), place of service (POS), diagnosis (dx or Dx), and procedures are recorded and transmitted in electronic format. Electronic signatures or codes are applied to documents when they are reviewed and authenticated by the creator. Insurance claims are compiled and transmitted in batches to a clearinghouse or to the insurance carrier. The revenue cycle is managed completely online.

Advantages of Electronic Health Records

An EHR system has several advantages over a paper-based system. The greatest advantage of the EHR is the accessibility of medical records between providers and health care organizations that in turn can improve quality of care and patient safety.

Cost savings and decreasing workplace inefficiencies are other advantages of the EHR. The EHR requires no physical space because the files remain in an electronic database and are available online. The health record is accessible from remote sites and retrieval of information at almost any work site is nearly immediate. Chart chasing is eliminated. The EHR can decrease charting time and charting errors, thus increasing the productivity and effectiveness of providers.

The need for staff to select information from a patient's electronic medical record for completion of an insurance claim (known as abstracting data) is often eliminated because data may be captured automatically from various documents via dictation or templates. The EHR is expected to increase patient safety through built-in safety features by use of medical alerts and reminders that can capture things such as medication allergies. The EHR reduces the likelihood of errors, since there is no illegible handwriting to decipher.

Disadvantages of Electronic Health Records

The greatest drawback to EHRs is startup costs, which can be extremely high. Usability can also be a major obstacle in implementation of an EHR, with learning curves that vary depending on the user's technical abilities and knowledge.

With increased accessibility comes greater concern with confidentiality and security issues. These issues are the primary focus of the Health Insurance Portability and Accountability Act (HIPAA) Privacy and Security Rules that call for practices to take on a higher level of integrity in these areas.

Although EHR is designed to save providers time and improve the quality and legibility of their documentation, the use of EHR has also led to a new problem with the medical record related to copied and templated documentation. These are referred to as **cloned notes.** The process may also be referred to as "cut and paste" or "carried over." Centers for Medicare and Medicaid Services (CMS) considers documentation to be cloned when each entry in the medical record for a patient is worded exactly alike or similar to the previous entries. Cloning also occurs when medical documentation is exactly the same from patient to patient. It would not be expected that every patient had the exact same problem or symptoms and required the exact same treatment. Cloned notes increase the risk for medical errors and can result in the loss of crucial clinical details that may be omitted from a patient's assessment or treatment plan. All documentation in the medical record must be specific to the patient and his or her situation at the time of the encounter. Payers are refusing to pay for services that appear to be cloned and this process has come under increased scrutiny by the Office of Inspector General (OIG). It is a red flag for fraud investigations.

INCENTIVE PROGRAMS FOR ADOPTION OF ELECTRONIC HEALTH RECORDS

Federal legislation established by the American Recovery and Reinvestment Act of 2009 (ARRA) established programs to help the health care industry change to electronic medical records. Legislation affecting Medicare and Medicaid programs was established to provide

ELECTRONIC SECURITY STANDARDS

The Medicare Modernization Act created the Commission on Systemic Interoperability to develop a strategy to make health care information available at all times to patients and physicians. To reach a goal of having electronic records for all Americans, adoption of health information standards and increase of funding demonstration projects has begun.

One provision of the Health Insurance Portability and Accountability Act (HIPAA) directs the adoption of national electronic standards for automatic transfer of certain health care data among health care payers, plans, and providers. This provision encourages medical practices to convert to an electronic record-keeping system or paperless office because this will help to transition insurance claim attachments from the paper world into the electronic world.

more than $27 billion in payout of incentives to eligible providers who implement electronic health records. These incentive programs will transition into disincentives for those who do not adopt EHR over the next several years in the form of adjusted or decreased payments. It is important for insurance billing specialists to be familiar with all incentive programs, as they will be involved in submission of qualifying data, collection of incentive payments, and analysis of incentive program outcomes as they affect the organization's accounts receivable.

Physician Quality Reporting System Incentive Program (PQRS)

PQRS was one of the initial incentive programs resulting from the Tax Relief and Health Care Act of 2006 (TRHCA). The Act established incentive payments for eligible providers who satisfactorily report data on quality measures for covered professional services furnished to Medicare beneficiaries. The program started in 2011 with incentives equal to 1.0% of the providers' allowed Medicare charges. Incentives declined in 2012 through 2014 to incentive payments equal to 0.5% of the allowed Medicare charges. Beginning in 2015, eligible providers who do not report PQRS measures satisfactorily will be subject to payment adjustments equal to 1.5% of their Medicare Physician Fee Schedule (MPFS) allowed charges. The payment adjustment increases to 2.0% in 2016 and beyond.

In Examples 4-1 to 4-3, the insurance specialist will need to confirm that the provider has in fact met the

Example 4-1	PQRS Quality Measure for Tobacco Use Screening and Cessation Intervention

Providers report the percentage of patients aged 18 years and older who were screened for tobacco use and received cessation counseling intervention if identified as a tobacco user.

Example 4-2	PQRS Quality Measure for Body Mass Index (BMI) Screening and Follow-Up

Providers report the percentage of patients aged 18 years and older with a documented BMI outside of the normal parameters. When the BMI is outside of normal parameters, a follow-up plan is documented.

Example 4-3	PQRS Quality Measure for Documentation of Current Medications in the Medical Record

Providers report the percentage of visits for patients aged 18 years and older for which the provider attests to documenting a list of current medications used by the patient on the date of the encounter.

documentation requirements of the quality measure being reported. They will also submit a Healthcare Common Procedure Coding System (HCPCS) code on the claim form associated with the services provided for that date of service; the HCPCS code will identify whether the requirement has been met.

E-Prescribing Incentive Program

The Electronic Prescribing (eRx) Incentive Program was another early incentive program that started in 2011 and used a combination of incentive payments and payment adjustments to encourage electronic prescribing. The eRx Incentive Program officially ended in January 2014; physicians who do not successfully e-prescribe will be penalized at a rate of 2.0% throughout 2014 and 2015. The only way that physicians can prevent such penalties at this point is for them to participate in the Medicare and Medicaid EHR meaningful use incentive programs.

Medicare and Medicaid Electronic Health Record (EHR) Incentive Programs

EHR incentive programs were established as part of the ARRA. The programs provide a reimbursement incentive for physician and hospital providers who adopt,

implement, upgrade, and demonstrate meaningful use (MU) of certified EHR technology. Eligible providers (EPs) will receive an incentive payment based on the criteria of the program under which they elect to receive payment (Medicare or Medicaid). If an EP qualifies for both the Medicare and the Medicaid EHR incentive program, it is limited to only one program and must choose which program to participate in.

Under the Medicare incentive program, EPs who began participation in this program prior to 2013 had the opportunity to earn incentive payments for up to 5 years (maximum total incentive of $44,000). EPs whose first year of participation is 2013 or later did not receive incentive payments and beginning in 2015, those providers who cannot demonstrate MU of certified EHR technology will be penalized through payment adjustments. The payment reduction starts at 1% and increases each year that an EP does not demonstrate MU, to a maximum of 5%.

Under the Medicaid incentive program, EPs have the opportunity to earn incentive programs for up to 6 years (maximum total incentive of $63,750). The last year in which an EP can begin participation in this program is 2016. However, EPs have 6 years to participate, with the last year of participation being 2021. There are currently no penalties for not demonstrating MU for Medicaid EPs.

Meaningful Use

Meaningful use (MU) involves demonstrating that the health care organization has the capabilities and processes in place so that the provider is actively using certified EHR technology to:
- Improve quality of care, patient safety, and efficiencies in health care and reduce health disparities.
- Engage patients and family in management of their care.
- Improve care coordination and the general public health.
- Maintain the privacy and security of patient health information.

Over time, it is anticipated that compliance with MU will result in better clinical outcomes, improved population health outcomes, increased transparency and efficiency, empowered individuals, and more robust research data on health systems.

To accomplish this, CMS has set specific criteria and objectives that EPs and hospitals must achieve to qualify for the incentive programs. The three specific criteria required to meet the definition of MU are as follows: (1) The EP must use "certified EHR technology" in a

---

Example 4-4   Meaningful Use Measure or Element

- Providers must maintain an up-to-date problem list of current and active diagnoses for each patient.
- Documentation must substantiate at least one entry or an indication that no problems are known for the patient.

Example 4-5   Meaningful Use Measure or Element

- Providers must maintain an active medication list for each patient.
- Documentation must substantiate at least one entry or an indication that the patient is not currently prescribed any medication.

Example 4-6   Meaningful Use Measure or Element

- Providers must record smoking status for patients aged 13 years and older.
- Documentation must substantiate smoking status of the patient.

---

meaningful manner, including electronic prescribing. (2) The EP must also demonstrate that the certified EHR technology is connected in a manner that provides for the electronic exchange of health information to improve the quality of health care, such as promoting care coordination. (3) Finally, the EP must submit information on clinical quality measures specified by the Department of Health and Human Services (DHHS). CMS established three stages to meet the objectives outlined for MU.

Stage 1

Stage 1 (2011, 2012, 2013) focused on data capture and sharing. The Stage 1 criteria for MU focused on electronically capturing health information in a coded format using that information to track key conditions, communicating that information for care coordination purposes, and initiating the reporting of clinical quality measures and public health information.

Stage 2

Stage 2 (2014, 2015) focused on advance clinical processes. Stage 2 expanded on Stage 1 criteria in the areas of disease management, clinical decision support, medication management support for patient access to their health information, transitions in care, quality measurement and

research, and bidirectional communication with public health agencies.

Stage 3

Stage 3 (2016) focuses on improved outcomes. Stage 3 will focus on achieving improvements in quality, safety, and efficiency, focusing on decision support for national high-priority conditions, patient access to self-management tools, access to **comprehensive** patient data, and improving population health outcomes.

Documentation is of utmost importance in all stages of the Meaningful Use programs (both Medicare and Medicaid). Providers must have the documentation to substantiate all elements required and attested to (Examples 4-4 to 4-6).

GENERAL PRINCIPLES OF HEALTH RECORD DOCUMENTATION

Documenters

All individuals providing health care services may be referred to as *documenters* because they chronologically record pertinent facts and observations about the patient's health. This process is called *documentation* (charting) and may be electronically handwritten, dictated and transcribed, or downloaded from a personal digital assistant (PDA) or smartphone using an electronic template. It is the health care physician's responsibility to either handwrite the medical information or dictate it for transcription. Some documenters use a speech recognition system, which is a computerized voice recognition system that makes it possible for a computer system to respond to spoken words. Two basic categories are (1) navigation or command control, which allows an individual to launch and operate software applications with spoken directions, and (2) *dictation software*, which makes it possible for a computer system to recognize spoken words and automatically convert them into text.

When a dictation software speech recognition system is used, many practices use a medical editor (*correctionist*) who proofreads and edits the computer-generated documents. Some practices use printed checklists for typical examinations. The physician notes his or her findings on the checklists and gives this document to an employee for input to the EMR system. The EMR system has access to these checklists to minimize typing costs.

The receptionist obtains the first document completed by the patient, called the *patient registration information form*, as shown in Figure 3-6. The medical assistant or a front desk staff member is often the one who records entries for no-show appointments, prescription refills, and telephone calls in the patient's health record. The insurance billing specialist uses the information in the health record for billing purposes and it is his or her responsibility to bring any substandard documentation to the physician's or office manager's attention, depending on office policy. In the hospital setting, a trained health information management (HIM) professional maintains the health record for completeness.

When referring to guidelines for documentation of the health record and completion of the insurance claim form, a physician's title may change, depending on the circumstances of each patient encounter. This can get confusing at times; to clarify the physician's various roles and the roles of the practitioners who work for the physician, some of these titles are defined as follows:

● Attending physician refers to the hospital staff member who is legally responsible for the care and treatment given to a patient.
● **Consulting physician** is a provider whose opinion or advice regarding evaluation or management of a specific problem is requested by another physician.
● **Non-physician practitioner (NPP)** is a nurse practitioner, clinical nurse specialist, licensed social worker, nurse midwife, physical therapist, speech therapist, audiologist, or physician assistant who furnishes a consultation or treats a patient for a specific medical problem, pursuant to state law, and who uses the results of a diagnostic test in the management of the patient's specific medical problem.
● **Ordering physician** is the individual in the hospital directing the selection, preparation, or administration of tests, medication, or treatment.
● **Primary care physician (PCP)** oversees the care of patients in a managed health care plan and refers patients to see specialists for services as needed.
● **Referring physician** is a provider who sends the patient for tests or treatment.
● **Resident physician** is a physician who has finished medical school and is performing one or more years of training in a specialty area on the job at a hospital (medical center). Residents perform the elements required for an evaluation and management (E/M) service in the presence of or jointly with the **teaching physician** and residents document the service.
● Teaching physician is a doctor who has responsibilities for training and supervising medical students, interns, or residents and who takes them to the bedsides of patients in a teaching hospital to review course and treatment. Teaching physicians must document that they supervised and were physically present during key portions of the service provided to the patient when performed by a resident.
● **Treating, or performing, physician** is the provider who renders a service to a patient. In the Medicare program, the definition of a treating physician

is a physician who furnishes a consultation or treats a beneficiary for a specific medical problem and who uses the results of a diagnostic test in the management of the beneficiary's specific medical problem. A radiologist performing a therapeutic intervention procedure is considered a treating physician. A radiologist performing a diagnostic intervention or diagnostic procedure is not considered a treating physician.

> **HIPAA Compliance Alert** **LEGIBLE DOCUMENTATION**
>
> If handwritten, entries in the patient's record must be legible. Illegible entries should be returned to the physician for clarification and/or rewritten.

Legible Documentation

Medical record documentation details pertinent facts, findings, and observations about an individual's health history, examinations, tests, treatments, and outcomes. It facilitates the health care professional in evaluating and planning the patient's immediate treatment and in monitoring the patient's health care over time. It is a basic and important element in providing the highest level of quality of care.

The documentation guidelines issued by the CMS states that the medical record should be complete and **legible.** The CMS definition of legible is that the data must be easily recognizable by someone outside of the medical practice who is unfamiliar with the handwriting. It is important that providers have comprehensive and legible documentation describing what occurred during the patient's visit for the following reasons:
● To avoid denial or delay of payments by insurance carriers
● To comply with insurance carrier payment policies requiring documentation to support procedural and diagnostic codes submitted on claims
● For subpoena of health records by state investigators or the court for review
● For defense of any professional liability claims
● For execution of the physician's written instructions to the patient or the caregiver

Common Documentation Errors

Understandably, health care providers put patient care first; documentation is a process that follows and is often times dashed off too quickly. Providing excellent patient care is frequently used as an excuse for very poor documentation. It is important to help physicians understand the link between quality care and documentation. The following is a list of common errors found in medical records:

- Medication lists are not updated with new or discontinued medications.
- Incorrect dosages of prescription medications are documented.
- Duplicate prescriptions are documented for both brand and generic medications
- Over-the-counter medications the patient is taking are not documented.
- Information related to medication allergies is not documented.
- Treatment outcomes are often incorrect. For example, a condition is noted as being resolved when it is still being treated.
- Lab information is missing or not updated.
- Important information related to the patient's illness and symptoms, as stated by the patient, are not documented.
- There are inaccuracies in diagnosis and incomplete documentation related to the plan of care for the condition.
- Information from other providers is missing.

HIPAA Compliance Alert

MEDICALLY NECESSARY

Third-party payers and federal programs have a responsibility to ensure that professional services provided to patients were medically necessary. Documentation must support the level of service and each procedure rendered.

Medical Necessity

Payment may be delayed, downcoded, or denied if the **medical necessity** of a treatment is questioned. As a rule, medical necessity is a criterion used by insurance companies, as well as federal programs such as Medicare, when making decisions to limit or deny payment. Some medical practices use electronic medical necessity software that verifies that the medical services or procedures are justified by the patient's symptoms and diagnosis. Medical treatment must be done in accordance with standards of good medical practice and the proper level of care provided in the most appropriate setting. However, insurers differ on this definition and may or may not cover the services depending on the benefits of the plan. Inform the patient of this situation with a letter, as shown in Figure 4-1. For Medicare patients, Chapter 12 discusses more about the Advance Beneficiary Notice of Noncoverage (ABN), also known as a *waiver of liability agreement* or *responsibility statement* that is used in this type of situation.

Legalities of Health Record Billing Patterns

Insurance carriers have become stricter in enforcing accurate coding substantiated by documentation. It is not uncommon for prepayment and postpayment random audits or reviews by Medicare carriers that monitor the accuracy of physicians' use of medical services and procedure codes. Medicare administrative contractors (fiscal intermediaries) have "walk-in rights" (access to a medical practice without an appointment or search warrant) that they may invoke to conduct documentation reviews, audits, and evaluations. Billing patterns that may draw attention to a medical practice for possible audit are as follows:

- Billing intentionally for unnecessary services
- Billing incorrectly for services of *physician extenders* (NPPs) (for example, nurse practitioner, midwife, physician assistant)
- Billing for diagnostic tests without a separate report in the health record
- Changing dates of service on insurance claims to comply with policy coverage dates
- Waiving copayments or deductibles or allowing other illegal discounts
- Ordering excessive diagnostic tests (for example, laboratory tests, x-ray studies)
- Using two different provider numbers to bill the same services for the same patient
- Misusing provider identification numbers, resulting in incorrect billing
- Using improper modifiers for financial gain
- Failing to return overpayments made by the Medicare program

DOCUMENTATION TERMINOLOGY

Terminology for Evaluation and Management Services

While learning the complexities of medical documentation and how important it is as it relates to coding and billing, you have discovered that you must have a good foundation of medical terminology. To use the diagnostic and procedure code books efficiently, you must become familiar with their language, abbreviations, and symbols.

In the early 1990s, the American Medical Association (AMA) modified the term "office visits" and replaced this phrase with "office and other outpatient services" when coding for those services; the AMA also adopted the phrase "evaluation and management (E/M)" for the name of the section of Current Procedural Terminology (CPT) in which those codes appear. This wording better reflects the components involved when performing an office visit. However, E/M services are also performed

COLLEGE CLINIC
4567 Broad Avenue
Woodland Hills, XY 12345-0001
Phone: 555/486-9002
Fax: 555/487-8976

September 20, 20XX

Dear ABC Managed Care Plan Participant:

This is a quick fact sheet to help our patients understand that some services may not be paid by ABC Managed Care Plan unless there is a *medical* reason to perform them.

The coverage provided by ABC Managed Care Plan, in most instances, includes payment for medically necessary services provided to treat a problem or illness. However, patients who wish their health care providers to perform services outside of those considered a "medical necessity" will be responsible for paying for those services out-of-pocket.

For example, many patients come to our office for the purpose of removing noncancerous facial moles. Although this procedure may be desired by the patient, ABC Managed Care Plan will not pay for the removal without a medical reason for it.

The patient's cost for noncancerous facial mole removal at our practice is approximately $75.

Please understand that, legally, we are required to submit our bill to ABC Managed Care Plan using accurate information about all of the services you received. Using a false medical reason to try to get insurance to pay for a service it otherwise would not cover is considered fraud, and our doctors will not do this. We regret that ABC Managed Care Plan may not wish to pay for a service you desire, but we must follow insurance regulations.

If you would like additional information about payment coverage for these services, you may refer to your ABC Managed Care Plan benefits handbook or call your ABC Managed Care Plan customer service representative at 555-271-0311.

Thank you for choosing us to assist you with your health care needs. As always, providing high-quality health care to you is and remains our primary purpose. If you have any questions about this information, please do not hesitate to telephone and ask our front office staff for more information.

Sincerely,

Mary Anne Mason, CPC

FIGURE 4-1 Letter to a patient who is a member of a managed care plan that provides important information about medical procedures or services that are not covered for payment unless there is a medical necessity.

in other settings, such as inpatient hospital facilities and nursing homes.

New versus Established Patient

In coding E/M services, two categories of patients are considered: the **new patient (NP)** and the established patient. An NP is one who *has not received* any professional services from the physician or another physician of the same specialty who belongs to the same group practice *within the past 3 years*. An **established patient** is one who *has received* professional services from the physician or another physician of the same specialty who belongs to the same group practice *within the past 3 years*. Refer to the decision tree in Figure 4-2 to help decide whether a patient is considered new or established.

A physician may provide a course of action to evaluate and manage a patient who is seeking medical care (that is, refer to a specialist for consultation, see a referral from another physician, give **concurrent care** as one of several physicians, render continuity of care for a doctor who is out of town, administer **critical care**, direct **emergency care**, or furnish **counseling** discussion to a patient's family).

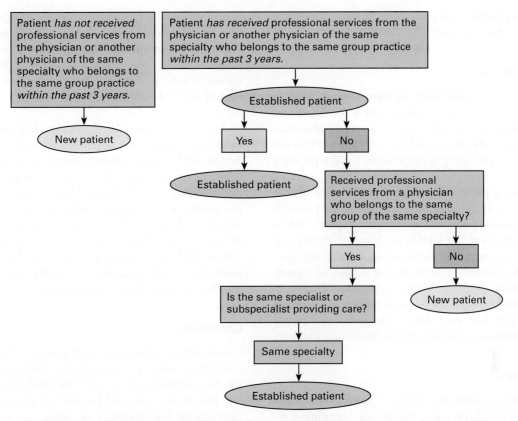

FIGURE 4-2 Decision tree for new patient (NP) versus established patient when selecting a CPT evaluation and management code.

Consultation

A consultation includes services rendered by a physician whose opinion or advice is requested by another physician or agency in the evaluation or treatment of a patient's illness or a suspected problem. The requesting physician must document the request in the patient's health record and the consulting physician should state: "Patient is seen at the request of Dr. John Doe for a ... reason." Consultations may occur in a home, office, hospital, extended care facility, or other location. A physician consultant recommends diagnostic or therapeutic services and may initiate these services if requested by the referring physician. The opinion must be in writing, documented in a consultation report, and communicated to the referring physician. The consultant may order a diagnostic or therapeutic service to formulate the opinion at an initial or subsequent visit.

Referral

A **referral** is the transfer of the total or specific care of a patient from one physician to another for known problems. It is not a consultation. For example, a patient is sent by a PCP to an orthopedist for care of a fracture.

However, when dealing with managed care plans, the term *referral* is also used when requesting an authorization for the patient to receive services elsewhere (for example, referral for laboratory tests, radiology procedures, or specialty care). In most cases, the PCP must obtain authorization for the referral to ensure that the managed care plan will pay for the specialist's services. Appropriate documentation of the referral and authorization is needed to substantiate approval of the referral.

Concurrent Care

Concurrent care is the providing of similar services (for example, hospital visits) to the same patient by more than one physician on the same day. For example, two internists (a general internist and a cardiologist) see the same patient in the hospital on the same day. The general internist admitted the patient for diabetes and requested that the cardiologist also follow the patient's periodic chest pain and arrhythmia. If the second doctor is not identified in carrier records as a cardiologist, the claim may be denied. This is because the services appear to be duplicated by physicians of the same specialty. When billing insurance companies, physicians providing concurrent care may be cross-referenced on the claim form. Medicare has a list that includes 62 specialties and subspecialties to help carriers more accurately judge whether concurrent care is necessary. Periodically, the physician should check with the carrier's provider service representative to determine whether the provider has updated its subspecialty status so that claims for concurrent care are not denied.

Continuity of Care

If a case involves **continuity of care** (for example, a patient who has received treatment for a condition and is then referred by the physician to a second physician for treatment for the same condition), both physicians are responsible for providing arrangements for the patient's continuing care. In such a case, records must be provided by the referring physician and the insurance billing specialist must obtain summaries or records of the patient's previous treatment and obtain hospital reports before coding if the patient was seen in the hospital, emergency department, or outpatient department. Contact the hospital's health records department for copies of reports after outpatient treatment or after a patient's discharge. In some cases, coding from hospital reports can increase reimbursement but can delay submission of claims because reports may not be available in a timely manner.

Critical Care

Critical care means the intensive care provided in a variety of acute life-threatening conditions requiring constant "full attention" by a physician. It can be provided in the critical care unit or emergency department (ED) of a hospital. A critical illness or injury acutely impairs one or more vital organ systems such that there is a high probability of imminent or life-threatening deterioration in the patient's condition. Examples of vital organ system failure include but are not limited to central nervous system failure; circulatory failure; shock; and renal, hepatic, metabolic, or respiratory failure. Critical care may sometimes, but not always, be rendered in a critical care area, such as a coronary care unit (CCU), intensive care unit (ICU), respiratory care unit (RCU), or ED (also called the emergency room [ER]).

Emergency Care

Emergency care differs from critical care in that it may be given by the physician in a hospital ED or in a physician's office setting. Emergency care is care provided to acutely ill patients that may or may not involve organ system failure but does require immediate medical attention. In physician-directed emergency care advanced life support, the physician is located in a hospital emergency or critical care department and is in two-way voice communication with ambulance or rescue personnel outside the hospital. The physician directs the performance of necessary medical procedures.

In the Medicare program, an emergency medical condition is currently defined as a medical condition manifesting itself by acute symptoms of sufficient severity (including severe pain) such that the absence of immediate medical attention could reasonably be expected to result in placing the patient's health in serious jeopardy, serious impairment to body functions, or serious dysfunction of any body organ or part.

Many states have adopted the prudent layperson definition of an emergency as defined in the Balanced Budget Act of 1997. This is similarly stated as "any medical condition of recent onset and severity, including but not limited to severe pain, that would lead a prudent lay person, possessing an average knowledge of medicine and health, to believe that his or her condition, sickness, or injury is of such a nature that failure to obtain immediate medical care could result in placing the patient's health in serious jeopardy, serious impairment to bodily functions, or serious dysfunction of bodily organ or part."

Counseling

Counseling is a discussion with a patient, family, or both concerning one or more of the following: diagnostic results, impressions, or recommended diagnostic studies; prognosis; risks and benefits of treatment options; instructions for treatment or follow-up; importance of compliance with chosen treatment options; risk factor reduction; and patient and family education.

Diagnostic Terminology and Abbreviations

Problems can occur with documentation because of missing or misused essential words. For example, if an entry says "heart failure due to diastolic dysfunction" instead of "diastolic dysfunction," the first statement gives more complete documentation of the medical condition. Always query the physician if in doubt about the documentation to obtain the most specific, accurate terminology for the record.

Some physicians document "imp" (impression) or "Dx" (diagnosis), which usually serves as the diagnosis when completing the claim. If the diagnosis is not in the health record and there is doubt about the diagnosis, always ask the physician to review it. If the patient has been in the hospital, request the electronic file of the discharge summary, which contains the admitting and discharge diagnoses.

The health care field uses many abbreviations and acronyms that can save time and aid in communication. However, they may be confusing in their interpretation. Frequently, an abbreviation can be translated into several meanings. Official American Hospital Association (AHA) policy states that "abbreviations should be totally eliminated from the more vital sections of the health

Table 4-1	Do Not Use Abbreviations	
DO NOT USE	**POTENTIAL PROBLEM**	**USE INSTEAD**
U, u (unit)	Mistaken for "0" (zero), the number 4 (four), or "cc"	Write "unit"
IU (International Unit)	Mistaken for IV (intravenous) or the number 10 (ten)	Write "International Unit"
Q.D, QD, q.d., qd (daily)	Mistaken for each other. Period after the Q mistaken	Write "daily"
Q.O.D., QOD, q.o.d., qod (every other day)	for "I" and the "O" mistaken for "I"	Write "every other day"
Trailing zero (X.O mg)	Decimal point is missed	Write X mg
Lack of leading zero (.X mg)		Write 0.X mg
MS	Can mean morphine sulfate or magnesium sulfate.	Write "morphine sulfate"
MSO4 and MgSO4	Confused for one another	Write "magnesium sulfate"

record, such as final diagnosis, operative notes, discharge summaries, and descriptions of special procedures." Many physicians are not aware of this policy and the final diagnosis may appear as an abbreviation in the patient's record.

The Joint Commission is an agency that provides accreditation status to health care organizations that comply with their standards of patient care. The Joint Commission has made it a mission to research what practices provide the best health care to patients and has hundreds of performance standards with which organizations must comply. Its National Patient Safety Goal was initiated to improve communication between caregivers and has stated that hospitals must take reasonable approaches to standardizing abbreviations, acronyms, and symbols. For example, hospitals can develop a standardized list of abbreviations or use a published reference source. When hospitals use multiple abbreviations, symbols, or acronyms for the same term, the hospitals must identify what they will use to eliminate any ambiguity.

In 2004, The Joint Commission created its "do not use" list of abbreviations (Table 4-1) for all organizations accredited with it.

Use your medical dictionary (most list abbreviations alphabetically with the unabbreviated words) to interpret an abbreviation or ask the physician when clarification is necessary.

Most medical practices create and retain a list of acceptable abbreviations with translations in their office policy manual to avoid misinterpretation. In the *Workbook*, refer to the detailed list of common medical abbreviations in Appendix A. Additional knowledge will be obtained when you complete each assignment involving a patient's health record in the *Workbook* because you must define all of the abbreviations.

If a lay term appears in a patient record, the correct medical term should be substituted to locate the correct diagnostic code (for example, "contusion" for "bruise").

Example 4-7	Eponyms and Medical Terms
EPONYM	**COMPARABLE MEDICAL TERM**
Buerger disease	Thromboangiitis obliterans
Graves disease	Exophthalmic goiter
Wilks syndrome	Myasthenia gravis

An **eponym** (a term including the name of a person; for example, Graves disease) should not be used when a comparable anatomic term can be used in its place (Example 4-7).

The word **acute** refers to a condition that runs a short (typically 3 to 5 days) but relatively severe course. The word **chronic** means a condition persisting over a long period of time. When the terms *acute* and *chronic* are listed in the diagnostic statement, always search for these terms in the code description. If the same condition is described as both acute (subacute) and chronic and separate subentries exist in the diagnostic code book alphabetic index at the same indentation level, code both and sequence the acute (subacute) code first. For proper documentation to support chronic conditions, two criteria are that the documentation actually states something about the chronic condition and that the conditions are pertinent to the patient's current treatment. For example, if a physician states "controlled diabetes," this is a fact. If the physician asks the patient about his or her sugar level and diet and documents the findings, then something specific has been identified about the chronic condition and this would pass an audit for correct documentation.

Whenever the words "question of," "suspected," or "rule out" or the abbreviation "R/O" are used in connection with a disease or illness, do not code these conditions as if they existed or were established. Instead, code the chief complaint, sign, or symptom. These are only a few of the many terms used in documentation.

An abnormal or unexpected finding without elaboration in the health record is insufficient documentation

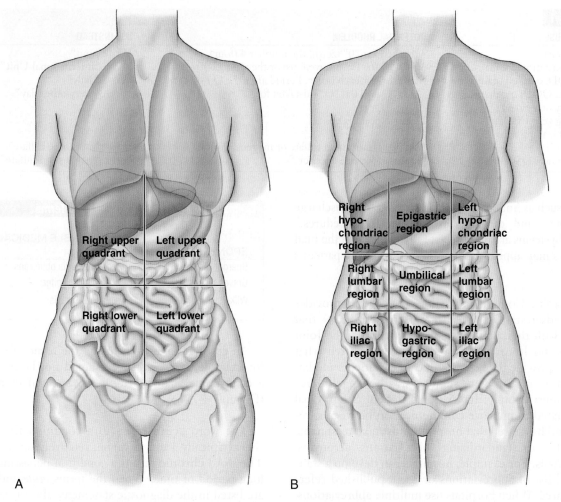

FIGURE 4-3 Regions of the abdomen. **A,** Four quadrants. **B,** Nine regions. *(From Herlihy B, Maebius NK: The human body in health and illness, ed 4, St Louis, 2011, Elsevier.)*

and should be described. Commonly used phrases or abbreviations that may not support billing of services are "WNL" (within normal limits), "noncontributory," "negative/normal," "other than the above, all systems were normal," and so on. For example, phrases used to document findings, such as "all extremities are within normal limits," do not indicate how many extremities or which ones were examined. Documentation must indicate exactly which limb was examined and abbreviated wording would not pass an external audit. If it is determined that such phrases are "canned" notes that can mean that no assessment was actually performed, this is fraud.

Another word commonly used when examining a patient and the findings are within normal limits is "negative" (for example, "ears, nose, and throat negative," "chest x-rays negative"). The physician needs to document that there were no abnormalities in the system being examined. Detailed documentation justifies billed services by providing verification and allows points when an external audit is performed. Thus it should be dictated "Chest film (or report) was reviewed" or "Chest x-ray report was read."

Directional Terms

The following terms are commonly used to describe location of pain and injuries to areas of the abdomen, as shown in Figure 4-3, *A* (four quadrants) and *B* (nine regions):

Right upper quadrant (RUQ) or right hypochondriac: Liver (right lobe), gallbladder, part of the pancreas, parts of the small and large intestines

Epigastric: Upper middle region above the stomach

Left upper quadrant (LUQ) or left hypochondriac: Liver (left lobe), stomach, spleen, part of the pancreas, parts of the small and large intestines

Right and left lumbar: Middle, right, and left regions of the waist

Umbilical: Central region near the navel

Right lower quadrant (RLQ) or right inguinal: Parts of the small and large intestines, right ovary, right uterine (fallopian) tube, appendix, and right ureter

Hypogastric: Middle region below the umbilical region contains urinary bladder and female uterus

Left lower quadrant (LLQ) or left inguinal: Parts of the small and large intestines, left ovary, left uterine tube, and left ureter

Surgical Terminology

Two frequently used terms are *preoperative* and *postoperative* (for example, preoperative diagnosis or postoperative care). Preoperative (preop) pertains to the period before a surgical procedure. Commonly, the preoperative period begins with the first preparation of the patient for surgery and ends with the introduction of anesthesia in the operating suite, whereas postoperative (PO) pertains to the period of time after surgery. It begins with the patient's emergence from anesthesia and continues through the time required for the acute effects of the anesthetic and surgical procedures to decrease.

Surgical procedures of the integumentary system, such as repair of lacerations, are listed in the procedure code book as *simple*, *intermediate*, or *complex* repairs. Simple lacerations are superficial, requiring one-layer closure. Intermediate lacerations require layered closure of one or more of the deeper layers of the skin and tissues. Complex lacerations require more than layered closure and may require reconstructive surgery. Documentation should list the length (in centimeters) of all incisions and layers of involved tissues (subcutaneous, fascia, muscle, and grafts) so that correct procedure codes for excision of lesions and type of repair can be determined.

If time is a factor in coding for reimbursement, documentation should list the length of time spent on the procedure, especially if of unusual duration, such as prolonged services, counseling, or team conferences. This should be stated somewhere in the report.

If state-of-the-art instruments or equipment are used, document the equipment as well as the time spent using it.

Therapeutic or cosmetic surgical procedures should be broken down into two categories—state how much of the procedure was functional and how much was cosmetic or therapeutic. Generally, the insurance carrier pays for the functional portion of the procedure even if there is no coverage for cosmetic or therapeutic procedures.

If you type reports to be submitted with insurance claims to help justify the claims, you should also become familiar with the terms for various operational incisions (Figure 4-4).

Terms such as *undermining* (cut in a horizontal fashion), *take down* (to take apart), or *lysis of adhesions* (destruction of scar tissue) appear in many operations but should not be coded separately. Note the *position* (for example, lithotomy, dorsal) of the patient during the operation and the *surgical approach* (for example, vaginal, abdominal). These help to determine the

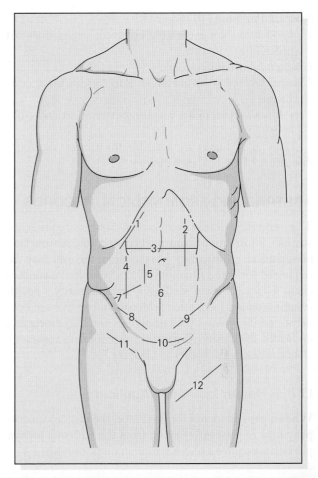

FIGURE 4-4 Operational incisions. Anterior (front) view: *1*, subcostal incision; *2*, paramedian incision; *3*, transverse incision; *4*, upper right rectus incision; *5*, midrectus incision; *6*, midline incision; *7*, lower right rectus incision; *8*, McBurney or right iliac incision; *9*, left iliac incision; *10*, suprapubic incision, *11*, hernia incision; *12*, femoral incision.

proper code selection. Major errors can occur when an insurance biller is not familiar with the medical terms being used. Ask the physician to clarify the case if there is a question because medical terminology is technical and can puzzle even the most knowledgeable insurance billing specialist. Additional key words to look for that may affect code selection and reimbursements are as follows:

Bilateral: Pertaining to both sides
Complete or total: Entire or whole
Complicated by: Involved with other situations at the same time
Hemorrhage: Escape of blood from vessels; bleeding
Initial: First procedure or service
Multiple: Affecting many parts of the body at the same time
Partial: Only a part, not complete
Prolonged procedure due to: Series of steps extended in time to get desired result
Simple: Single and not compound or complex
Subsequent: Second or more procedures or services

Surgical: Pertaining to surgery

Uncomplicated: Not intricately involved; straightforward (procedure)

Unilateral: Pertaining to one side

Unusual findings or circumstances: Rare or not usual conclusion

Very difficult: Hard to do, requiring extra effort and skill

Many good books are available for a more thorough discussion of medical terminology.*

ABSTRACTING FROM MEDICAL RECORDS

The insurance billing professional may be required to abstract information from medical records. Abstraction of technical information from patient records may be requested for three situations: (1) to complete insurance claim forms; (2) when sending a letter to justify a health insurance claim form after professional services are rendered; or (3) when a patient applies for life, mortgage, or health insurance. Abstracting to complete insurance claims is discussed further in Chapter 7.

Life or Health Insurance Applications

When a patient applies for insurance, the insurance company may request information from the patient's private physician, require a physical examination, or both.

On some application forms, the release of medical information signed by the patient may be separate or may be included with the rest of the application. In the latter case, the first section is completed by the insurance agent when interviewing the client; the second section is completed by the physician at the time of the physical examination of the prospective insured. Sometimes a form is sent to the client's attending physician along with a check requesting medical information. The amount of the check may vary, depending on how much information is requested. If the check is not included, the physician should request a fee on the basis of the length of the report before sending in the completed report form. The fee is required before completion of the form or payment may not be received. Be extremely accurate when abstracting medical information from the patient's record. Abbreviations on the chart must be understood and only the requested information should be provided. If the form has questions about high blood pressure, kidney infection, or heart problems, the patient could be prohibited from obtaining life, health, or mortgage insurance if the answers are derogatory. If a patient tests positive for human immunodeficiency virus (HIV), legal counsel may

be necessary because some state laws allow information on HIV infection and acquired immunodeficiency syndrome (AIDS) to be given only to the patient or to the patient's spouse. In some states it is illegal to require a blood test for HIV antibodies, a urinalysis for HIV, or an HIV antigen test as a condition of coverage. It also may be illegal to question applicants about HIV status or prior symptoms of and treatment for AIDS or other forms of immune deficiency. A separate release of information is necessary before any information can be released regarding an HIV/AIDS patient.

In some situations, it is preferable to submit a narrative report dictated by the physician instead of completing the form, which has numerous check-off columns and no space for comments. It may be necessary to attach a copy of an operative, pathology, laboratory, or radiology report and an electrocardiogram (ECG) tracing.

A "Please Read" note should be placed on the insurance questionnaire to have the physician check it over thoroughly before signing it and to ensure that the information is accurate and properly stated.

An insurance company may ask a copy service to visit your office to photocopy the patient's record. Usually this is done at the convenience of the office staff and an appointment should be made. The insurance company should be reminded that an authorization form signed by the patient is necessary to release medical information. An appropriate fee for this service is charged and quoted at the time of the telephone request. The physician should review the records in advance to ensure that they are in proper order.

REVIEW AND AUDIT OF HEALTH RECORDS

Internal Review

Prospective Review

The first type of internal review is a **prospective review,** also termed *prebilling audit* or *review,* which is done *before* billing is submitted. This may be done by some medical practices daily, weekly, or monthly.

Stage 1 of a prospective review is done to verify that completed encounter forms match patients seen according to the appointment schedule and have been posted on the daysheet. A prospective review is begun by obtaining the encounter forms and locating the dates in question for the review in the appointment schedule, printing the schedule as verification. The appointment schedule is then compared with the encounter forms to match patients for the date in question. Next, check to see if all charges (procedures or services) have been posted on the daysheet or daily transaction register.

---

*Chabner D-E: *The language of medicine,* ed 10, St Louis, 2014, Saunders; Leonard PC: *Building a medical vocabulary,* ed 8, St Louis, 2012, Elsevier.

Stage 2 of a prospective review is done to verify that all procedures or services and diagnoses listed on the encounter form match data on the insurance claim form. To perform this stage, use the completed claim form or print an insurance billing worksheet. Match the information on the claim or worksheet with the date of service, procedure or service, and diagnosis on the encounter form. It is possible that one or more diagnoses may not match. A common reason is because an active diagnosis has not been entered in the computer system and the computer defaults to the last diagnosis given for an established patient. Another problem occurs when the diagnosis is not linked to the procedure. Such problems must be found before billing and corrected before claims are printed.

Retrospective Review

The second type of internal review is called a **retrospective review,** which is done after billing insurance carriers. A coder or insurance billing specialist may be asked to perform a retrospective review to determine whether there is a lack of documentation. To accomplish this, pull 15 to 20 health records per provider from the past 2 to 4 months at random. The following are recommended internal audit tools:
- Internal record review worksheets
- Current procedure code book
- Current diagnostic code book
- Current Healthcare Common Procedure Coding System (HCPCS) code book
- Medical dictionary
- Abbreviation reference book
- Drug reference book (for example, *Physicians' Desk Reference* or drug reference for nurses)
- Laboratory reference book
- Provider's manual for insurance program or plan
- Insurance carrier's newsletters

Forms similar to the Internal Record Review Form shown in Figures 4-13 to 4-18 later in this chapter may be used as tools to gather information from the patient's record, laboratory reports, pathology reports, radiology reports, operative reports, and other diagnostic tests. If the physician's documentation is inadequate, errors or deficiencies will appear as the review is being conducted. You will discover that doing an internal review of this type is not an exact science and critical thinking skills are put to use. Because documentation guidelines and code policies are updated and refined periodically, it is extremely important to read and keep bulletins from all insurance carriers, especially those from the local fiscal Medicare intermediary. Advise the physician of any new requirements. This resource may be the only notification of changes unless you routinely attend local or national workshops.

EXTERNAL REVIEWS

An external review is an audit of medical and financial records at the request of a physician, outside contractor, insurance company, or external reviewer as part of the practice's compliance plan. It may be done by a Medicare representative to investigate suspected fraud or abusive billing practices.

External audits can be performed as **prepayment audits** (prospective) or as retrospective audits. When a physician is placed on a prepayment audit review by an insurance company, each time the physician submits a claim, the claim is pended by the insurance carrier and there is a request that the physician submit a copy of his or her medical record to support the claim. Upon receipt of the medical record, the insurance carrier will review the record and determine whether the claim should be paid or not. This process can be very timely and can have a significant impact on the practice's cash flow.

Retrospective audits are performed by insurance carriers after a claim has been paid. If it is determined that incorrect payment was made, a request will be made for monies to be refunded.

Most insurance companies perform routine audits on unusual billing patterns, such as the same diagnosis code for every visit or billing the same procedure code repeatedly. Additional red flags to auditors are lack of documentation for hospital admissions, canned template documentation, illegible documentation, blank documentation, or tests documented but not performed. Insurance companies have computer software programs capable of editing and screening insurance claims to identify billing excesses or potential abuses before payment is rendered. Insurance carriers may hire undercover agents who visit physicians' offices if overuse and abuse of procedure codes are suspected. Physicians who charge excessive fees are routinely audited by most carriers. Carriers spot-check by sending questionnaires to patients and asking them if they received medical care from Dr. Doe to verify the services rendered. The answers are then compared with what the physician billed. Many insurance companies have installed antifraud telephone hotlines or billing question telephone lines for patients. Investigations can result from such calls, depending on the circumstances. Tips also come from peer review organizations, state licensing boards, whistle-blowing physicians, former staff members, and patients. If there is any suspicion of fraud, the insurance company will notify the medical practice, specify a date and time at which they will come to the office, and indicate which records they wish to audit (Figure 4-5).

Investigators question the patient, look at the documentation in the medical record, and interview the staff and all

Continued

EXTERNAL REVIEWS—cont'd

physicians who have participated in the care of the patient. Points are awarded if documentation is present. Auditors also look at appointment books and add up the hours the physician sees patients on any given day when a medical practice uses time-based procedure codes when submitting insurance claims.

Audit Prevention

Health Insurance Portability and Accountability Act (HIPAA) Compliance Program

As discussed in Chapter 2, HIPAA was created in 1996 by the Department of Health and Human Services (DHHS) Office of the Inspector General (OIG) to combat fraud and abuse, to protect workers so they could obtain and maintain health insurance if changing or losing a job, and to establish a medical savings account. The Act also developed the concept of compliance planning as related to clinical documentation. OIG and DHHS, as well as the Health Care Compliance Association (HCCA) and many other health care agencies, have asked physicians to voluntarily develop and implement compliance programs. OIG published guidelines to assist a physician and his or her staff in establishing a medical practice's compliance program to enhance documentation for Medicare cases as well as for all patients seen by the physician. The purposes of a compliance program are to reduce fraudulent insurance claims and to provide quality care to patients.

A *compliance program* is composed of policies and procedures to accomplish uniformity, consistency, and conformity in medical record keeping that fulfills official requirements. If a medical practice experiences an external Medicare audit, DHHS OIG and the Department of Justice (DOJ) consider that the medical practice made a reasonable effort to avoid and detect misbehavior if a compliance plan has been in place. When errors are found and a determination is made that fraud did occur, an existing compliance program shows a good faith effort that the medical practice is committed to ethical and legal business. There is no single best compliance program because every medical practice is different. The components of a compliance program are outlined in Chapter 2. A compliance program must be tailored to fit the needs of each medical practice depending on its corporate structure, mission, size, and employee composition. The statutes, regulations, and guidelines of the federal and state health insurance programs, as well as the policies and procedures of the private health plans, should be integrated into every medical practice's compliance program. The ultimate goals are to improve quality of services and control of claims submission and to reduce fraud, waste, abuse, and the cost of health care to federal, state, and private health insurers.

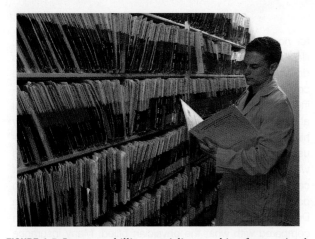

FIGURE 4-5 Insurance billing specialist searching for a patient's chart in the files to pull records for an external audit.

Software Edit Checks

An *edit check* is a good audit prevention measure to have in place because the software program automatically screens transmitted insurance claims and electronically examines them for errors and conflicting code entries. There must be correct use of diagnostic and procedural codes. If the diagnosis does not match the service provided, the claim will be thrown out by the edit check of the computer

program. It is equally important that everything involved in patient care be well documented so that selected diagnostic and procedural codes are supported.

In subsequent chapters, you will obtain further knowledge on what needs to be documented in relation to diagnostic and procedure codes.

Subpoena

Subpoena literally means "under penalty." In legal language, it is a writ requiring the appearance of a witness at a trial or other proceeding. Strictly defined, a **subpoena duces tecum** requires the witness to appear and bring or send certain records "in his possession." For a *subpoena duces tecum* for health information to be valid under the HIPAA Privacy Rule, it must be accompanied by a court order or the covered entity must receive satisfactory assurance from the party seeking the information that reasonable efforts have been made to ensure that the individual who is the subject of the protected health information (PHI) requested has been given notice of the request or that the party seeking the information has made reasonable efforts to secure a qualified protective order that meets the requirements of the HIPAA Privacy Rule. A subpoena is a legal document signed by a judge or an attorney in the name of a judge. In cases in which a pretrial of evidence or deposition is set up, the subpoena may be issued by a notary public, in which event it is called a *notary subpoena*. If an attorney signs it, he or she must attest it in the name of a judge, the court clerk, or other proper officer.

It is possible for a state investigator to subpoena patient records and then file administrative charges against the physician, not because of the practice of shoddy medicine but rather because the case was inadequately documented for the treatment provided. Health records also may be subpoenaed as proof in a medical malpractice case. Complete documentation and well-organized patient records help to establish a strong defense in a medical professional liability claim.

Subpoena Process

A subpoena must be personally served or handed to the prospective witness or keeper of the health records. The acceptance of a document by someone authorized to accept it is the equivalent of personal service. The subpoena cannot be left on a counter or desk. Never accept a subpoena or give records to anyone without the physician's prior authorization. The medical office should designate one person as keeper of the health records. If the subpoena is only for health records or financial data, the representative for the specific doctor can usually accept it and the physician will not be called to court.

If a physician is on vacation and there is no designated keeper of the records, tell the deputy that the physician is not in and cannot be served. Suggest that the deputy contact the physician's attorney and relay this information.

The medical office is given a prescribed time in which to produce the records. It is not necessary to show them at the time the subpoena is served unless the court order so states. The attorney usually employs a person or copy service to copy records that are under subpoena. At the time the subpoena is served, a date is usually agreed on when the representative will return and copy the portion of the record that is named in the subpoena. Often only the portion of the health record requested is removed from the original chart and put in a copy folder. Items such as the patient registration information sheet, encounter form, and explanation of benefits should not be included. You may also telephone the attorney who sent the subpoena and ask whether the records can be mailed. If so, mail them by certified mail with return receipt requested. Retain a copy of the records released. You will have to appear in court if specified in the subpoena. Verify with the court that the case is actually on the calendar. If you do not appear, you are in contempt of court and subject to a penalty, possibly several days in jail.

Retention of Records

In an electronic system, health records are stored in the computer. Paper-based records either are stored in color-coded file folders containing a collection of paper documents or reside in multiple electronic databases displayed in a variety of formats via computer access. Many practices have a combination of both paper records and electronic records to consider when they are creating a records retention policy. Regardless of the system used, general guidelines must be followed to record information correctly, use it according to law, and retain it.

Health Records

Preservation of health records is governed by federal, state, and local laws. The HIPAA Administrative Simplification Rules require a covered entity to retain required documentation for 6 years from the date of its creation or the date when it last was in effect, whichever is later. HIPAA requirements preempt state laws if they require shorter periods. Your state may require a longer retention period; the law that is most stringent is the law that should be adhered to.

Although the HIPAA Privacy Rule does not include medical record retention requirements, it does require that covered entities apply appropriate administrative, technical, and physical safeguards to protect the privacy of medical records and other PHI for whatever period is maintained by a covered entity, including through disposal.

The CMS does not have requirements for EMRs and retention periods may vary depending on state law. However, the CMS does maintain that the medical record needs to be in its original form or in a legally reproduced form, which may be electronic, so that medical records may be reviewed and audited by authorized entities. Providers must have a medical record system that ensures that the record may be accessed and retrieved promptly. Guidance concerning record retention after these time periods should be obtained through legal advice based on laws applicable to the state in which the practice resides.

Effective December 1, 2006, changes to the Federal Rules of Civil Procedure make requests for electronic data a standard part of the discovery process during federal lawsuits. This includes health records, accounting documents, cellphone records, instant messaging, and electronic mail that might be needed for future litigation.

Under the federal False Claims Act, proof materials for the establishment of evidence, such as x-ray films, laboratory reports, and pathologic specimens, probably should be kept indefinitely in the event of a legal inquiry. Calendars, appointment books, and telephone logs also

Table 4-2	Records Retention Schedule	
TEMPORARY RECORD	**RETENTION PERIOD (YR)**	**PERMANENT RECORD (RETAINED INDEFINITELY)**
Accounts receivable (patient ledger)	7	
Appointment sheets	3	Accounts payable records
Bank deposit slip (duplicate)	1	Bills of sale for important purchases (or until you no longer own them)
		Canceled checks and check registers
Bank statements and canceled checks	7	Capital asset records
		Cash books
Billing records (for outside service)	7	Certified financial statements
Cash receipt records	6	Contracts
		Correspondence, legal
Contracts (expired)	7	Credit history
Correspondence, general	6	Deeds, mortgages, contracts, leases, and property records
Daysheets (balance sheets and journals)	5	Equipment guarantees and records (or until you no longer own them)
Employee contracts	6	Income tax returns and documents
Employee time records	5	Insurance policies and records
Employment applications	4	Journals (financial)
Insurance claim forms (paid)	3	
Inventory records	3	
Invoices	6	Health records (active patients)
Health records (expired patients)	5	Health records (inactive patients)
Medicare financial records	7	
Remittance advice documents	8	Mortgages
Payroll records	7	Property appraisals and records
Petty cash vouchers	3	Telephone records
Postal and meter records	1	X-ray films
Tax worksheets and supporting documents	7	Year-end balance sheets and general ledgers

should be filed and stored. Cases that involve radiologic injury claims (for example, leukemia from radiation) may begin running the statute of limitations after discovery of the injury, which may occur 20 or 30 years after radiation exposure. Recommended retention periods for paper files are shown in Table 4-2.

A person's health record may be of value not only to himself or herself in later years but also to the person's children. In some states, a minor may file suit after he or she has attained legal age, for any act performed during childhood that the person believes to be wrong or harmful. Sometimes a suit may be permitted even 2 to 3 years after the child has reached legal age. Thus it is important to keep records until patients are 3 to 4 years beyond the age of majority. Under HIPAA, records must be retained for 2 years after a patient's death. However, the Medicare Conditions of Participation states that all hospitals must retain medical records in their original or legally produced form for a period of 5 years. Therefore it is advised that deceased patients' charts be kept for at least 5 years.

In a paper-based system, it is recommended that documents that are no longer needed be shredded. Electronic storage media, such as CD-ROMs, floppy disks, or flash drives, containing confidential or sensitive information may be disposed of only by approved destruction methods. These methods should be outlined in the practice's HIPAA Security Plan and may include burning, shredding, pulverizing, or some other approach that renders the media unusable, such as **degaussing,** which uses electromagnetic fields to erase data, or **zeroization** programs (a process of writing repeated sequences of ones and zeros over the information). CD-ROMs and other media storage devices must be physically destroyed.

Some practices prefer to use medical record storage companies. When records are disposed of by a professional company, be sure to obtain a certificate of destruction verifying the method of disposal. This document should be indefinitely retained in the office. Maintain a log of destroyed records showing the patient's name, Social Security number, date of last visit, and treatment.

Financial Documents

According to income tax regulations on record retention, accounting records should be kept a minimum of 4 to 7 years (following the due date for filing the tax return or the date the tax is paid, whichever is later). Always contact an accountant before discarding records that may determine tax liability. Suggested retention periods are listed in Table 4-2.

A federal regulation mandates that assigned claims for Medicaid and Medicare be kept for 7 years; the physician

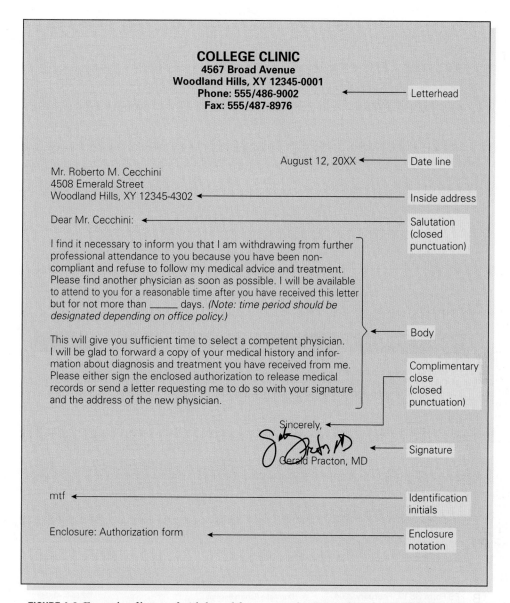

FIGURE 4-6 Example of letter of withdrawal from a case that is typed in modified block style with closed punctuation and special notations (placement of parts of letter).

is subject to auditing during that period. The federal False Claims Amendments Act of 1986 allows a claim of fraud to be made up to 10 years from the date a violation was committed. Documentation must be available for inspection and copying by the investigator of the false claim (31 US Code §3729–3733).

HIPAA Documents

Under HIPAA guidelines, Notice of Privacy Practices (NPP) acknowledgements signed by patients must be kept on file for at least 6 years from the date of the creation or the date it was last in effect.

Termination of a Case

A physician may wish to withdraw formally from further care of a patient because of patient noncompliance (for example, the patient discharged the physician, did not follow instructions, did not take the recommended medication, failed to return for an appointment, discontinued payment on an overdue account). A physician may terminate a contract by doing the following:

● Sending a letter of withdrawal (Figure 4-6) to the patient by certified mail with return receipt (Figure 4-7) so that proof of termination is in the patient's health record.

● Sending a letter of confirmation of discharge when the patient states that he or she no longer desires care (Figure 4-8). This should also be sent certified mail with return receipt requested.

● Sending a letter confirming that the patient left the hospital against medical advice or the advice of the physician. If there is a signed statement in the patient's hospital records to this effect, it is not necessary to

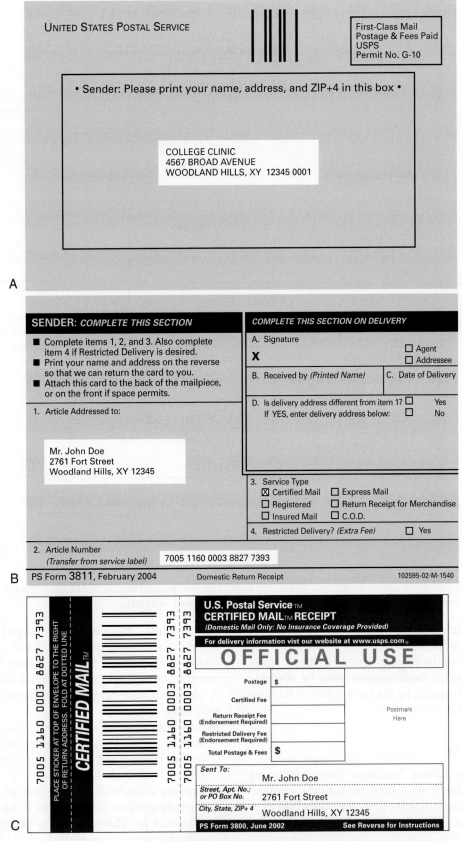

FIGURE 4-7 A and **B** (front and back), A domestic return receipt Postal Service Form 3811. **C,** Receipt for certified mail Postal Service Form 3800 (US Government Printing Office) shown completed.

COLLEGE CLINIC
4567 Broad Avenue
Woodland Hills, XY 12345-0001
Phone: 555/486-9002
Fax: 555/487-8976

September 3, 20XX

Mrs. Gregory Putnam
4309 North E Street
Woodland Hills, XY 12345-4398

Dear Mrs. Putnam:

This will confirm our telephone conversation today during which you discharged me from attending you as your physician in your present illness. In my opinion, your medical condition requires continued treatment by a physician. If you have not already obtained the services of another physician, I suggest you do so without further delay.

You may be assured that, upon your written authorization, I will furnish your new physician with information regarding the diagnosis and treatment you have received from me.

Very truly yours,

Gerald Procton, MD

mtf

FIGURE 4-8 Letter to confirm discharge by patient. Letter typed in modified block style (dateline, complimentary close, and signature indented) with open punctuation (no commas after salutation or complimentary close).

send a letter. If a letter is sent, a copy of the letter and return signature card from the post office must be filed with the patient's records.

If a noncompliant patient refuses a certified dismissal letter and it is returned unopened, file the returned letter and refusal notice in the patient's chart. Then, in a plain envelope, send another copy of the letter to the patient. Document the date and time it was posted and the location of the mailbox used. Place these data in the patient's chart and initial them; after 10 days, telephone the patient to confirm receipt of the correspondence. If the patient denies receiving it, read it over the telephone. In most regions, this will provide immunity against abandonment of a case, which is the discontinuance of medical care by a provider without proper notice.

Prevention of Legal Problems

After reading Chapters 1 through 4, you have discovered there are many instances in which an insurance billing specialist must be careful in executing job duties to avoid the possibility of a lawsuit. A summary of guidelines for prevention of lawsuits is shown in Box 4-1.

DOCUMENTATION GUIDELINES FOR EVALUATION AND MANAGEMENT SERVICES

Earlier in this chapter, E/M services were introduced. The following information is a more extensive look at the documentation requirements for those services. As the insurance billing specialist gains experience, an additional task that he or she may be faced with is auditing of E/M services to ensure that the guidelines for the services are met. Understanding the documentation requirements for E/M services is essential in effectively carrying out that task.

The AMA and CMS developed documentation guidelines for CPT E/M services. These were released to Medicare carriers by CMS in 1995 and then modified and released again in 1997. The guidelines were

---

Box 4-1   Prevention of Lawsuits: Guidelines for Insurance Billing Specialists

1. Keep information about patients strictly confidential.
2. Obtain proper instruction and carry out responsibilities according to the employer's guidelines.
3. Keep abreast of general insurance program guidelines, annual coding changes, and medical and scientific progress to help when handling insurance matters.
4. Secure proper written consent in all cases before releasing a patient's protected health information (PHI) for purposes other than treatment, payment, or routine health care operations (TPO).
5. Do not refer to consent or acknowledgment forms as "releases." Use the word "consent" or "authorization" forms as required by law. This also produces a better understanding of the document to be signed.
6. Ensure that documentation of patient care in the health record corresponds with billing submitted on the insurance claim.
7. Exercise good judgment in what you write and how you word e-mails because they do not give security against confidentiality.
8. Make every effort to reach an understanding with patients in the matter of fees by explaining what services will be received and what the "extras" may be. For hospital cases, it is advisable to explain that the fee the physician charges is for his or her services only and that charges for the bed or ward room, operating room, laboratory tests, and anesthesia will be billed separately in addition to the physician's charges.
9. Do not discuss other physicians with the patient. Patients sometimes invite criticism of the methods or results of former physicians. Remember that you are hearing only one side of the story.
10. Tell the physician immediately if you learn that a new patient (NP) is still under treatment by another physician and did not give this information to the physician during the initial interview.
11. Do not compare the respective merits of various forms of therapy and refrain from discussing patients' ailments with them. Patients come to talk to the physician about their symptoms and you may give them incorrect information. Let the physician make the diagnosis. Otherwise, you may seriously embarrass the physician, yourself, or both of you.
12. Report a physician who is doing something illegal that you are aware of. You can be held responsible for being silent and failing to report an illegal action.
13. Say nothing to anyone except as required by the attorney of the physician or by the court if litigation is pending.
14. Be alert to hazards that may cause injury to anyone in the office and report such problems immediately.
15. Consult the physician before turning over a delinquent account to a collection agency.
16. Be courteous in dealing with patients and always act in a professional manner.

---

developed because Medicare has an obligation to those enrolled to ensure that services paid for have been provided and are medically necessary. Auditors determined that some medical practices should improve their quality of documentation.

Some physicians have adopted the 1995 guidelines and others use those introduced in 1997. A modification of the 1997 guidelines is under consideration but has not been released as of this edition. Insurance claims processors and auditors may use the 1995 or 1997 guidelines when doing an internal or external chart audit to determine whether the reported services were actually rendered and the level of service was warranted. When significant irregular reporting patterns are detected, a review is conducted.

The following is a brief overview of documentation guidelines for medical services.
1. The health record should be accurate, complete **(detailed),** and legible.
2. The documentation of each patient encounter should include or provide reference to the following:
   a. **Chief complaint** or reason for the encounter
   b. Relevant history
   c. Examination
   d. Findings
   e. Prior diagnostic test results
   f. Assessment, clinical impression, or diagnosis
   g. Plan for care
   h. Date and legible identity of the health care professional
3. The reason for the encounter or chief complaint should be stated and the rationale should be documented or inferred for ordering diagnostic and other ancillary services (x-rays or laboratory tests).
4. Past and present diagnoses, including those in the prenatal and intrapartum period that affect the newborn, should be accessible to the treating or consulting physician.
5. Appropriate health risk factors should be identified.
6. The patient's progress, response to, and changes in treatment, planned follow-up care and instructions, and diagnosis should be documented.
7. Patient refusal to follow medical advice should be documented and a letter sent to the patient about this noncompliance. Information on termination of a case is discussed earlier in this chapter.
8. Procedure and diagnostic codes reported on the health insurance claim form or billing statement should be supported by the documentation in the health record and be at a level sufficient for a clinical peer to determine whether services have been coded accurately.
9. The confidentiality of the health record should be fully maintained, consistent with the requirements of medical ethics and the law.

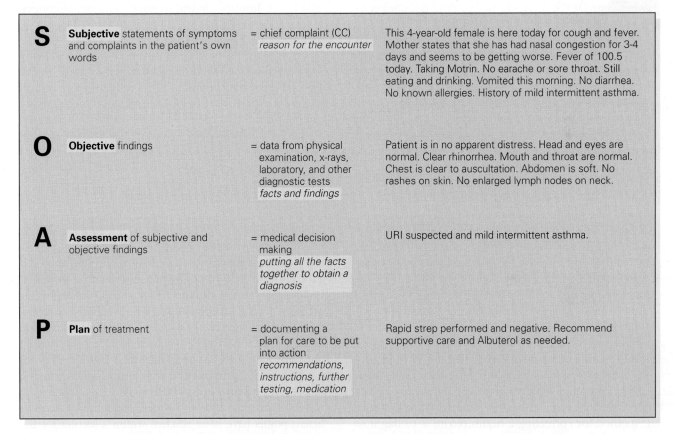

SIGNATURE LOG

Name	Position	Signature or Initials	
Ann M. Arch	Receptionist	*Ann M. Arch*	*AMA*
John Bortolonni	Office manager	*John Bortolonni*	*JB*
Gerald Practon, MD	Provider	*Gerald Practon, MD*	*GP*
Rachel Vasquez, CPC	Insurance billing specialist	*Rachel Vasquez, CPC*	*RV*
Mary Ann Worth	Clinical medical assistant	*Mary Ann Worth*	*MAW*

FIGURE 4-9 Example of a signature log for paper-based records.

S	**Subjective** statements of symptoms and complaints in the patient's own words	= chief complaint (CC) *reason for the encounter*	This 4-year-old female is here today for cough and fever. Mother states that she has had nasal congestion for 3-4 days and seems to be getting worse. Fever of 100.5 today. Taking Motrin. No earache or sore throat. Still eating and drinking. Vomited this morning. No diarrhea. No known allergies. History of mild intermittent asthma.
O	**Objective** findings	= data from physical examination, x-rays, laboratory, and other diagnostic tests *facts and findings*	Patient is in no apparent distress. Head and eyes are normal. Clear rhinorrhea. Mouth and throat are normal. Chest is clear to auscultation. Abdomen is soft. No rashes on skin. No enlarged lymph nodes on neck.
A	**Assessment** of subjective and objective findings	= medical decision making *putting all the facts together to obtain a diagnosis*	URI suspected and mild intermittent asthma.
P	**Plan** of treatment	= documenting a plan for care to be put into action *recommendations, instructions, further testing, medication*	Rapid strep performed and negative. Recommend supportive care and Albuterol as needed.

FIGURE 4-10 In a paper-based system, explanation of the acronym SOAP used as a format for progress notes defining subjective and objective information, the assessment, and the treatment plan.

10. Each chart entry must have a date and signature or electronic validation, including the title or position of the person verifying the documentation. If a signature log has been established for paper-based records, initials are acceptable, because these would be defined in the log (Figure 4-9). A *signature log* is a list of all staff members' names, job titles, signatures, and initials. In regard to paperless documents, if passwords are used for restricted access, electronic or digital signatures may be acceptable.

11. Charting procedures for progress notes should be standardized. For office visits, the majority of physicians in a paper-based system use a method called the *SOAP style of documentation* (Figure 4-10). Some physicians prefer to document using a narrative or more detailed descriptive style when creating a medical report such as history and physical report, operative report, radiologic report, or pathology report. Whatever method is used, the provider must ensure that it is detailed enough to support current documentation requirements.

12. Treatment plans should be written. Include patient and family education and specific instructions for follow-up. Treatment must be consistent with the working diagnosis.

13. Medications prescribed and taken should be listed, specifying frequency and dosage.

14. *Request* for a consultation from the attending or treating physician and the *need* for consultation must be documented. The consultant's opinion and any services ordered or performed must be documented and communicated to the requesting physician. Remember the four Rs: There must be a *requesting* physician and the consultant must *render* an opinion and send a *report*. The requesting physician must document the *reason* for a consult in the patient's medical record. A possible fifth R of consultations is *return*. The consulting physician must return the patient to the requesting physician for treatment of the problem so that no transfer of care is shown.

HIPAA Compliance Alert **SIGNATURE REQUIREMENTS**

Ensure that all health record entries are signed or electronically verified by the physician (author) with his or her title or position. This provides clear evidence that the physician reviewed the note and/or ensures that he or she is aware of all test results (normal and abnormal). Documented physician review of test results can be factored when determining appropriate coding levels for services.

15. Record a patient's failure to return for needed treatment by noting it in the health record, in the appointment book, and on the financial record or ledger card. Follow up with a telephone call or send a letter to the patient advising him or her that further treatment is indicated.

16. Corrections: For electronic health records, the software program should make an electronic record entry permanent when originally completed and authenticated. To make a correction, note that a section is in error with the date and time and enter the correct information with a notation of when and why the physician changed the entry. Authenticate the correction via electronic signature and date. Never delete or key over incorrect data in a computerized file. Another method for correcting a health record is to flag it as amended or obsolete and create an addendum either typed as a separate document or for a chart note inserted below in the next space available. For paper-based records, use a permanent, not water-soluble, ink pen (legal copy pen) to cross out an incorrect entry on a patient's record. Mark it with a single line and write the correct information, then date and initial the entry. Never erase, white out, or use self-adhesive paper over any information recorded on a patient record.

17. Document all laboratory tests ordered in the health record. When the report is received, the physician should initial the report, indicating that it has been read. Each documentation is considered an element and allows a point if the record undergoes an **external audit.**

18. Ask the physician for approval for a different code before transmitting the claim to the insurance carrier

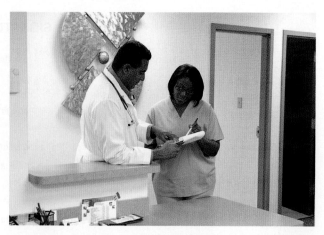

FIGURE 4-11 Insurance billing specialist checking information with the physician before recording it on the insurance claim.

when the insurance billing specialist questions any procedure or diagnostic codes marked on the encounter form (Figure 4-11). Retain all records until you are positive that they are no longer necessary by conforming to federal and state laws as well as to the physician's wishes.

Audit Point System

As discussed in Chapter 2, if a provider has submitted insurance claims for payments that are deemed to be fraudulent or inappropriate by the government, an investigation may be conducted in the form of an audit of the practice's financial records. A point system is used while reviewing each patient's health record during the performance of an audit. Points are awarded only if documentation is present for elements required in the health record. Each provider of service documents every health record differently; therefore a patient's history may contain details for more than one body area or organ system. Thus when gathering points, it is possible that the auditor may shift the points from the **history of present illness (HPI)** to those required for the review of the patient's body systems. In addition, when sufficient points have been reached within a section for the level of code used in billing, no further documentation is counted for audit purposes, even though there may be additional comments for other body systems. This point system is used to show where deficiencies occur in health record documentation. It is also used to evaluate and substantiate proper use of diagnostic and procedural codes.

Health maintenance organizations, preferred provider organizations, and all private carriers have the right to claim refunds in the event of accidental (or intentional) miscoding. However, Medicare has the power to levy fines and penalties and exclude providers from the Medicare program. If improper coding patterns exist and are not corrected, the provider of service will be penalized. Insurance carriers go by the rule "If it is not documented, then it was not performed" and they have the right to deny reimbursement.

Hospital number: 00-83-06

Scott, Aimee

Rex Rumsey, MD

HISTORY

CHIEF COMPLAINT: Pain and bleeding after each bowel movement
for the past 3 to 4 months.

PRESENT ILLNESS: This 68-year-old white female says she usually has three
bowel movements a day in small amounts, and there
has been a change in the last 3 to 4 months in frequency, size,
and type of bowel movement. She has slight burning pain
and irritation in the rectal area after bowel movements. The
pain lasts for several minutes, then decreases in intensity. She
has had no previous anorectal surgery or rectal infection.
She denies any blood in the stool itself or associated
symptoms. Bright red blood occurs after stools have passed.

PAST HISTORY:
ILLNESSES: The patient had polio at age 8 from which she has made a
remarkable recovery. Apparently, she was paralyzed in both
lower extremities and now has adequate use of these. She
has no other serious illnesses.

ALLERGIES: ALLERGIC TO PENICILLIN. She denies any other drug
or food allergies.
MEDICATIONS: None.
OPERATIONS: Right inguinal herniorrhaphy 25 years ago.

SOCIAL HISTORY: She does not smoke or drink. She lives with her husband
who is an invalid and for whom she cares. She is a retired
former municipal court judge.

FAMILY HISTORY: One brother died of cancer of the throat (age 59), and
another has cancer of the kidney (age 63).

REVIEW OF SYSTEMS:
SKIN: No rashes or jaundice.
HEENT: Head normocephalic. Normal TMs. Normal hearing. Pupils
equal, round, reactive to light. Deviated septum. Oropharynx
clear.
CR: No history of chest pain, shortness of breath, or pedal
edema. She has had some mild hypertension in the past but
is not under any medical supervision nor is she taking any
medication for this.
GI: Weight is stable. See present illness.
OB-GYN: Gravida II Para II. Climacteric at age 46, no sequelae.
EXTREMITIES: No edema.
NEUROLOGIC: Unremarkable.

mtf
D: 5-17-20XX
T: 5-20-20XX

_____
Rex Rumsey, MD

FIGURE 4-12 Example of medical report done in modified block format showing the six components of a history.

Documentation of History

The following documentation information for the history and physical examination is based on the 1997 Medicare guidelines. The history includes the chief complaint (CC); history of present illness (HPI); **review of systems (ROS);** and past, family, or social history (PFSH).* The extent of the history depends on clinical judgment and the nature of the presenting problems. Each history includes some or all of the elements shown in Figure 4-12.

_____
*These abbreviations in the history portion of the report may vary, depending on the physician who is dictating (for example, PI for present illness, PH for past history, FH for family history).

Chief Complaint

The CC is a concise statement, usually in the patient's own words, describing the symptom, problem, condition, diagnosis, physician-recommended return, or other factor that is the reason for the encounter. *The CC is a requirement for all levels of history:* **problem focused (PF), expanded problem focused (EPF),** detailed, and comprehensive; these are described below.

History of Present Illness

The HPI is a chronologic description of the development of the patient's present illness from the first sign or symptom or from the previous encounter to the present. If the physician is unable to obtain a sufficient diagnosis for the patient's condition, the health record documentation must reflect this. The history may include one or more of the following eight descriptive elements:

1. Location—Area of the body where the symptom is occurring
2. Quality—Character of the symptom or pain (burning, gnawing, stabbing, fullness)
3. Severity—Degree of symptom or pain on a scale from 1 to 10 (Severity also can be described with terms such as *severe, slight,* and *persistent.*)
4. Duration—How long the symptom or pain has been present and how long it lasts when the patient has it
5. Timing—When the pain or symptom occurs (for example, morning, evening, after or before meals)
6. Context—The situation associated with the pain or symptom (for example, dairy products, big meals, activity)
7. Modifying factors—Things done to make the symptom or pain worse or better (for example, "If I eat spicy foods I get heartburn but if I drink milk afterward the pain is not as bad.")
8. Associated signs and symptoms—The symptom or pain and other things that happen when the symptom or pain occurs (for example, chest pain leads to shortness of breath)

Medicare Conditions for History of Present Illness (HPI) for Evaluation and Management Services		
Brief HPI		Documentation of one to three of the eight elements
Extended HPI	1995	Documentation of four or more elements
	1997	Documentation of four or more elements or the status of at least three chronic or inactive conditions

Review of Systems

An ROS is an inventory of body systems obtained through a series of questions that is used to identify signs or symptoms that the patient might be experiencing or has experienced. Checklists are permitted but if a body system is not considered, it should be crossed out. For an ROS, the following systems are recognized: constitutional symptoms (for example, fever, weight loss), eyes, ears, nose, mouth, throat, cardiovascular, respiratory, gastrointestinal, genitourinary, musculoskeletal, integumentary (skin or breast), neurologic, psychiatric, endocrine, hematologic and lymphatic, and allergic and immunologic.

Medicare Conditions for Review of Systems (ROS) for Evaluation and Management Services		
Problem-pertinent ROS		Positive and pertinent negatives for the system related to the problem
Extended ROS		Positive and pertinent for two to nine systems
Complete ROS	1995	Review 10 or more systems or a problem-pertinent ROS plus a notation that all other systems appear negative
	1997	Review of at least 10 systems

Past, Family, and Social Histories

The PFSH consists of a review of three areas:

1. **Past history (PH)**—The patient's past experiences with illnesses, operations, injuries, and treatments
2. **Family history (FH)**—A review of medical events in the patient's family, including diseases that may be hereditary or place the patient at risk
3. **Social history (SH)**—An age-appropriate review of past and current activities (for example, smokes, consumes alcohol)

Medicare Conditions for Past, Family, or Social History (PFSH) for Evaluation and Management Services		
Pertinent PFSH		Specific information for one of the history areas directly related to the problem identified in the history of present illness (HPI)
Complete PFSH	1995	Specific information for two or three history areas
	1997	Specific information for one specific item from two of the three history areas for established patient services (office, home care) and emergency room (ER) services. One specific item from each of the three history areas for new patient services (office, home care); hospital observation, inpatient services, initial care; consults; comprehensive nursing facility assessments

Documentation Review or Audit Worksheet

The documented history elements are counted and totaled (Figure 4-13, *A*). The health record should describe one to three elements of the present illness for a brief level of HPI. At least four elements of the HPI or the status of at least three chronic or inactive conditions is required for the extended level of HPI. Only two of three history elements are required for certain types of cases, such as newborns or subsequent hospital care. Figure 4-13, *B*,

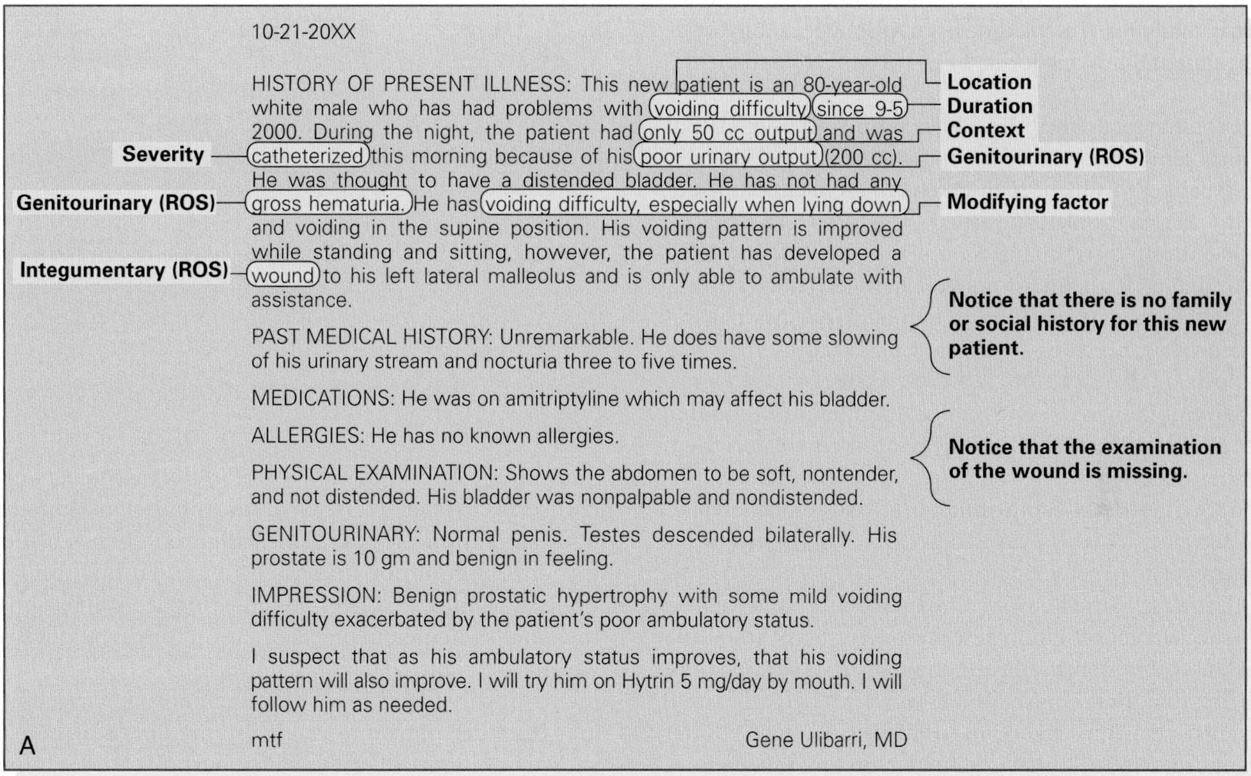
10-21-20XX

HISTORY OF PRESENT ILLNESS: This new patient is an 80-year-old white male who has had problems with voiding difficulty since 9-5 2000. During the night, the patient had only 50 cc output and was catheterized this morning because of his poor urinary output (200 cc). He was thought to have a distended bladder. He has not had any gross hematuria. He has voiding difficulty, especially when lying down and voiding in the supine position. His voiding pattern is improved while standing and sitting, however, the patient has developed a wound to his left lateral malleolus and is only able to ambulate with assistance.

PAST MEDICAL HISTORY: Unremarkable. He does have some slowing of his urinary stream and nocturia three to five times.

MEDICATIONS: He was on amitriptyline which may affect his bladder.

ALLERGIES: He has no known allergies.

PHYSICAL EXAMINATION: Shows the abdomen to be soft, nontender, and not distended. His bladder was nonpalpable and nondistended.

GENITOURINARY: Normal penis. Testes descended bilaterally. His prostate is 10 gm and benign in feeling.

IMPRESSION: Benign prostatic hypertrophy with some mild voiding difficulty exacerbated by the patient's poor ambulatory status.

I suspect that as his ambulatory status improves, that his voiding pattern will also improve. I will try him on Hytrin 5 mg/day by mouth. I will follow him as needed.

mtf Gene Ulibarri, MD

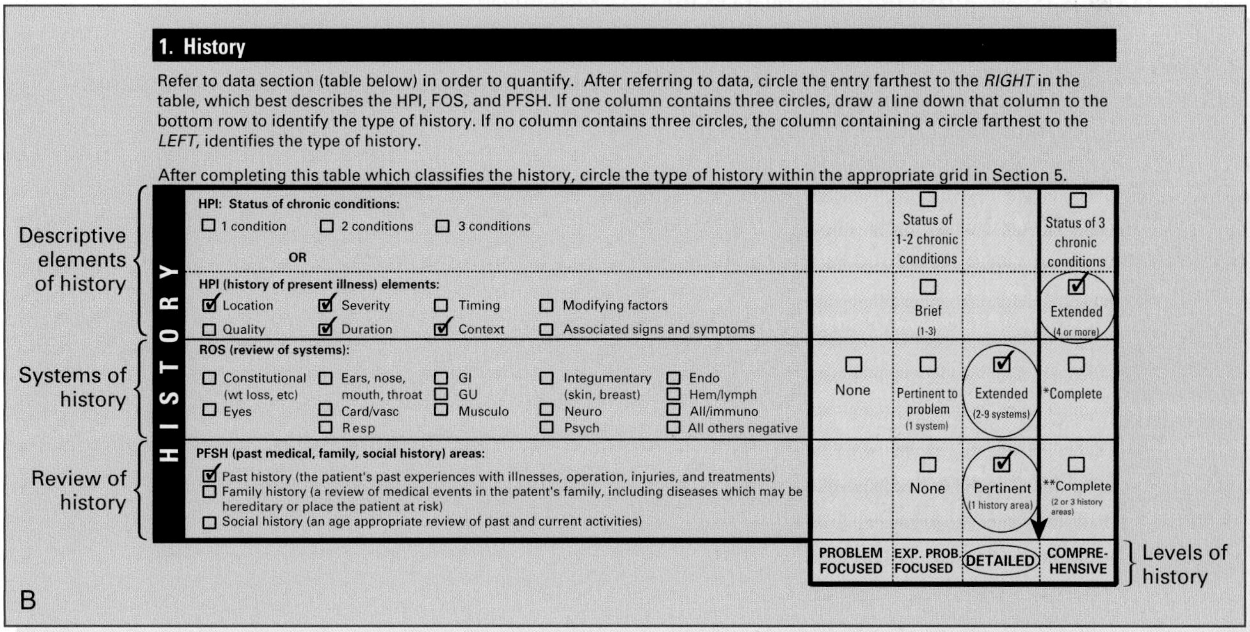
1. History

Refer to data section (table below) in order to quantify. After referring to data, circle the entry farthest to the *RIGHT* in the table, which best describes the HPI, FOS, and PFSH. If one column contains three circles, draw a line down that column to the bottom row to identify the type of history. If no column contains three circles, the column containing a circle farthest to the *LEFT*, identifies the type of history.

After completing this table which classifies the history, circle the type of history within the appropriate grid in Section 5.

HISTORY				
HPI: Status of chronic conditions: ☐ 1 condition ☐ 2 conditions ☐ 3 conditions OR		☐ Status of 1-2 chronic conditions		☐ Status of 3 chronic conditions
HPI (history of present illness) elements: ☑ Location ☑ Severity ☐ Timing ☐ Modifying factors ☐ Quality ☑ Duration ☑ Context ☐ Associated signs and symptoms		☐ Brief (1-3)		☑ Extended (4 or more)
ROS (review of systems): ☐ Constitutional (wt loss, etc) ☐ Eyes ☐ Ears, nose, mouth, throat ☐ Card/vasc ☐ Resp ☐ GI ☐ GU ☐ Musculo ☐ Integumentary (skin, breast) ☐ Neuro ☐ Psych ☐ Endo ☐ Hem/lymph ☐ All/immuno ☐ All others negative	☐ None	☐ Pertinent to problem (1 system)	☑ Extended (2-9 systems)	☐ *Complete
PFSH (past medical, family, social history) areas: ☑ Past history (the patient's past experiences with illnesses, operation, injuries, and treatments) ☐ Family history (a review of medical events in the patent's family, including diseases which may be hereditary or place the patient at risk) ☐ Social history (an age appropriate review of past and current activities)		☐ None	☑ Pertinent (1 history area)	☐ **Complete (2 or 3 history areas)
	PROBLEM FOCUSED	EXP. PROB. FOCUSED	DETAILED	COMPRE-HENSIVE

FIGURE 4-13 **A,** Documentation from a health record highlighting elements required for the history. **B,** Review or audit sheet Section I with check marks and circled elements shows how the history in the example is declared as detailed. This shows two of three history components *(arrow)* used for the purpose of determining the assignment of a procedure code at the appropriate level of service.

shows Section I of the review or audit sheet that depicts the history containing the HPI, ROS, and PFSH. The check marks and circled element in the HPI (Section I) of the figure relate to the case illustrated.

The types of E/M services for the history are based on four levels of history. However, the ROS and PFSH must be totaled before the final decision on the level of service is assigned. The four levels of history may be defined as follows:

1. Problem focused (PF)—Chief complaint; brief HPI or problem
2. Expanded problem focused (EPF)—Chief complaint; brief HPI; problem-pertinent system review
3. Detailed (D)—Chief complaint; extended HPI; problem-pertinent system review extended to include a review of a limited number of additional systems; *pertinent* PFSH directly related to the patient's problems
4. Comprehensive (C)—Chief complaint; extended HPI; ROS that is directly related to the problem identified in the history of the present illness, plus a review of all additional body systems; *complete* PFSH

In the ROS, the body systems are counted and totaled. The health record should describe one system of the ROS for a *pertinent to problem level*. For an *extended level*, two to nine systems are required. For a *complete level*, at least 10 organ systems must be reviewed and documented. Refer to Figure 4-13, *B*, for a visual understanding of Section I of the review or audit sheet. The check marks and circled element in the ROS (Section I) of the figure relate to the case illustrated.

The PFSH review areas are counted and totaled. The health record must contain at least one history area for a *detailed extended level* and specific items from two of the three history areas for a *comprehensive level* of PFSH. Refer to Figure 4-13, *B*, for a visual guide of the PFSH in Section I of the review or audit sheet. Note the difference in the number of required elements for new versus established patients and the circled element for the case in question.

A vertical line is drawn down the right four columns that contain the most elements to determine the history level. The elements of HPI, ROS, and PFSH must at least be met or may exceed the criteria determined for a PF, EPF, D, or C history level.

Figure 4-14 shows a gradual advancement of the elements that are required for each level of history. One to three elements must be met to qualify for a given level of history.

Elements Required for Each Level of History			
Present History	Review of Systems	Past, Family, or Social History	Levels of History
Brief	N/A	N/A	Problem focused
Brief problem	Problem pertinent	N/A	Expanded focused
Extended	Extended	Pertinent	Detailed
Extended	Complete	Complete	Comprehensive

FIGURE 4-14 Elements required for each type of history. One to three elements must be met to qualify for a given level of history.

Documentation of Examination
Physical Examination

The physical examination (PE or PX) is objective in nature; that is, it consists of the physician's findings by examination or test results. Figure 4-15 is an illustration of a multiorgan system examination from the CMS Documentation Guidelines for 1997 that shows the details (elements) of examination for each body area within the genitourinary system. The three circled elements of the genitourinary system and one circled element of the gastrointestinal system relate to the case shown in Figure 4-13, *A*. For purposes of examination, the following body areas and organ systems are recognized.

Organ Systems and Body Areas—Elements of Examination

Constitutional (vital signs, general appearance)
Eyes
Ears, nose, mouth, and throat
Neck
Respiratory
Cardiovascular
Chest, including breasts and axillae
Gastrointestinal (abdomen)
Genitourinary (male)
Genitourinary (female)
Lymphatic
Musculoskeletal
Skin
Neurologic
Psychiatric

Note: In addition, any reasons for not examining a particular body area or system should be listed.

MULTIORGAN SYSTEM EXAMINATION REQUIREMENTS (SHADED)
CONTENT and DOCUMENTATION

Level of Exam	Perform and Document
Problem Focused	One to five elements identified by a bullet.
Expanded Problem Focused	At least six elements identified by a bullet.
Detailed	At least twelve elements identified by a bullet.
Comprehensive	Perform all elements identified by a bullet; document every element in every shaded box and at least one element in every unshaded box.

Genitourinary

System/Body Area	Elements of Examination
Constitutional	• Measurement of **any three of the following seven** vital signs: 1) sitting or standing blood pressure, 2) supine blood pressure, 3) pulse rate and regularity, 4) respiration, 5) temperature, 6) height, 7) weight (may be measured and recorded by ancillary staff) • General appearance of patient *(e.g., development nutrition, body habitus, deformities, attention to grooming)*
Neck	• Examination of neck *(e.g., masses, overall appearance, symmetry, tracheal position, crepitus)* • Examination of thyroid *(e.g., enlargement, tenderness, mass)*
Respiratory	• Assessment of respiratory effect *(e.g., intercostal retractions, use of accessory muscles, diaphragmatic movement)* • Auscultation of lungs *(e.g., breath sounds, adventitious sounds, rubs)*
Cardiovascular	• Auscultation of heart with notation of abnormal sounds and murmurs • Examination of peripheral vascular system by observation *(e.g., swelling, varicosities)* and palpation *(e.g., pulses, temperature, edema, tenderness)*
Chest (breasts)	See genitourinary (female)
Gastrointestinal (abdomen)	⊙ Examination of abdomen with notation of presence of masses or tenderness • Examination for presence or absence of hernia • Examination of liver and spleen • Obtain stool sample for occult blood test when indicated
Genitourinary (male)	• Inspection of anus and perineum Examination (with or without specimen collection for smears and cultures) of genitalia including: • Scrotum *(e.g., lesions, cysts, rashes)* • Epididymides *(e.g., size, symmetry, masses)* ⊙ Testes *(e.g., size, symmetry, masses)* • Urethral meatus *(e.g., size, location, lesions, discharge)* ⊙ Penis *(e.g., lesions, presence or absence of foreskin, foreskin retractability, plaque, masses, scarring, deformities)* Digital rectal examination including: ⊙ Prostate gland *(e.g., size, symmetry, nodularity, tenderness)* • Seminal vesicles *(e.g., symmetry, tenderness, masses, enlargement)* • Sphincter tone, presence of hemorrhoids, rectal masses
Genitourinary (female) Includes at least seven of the eleven elements to the right identified by bullets:	• Inspection and palpation of breasts *(e.g., masses or lumps, tenderness, symmetry, nipple discharge)* • Digital rectal examination including sphincter tone, presence of hemorrhoids, rectal masses Pelvic examination (with or without specimen collection for smears and cultures) including: • External genitalia *(e.g., general appearance, hair distribution, lesions)* • Urethral meatus *(e.g., size, location, lesions, prolapse)* • Urethra *(e.g., masses, tenderness, scarring)* • Bladder *(e.g., fullness, masses, tenderness)* • Vagina *(e.g., general appearance, estrogen effect, discharge, lesions, pelvic support, cystocele, rectocele)* • Cervix *(e.g., general appearance, lesions, discharge)* • Uterus *(e.g., size, contour, position, mobility, tenderness, descent or support)* • Adnexa/parametria *(e.g., masses, tenderness, organomegaly, nodularity)* • Anus and perineum

Genitourinary (continued)

System/Body Area	Elements of Examination
Lymphatic	• Palpation of lymph nodes in neck, axillae, groin and/or other location
Skin	• Inspection and/or palpation of skin and subcutaneous tissue *(e.g., rashes, lesions, ulcers)*
Neurological/psychiatric	Brief assessment of mental status including: • Orientation to time, place, and person • Mood and affect *(e.g., depression, anxiety, agitation)*

Skin

System/Body Area	Elements of Examination
Constitutional	• Measurement of **any three of the following seven** vital signs: 1) sitting or standing blood pressure, 2) supine blood pressure, 3) pulse rate and regularity, 4) respiration, 5) temperature, 6) height, 7) weight (may be measured and recorded by ancillary staff) • General appearance of patient *(e.g., development, nutrition, body habitus, deformities, attention to grooming)*
Eyes	• Inspection of conjunctivae and lids
Ears, nose, mouth, and throat	• Inspection of lips, teeth and gums • Examination of oropharynx *(e.g., oral mucosa, hard and soft palates, tongue, tonsils, and posterior pharynx)*
Neck	• Examination of thyroid *(e.g., enlargement, tenderness, mass)*
Gastrointestinal (abdomen)	• Examination of liver and spleen • Examination of anus for condyloma and other lesions
Lymphatic	• Palpation of lymph nodes in neck, axillae, groin and/or other location
Extremities	• Inspection and palpation of digits and nails *(e.g., clubbing, cyanosis, inflammation, petechiae, ischemia, infections, nodes)*
Skin	• Palpation of scalp and inspection of hair of scalp, eyebrows, face, chest, pubic area (when indicated) and extremities • Inspection and/or palpation of skin and subcutaneous tissue *(e.g., rashes, lesions, ulcers, susceptibility in and presence of photo damage)* in **eight of the following ten areas:** 1) head including face, 2) neck, 3) chest including breasts and axilla, 4) abdomen, 5) genitalia, groin, buttocks, 6) back, 7) right upper extremity, 8) left upper extremity, 9) right lower extremity, 10) left lower extremity Note: For the comprehensive level, the examination of all eight anatomic areas must be performed and documented. For the three lower levels of examination, each body area is counted separately. For example, inspection and/or palpation of the skin and subcutaneous tissue of the head and neck extremities constitutes two areas. • Inspection of eccrine and apocrine glands of skin and subcutaneous tissue with identification and location of any hyperhidrosis, chromhidroses or bromhidrosis
Neurological/psychiatric	Brief assessment of mental status including: • Orientation to time, place and person • Mood and affect *(e.g., depression, anxiety, agitation)*

FIGURE 4-15 Review or audit worksheet of a general multiorgan system physical examination that shows the details (elements) of examination for each body area and system. Circled bullets relate to the example case shown in Figure 4-13, *A. (Audit Tool format developed by Iowa Medical Society, IMS Services, West Des Moines, Iowa, 1998.)*

SECTION II

Four elements identified

	General Multisystem Exam		Single Organ System Exam
E X A M	1-5 elements identified by •	⟨PROBLEM FOCUSED⟩	1-5 elements identified by •
	≥6 elements identified by •	EXPANDED PROBLEM FOCUSED	≥6 elements identified by •
	≥2 elements identified by •	DETAILED	≥12 elements identified by • EXCEPT
	from 6 areas/systems OR		≥9 elements identified by •
	≥12 elements identified by •		for eye and psychiatric exams
	from at least 2 areas/systems		
	≥2 elements identified by •	COMPREHENSIVE	Perform all elements identified by • ;
	from 9 areas/systems		document all elements in shaded
			boxes; document ≥1 element in
			unshaded boxes.

FIGURE 4-16 Review or audit worksheet Section II for a general multisystem physical examination and single organ system examination. The circled item relates to a problem-focused examination for the example case (see Figure 4-13, *A*) for coding purposes. (*Audit Tool format developed by Iowa Medical Society, IMS Services, West Des Moines, Iowa, 1998.*)

Types of Physical Examination

When performing an **internal review** of a patient's health record, the number of elements identified by bullets is counted for each system and a total is obtained. The total is circled on Section II of the review or audit sheet as shown in Figure 4-16 for the case illustrated.

The levels of evaluation and management services are based on four types of physical examination (PE):
1. Problem focused (PF)—A limited examination of the affected body area or organ system. The health record should describe one to five elements identified by a bullet in Figure 4-16 for a problem-focused level of PE.
2. Expanded problem focused (EPF)—A limited examination of the affected body area or organ system and other symptomatic or related organ systems. At least six elements identified by a bullet in Figure 4-16 are required for an expanded problem focused level of PE.
3. Detailed (D)—An extended examination of the affected body areas and other symptomatic or related organ systems. At least two elements identified by a bullet in Figure 4-16 from each of six areas and body systems *or* at least 12 elements identified by a bullet in two or more areas and body systems are required for a detailed level of PE.
4. Comprehensive (C)—A general multisystem examination or complete examination of a single organ system. For a comprehensive level of PE, all elements must be identified by a bullet in Figure 4-16 and documentation must be present for at least two elements identified by a bullet from each of nine areas and body systems.

The extent of the examination and what is documented range from limited examinations of single body areas to general multisystem or complete single-organ system examinations, depending on clinical judgment and the nature of the presenting problem.

1995 Medicare Conditions for the Physical Examination for Evaluation and Management Services

Problem focused (PF)	Documentation of only one body area or organ system
Expanded problem focused (EPF) or detailed	Documentation of up to seven systems (the affected body area or system plus up to six additional systems)
Comprehensive	Documentation of eight or more systems

1997 Medicare Conditions for General Multisystem Examination

PF	One to five elements identified by a bullet in one or more body or system areas
EPF	At least six elements identified by a bullet in one or more body or system areas
Detailed	At least two elements identified by a bullet from each of six body areas or systems or at least 12 elements in two or more body or system areas
Comprehensive	Perform all elements for each selected system or body area; document at least two elements identified by a bullet from each of at least nine body or system areas

Documentation of Medical Decision Making

Medical decision making (MDM) is a health care management process done after performing a history and physical examination on a patient that results in a plan of treatment. It is based on establishing one or more diagnoses and/or selecting a management or treatment option, amount or complexity of data reviewed, and risk of complications or associated morbidity or mortality. *Morbidity* is a diseased condition or state, whereas *mortality* has to do with the number of deaths that occur in a given time or place.

Number of diagnoses or management options is based on the number and types of problems addressed during the visit, the complexity of establishing a diagnosis, and the number of management options that must be considered by the physician. For the case illustrated, the number of problems is 1, which equals 3 points (Figure 4-17, *top section*).

Amount or complexity of data to be reviewed is based on the types of diagnostic tests ordered or reviewed. A decision to obtain and review old health records or obtain history from sources other than the patient increases the amount and complexity of data to be analyzed. For the case illustrated, no points apply (see Figure 4-17, *middle section*).

Risk of complications, morbidity, or mortality is based on other conditions associated with the presenting problem known as the risk of complications, morbidity, or mortality as well as comorbidities, the diagnostic procedures, or the possible management options (treatment rendered—surgery, therapy, drug management, services, and supplies). **Comorbidity** means underlying disease or other conditions present at the time of the visit. In determining the level of risk, the element (presenting problem, diagnostic procedure ordered, or management options selected) that has the highest level (minimal, low, moderate, or high) is used.

To discover whether the level of risk is minimal, low, moderate, or high, bulleted elements are marked on the review or audit sheet (Figure 4-18). For the case illustrated, the elements fall within the moderate level of risk category.

To conclude the internal review of a patient's health record, a level must be determined by the health care provider from one of four types of MDM: **straightforward (SF), low complexity (LC), moderate complexity (MC),** and **high complexity (HC).** The bottom portion of Figure 4-18 shows the results obtained from Parts A, B, and C highlighted. For the case illustrated, the number of diagnoses is declared *multiple*, there are no *data to review*, and the risk of complications is *moderate;* therefore a *moderately complex* level of decision making has been assigned to be used for coding and billing purposes.

COMPLEXITY

SECTION III A AND B

A

NUMBER OF DIAGNOSES OR TREATMENT OPTIONS

Problems to exam physician	Number X points = Result		
Self-limited or minor (stable, improved, or worsening)	Max = 2	1	
Est. problem (to examiner); stable, improved		1	
Est. problem (to examiner); worsening		2	
New problem (to examiner); no additional workup planned	Max = 1 1	3	3
New prob. (to examiner); add. workup planned		4	
	TOTAL	3	

Bring total to line A in final result for complexity.

B

AMOUNT AND/OR COMPLEXITY OF DATA TO BE REVIEWED

Data to be reviewed	Points
Review and/or order of clinical lab tests	1
Review and/or order of tests in the radiology section of CPT	1
Review and/or order of tests in the medicine section of CPT	1
Discussion of test results with performing physician	1
Decision to obtain old records and/or obtain history from someone other than patient	1
Review and summarization of old records and/or obtaining history from someone other than patient and/or discussion of case with another health care provider	2
Independent visualization of image, tracing or specimen itself (not simply review of report)	2
TOTAL	0

Bring total to line B in final result for complexity.

Draw a line down the column with 2 or 3 circles and circle decision making level OR draw a line down the column with the center circle and circle the decision making level.

A	Number diagnoses or treatment options	≤1 Minimal	2 Limited	3 Multiple	≥4 Extensive
B	Amount and complexity of data	≤1 Minimal or low	2 Limited	3 Moderate	≥4 Extensive
C	Highest risk	Minimal	Low	Moderate	High
	Type of decision making	Straight-forward	Low complex	Moderate complex	High complex

Note: The wound was not a considering factor in the medical decision making.

FIGURE 4-17 Section III of the review or audit worksheet. *Part A:* Number of diagnoses or treatment options. *Part B:* Amount or complexity of data to be reviewed. *Lower one third:* Used to compile the results obtained from Parts A, B, and C (see Figure 4-16) to determine the level of medical decision making (MDM). In Figure 4-13, *A and B,* for the example case, circled points and words relate to a moderately complex level of decision making for coding and billing purposes. (*Audit Tool format developed by Iowa Medical Society, IMS Services, West Des Moines, Iowa, 1998.*)

SECTION III

C

RISK OF COMPLICATIONS AND/OR MORBIDITY OR MORTALITY

Level of risk	Presenting problem(s)	Diagnostic procedure(s) ordered	Management options selected
MINIMAL	• One self-limited or minor problem *(e.g., cold, insect bite, tinea corporis)*	• Laboratory tests requiring venipuncture • Chest x-rays • KOH prep • EKG/EEG • Urinalysis • Ultrasound *(e.g., echo)*	• Rest • Gargles • Elastic bandages • Superficial dressings
LOW	• Two or more self-limited or minor problems • One stable chronic illness *(e.g., well-controlled hypertension, non-insulin dependent diabetes, cataract, BPH)* • Acute uncomplicated illness or injury *(e.g., cystitis, allergic rhinitis, simple sprain)*	• Physiologic test not under stress *(e.g., pulmonary function tests)* • Non-cardiovascular imaging studies with contrast *(e.g., barium enema)* • Superficial needle biopsies • Clinical laboratory tests requiring arterial puncture • Skin biopsies	• Over-the-counter drugs • Minor surgery with no identified risk factors • Physical therapy • Occupational therapy • IV fluids without additives
MODERATE	• *One* or more *chronic illnesses* with mild exacerbation, progression or side effects of treatment • Two or more stable chronic illnesses • Undiagnosed new problem with uncertain prognosis *(e.g., lump in breast)* • Acute illness with systemic symptoms *(e.g., pyelonephritis, pneumonitis, colitis)* • Acute complicated injury *(e.g., head injury with brief loss of consciousness)*	• Physiologic test under stress *(e.g., cardiac stress test, fetal contraction stress test)* • Diagnostic endoscopies with no identified risk factors • Deep needle or incisional biopsy • Cardiovascular imaging studies with contrast and no identified risk factors *(e.g., arteriogram, cardiac cath)* • Obtain fluid from body cavity *(e.g., lumbar puncture, thoracentesis, culdocentesis)*	• Minor surgery with identified risk factors • Elective major surgery (open percutaneous or endoscopic) with no identified risk factors • *Prescription drug management* • Therapeutic nuclear medicine • IV fluids with additives • Closed treatment of fracture or dislocation without manipulation
HIGH	• One or more chronic illnesses with severe exacerbation, progression or side effects of treatment • Acute or chronic illnesses or injuries that may pose a threat to life or bodily function *(e.g., multiple trauma, acute MI, pulmonary embolus, severe respiratory distress, progressive severe rheumatoid arthritis, psychiatric illness with potential threat to self or others, peritonitis, acute renal failure)* • An abrupt change in neurological status *(e.g., seizure, TIA, weakness, sensory loss)*	• Cardiovascular imaging studies with contrast with identified risk factors • Cardiac electrophysiological tests • Diagnostic endoscopies with identified risk factors • Discography	• Elective major surgery (open, percutaneous, or endoscopic) with identified risk factor • Emergency major surgery (open, percutaneous, or endoscopic) • Parenteral controlled substances • Drug therapy requiring intensive monitoring for toxicity • Decision not to resuscitate or de-escalate care because of poor prognosis

FIGURE 4-18 Section III, Part C, of the review or audit worksheet used for determining the level of risk. The highlighted areas relate to a moderate level of risk for the example case (see Figure 4-13, *A*) for coding purposes. *(Audit Tool format developed by the Iowa Medical Society, IMS Services, West Des Moines, Iowa, 1998.)*

PROCEDURE 4-1

Abstract Data from a Health Record

OBJECTIVE: To abstract data from a health record for composing a letter or completing an insurance claim form or other related billing document

EQUIPMENT/SUPPLIES: Patient's health record, form to insert abstracted data, and pen or pencil

DIRECTIONS: Follow these steps, including rationales to learn this skill, and practice it by completing the *Workbook* assignment.

1. What is the patient's diagnosis? This gives the reason for the visit.
2. What professional services were provided?
3. Did the patient undergo surgery? What surgical procedure was performed?
4. Read and review the patient's health record thoroughly to learn all parts of the case. In the *Workbook* assignment, use the check-off list and answer the questions to assist you in understanding all aspects of the patient's health record.
5. What medication was prescribed, if any?
6. Does the patient have any past history (PH) indicating anything of importance?
7. Does the patient have any food or drug allergies? If so, what are they?
8. What is the etiology (cause) of the present disease, injury, or illness?
9. What is the prognosis (prediction) for this patient's medical condition?
10. What laboratory tests were ordered or performed?
11. What x-rays were ordered or obtained?
12. Define every abbreviation listed in the patient's chart notes or history and physical examination.
13. What documents assisted you in locating the answers to these questions?

PROCEDURE 4-2

Compose, Format, Key, Proofread, and Print a Letter

OBJECTIVE: To compose, format, key, proofread, and print a letter using common business letter style guidelines

EQUIPMENT/SUPPLIES: Computer, printer, letterhead stationery, envelope, attachments (documents, if necessary), thesaurus, English dictionary, medical dictionary, and pen or pencil

DIRECTIONS: Follow these steps, including rationales to learn this skill, and practice it by completing the *Workbook* assignments.

1. Assemble materials, determine the recipient's address, and decide on modified or full block letter style or format.
2. Turn on the computer and select the word processing program. Open a blank document.
3. Key the date line beginning at least three lines below the letterhead and make certain it is in the proper location for the chosen style.
4. Double-space down, insert the inside address, and make certain it is in the proper location for the chosen style. Select a style to insert an attention line, if necessary.
5. Double-space down and key the salutation. Use either open or mixed punctuation. A business letter should include a title and the person's last name.
6. Double-space down and enter the reference line ("Re:" or "Subject:") in the location for the chosen letter style. This assists the recipient in identifying the contents of the letter immediately.
7. Double-space down and key the body (content) of the letter in single-space. Make certain the paragraph style is proper for the format chosen. Double-space between paragraphs. Save the letter to the computer hard drive every 15 minutes.
8. Proofread the letter on the computer screen for composition and format.
9. Proofread the letter on the computer screen for typographic, spelling, grammatical, and mechanical errors. Use the spell-check feature of the word processing program and reference books to check for correct spelling, meaning, or usage.
10. Key the second page heading (name, page number, and date) in vertical or horizontal format if a second page is necessary.
11. Key a complimentary close and make certain it is in the proper location for the chosen style.
12. Drop down four spaces and key the sender's name and title or credentials as printed on the letterhead because handwritten signatures may be difficult to read.
13. Double-space down and insert the sender's reference initials in uppercase letters and the typist's initials in lowercase letters, separating the two sets of initials with either a colon or a slash (for example, DLJ:md or DLJ/md).
14. Single- or double-space down to insert copy ("CC"), enclosure ("Enclosure" or "En"), or attachment notations.

PROCEDURE 4-2—cont'd

15. Double-space down to insert a postscript ("PS"), if necessary.
16. Save the file before printing a hard copy and proofread the letter once more. Make corrections, if necessary.
17. Print the final copy to be sent and proofread. Make a copy to be retained in the files in case it is necessary for future reference.
18. Save the file to a CD-ROM to be stored for future reference.

19. Prepare an envelope and use the format for optical scanning recommended by the US Postal Service. Insert special mailing instructions in the correct location on the envelope if sending by certified mail.
20. Clip attachments to the letter and give it to the physician for review and signature.

KEY POINTS

This is a brief chapter review, or summary, of the key issues presented. To further enhance your knowledge of the technical subject matter, review the key terms and key abbreviations for this chapter by locating the meaning for each in the Glossary at the end of this text, which appears in a section before the Index.

1. The key to substantiating procedure and diagnostic code selection for appropriate reimbursement is supporting documentation in the health record.
2. Paper-based offices are fading into the past and the EHR is gradually becoming the norm as the ability to share patient health records among other professionals who constitute the patient's health care team has become increasingly important.
3. Federal legislation has established programs to help the health care industry change to EMRs and has offered incentives to those who participate in the programs. These incentive programs will transition to disincentives for those who do not adopt EHRs over the next several years in the form of adjusted payments.
4. Every patient seen by the physician must have comprehensive legible documentation about what occurred during the visit for the following reasons: (1) avoidance of denied or delayed payments by insurance carriers investigating the medical necessity of services; (2) enforcement of medical record-keeping rules by insurance carriers requiring accurate documentation that supports procedure and diagnostic codes; (3) subpoena of health records by state investigators or the court for review; (4) defense of a professional liability claim.
5. Consultation and referral are not the same. A consultation service is rendered at the request of opinion or advice by another physician, whereas a referral is the transfer of the total or specific care of a patient for a known problem.

6. External and internal audit of medical records shows where deficiencies occur in health record documentation and substantiates proper use of diagnostic and procedural codes.
7. Health record abbreviations should be eliminated from the more vital sections, such as final diagnosis, operative notes, discharge summaries, and descriptions of special procedures.
8. An eponym should not be used when a comparable anatomic term can be used in its place.
9. Abstraction of technical information from patient records may be requested to complete insurance claim forms; when sending letters to justify a health insurance claim form; or when a patient applies for life, mortgage, or health insurance.
10. The two types of internal and external review of records are (1) prospective (prepayment) review (before billing insurance carrier) and (2) retrospective review (after billing insurance carrier).
11. An edit check is a good audit prevention measure because the software program automatically screens transmitted insurance claims and electronically examines them for errors and/or conflicting code entries.
12. When health records are subpoenaed, produce only the records requested and nothing more. Retain a copy of the records released.
13. HIPAA requires documents to be retained for 6 years from the date of creation or the date when it was last in effect, whichever is later. However, if your state requires a longer retention period, the law that is most stringent should be adhered to.
14. When a patient does not comply with physician or office policy, the physician may wish to withdraw formally from further care of the patient. The physician must send a formal letter of termination, or

withdrawal, by certified mail with return receipt to the patient.

15. In 1995 and 1997, the CMS introduced documentation guidelines to Medicare carriers to ensure that services paid for have been provided and were

medically necessary. Documentation must support the level of service and each procedure rendered.

16. The levels of E/M services selected by the provider must be supported through documentation of the chief complaint, HPI, ROS, PFSH, examination, and MDM.

💻 STUDENT ASSIGNMENT

✔ Study Chapter 4.

✔ Answer the fill-in-the-blank, multiple-choice, and true/false questions in the *Workbook* to reinforce the theory learned in this chapter and help prepare you for a future test.

✔ Complete the assignments in the *Workbook* to give you experience in reviewing patients' medical reports and records.

✔ Turn to the Glossary at the end of this text for a further understanding of the key terms and key abbreviations used in this chapter.

5

Diagnostic Coding

Linda Smith

OBJECTIVES

After reading this chapter, you should be able to:

1. Explain the reasons for and importance of coding diagnoses.
2. Describe the importance of matching the correct diagnostic code to the appropriate procedural code.
3. Differentiate between primary (first listed), principal, and secondary diagnoses and discuss admitting diagnoses.
4. Describe how medical necessity is supported by the diagnosis code.
5. Discuss the history of diagnostic coding.
6. Describe the transition from ICD-9-CM to ICD-10-CM, compare the processes for locating a code, and discuss the need for GEMs.
7. Discuss the benefits of the ICD-10 coding system and differentiate between ICD-10-CM and ICD-10-PCS.
8. Identify and describe the Alphabetic and Tabular Index of the ICD-10-CM coding manual.
9. Define and demonstrate an understanding of diagnostic code conventions, symbols, and terminology.
10. Apply general coding guidelines to translate written descriptions of conditions into diagnostic codes.
11. Apply chapter-specific coding guidelines to reporting of specific illnesses and conditions.
12. Relate additional coding guidelines specific to reporting of outpatient services.
13. Describe methods of becoming more familiar with codes commonly encountered in your office and discuss computer-assisted coding.
14. Anticipate future changes to the diagnosis coding system, known as ICD-11.

KEY TERMS

adverse effect
benign tumor
carcinoma in situ
chief complaint
combination code
computer-assisted coding
conventions
eponym
essential modifiers
etiology
Excludes 1
Excludes 2
external causes of morbidity

International Classification of Diseases, Ninth Revision, Clinical Modification
International Classification of Diseases, Tenth Revision, Clinical Modification
International Classification of Diseases, Tenth Revision, Procedure Coding System
intoxication
late effect
malignant tumor
medical necessity
metastasis

neoplasm
nonessential modifiers
not elsewhere classifiable
not otherwise specified
Official Guidelines for Coding and Reporting
placeholder
poisoning
primary diagnosis
principal diagnosis
secondary diagnosis
sequela
syndrome
Uncertain Behavior
Z codes

KEY ABBREVIATIONS

AHA	CPT	ICD-10-PCS	NOS
AHIMA	DM	ICD-11	WHO
CAC	GEM	MRI	
CC	ICD-9-CM	NCHS	
CM	ICD-10-CM	NEC	

Service to Patients

Good customer service to the patient involves knowing the diagnostic coding guidelines in both inpatient and outpatient settings to obtain the proper payment from third-party payers.

Two basic principles are as follows:
- Diagnostic coding must be accurate because payment for inpatient services rendered to a patient may be based on the diagnosis.
- In the outpatient setting, the diagnosis code must correspond to the treatment or services rendered to the patient or payment may be denied.

DIAGNOSIS CODING FOR OUTPATIENT PROFESSIONAL SERVICES

This chapter deals with diagnostic coding for outpatient professional services. The rules for coding inpatient cases can differ and are covered more thoroughly in Chapter 17 of this text. Medical practices and outpatient facilities use diagnostic codes on insurance claims to explain the reason the patient has sought health care services from a provider. Using a code eliminates the need to write out the diagnostic description on the claim form.

Diagnostic codes must be used on all claims and must be accurately assigned. Appropriate diagnosis coding can mean the financial success or failure of a medical practice. To assign diagnosis codes accurately, the insurance billing specialist must have knowledge of the current approved coding guidelines and a working knowledge of medical terminology. This includes having knowledge of anatomy and physiology, clinical disease processes, and pharmacology words. The consequences of inaccurate assignment of diagnostic codes are many. For example, claims can be denied, fines or penalties can be levied, sanctions can be imposed, and the physician's level of reimbursement for claims may be affected.

Assigning a Diagnosis Code

All documented diagnoses that affect the current status of the patient may be assigned a code. This includes conditions that exist at the time of the patient's initial contact with the physician as well as conditions that develop subsequently and affect the treatment received. Diagnoses that relate to a patient's previous medical problem but have no bearing on the patient's present condition are not coded. The Centers for Medicare and Medicaid Services (CMS) and the National Center for Health Statistics (NCHS), two departments within the Department of Health and Human Services (DHHS), provide a set of Official Guidelines for Coding and Reporting. These guidelines are a set of rules that have been developed to provide instructions. Adherence to the guidelines when assigning diagnosis codes is required under the Health Insurance Portability and Accountability Act (HIPAA).

Sequencing of Diagnostic Codes

Diagnosis codes must be sequenced correctly on an insurance claim so that the chronology of patient care events (main reason for the office visit) and the severity of the disease can be understood. The primary surgical procedure code must always be listed first on the claim form for full reimbursement and the secondary procedures, which are paid at less than 100% of allowable, must be listed in succession. The correct diagnostic code must be matched to the appropriate surgical or medical procedure code for third-party reimbursement.

When submitting insurance claims for patients seen in a physician's office or an outpatient hospital setting, the **primary diagnosis** (first listed condition) is the main reason for the encounter. In an office setting, this is related to the **chief complaint (CC).** The **secondary diagnosis,** listed subsequently, may contribute to the condition or define the need for a higher level of care but is not the underlying cause. The underlying cause of a disease is referred to as the **etiology** and is sequenced in the first position. The **principal diagnosis,** used in inpatient hospital coding, is the diagnosis obtained after study that prompted the hospitalization. It is possible for the primary and principal diagnosis codes to be the same. The concept of a "principal diagnosis" is only applicable to inpatient hospital claims or cases. Box 5-1 outlines the important considerations when you come across the same or similar phrases related to the diagnosis because these represent two very different coding scenarios in the outpatient versus inpatient settings.

Box 5-1 Primary versus Principal Diagnosis

	PRIMARY DIAGNOSIS	PRINCIPAL DIAGNOSIS
Definition	Main reason (diagnosis, condition, chief complaint) for the encounter/visit in the health record that is responsible for services provided.	Condition established after study that prompted the hospitalization.
Location	Outpatient setting only (physician office visits and hospital-based outpatient services).	Inpatient setting only.
"Probable," "Suspected," "Questionable," "Rule Out," or "Working Diagnosis"	May not report "Probable," "Suspected," "Questionable," "Rule Out," or "Working Diagnosis." Codes that describe symptoms and signs, as opposed to diagnoses, are acceptable for reporting purposes when a related definitive diagnosis has not been established (confirmed) by the provider.	Code the condition as if it existed or was established at the time of discharge if it is documented on the final diagnostic statement as "Probable," "Suspected," "Questionable," "Rule Out," or "Working Diagnosis."

Admitting Diagnoses

Some diagnostic codes are considered questionable when used as the first diagnosis on admission of a patient to the hospital (for example, obesity, benign hypertension, controlled diabetes). The inpatient admission diagnosis may be expressed as one of the following:

1. One or more significant findings (symptoms or signs) representing patient distress or abnormal findings on examination.
2. A diagnosis established on an ambulatory care basis or previous hospital admission.
3. An injury or poisoning.
4. A reason or condition not classifiable as an illness or injury, such as pregnancy in labor or follow-up inpatient diagnostic tests.

When a physician makes hospital visits, code the reason for the visit, which might not necessarily be the reason the patient was admitted to the hospital (Example 5-1).

Medical Necessity

Medical necessity is defined as the "performance of services, supplies or procedures that are needed by the patient for the diagnosis or treatment of a medical condition. The services must be consistent with the diagnosis and in accordance with standards of medical practice, performed at the proper level of care and provided in the most appropriate setting."

Most health plans will not pay for health care services that they deem to be not medically necessary. The most common example is a cosmetic procedure, such as the injection of medications (such as Botox) to decrease facial wrinkles or tummy-tuck surgery. In those cases, an insurance company may reply to a claim submission with an explanation of benefits or remittance advice stating, "This procedure or item is not payable for the

Example 5-1

A patient is admitted to the hospital with chest pains and is being monitored in the cardiac telemetry unit. Upon examination, it is noted that the patient has an enlarged thyroid and an endocrinologist is asked to see the patient in consultation.

Reason for Hospital Admission	Reason for Hospital Visit by Endocrinologist
Chest pain	Enlarged thyroid

diagnosis as reported for lack of medical necessity." In addition to certain surgical procedures, other services have medical necessity restrictions and include most imaging services (for example, radiography, computed tomography, or magnetic resonance imaging [MRI]), cardiovascular services (for example, electrocardiograms, Holter monitors, echocardiography, Doppler imaging, or stress testing), neurologic services (for example, electroencephalography, noninvasive ultrasonography), many laboratory services, and vitamin B_{12} injections. It is important to know which procedures are diagnosis related and exactly which diagnosis relates to the procedure being billed. A reference book may be helpful in this situation and a number of manuals are available from commercial publishers. For cases dealing with the CMS, consult the regional fiscal intermediary's website for local coverage determinations (LCDs) and the federal government's website for national coverage determinations (NCDs), or download the manual that is updated quarterly.

INTERNATIONAL CLASSIFICATION OF DISEASES

Diagnosis coding is performed using the World Health Organization's (WHO's) International Classification of Diseases (ICD). The coding system classifies morbidity and mortality information for statistical purposes, indexing of hospital records by disease and operations, and data storage and retrieval.

History

From the earliest days of medical treatment, people have tried to name and classify diseases. The ICD had its beginning in England during the seventeenth century.

In 1948 the WHO developed the official version of the ICD in Geneva, Switzerland. The system was designed to compile and present statistical data on morbidity (disease) and mortality (death) rates and frequency. WHO assumed responsibility for preparing and publishing revisions to the coding system every 10 years. The United States began using the ICD to report causes of death and prepare mortality statistics in the latter half of the nineteenth century and hospitals began using the ICD in 1950 to classify and index diseases.

The eighth revision of the ICD was constructed in 1966 and was adapted for use in the United States in 1968 by the United States Public Health Service. This became known as ICDA-8 and served as the basis for coding diagnostic data for both official morbidity and mortality statistics in the United States.

In 1979 the ninth revision of the *International Classification of Diseases* (ICD-9) was published by the WHO. Passage of the Medicare Catastrophic Coverage Act in 1988 then placed requirements on physicians to submit appropriate diagnosis codes on all claims when billing for services provided to Medicare beneficiaries on or after April 1, 1989. The CMS designated **International Classification of Diseases, Ninth Revision, Clinical Modification (ICD-9-CM)** as the coding system physicians must use.

In 1992 the WHO published the tenth revision of the *International Classification of Diseases* (ICD-10). The NCHS further developed a clinical modification to the WHO's system, which is referred to as **International Classification of Diseases, Tenth Revision, Clinical Modification (ICD-10-CM)**. On January 16, 2009, the DHHS published the final rule in the *Federal Register* for adoption of the ICD-10 code set with an implementation date of October 1, 2015.

Transition from ICD-9-CM to ICD-10-CM

Because this is a transition period and some insurance programs may not adopt ICD-10-CM, the insurance billing specialist must be familiar with both ICD-9-CM and ICD-10-CM coding systems. The date of service will determine which coding system is used for reporting purposes. Additionally, any noncovered entities (those not covered by HIPAA, such as workers' compensation and

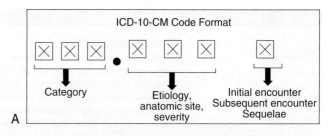

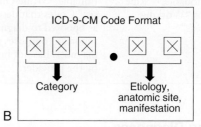

FIGURE 5-1 ICD-10-CM versus ICD-9-CM diagnostic code format. *(From Fordney MT: Fordney's medical insurance dictionary for billers and coders, St Louis, 2010, Elsevier.)*

auto insurance companies) are not required to implement ICD-10. However, it is in the noncovered entities' best interest to use the ICD-10 coding system due to the significant value of the increased detail of diseases.*

The process for locating a diagnosis code is the same in both coding systems. Coding manuals for both systems are organized similarly with an alphabetic index for locating the main term or condition treated. Both coding systems have a neoplasm and table of drugs and chemicals included in the alphabetic index. A tabular index is provided in both coding systems to verify the selected code.

The ICD-10-CM coding system exceeds previous versions of the ICD in the number of concepts and codes provided. The disease classification was expanded to include health-related conditions and to provide greater specificity through reporting at a sixth-digit level with a seventh-digit extension. The sixth and seventh characters are not optional and are required for use in recording the information documented in the clinical record. ICD-10-CM allows more code choices and requires greater documentation in the medical record (Figure 5-1).

The insurance billing specialist should maintain coding manuals for both ICD-9-CM and ICD-10-CM coding systems as reference. Many of the conventions and guidelines are the same for both coding systems; however, there are more extensive guidelines for ICD-10-CM. The appropriate conventions and Official Guidelines for the specific coding system (ICD-9-CM versus ICD-10-CM) being used should be referenced any time codes are selected to ensure accurate reporting.

---

*As of this printing, 39 states will accept ICD-10-CM codes on workers' compensation claims on October 1, 2015.

Crosswalks

To facilitate the coding process between ICD-9-CM and ICD-10-CM systems, a common translation tool referred to as general equivalence mappings (GEMs) was developed by CMS and the Centers for Disease Control and Prevention (CDC).

GEMs is a comprehensive translation tool that can be used to translate codes accurately and effectively. GEMs can be used to convert data from ICD-9 to ICD-10 and vice versa in a manner similar to foreign-language translation dictionaries (such as English to Spanish translation and Spanish to English translation). Mapping from ICD-10 to ICD-9 is referred to as *backward mapping*. Mapping from ICD-9 to ICD-10 is referred to as *forward mapping*.

Many software vendors have used GEMs to create crosswalk publications and software that are available and will facilitate cross-referencing between the two coding systems. Crosswalks are not exact but they can assist in finding appropriate code ranges for reporting purposes (Example 5-2).

ICD-10 DIAGNOSIS AND PROCEDURE CODES

There are many benefits associated with the adoption of the ICD-10 coding system. Benefits include:
● Much greater specificity, including laterality (which side of the body is affected) or ordinality of encounter (whether the care encounter is the patient's first for the condition)
● Expansion of clinical information and reduced cross-referencing
● Flexibility and ease of expandability of the coding system
● Updated medical terminology and classification of diseases
● The ability to compare mortality and morbidity data
● Fewer nonspecific codes than in ICD-9-CM

The ICD-10 coding system consists of two code sets, ICD-10-CM and ICD-10-PCS.

Example 5-2	Forward Mapping from ICD-9-CM to ICD-10-CM
ICD-9-CM	**ICD-10-CM**
461.9 Acute sinusitis, unspecified	J01.80 Other acute sinusitis
	J01.90 Acute sinusitis, unspecified
	J01.91 Acute recurrent sinusitis, unspecified
470 Deviated nasal septum	J34.2 Deviated nasal septum
Crosswalks are not exact and may not always provide a one-to-one correlation but can assist in finding appropriate code ranges for reporting purposes.	

ICD-10-CM	Used to report diagnosis codes in all health care settings.	To replace ICD-9-CM, Volumes 1 and 2.
ICD-10-PCS	Used for hospitals to report procedural codes.	To replace ICD-9-CM, Volume 3.

ICD-10-CM

ICD-10 was published by the WHO in 1992, and then clinically modified by the NCHS before code adoption. The Clinical Modification (CM) provides the specifics that the United States needs for collecting data on health status. This became known as the *International Classification of Diseases*, Tenth Revision, Clinical Modification (ICD-10-CM) and is used for reporting of diagnoses treated during encounters in all health care settings.

Additional information on using ICD-10-CM is included in this chapter.

ICD-10-PCS

Subsequently, the ***International Classification of Diseases, Tenth Revision, Procedure Coding System (ICD-10-PCS)*** was developed in mid-1992 by 3M Health Information Systems under contract with the CMS. This replaced Volume 3 of ICD-9-CM, which was previously used for coding of procedures in hospital billing.

Additional information on using ICD-10-PCS is included in Chapter 17.

HIPAA Compliance Alert — ICD-10-CM AND ITS COMPLIANCE WITH HIPAA

ICD-10-CM meets HIPAA criteria by providing specific information for outpatient and inpatient procedures; describing medical services using terminology in today's environment; expanding injury and disease codes and categories; and giving a more precise, clear, and clinical picture of the patient.

Organization and Format of ICD-10-CM

ICD-10-CM is updated annually and contains a Tabular List of Diseases, each disease having an assigned number (Figure 5-2), and an Alphabetic Index to Diseases and Injuries (Figure 5-3). The systematized arrangement in these books makes it possible to encode, computerize, store, and retrieve large volumes of information from the patient's medical record.

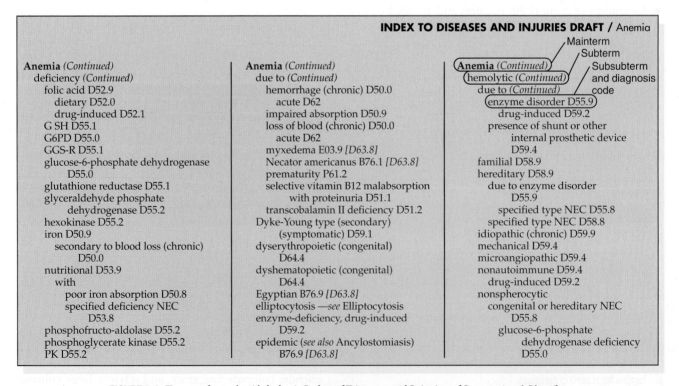

D55   **PART III /** Tabular List of Diseases and Injuries   **D57.1**

HEMOLYTIC ANEMIAS (D55-D59)

● **D55 Anemia due to enzyme disorders**

> **Excludes 1**   drug-induced enzyme deficiency anemia
> (D59.2)

D55.0 Anemia due to glucose-6-phosphate dehydrogenase [G6PD] deficiency
Favism
G6PD deficiency anemia

D55.1 Anemia due to other disorders of glutathione metabolism
Anemia (due to) enzyme deficiencies, except G6PD, related to the hexose monophosphate [HMP] shunt pathway
Anemia (due to) hemolytic nonspherocytic (hereditary), type I

D55.2 Anemia due to disorders of glycolytic enzymes
Hemolytic nonspherocytic (hereditary) anemia, type II
Hexokinase deficiency anemia
Pyruvate kinase [PK] deficiency anemia
Triose-phosphate isomerase deficiency anemia

> **Excludes 1**   disorders of glycolysis not associated with anemia (E74.8)

D55.3 Anemia due to disorders of nucleotide metabolism

D55.8 Other anemias due to enzyme disorders

■ **D55.9 Anemia due to enzyme disorder, unspecified**

Diagnosis code verified
Complete description

D56.3 Thalassemia minor
Genetic disorders that have in common defective production of hemoglobin
Alpha thalassemia minor
Alpha thalassemia silent carrier
Alpha thalassemia trait
Beta thalassemia minor
Beta thalassemia trait
Delta-beta thalassemia minor
Delta-beta thalassemia trait
Thalassemia trait NOS

> **Excludes 1**   alpha thalassemia (D56.0)
> beta thalassemia (D56.1)
> delta-beta thalassemia (D56.2)
> hemoglobin E-beta thalassemia (D56.5)
> sickle-cell trait (D57.3)

D56.4 Hereditary persistence of fetal hemoglobin [HPFH]
Persistent production of hemoglobin

D56.5 Hemoglobin E-beta thalassemia

> **Excludes 1**   beta thalassemia (D56.1)
> beta thalassemia minor (D56.3)
> beta thalassemia trait (D56.3)
> delta-beta thalassemia (D56.2)
> delta-beta thalassemia trait (D56.3)
> hemoglobin E disease (D58.2)
> other hemoglobinopathies (D58.2)
> sickle-cell beta thalassemia (D57.4-)

FIGURE 5-2 Excerpt from the Tabular List of *International Classification of Diseases,* Tenth Revision, Clinical Modification (ICD-10-CM), Volume 1.

INDEX TO DISEASES AND INJURIES DRAFT / Anemia

Mainterm
Subterm
Subsubterm and diagnosis code

Anemia *(Continued)*
deficiency *(Continued)*
folic acid D52.9
dietary D52.0
drug-induced D52.1
G SH D55.1
G6PD D55.0
GGS-R D55.1
glucose-6-phosphate dehydrogenase D55.0
glutathione reductase D55.1
glyceraldehyde phosphate dehydrogenase D55.2
hexokinase D55.2
iron D50.9
secondary to blood loss (chronic) D50.0
nutritional D53.9
with
poor iron absorption D50.8
specified deficiency NEC D53.8
phosphofructo-aldolase D55.2
phosphoglycerate kinase D55.2
PK D55.2

Anemia *(Continued)*
due to *(Continued)*
hemorrhage (chronic) D50.0
acute D62
impaired absorption D50.9
loss of blood (chronic) D50.0
acute D62
myxedema E03.9 *[D63.8]*
Necator americanus B76.1 *[D63.8]*
prematurity P61.2
selective vitamin B12 malabsorption with proteinuria D51.1
transcobalamin II deficiency D51.2
Dyke-Young type (secondary) (symptomatic) D59.1
dyserythropoietic (congenital) D64.4
dyshematopoietic (congenital) D64.4
Egyptian B76.9 *[D63.8]*
elliptocytosis —*see* Elliptocytosis
enzyme-deficiency, drug-induced D59.2
epidemic (*see also* Ancylostomiasis) B76.9 *[D63.8]*

Anemia *(Continued)*
hemolytic *(Continued)*
due to *(Continued)*
enzyme disorder D55.9
drug-induced D59.2
presence of shunt or other internal prosthetic device D59.4
familial D58.9
hereditary D58.9
due to enzyme disorder D55.9
specified type NEC D55.8
specified type NEC D58.8
idiopathic (chronic) D59.9
mechanical D59.4
microangiopathic D59.4
nonautoimmune D59.4
drug-induced D59.2
nonspherocytic
congenital or hereditary NEC D55.8
glucose-6-phosphate dehydrogenase deficiency D55.0

FIGURE 5-3 Excerpt from the Alphabetic Index of Diseases and Injuries of *International Classification of Diseases,* Tenth Revision, Clinical Modification (ICD-10-CM).

ICD-10-CM is used by hospitals, physicians, and other health care providers to code and report diagnostic information necessary for participation in various government programs such as Medicare, Medicaid, quality improvement organizations, and professional review organizations.

Annual updates of ICD-10-CM are published in three publications: *Coding Clinic*, published by the American Hospital Association (AHA); *American Health Information Management Association Journal*, published by American Health Information Management Association (AHIMA); and the *Federal Register*, published by the US Government Printing Office. Coding from an out-of-date manual can delay payment, result in denied claims, or cause costly mistakes that can lead to financial disaster. Annual ICD-10-CM code revisions must be in place and in use by October 1 each year.

Standard Transaction Code Sets

HIPAA Compliance Alert ICD-10-CM STANDARD CODE SET

As discussed in Chapter 2, a code set is any set of codes with their descriptions used to encode data elements, such as tables of terms, medical concepts, medical diagnostic codes, or medical procedure codes. Each transaction must include the use of medical and other code sets. The ICD-10-CM official guideline for coding and reporting is the standard code set outlined under HIPAA and must be used when assigning diagnostic codes. HIPAA does not require health insurance plans to change their business rules regarding payment based on the codes. However, insurance payers cannot reject an insurance claim because it includes a valid HIPAA standard code that the payer system does not yet recognize.

Alphabetic Index to Diseases and Injuries

The Alphabetic Index to Diseases and Injuries is placed first in most ICD-10-CM coding manuals. The Alphabetic Index contains the Tables of Drugs and Chemicals, Neoplasm Table, and Index to External Cause. Main code descriptor items are in alphabetic order and indented subterms and applicable additional qualifiers, descriptors, or modifiers are beneath the main terms.

Alphabetic Index elements are structured as follows:
- Main terms are classifications of diseases and injuries and appear as headings in bold type.
- Subterms are listings under main terms and are indented two spaces to the right under main terms. These are referred to as **essential modifiers** because their presence changes the code assignment.
- Modifiers (often referred to as **nonessential modifiers** because their presence or absence does not affect the code assigned) provide additional description and are enclosed in parentheses.
- Carryover lines continue the text and are indented more than two spaces from the level of the preceding line.
- Subterms of subterms are additional listings and are indented two spaces to the right under the subterm (Box 5-2).

Special Points to Remember in the Alphabetic Index

1. Notice that appropriate sites or modifiers are listed in alphabetic order under the main terms with further subterm listings as needed.
2. Examine all nonessential modifiers that appear in parentheses next to the main term. Check for nonessential modifiers that apply to any of the qualifying terms used in the statement of the diagnosis found in the patient's medical record (Figure 5-4).

Box 5-2   Illustration of Main Terms, Subterms, and Nonessential Modifiers

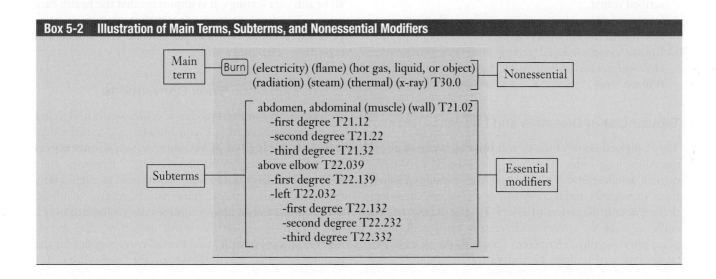

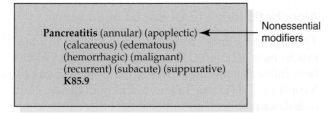

FIGURE 5-4 Coding with modifiers in parentheses.

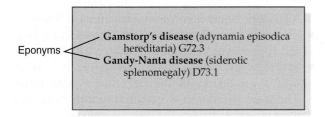

FIGURE 5-5 Coding diagnoses associated with an eponym.

```
Inflammation, inflamed, inflammatory
    (with exudation)

Spider
    bite—see Toxicity, venom, spider
    fingers—see Syndrome, Marfan's
    nevus I78.1
    toes—see Syndrome, Marfan's
    vascular I78.1
```

FIGURE 5-6 Cross-referencing synonyms, closely related terms, and code categories from the Alphabetic Index of *International Classification of Diseases*, Tenth Revision, Clinical Modification (ICD-10-CM).

3. Notice that eponyms appear as both main term entries and modifiers under main terms such as "disease" or "syndrome" and "operation." As mentioned in Chapter 4, an **eponym** is the name of a disease, structure, operation, or procedure, usually derived from the name of a place or a person who discovered or described it first.
4. Look for sublisted terms in parentheses that are associated with the eponym (Figure 5-5).
5. Locate closely related terms, code categories, and cross-referenced synonyms indicated by *see* and *see also* (Figure 5-6).

Tabular List of Diseases and Injuries

The Tabular List of Diseases and Injuries is placed after the Alphabetic Index (Volume 2) in most ICD-10-CM manual publications. The Tabular List contains Chapters 1 through 21 and is composed of alphanumeric codes that represent diagnoses (Table 5-1). The ICD-10-CM codes contain up to seven characters, with a decimal point after the third character. This is shown as digit #1 (alpha character), digits #2 and #3 (numeric character),

and digits #4 to #7 (alpha or numeric character). The first three characters are placed to the left of the decimal point and indicate the category. The remaining digits to the right of the decimal point indicate the etiology, anatomic site, and severity. The sixth character can signify laterality, the intent of a drug poisoning (intentional self-harm, assault), "with" or "without" a given manifestation, the trimester of a pregnancy, the depth of a skin ulcer, or the nature of an injury. An "X" is used as a **placeholder** to save a space for future code expansion and/or to meet the requirement of coding to the highest level of specificity (Figure 5-7).

Special Points to Remember in the Tabular List

1. Use two or more codes when necessary to describe a given diagnosis completely (for example, arteriosclerotic cardiovascular disease I25.10 with congestive heart failure I50.9).
2. Search for one code when two diagnoses or a diagnosis with an associated secondary process (manifestation) or complication is present. There are instances when two diagnoses are classified with a single code number called a *combination code* (for example, diabetic retinopathy E11.319).
3. Use category codes only if there are no subcategory codes (for example, hypertension I10).
4. Read all instructional notes provided.

OFFICIAL GUIDELINES FOR ICD-10-CM

The **Official Guidelines for Coding and Reporting** is a set of rules developed to accompany and complement the official conventions and instructions provided in the ICD-10-CM coding manual. The guidelines include definitions, standards, rules, general coding guidelines, and 21 chapter-specific coding guidelines. Adherence to the guidelines when assigning an ICD-10-CM diagnosis code is required under HIPAA and has been adopted for all health care settings. It is important that the health care provider and the coder work together to achieve complete and accurate documentation, code assignment, and reporting of diagnosis codes.

Diagnostic Code Book Conventions

To become a proficient coder, it is important to develop an understanding of the conventions and terminology related to the ICD-10-CM coding system. **Conventions** are rules or principles for determining a diagnostic code when using diagnostic code books such as each space, typefaces, indentations, punctuation marks, symbols, instructional notes, abbreviations, cross-reference notes, and specific usage of the words *and*, *with*, and *due to*. These rules assist in the selection of correct codes for the diagnoses encountered. Some of the conventions for

Table 5-1	Outline of Tabular List and Alphabetic Index of ICD-10-CM	
TABULAR LIST	**CHAPTER HEADINGS**	**CODES**
1	Certain Infectious and Parasitic Diseases	A00-B99
2	Neoplasms	C00-D49
3	Diseases of the Blood and Blood-Forming Organs and Certain Disorders Involving the Immune Mechanism	D50-D89
4	Endocrine, Nutritional, and Metabolic Diseases	E00-E89
5	Mental and Behavioral Disorders	F01-F99
6	Diseases of the Nervous System	G00-G99
7	Diseases of the Eye and Adnexa	H00-H59
8	Diseases of the Ear and Mastoid Process	H60-H95
9	Diseases of the Circulatory System	I00-I99
10	Diseases of the Respiratory System	J00-J99
11	Diseases of the Digestive System	K00-K95
12	Diseases of the Skin and Subcutaneous Tissue	L00-L99
13	Diseases of the Musculoskeletal System and Connective Tissue	M00-M99
14	Diseases of the Genitourinary System	N00-N99
15	Pregnancy, Childbirth, and the Puerperium	O00-O9A
16	Certain Conditions Originating in the Perinatal Period	P00-P96
17	Congenital Malformations, Deformations, and Chromosomal Abnormalities	Q00-Q99
18	Symptoms, Signs, and Abnormal Clinical and Laboratory Findings, Not Elsewhere Classifiable	R00-R99
19	Injury, Poisoning, and Certain Other Consequences of External Causes	S00-T88
20	External Causes of Morbidity	V00-Y99
21	Factors Influencing Health Status and Contact with Health Services	Z00-Z99
Alphabetic Index		
Section 1	Index to Diseases, Alphabetic	
Section 2	Table of Drugs and Chemicals	
Section 3	Alphabetic Index to External Causes	

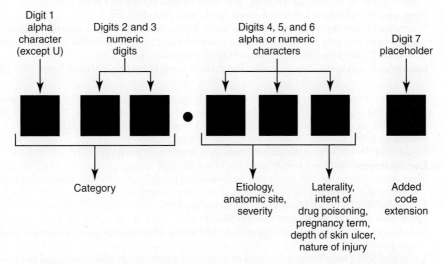

FIGURE 5-7 Explanation of the seven character positions in ICD-10-CM.

ICD-10-CM are listed on the next page; however, the insurance billing specialist should read all of the information included in the introduction section of the coding manual, which will provide a complete outline of all conventions used in the manual.

Abbreviations, Punctuation, and Symbols

ICD-10-CM's Alphabetic Index and Tabular List make use of certain abbreviations, punctuation, symbols, and other conventions, as shown in Box 5-3.

Box 5-3   Official ICD-10-CM Code Book Conventions

Punctuation

[ ]
    Brackets are used in the Tabular List to enclose synonyms, alternative wording, or explanatory phrases.
Example: J95.85 Mechanical complication of respirator [ventilator]

:
    Colons are used in the Tabular List after an incomplete term, which needs one or more of the modifiers following the colon to make it assignable to a given category.
Example: L99 Other disorders of skin and subcutaneous tissue in diseases classified elsewhere
Code first underlying disease, such as: amyloidosis (E85.-)

-
    Dashes are used in both the ICD-10-CM Indexes and the Tabular List. The Indexes use the dash to show the level of indentation. A symbol (-) at the end of an index entry indicates an incomplete code, so additional characters are needed. Locate the referenced category or subcategory elsewhere in the Tabular List, review the options, and assign the code.
Example:
Excludes 2: cellulitis of fingers (L03.01-)

( )
    Parentheses are used in the Tabular List to enclose supplementary words (nonessential modifiers) that may be present or absent in the statement of a disease or condition without affecting the code number to which it was assigned.
Example: N39.3 Stress incontinence (female) (male)

Abbreviations

NEC
    Not elsewhere classifiable (NEC) in the Tabular List under a code identifies it as an "other specified" code.
Example: A85 Other viral encephalitis, not elsewhere classifiable
Includes: specified viral encephalomyelitis **NEC**

NOS
    Not otherwise specified (NOS) is equivalent to an unspecified code.
Example: Q66.8 Other congenital deformities of feet
Congenital clubfoot **NOS**

Cross-Reference Terms

and
    This word represents and/or when used in a narrative statement.
Example: B35.0 Tinea barbae **and** tinea capitis

with/without
    When a condition may have two versions—*with* or *without* a specific sign, symptom, or manifestation—this is indicated by a change in one of the code characters. These words in the Alphabetic Index are sequenced following the main term, not in alphabetical order.
Example: Epilepsy, epileptic, epilepsia intractable G40.919
with status epilepticus G40.911
without status epilepticus G40.919

see
    Instruction that follows a main term in the Index indicating that another term should be referenced. Go to the main term referenced with the "see" note to find the correct code.
Example: Postphlebitic syndrome—**see** Syndrome, postphlebitic

see also
    Instruction following a main term in the Index to indicate that there is another main term that may also be referenced and may provide additional index entries that may be useful. It is not necessary to follow the "see also" note when the original main term gives the code.
Example: Preterm delivery (**see also** Pregnancy, complicated by, preterm labor) 060.10

Instructional Notes

Code first/use
  additional code
    Notes that certain conditions have both an underlying etiology and multiple body system manifestations due to the underlying etiology. Manifestation code titles have a phrase, "in diseases classified elsewhere." The underlying condition must be sequenced first followed by the manifestation.
Example: E08 Diabetes mellitus due to underlying condition
Code first the underlying condition, such as: Congenital rubella (P35.0)
Use additional code to identify any insulin use (Z79.4)

Code also
    Note instructions that two codes may be needed to completely describe a condition dependent on the severity of the conditions and the reason for the encounter.
Example: S85 Injury of blood vessels at lower leg level
Code also any associated open wound (S81.-)

Includes
    Includes appears under certain categories to add to the definition or give an example of the content of the category.
Example: S93 Dislocation and sprain of joints and ligaments at ankle, foot, and toe level
Includes: avulsion of joint or ligament of ankle, foot, and toe

Inclusion terms
    List of terms included under some codes, such as conditions for which that code is to be used, synonyms, or various specified conditions assigned to "other specified" codes.
Example: C46.1 Kaposi's sarcoma of soft tissue
Kaposi's sarcoma of blood vessel
Kaposi's sarcoma of connective tissue
Kaposi's sarcoma of fascia
Kaposi's sarcoma of ligament

Box 5-3	Official ICD-10-CM Code Book Conventions—cont'd
Excludes 1	An *Excludes 1* note very simply indicates "not coded here." An Excludes 1 note should never be used at the same time as the code above the Excludes 1 note. It is used when two conditions cannot occur together, such as a congenital form versus an acquired form of the same condition. **Example: E20 Hypoparathyroidism** **Excludes 1:** Di George's syndrome (D82.1)
Excludes 2	An *Excludes 2* note very simply indicates "not included here." An Excludes 2 note indicates that the condition excluded is not part of the condition represented by the code but that a patient may have both conditions at the same time. When an Excludes 2 note appears under a code, use both the code and the excluded code together. **Example: I10 Essential (primary) hypertension** **Excludes 2:** Essential (primary) hypertension involving vessels of brain (I60-I69)

Example 5-3

T55.0X1A	Toxic effects of soap, unintentional; Initial encounter

Example 5-4

S01.312A	Laceration without foreign body of left ear; Initial encounter
T36.0X2A	Poisoning by penicillin, intentional, self-harm; Initial encounter

Example 5-5

K63.0	Abscess, intestine, intestinal, NEC

Example 5-6

J32.9	Chronic sinusitis, unspecified Sinusitis (chronic) NOS

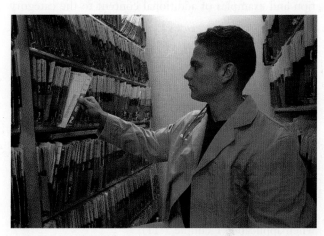

FIGURE 5-8 Insurance billing specialist looking up a patient's medical record file to verify documentation for a diagnostic code.

Placeholder Character

ICD-10-CM uses the placeholder character "X" when reporting certain codes to allow for future expansion of the code. When a placeholder is indicated, the X must be used in order for the code to be valid (Example 5-3).

Seventh Characters

Certain ICD-10-CM codes must be reported with seven characters. If a code that requires a seventh character is not six characters, a placeholder X must be used to fill in the empty characters (Example 5-4).

Other and Unspecified Codes

The abbreviation NEC represents codes that are **"not elsewhere classifiable."** The Alphabetic Index will direct the coder to an "other specified" code in the Tabular List. Alphabetic Index entries with NEC in the line designate "other" codes in the Tabular List. These Alphabetic Index entries represent specific disease entities for which no specific code exists, so the term is included within an "other" code (Example 5-5).

The abbreviation NOS represents **"not otherwise specified"** and is the equivalent of unspecified. In ICD-10-CM, a code with a fourth digit 9 or fifth digit 0 for diagnosis codes titled "unspecified" is used when the information in the medical record is insufficient to assign a more specific code. For those categories for which an unspecified code is not provided, the "other specified" code may represent both other and unspecified. "Other specified" and "unspecified" subcategories are referred to as *residual subcategories* (Example 5-6).

Residual subcategories are used for conditions that are specifically named in the medical record but not specifically listed under a code description. If there is a lack of details in the medical record and you cannot match to a specific subdivision, research the medical record for a qualifying statement in the physician's progress notes or history and physical examination report that will allow you to use a more specific diagnostic code (Figure 5-8).

Brackets, [ ], are used in the Tabular List to enclose synonyms or alternative wording or to provide explanatory phrases (Example 5-7).

Parentheses, ( ), are used in the Alphabetic Index and Tabular List to enclose supplementary words that may further define the condition but do not affect the code number assigned. These are referred to as *nonessential modifiers* (Example 5-8).

Colons, :, are used in the Tabular List after an incomplete term that requires additional modifiers to appropriately assign the code (Example 5-9).

Includes Notes

A note appears immediately under the three-character code title in the Tabular List and provides further definition and examples of additional content to the category (Example 5-10).

Excludes Notes

There are two types of excludes notes used in the Tabular List of ICD-10-CM. An **Excludes 1** note indicates certain codes that should never be used at the same time as the code selected and is used when two conditions could not possibly occur at the same time. **Excludes 2** notes indicate that the condition selected is not part of the excluded condition; however, it is possible for the patient to have both conditions at the same time. It is acceptable to report both the code and the excluded code together, when applicable (Example 5-11).

Default Code

A default code is shown next to a main term in the Alphabetic Index and represents the condition that is commonly associated with the main term or is the unspecified code for the condition. For example, if the electronic health record (EHR) documents appendicitis but does not list acute or chronic, then the default code should be assigned (Example 5-12).

Gender and Age Codes

Diagnostic codes must match the age and gender of the patient. If an adult female patient with breast cancer is seen (excluding carcinoma in situ and skin cancer of breast), a code from the ICD-10-CM Neoplasm Table must be used (Example 5-13).

Selection of a Coding Manual

Many companies publish the ICD-10-CM coding manuals. Publishers very often use different styles and formats, so it is important to study and compare the features of several books before making a decision to purchase. When choosing a book, the following questions should be asked: Are colors used for emphasis in locating items quickly? Are definitions or notes included to help one interpret and gain a better understanding of difficult medical terms and phrases? Are coding guidelines boxed for easy reference? Are icons or symbols used? Are fonts and type styles used that can be read easily? Is print large enough to allow accurate coding? All of these benefit the coder.

Example 5-7

B01	Varicella [chickenpox]

Example 5-8

E05.90	Hyperthyroidism (latent) (pre-adult) (recurrent)

Example 5-9

D59.3 Hemolytic-uremic syndrome
    Use additional code to identify associated:
    E. coli infection (B96.2-)
    Pneumococcal pneumonia (J13)
    Shigella dysenteriae (A03.9)

Example 5-10

R18.- Ascites
    Includes: fluid in the peritoneal cavity

Example 5-11

R07.- Pain in throat and chest
    Excludes 1: epidemic myalgia (B33.0)
    Excludes 2: jaw pain (R68.84)
             pain in breast (N64.4)

Example 5-12

K03.81	Cracked tooth

Example 5-13

C50.421	Malignant neoplasm of upper-outer quadrant of right *male* breast
P70.2	*Neonatal* diabetes mellitus

General Coding Guidelines
Locating a Code in the ICD-10-CM

To select a code that corresponds to a diagnosis or reason for a visit that is documented in a medical record, the coder should first locate the term in the Alphabetic Index and then verify the code in the Tabular List. Step-by-step procedures for selecting ICD-10-CM diagnostic codes are presented at the end of this chapter.

A dash (-) at the end of an Alphabetic Index entry indicates that an additional character is required and can be determined by referencing the Tabular List. Even if a dash is not present, the coder must always consult the Tabular List to refer to all additional instructional notes (Example 5-14).

Level of Detail in Coding

ICD-10-CM codes are composed of 3, 4, 5, 6, or 7 characters. Some conditions may be reported with a three-character code. However, if the code is further subdivided, it should be reported at the highest number of characters assigned. This is commonly referred to as coding to the highest level of specificity. A code is invalid if it has not been coded to the full number of characters required for that condition.

Signs and Symptoms

Codes that describe signs and symptoms are acceptable for reporting purposes when a related definitive diagnosis has not been established. This is reported using codes from Chapter 18 of the ICD-10-CM coding manual (for example, symptoms, signs, and abnormal clinical and laboratory findings, not elsewhere classified). When coding for office or outpatient services, if the final diagnosis at the end of the encounter is qualified by any of the following terms—apparent, likely, might, possible, probably, questionable, rule out, suspected, or suspicion of—do not code these conditions as if they existed or were established. Instead, document the condition to the highest degree of certainty for each encounter or visit (for example, signs, symptoms, abnormal test results, or other reason for the visit) and code the chief complaint (CC), sign, or symptom.

This is contrary to coding practices used by hospital health information management departments for coding the diagnoses of hospital inpatients. If you were to follow guidelines used for hospital coding and the patient was suspected of having a heart attack, this would be coded as a confirmed case of myocardial infarction. The same holds true for "possible epilepsy." If the patient had a convulsion and epilepsy was the probable cause but had not been proved, you would code the convulsion.

The following are instances in which sign and symptom codes can be used.

- No precise diagnosis can be made (Examples 5-15 and 5-16).
- Signs or symptoms are transient and a specific diagnosis was not made (Example 5-17).
- Provisional diagnosis is made for a patient who does not return for further care (Example 5-18).
- A patient is referred for treatment before a definite diagnosis is made (Example 5-19).

Example 5-14

Conjunctivitis, acute   H10.3-

Example 5-15   No Precise Diagnosis

The patient has an enlarged liver and further diagnostic studies may or may not be done. **Use code R16.0 for hepatomegaly.**

Example 5-16   No Precise Diagnosis

The patient complains of painful urination and urinalysis is negative. **Use code R30.0 for dysuria.**

Example 5-17   Transient Sign and Symptom Code

The patient complains of chest pain on deep inspiration. On examination, the physician finds nothing abnormal and tells the patient to return in 1 week. When the patient returns, the pain has ceased. **Use code R07.1 for painful respiration.**

Example 5-18   Provisional Diagnosis

On examination, the physician documents abnormal percussion of the chest. The patient is sent for a chest x-ray and is asked to return for a recheck. The patient does not have the x-ray and fails to return. **Use code R09.89 for abnormal chest sounds.**

Example 5-19   Sign and Symptom Code before Definite Diagnosis

A patient complains of nausea and vomiting and is referred to a gastroenterologist. **Use code R11.2 for nausea with vomiting.**

Conditions That Are an Integral Part of a Disease Process

Signs and symptoms that are typically associated with a disease process should not be assigned as additional codes (Example 5-20).

Conditions That Are Not an Integral Part of a Disease Process

Signs and symptoms that are not typically associated with a disease process should be reported when documented (Example 5-21).

Multiple Coding for a Single Condition

In some cases, two codes will be required to describe a single condition. "Use additional code" notes from the Tabular List will guide the coder as to when it is appropriate to report a secondary code. When determining which code to sequence first, the additional code would be reported as a secondary code (Example 5-22).

"Code first" notes are also indicated in the Tabular List and are typically used to identify an underlying condition. The underlying condition is always reported as the primary code (Example 5-23).

Acute, Subacute, and Chronic Conditions

When the documentation mentions that a condition is both acute (subacute) and chronic and separate codes exist in the Alphabetic Index, both are coded with the acute (subacute) sequence first followed by the code for the chronic condition (Example 5-24).

Combination Code

A **combination code** is a situation in which a single code is used to classify two diagnoses or a diagnosis with an associated secondary process (manifestation) or a diagnosis with an associated complication. Identify a combination code by referring to subterm entries in the Alphabetic Index and by reading the inclusion and exclusion notes in the Tabular List. If the combination code does not specifically describe the manifestation or complication, use a secondary code (Example 5-25).

Example 5-20

The provider documents asthma with wheezing. Wheezing is a sign and symptom typically associated with asthma; therefore the code for asthma is all that should be reported.

The provider documents nausea and vomiting due to gastroenteritis. Nausea and vomiting are signs and symptoms typically associated with gastroenteritis; therefore only the code for gastroenteritis should be reported.

Example 5-21

The provider documents diverticulosis with abdominal pain. Patients can have diverticulosis without having abdominal pain. By reporting abdominal pain in addition to diverticulosis, the severity of the condition is better described. Medical necessity for further study is also supported by reporting abdominal pain with diverticulosis.

The provider documents benign prostatic hypertrophy with urinary frequency. Patients can have benign prostatic hypertrophy without urinary frequency. By reporting urinary frequency in addition to benign prostatic hypertrophy, the severity of the condition is better described. Medical necessity for further study is also supported by reporting urinary frequency with benign prostatic hypertrophy.

Example 5-22

Alzheimer's disease (G30.-)	Use additional code to identify: Delirium, if applicable (F05) Dementia with behavioral disturbance (F02.81) Dementia without behavioral disturbance (F02-80)

Example 5-23

Maternal care for abnormality of pelvic organ (O34.-)	Code first any associated obstructed labor (O65.5)

Example 5-24

Appendicitis (pneumococcal) (retrocecal) K37
  acute (catarrhal) (fulminating) (gangrenous) (obstructive) (retrocecal) (suppurative) K35.80
  subacute (adhesive) K36
  chronic (recurrent) K36

Example 5-25

J44.0	Chronic obstructive pulmonary disease with acute lower respiratory infection Use additional code to identify the infection.
G03	Meningitis due to other and unspecified causes Includes: arachnoiditis NOS Excludes 1: meningomyelitis (G04.-)

Sequela

A **sequela** is a **late effect** or condition produced after the acute phase of an illness. There is no time limit on when a late effect code can be used. Coding of sequela generally requires two codes. The nature of the sequela is sequenced first; the sequela code is sequenced second (Example 5-26).

Impending or Threatened Condition

Codes that are described as "impending" or "threatened" should be referenced as such in the Alphabetic Index and reported accordingly. If there is no subterm under "impending" or "threatened" for the condition described, report the existing underlying condition(s) (Example 5-27).

Reporting the Same Diagnosis Code More Than Once

Each unique ICD-10-CM diagnosis code may be reported only once for an encounter. This applies to bilateral conditions where there are no distinct codes to identify laterality or two different conditions are classified to the same diagnosis code.

Laterality

When reporting bilateral sites, the final character of the code in ICD-10-CM should be selected to indicate laterality. The right side is always character 1 and the left side character 2. In those situations when a bilateral code is given, the bilateral character is always 3. If the side is not identified, an unspecified code is provided, which is either 0 or 9, depending on whether it is a fifth or sixth character (Example 5-28).

Documentation for BMI and Pressure Ulcer Stages

Information documented by clinicians who are not the patient's provider in the medical record to indicate body mass index (BMI) or pressure ulcer stage codes can be coded. However, the patient's provider must document the associated diagnosis (obesity, pressure ulcer).

Syndromes

A **syndrome** is another name for a symptom complex, which is a set of complex signs, symptoms, or other manifestations resulting from a common cause or appearing in combination, presenting a distinct clinical picture of a disease or inherited abnormality. Syndromes should be reported by following the Alphabetic Index (Example 5-29).

Documentation of Complications of Care

Complications of care codes are assigned based on provider's documentation of the relationship between the condition and the care or procedure (Example 5-30).

Chapter-Specific Coding Guidelines

In addition to general diagnosis coding guidelines, there are guidelines specific to the 21 chapters of the Tabular Index. Some of the most frequently referenced chapter-specific coding guidelines are provided in this text; however, the insurance billing specialist must be familiar with the entire contents of the Official Guidelines for Coding and Reporting and refer to them when reporting all conditions. The chapter-specific guidelines are located in Section I, Subsection C of the Official Guidelines.

Human Immunodeficiency Virus

Human immunodeficiency virus (HIV) is a disease of the immune system characterized by increased susceptibility

---

Example 5-26

R13.1-	Dysphagia
I69.991	Dysphagia due to late effect (sequela) of cerebrovascular disease
	(Instructional note states: "Use additional code to identify the type of dysphagia, if known [R13.1-]".)

Example 5-27

I20.0	Impending myocardial infarction
O20.0	Threatened abortion

Example 5-28

S67.0-	Crushing injury of thumb
S67.00-	Crushing injury of thumb of unspecified side
S67.01-	Crushing injury of right thumb
S67.02-	Crushing injury of left thumb

Example 5-29

Q90.9	Down syndrome
I45.9	Adams-Stokes syndrome

Example 5-30

T88.59-	Complication of anesthesia
K94.00	Complication of colostomy

Table 5-2	Coding for Neoplasms					
	Malignant					
	PRIMARY	**SECONDARY**	**CARCINOMA IN SITU**	**BENIGN**	**UNCERTAIN BEHAVIOR**	**UNSPECIFIED**
Neoplasm, neoplastic	C80.1	C79.9	D09.9	D36.9	D48.9	D49.9
abdomen, abdominal	C76.2	C79.8-	D09.8	D36.7	D48.7	D49.89
cavity	C76.2	C79.8-	D09.8	D36.7	D48.7	D49.89
organ	C76.2	C79.8-	D09.8	D36.7	D48.7	D49.89
viscera	C76.2	C79.8-	D09.8	D36.7	D48.7	D49.89
wall	C44.509	C79.2-	D04.5	D23.5	D48.5	D49.2
connective tissue	C49.4	C79.8-	—	D21.4	D48.1	D49.2
abdominopelvic	C76.8	C79.8-	—	D36.7	D48.7	D49.89
accessory sinus—see Neoplasm, sinus						
acoustic nerve	C72.4-	C79.49	—	D33.3	D43.3	D49.7
adenoid (pharynx) (tissue)	C11.1	C79.89	D00.08	D10.6	D37.05	D49.0
adipose tissue (see also Neoplasm, connective tissue)	C49.4	C79.89	—	D21.9	D48.1	D49.2
adnexa (uterine)	C57.4	C79.89	D07.39	D28.7	D39.8	D49.5
adrenal	C74.9-	C79.7-	D09.3	D35.0-	D44.1-	D49.7
capsule	C74.9-	C79.7-	D09.3	D35.0-	D44.1-	D49.7
cortex	C74.0-	C79.7-	D09.3	D35.0-	D44.1-	D49.7
gland	C74.9-	C79.7-	D09.3	D35.0-	D44.1-	D49.7
medulla	C74.1-	C79.7-	D09.3	D35.0-	D44.1-	D49.7
ala nasi (external)	C44.301	C79.2-	D04.39	D23.39	D48.5	D49.2
alimentary canal or tract NEC	C26.9	C78.80	D01.9	D13.9	D37.9	D49.0

NEC, Not elsewhere classifiable.

to opportunistic infections, certain cancers, and neurologic disorders. Specific guidelines for reporting HIV infections are provided in Section I, Chapter 1, Subsection C of the Chapter-Specific Coding Guidelines. Only confirmed cases of HIV infection or illness should be reported. The provider's documentation that the patient is HIV positive would serve as confirmation. The diagnosis code B20 is used to report HIV disease whereas an asymptomatic HIV infection status is reported as Z21. Patients who present for testing for HIV are coded as Z11.4, encounter for screening for HIV.

Neoplasms

Section I, Chapter 2, Subsection C of the Chapter-Specific Coding Guidelines provides guidelines for neoplasm coding. A **neoplasm** is a spontaneous new growth of tissue forming an abnormal mass that is also known as a *tumor.* It may be benign or malignant. A table is provided in the Alphabetic Index to look up the condition using the main entry "Neoplasm." The table has the column headings Malignant, Benign, Uncertain Behavior, and Unspecified (Table 5-2).

First, check the index; if you are not able to locate the word (area in active treatment) you are searching for, then go to the table. Often the index entry will produce the correct code and tell you what area of the table to look at. If you search the table first, you may end up obtaining an incorrect code. Code numbers for neoplasms are given by anatomic site. For each site, there are six possible code numbers, indicating whether the neoplasm in question is malignant (primary, secondary, or carcinoma in situ), benign, of uncertain behavior, or of unspecified nature. The description of the neoplasm often indicates which of the six code numbers is appropriate (for example, malignant melanoma of skin, benign fibroadenoma of breast, or carcinoma in situ of cervix uteri) (Example 5-31).

A **benign tumor** is one that does not have the properties of invasion and **metastasis** (that is, spread or transfer of tumor cells from one organ to another site) and is usually surrounded by a fibrous capsule. Cysts and lesions are not neoplasms. A **malignant tumor** has the properties of invasion and metastasis. The term *carcinoma* refers to a cancerous or malignant tumor. **Carcinoma in situ** means cancer confined to the site of origin without invasion of neighboring tissues. A *primary malignancy* means the original neoplastic (malignant) site. A *secondary neoplasm* or malignancy is the site or location to which the original malignancy has spread or metastasized. If the diagnosis does not mention metastasis, code the case as a primary neoplasm (Example 5-32). Lymphomas and leukemias are not classified using the primary and secondary terminology.

The diagnostic statement "metastatic from" indicates primary stage carcinoma whereas "metastatic to" indicates secondary stage carcinoma. If the diagnostic statement is "malignant neoplasm spread to," code it as the primary site spread to the secondary site. The phrase

Example 5-31	Adenocarcinoma of the Breast with Metastases to the Pelvic Bone
Step 1	Look up adenocarcinoma in the Alphabetic Index. Notice it states: "*see also* Neoplasm, by site, malignant."
Step 2	Locate neoplasm in the table in the Alphabetic Index. At the top of the page, notice the Malignant heading with the subheadings Primary, Secondary, and Ca In Situ. *Primary* means the first site of development of the malignancy. *Secondary* means metastasis from the primary site to a second site. *Ca In Situ* means cancer confined to the epithelium of the site of origin without invasion of the basement membrane tissue of the site.
Step 3	Find the site of the adenocarcinoma (in this case the breast) and look under the Malignant and Primary headings. Note that the code given is C50.919.
Step 4	Next, find bone as a subterm in the Neoplasm Table and look for the subterm *pelvic*. Then look at the three columns under Malignant and using the Secondary column, find the correct code number C79.51. In listing these diagnoses on the insurance claim, you give the following: C50.919 and C79.51.

Example 5-32	Primary and Secondary Cancerous Tumors
Primary	**C64** **Malignant neoplasm of kidney and other and unspecified urinary organs**
	C64.9 **Kidney, except pelvis**
	Kidney NOS
	Kidney parenchyma
Secondary	**C79** **Secondary malignant cancerous neoplasm of other tumor specified sites**
	Excludes lymph node metastasis (C77.0)
	C79.00 **Kidney**

"recurrent malignancy" is new and is coded as a primary neoplasm.

The column of the neoplasm table labeled **"Uncertain Behavior"** is used when the lesion's behavior cannot be predicted. The pathologist has examined the specimen and found it to be benign at the present time but there is a chance it could undergo malignant transformation over time. These are histomorphologically well-defined neoplasms, the subsequent behavior of which cannot be predicted from the present appearance. These codes should be reported only if the pathology reports the neoplasm as

Example 5-33	
Congenital giant pigmented nevus (D48.5)	See also Neoplasm, skin, uncertain behavior

Table 5-3	Features of Type I and Type II Diabetes
TYPE I DIABETES	**TYPE II DIABETES**
Insulin-dependent diabetes mellitus	Non–insulin-dependent diabetes mellitus
Patients must be treated with insulin	Patients may be treated with insulin
Insulin levels are very low	Insulin levels may be high, "normal," or low
Ketosis prone	Non-ketosis prone
Patients usually are lean	Patients usually are obese
Usually "juvenile onset" (peak onset at early puberty)	Usually "adult onset," although occasionally seen in children
Often little family history of diabetes mellitus	Often strong family history of diabetes mellitus

"Uncertain Behavior" or an instructional note in the Alphabetic Index guides you to an "Uncertain Behavior" code (Example 5-33).

If a neoplasm has been excised but no pathology report is available, it is not reported as "Uncertain Behavior"; it would be reported using the "Unspecified Behavior" column of the table. Reporting a lesion of unknown diagnosis as a lesion of uncertain behavior is a common coding error.

It is always recommended that the coder wait for the final pathology report, following excision of a neoplasm. Although waiting for the final diagnosis may mean a delay in submission of the bill for payment, it is preferable to submit with the correct diagnosis.

Coding of Diabetes Mellitus

Diabetes mellitus (DM) is an endocrine disease; guidelines for coding DM are found in Section 1, Subsection C, Chapter 4 of the Chapter-Specific Coding Guidelines.

DM is categorized as either type I or type II and should be identified in the provider's documentation for accurate reporting of the condition. Table 5-3 outlines the clinical features important in the classification of diabetes.

Type I DM is juvenile diabetes that develops before the individual reaches puberty; however, the age of the patient should not be the sole determining factor. In type I diabetes, the patient's pancreas does not function and produce the necessary insulin. Thus this patient's body is dependent on insulin. Do not assume that because a patient is taking insulin, he or she has an insulin-dependent diabetes; look to the physician's documentation for clarification.

Type II DM is referred to as adult onset. In type II diabetes, the patient's pancreas produces some insulin but the insulin is ineffective in doing its job, which is to remove sugar from the bloodstream. This type of diabetes may be controlled with diet, oral medication, or insulin. If the type of diabetes is not documented in the medical record, the default is E11.-, type II diabetes.

Patients with DM frequently encounter complications that affect other body systems. The diabetes codes are combination codes that include the type of diabetes, the body system affected, and the complications affecting that body system. The coder should assign as many codes from categories E08-E13 as needed to identify all of the associated conditions the patient has. They should be sequenced based on the reason for the particular encounter (Example 5-34).

Diabetes code categories (E08, E09, E11, and E13) have an associated instructional note in the Tabular Index that advises the coder to "Use additional code to identify any insulin use (Z79.4)." If the patient routinely takes insulin, use diagnosis code Z79.4, long-term (current) use of insulin, but do not use this code if the patient takes insulin temporarily to control blood sugar.

If the patient receives an underdose because of pump failure, assign a code from subcategory T85.6, mechanical complication of other specified internal and external prosthetic devices, implants and grafts, followed by code T38.3X6-, with the appropriate code for the type of DM and any associated complications. If the pump failure causes an insulin overdose, the second diagnosis code should be T38.3X1-, poisoning by insulin and oral hypoglycemic drugs, accidental, with the appropriate code for the type of DM and related complications.

Diabetes is a significant complicating factor in pregnancy. When coding DM in pregnancy, assign a code from category O24, DM in pregnancy, childbirth and the puerperium, as the primary code. The appropriate diabetes code from the category E08-E13 should be reported as a secondary code.

Gestational diabetes occurs when the diabetes was induced by the pregnancy. This can occur during the second or third trimester of pregnancy in women who were not diabetic prior to pregnancy. Codes from subcategory O24.4, gestational DM, are reported when this condition is documented.

Circulatory System Conditions

Diseases of the circulatory system are difficult to code because of the variety and lack of specific terminology used by physicians in stating the diagnoses. The insurance billing specialist should refer to Section 1, Subsection C, Chapter 9 of the Chapter-Specific Coding Guidelines for assistance in coding circulatory system conditions. When selecting codes, carefully read all inclusion, exclusion, and "use additional code" notations contained in the Tabular List.

Hypertension

The lay term "high blood pressure" is medically termed *hypertension (HTN)*. Hypertension may be documented as *malignant*, which has nothing to do with tumor formation. Malignant hypertension is a condition of very high blood pressure with poor prognosis. It is a symptom complex of markedly elevated blood pressure (that is, diastolic pressure greater than 140 mm Hg) associated with papilledema. In this disease, the term *malignant* denotes "life threatening." *Benign hypertension* refers to high blood pressure that runs a relatively long and symptomless course. In ICD-10-CM, hypertension is reported with the code I10, regardless of whether the hypertension is documented as benign or malignant.

Hypertension can cause various forms of heart and vascular disease or it can accompany some heart conditions. There are code categories used to report these conditions as combination codes.

Code Category I11	Hypertensive heart disease
Code Category I12	Hypertensive chronic kidney disease
Code Category I13	Hypertensive heart and chronic kidney disease

When the diagnostic statement indicates a cause by stating "heart condition *due to* hypertension" or "hypertensive heart disease," assign a code from category I11. If the diagnostic statement reads "*with* hypertension" or "cardiomegaly *and* hypertension," you need two separate codes.

Elevated blood pressure without mention of hypertension is coded R03.0. Secondary hypertension is due to an underlying condition and is reported from the code category I15. An additional code is required to report

Example 5-34	**Complications Related to Diabetes**
E11.40	Diabetic neuropathy
E11.36	Diabetic cataracts

secondary hypertension to identify the cause of the hypertension when specified.

Myocardial Infarctions

A myocardial infarction (MI) is commonly referred to as a heart attack. During an MI, there is death to a segment of heart muscle caused by a blood clot in the coronary artery that interrupts the heart's blood supply. An MI of 4 weeks' duration or less is considered acute and is reported with codes from category I21. If the patient is still receiving care related to the MI after the four-week time frame, the appropriate aftercare code should be assigned. If the patient suffers an acute MI during the four-week time frame, the incident should be reported with a code from category I22 to indicate a subsequent acute MI. The code I25.2 is reported for old or healed myocardial infarctions that do not require further care.

Pregnancy, Delivery, or Abortion

Section 1, Subsection C, Chapter 15 of the Chapter-Specific Coding Guidelines provides guidelines for reporting pregnancy, delivery, or abortion cases. Chapter 15 codes have sequencing priority over codes from other chapters. When the provider has treated a condition unrelated to the pregnancy but the pregnancy has been documented as incidental to the encounter, code Z33.1, pregnant state, incidental, should be used in place of a Chapter 15 code.

The following main sections are included:
O00-O08 Pregnancy with abortive outcome
O09 Supervision of high-risk pregnancy
O10-O16 Edema, proteinuria, and hypertensive disorders in pregnancy, childbirth, and the puerperium
O20-O29 Other maternal disorders predominately related to pregnancy
O30-O48 Maternal care related to the fetus and amniotic cavity and possible delivery problems
O60-O77 Complications of labor and delivery
O80-O82 Encounter for delivery
O85-O92 Complications predominantly related to the puerperium
O94-O9A Other obstetric conditions, not elsewhere classifiable

An entire section of the Chapter-Specific Coding Guidelines is devoted to reporting obstetric cases, which are not limited to but include the following:
1. Chapter 15 codes are reported only on the maternal record, never on the newborn record.
2. Codes in Chapter 15 have a final character to indicate the trimester of pregnancy. Trimesters are counted from the first day of the last menstrual period and defined as first trimester (less than 14 weeks, 0 days), second trimester (14 weeks, 0 days to less than 28 weeks, 0 days), and third trimester (28 weeks, 0 days until delivery). Assignment of the final character should be based on the provider's documentation of the trimester. If documentation in the record is insufficient to clarify trimester, report the final character for "unspecified trimester."
3. When reporting complications in pregnancy or childbirth, a seventh character may be required in some instances to identify the fetus affected by the complications. A seventh character of "0" is reported for single gestations when the document in the record is insufficient or when it is not possible to clinically determine which fetus is affected (Example 5-35).
4. Routine outpatient prenatal visits are reported with a code from category Z34 when no complications are present.
5. Outpatient prenatal visits for high-risk patients are reported with a code from category O09.
6. Full-term uncomplicated vaginal delivery should be reported with code O80. Code O80 is always a principal diagnosis and is not reported with any other code from Chapter 15.
7. A code from category Z37 is reported on every maternal record to report the outcome of delivery.

Injury, Poisoning, and Other Consequences of External Causes

Section 1, Subsection C of Chapter 19 of the Chapter-Specific Coding Guidelines is a large section of rules for coding of injuries, fractures, burns, poisoning, adult and child abuse, and complications of care that should be referred to ensure accuracy of coding.

Most categories in Chapter 19 require a seventh character extension to indicate whether the encounter is an initial encounter (identified with an "A"), a subsequent encounter (identified with a "D"), or a sequela or late effect (identified with an "S").

Injuries and Late Effects

Diagnostic codes for injuries are listed in the Alphabetic Index by the type of injury and are broken down by anatomic site. To code multiple injuries, a separate code should be assigned for each injury, unless a combination code is assigned. List the diagnosis for the conditions treated in order of importance, with the diagnosis for the

Example 5-35	Complications Related to Pregnancy
O10.919	Preexisting hypertension complicating pregnancy
O36.5910	Pregnancy complicated by poor fetal growth, third trimester

most severe problem listed first. If surgery is involved, the diagnostic code for the surgical problem should be listed first unless there is a severe injury of another part of the body (Example 5-36).

The most difficult part of assigning injury codes is to know what main terms to look for in the Alphabetic Index. Codes S00-T88 include fractures, dislocations, sprains, and other types of injury. Injuries are coded according to the general type of injury and broken down within each type by anatomic site. A list of common injury medical terms and the types of injuries included for each is shown in Table 5-4.

Use the following guidelines for coding injuries:
1. Decide whether a diagnosis represents a current injury or a late effect of an injury (Example 5-37).
2. Fractures are coded as "closed" if there is no indication of whether the fracture is open or closed.
3. The word "with" indicates involvement of both sites and the word "and" indicates involvement of either one or two sites when multiple injury sites are given.

A sequela describes the residual effect (condition produced) after the acute phase of an illness or injury has terminated. An injury may have a residual effect, which must be coded in a different fashion. An effect is considered to be a sequela if the diagnosis reads "due to an old injury," "late," "due to" or "following" (previous illness or injury), or "due to an injury or illness that occurred 1 year or more before the current admission of encounter." Residual effects can be found under the main term "sequelae." The condition or nature of the residual effect is sequenced first and the sequela is listed second (Example 5-38).

Example 5-37	Current Injury
S82.92XA	**Current injury:** Fracture, left ankle; Initial encounter
	or
M12.572 and S82.92XS	**Late effect:** Traumatic arthritis, due to old fracture, left ankle

Example 5-36	Injuries
Case: An intracranial injury, managed medically, and a fractured middle phalanx of the right hand, managed surgically	
S06.9X0A	Intracranial injury, Initial encounter (first-listed primary diagnosis)
S62.602A	Fractured middle phalanx, Initial encounter (secondary diagnosis)

Example 5-38	Late Effects
A. Unilateral posttraumatic osteoarthritis (M17.31), **due to crushing injury of right knee (S87.01XS)**	
B. Osteoporosis (M81.8), **due to late effect of calcium deficiency (E64.8)**	
C. Anemia of the puerperium (O90.81), **sequela of pregnancy, childbirth and the puerperium (O94)**	

Table 5-4	Common Injury Medical Terms
MAIN TERM	**EXPLANATION**
Contusion	Bruise and hematoma without a fracture or open wound.
Crush	Crushing injury not complicated by concussion, fractures, injury to internal organs, or intracranial injury.
Dislocation	Displacement and subluxation. Dislocation may be open or closed. Closed dislocation may be complete, partial, simple, or uncomplicated. Open dislocation may be compound, infected, or with foreign body. A dislocation not indicated as closed or open is classified as closed.
Fracture	Fractures may be open or closed. A fracture not indicated as open or closed is classified as closed. An injury described as fracture dislocation is coded as a fracture. Open fractures may be described as compound, infected, missile, puncture, or with foreign body. Closed fractures may be described as comminuted, depressed, elevated, fissured, greenstick, impacted, linear, march, simple, slipped, epiphyseal, or spiral.
Injury, blood vessel	Described as arterial hematoma, avulsion, laceration, rupture, traumatic aneurysm, or traumatic fistula.
Injury, internal	Includes all injuries to internal organs such as the heart, lung, liver, kidney, and pelvic organs. Types of injuries to internal organs include laceration, tear, traumatic rupture, penetrating wound, blunt trauma, crushing, blast injury, or open wound to internal organs with or without fracture in the same region.
Injury, intracranial	Includes concussion, cerebral laceration and contusion, or intracranial hemorrhage. These injuries may be open or closed. Intracranial injuries with skull fractures may be found under fracture.
Injury, superficial	Includes abrasion, insect bite (nonvenomous), blister, or scratch.
Sprain or strain	Injury to the joint capsule, ligament, muscle, or tendon described by the following terms: avulsion, hemarthrosis, laceration (closed), rupture, or tear. Open laceration of these structures should be coded as open wounds.
Wound, open	Includes open wounds not involving internal organs. Wounds may be to skin, muscle, or tendon, described as animal bite, avulsion, cut, laceration, puncture wound, or traumatic amputation. Open wounds may be complicated or uncomplicated. Complicated includes injuries with mention of delayed healing, delayed treatment, foreign body, or major infection.

Use the following guidelines for coding a sequela:
1. Refer to the main term "sequela—*see also* condition" in ICD-10-CM's Alphabetic Index when coding a case with a sequela.
2. Look for the condition.
3. The Tabular Index will provide instructional notes that may indicate that two codes must be reported; code first the condition resulting from the sequela.

Burns and Corrosions

Burn codes are used for reporting thermal burns, except burns that come from a heat source, such as a fire or hot appliance, or those that result from electricity or radiation. Corrosions are defined as burns caused by chemicals.

Burns are classified by depth, extent, and agent. When multiple burns are reported, a separate code for each burn site is reported. The code that reflects the highest degree of burn should be sequenced first using a code from the range T20-T25. An additional code from category T31 or T32 should be reported to identify the total body surface area (TBSA) for all sites. Think of the body as a whole and not the body parts as a whole. The adult body is divided into regions: head, 9%; arms, 9% each; trunk, 18% front and 18% back; legs, 18% each; and perineum, 1% (Figure 5-9). Children's and infants' bodies have different regional percentages.

Adverse Effects, Poisoning, Underdosing, and Toxic Effects

Adverse effects, poisoning, underdosing, and toxic effects are reported using combination codes from the range T36-T65. No additional external cause code is required.

The Table of Drugs and Chemicals is found after the Alphabetical Index, Section 2 (see Table 5-2) and contains a classification of drugs and other chemical substances for identifying poisoning states and external causes of adverse effects.

Adverse effect is defined as an adverse or pathologic reaction to a drug that occurs when appropriate doses are given to humans for prophylaxis (prevention of disease), diagnosis, and therapy (Example 5-39). When an adverse effect occurs (for example, drug reaction, hypersensitivity, drug intolerance, or idiosyncratic reaction), a code is assigned to the diagnosis that classifies the specific reaction or symptom (for example, dermatitis, syncope, tachycardia, or urticaria). The specific reaction or symptom from use of the drug is reported as the primary code, followed by a code from the table for the correct code assignment for the adverse effect of the drug (T36-T50). The code for the drug should have a fifth or sixth character.

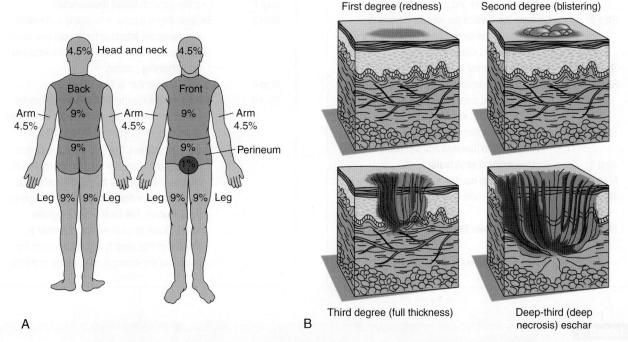

FIGURE 5-9 A, The rule of nines estimation of total body surface area (TBSA) burned. **B,** The degrees of burn involving the layers of the skin: first-degree burns include the epidermis (redness), second-degree burns include the epidermis and dermis (blistering), third-degree burns include the first two layers and the subcutaneous tissues (full thickness), and deep-third burns involve all layers of the skin with resulting eschar (deep necrosis).

Poisoning is defined as a condition resulting from an intentional overdose of drugs or chemical substances or from the drug or agent given or taken in error. The following situations occur and are documented in the medical record to indicate poisoning:

- Taking the wrong medication
- Receiving the wrong medication
- Taking the wrong dose of the right medication
- Receiving the wrong dose of the right medication
- Ingesting a chemical substance not intended for human consumption
- Overdose of a chemical substance (drug)
- Prescription drug taken with alcohol
- Mixing prescription drugs and over-the-counter medications without the physician's advice or consent

Each of the substances listed in Table 5-5 is assigned a code according to the poisoning classification (categories T36-T50). These adverse effect codes are used when there is a state of poisoning, overdose, wrong substance given or taken, or **intoxication.** Intoxication is defined as an adverse effect rather than a poisoning when drugs such as digitalis and steroid agents are involved. However, whenever the term *intoxication* is used, the insurance billing specialist should clarify with the physician the circumstances surrounding the administration of the drug or chemical before assigning the appropriate code. This must be documented in the health record. If a diagnosis is stated as possible or suspected suicide attempt, go to the column titled "Undetermined" and not to "Suicide Attempt."

Example 5-40 shows the steps for coding a case that involves poisoning.

External Causes of Morbidity

External causes of morbidity codes are a classification of codes in which you look for external causes of injury rather than disease. The code description refers to the circumstances that caused an injury rather than the nature of the injury. The codes are also used in coding adverse reactions to medications (Figure 5-10).

Example 5-39   Coding an Adverse Effect

An inpatient had an adverse effect (ventricular fibrillation) to the medication digoxin, which was prescribed by her physician and taken correctly.

Step 1	Refer to the Table of Drugs and Chemicals in the Alphabetic Index and look up **digoxin.**
Step 2	Because this medication was for therapeutic use, locate the correct code number under the adverse effect column.
Step 3	The correct number is **T46.0X5.**
Step 4	Verify the code number T46.0X5 in the Tabular List. Note that a seventh character is required to indicate initial encounter **T46.0X5A.**
Step 5	Locate the main term **fibrillation** in the Alphabetic Index to Diseases and Injuries.
Step 6	Find the subterm **ventricular.**
Step 7	The correct code number is **I49.01.**
Step 8	Verify the code number I49.01 in the Tabular List.
Sequencing	**I49.01 Ventricular fibrillation (chief complaint)**
	T46.0X5A Therapeutic use, Digoxin

Example 5-40   Coding a Poisoning

Baby Kathy got into the kitchen cabinet and ingested liquid household ammonia. She was taken to the emergency room for immediate treatment.

Step 1	Refer to the Table of Drugs and Chemicals in the Alphabetic Index and look up **ammonia.**
Step 2	Find the subterm **liquid (household).**
Step 3	Because this is a case of ingesting a chemical substance not intended for human use, locate the correct code number under the **Accidental Poisoning** column.
Step 4	The correct number is **T54.3X1.**
Step 5	Verify the code number T54.3X1 in the Tabular List. Note that a seventh character is required to indicate initial encounter **T54.3X1A.**
Sequencing	Codes in categories T36-T65 are combination codes that include the substances related to the poisoning as well as the external cause. No additional external cause code is required for poisoning. The code from categories T36-T65 are sequenced first, followed by any codes that specify any outcomes of the poisoning (for example, nausea and vomiting).

Table 5-5   Table of Drugs and Chemicals

SUBSTANCE	POISONING, ACCIDENTAL	POISONING, INTENTIONAL SELF-HARM	POISONING, ASSAULT	POISONING, UNDETERMINED	ADVERSE EFFECT	UNDERDOSING
Acetylsalicylic acid (salts)	T39.011	T39.012	T39.013	T39.014	T39.015	T39.016

External cause codes are listed in a separate section of the Tabular List and are included in the code range V01-Y99. To look up external cause codes, use Section III in the Alphabetic Index. The external cause codes are also in a separate section, Index to External Causes of Injury and Poisoning, which follows the regular Alphabetic Index.

Use of an external cause code after the primary or other acute secondary diagnosis explains the mechanism for the injury. For example, if a patient falls and fractures a finger, the fracture code is primary and an external cause code following it helps to explain how the accident or injury occurred (Example 5-41). This can help to speed the reimbursement process because a payer will see an acute injury code and know that a third party is responsible for payment, as in a workers' compensation injury or motor vehicle accident. External cause codes

also play a role in gathering data, such as in statistical reporting, credentialing, utilization, review, and state injury prevention programs. On the negative side, however, many payers require that chart notes accompany external cause code claims, which means generating a paper claim rather than sending it electronically. External cause codes often trigger a questionnaire that is sent to the beneficiary. This may lead to a delay in reimbursement. Although external cause codes do not generate revenue, it is recommended that they be reported in addition to the appropriate procedural and diagnostic codes. This ensures that the most specific information possible is provided regarding the patient's injury. External cause codes are billed by the initial entity seeing the patient. If the patient visits the physician's office after hospitalization for injuries sustained in a motor vehicle accident, the hospital assigns an external cause code and there is no requirement for repeating it for the office visit. An external cause code may never be sequenced as the primary diagnosis in the first position. When using external cause codes, be sure to list them last on the claim form.

External cause codes must be reported with appropriate seventh character (initial encounter, subsequent encounter, or sequela) for each encounter for which the injury or condition is being treated. As many external cause codes as are necessary to fully explain each cause should be reported.

Codes from category Y92, place of occurrence, should be reported to identify the location of the patient at the time of injury or other condition. The place of occurrence code is reported only at the initial encounter for treatment. It should not be reported if not stated in the provider's documentation.

Factors Influencing Health Status and Contact with Health Services

Factors influencing health status and contact with health services are reported with the code range Z00-Z99 and are referred to as **Z codes**. All guidelines for reporting Z codes can be found in Section 1, Subsection C of Chapter 21 of the Chapter-Specific Coding Guidelines.

Z codes are included in the major section of the Alphabetic Index to Diseases and Injuries. They are used for the following four primary circumstances:
1. When a person who is not currently sick encounters health services for some specific purpose, such as to act as a donor of an organ or tissue, receive a vaccination, discuss a problem that is not in itself a disease or injury, seek consultation about family planning, request sterilization, or obtain supervision of a normal pregnancy (Example 5-42).

INDEX TO EXTERNAL CAUSES

Fall, falling (accidental) W19
  building W20.1
    burning (uncontrolled fire) X00.3
  down
    embankment W17.81
    escalator W10.0
    hill W17.81
    ladder W11
    ramp W10.2
    stairs, steps W10.9
  due to
    bumping against
      object W18.00
        sharp glass W18.02
        specified NEC W18.09
        sports equipment W18.01
      person W03
        due to ice or snow W00.0
        on pedestrian conveyance —
          see Accident, transport,
            pedestrian, conveyance
      collision with another person W03
      due to ice or snow W00.0
      involving pedestrian conveyance —
        see Accident, transport,
          pedestrian, conveyance

FIGURE 5-10 External cause coding.

Example 5-41	External Cause Codes
26720	Closed treatment of phalangeal shaft fracture, proximal phalanx, finger; without manipulation, each
S62.649A	Nondisplaced fracture of proximal phalanx of finger, Initial encounter
W10.1XXA	Fall from sidewalk curb

Note: Code 26720 is a Current Procedural Terminology (CPT) code; CPT is discussed in Chapter 6.

Example 5-42	Supervision of First Pregnancy, Normal, First Trimester

Step 1   Find the heading **Pregnancy** in the Alphabetic Index.
Step 2   Look for the subheading **supervision.**
Step 3   Look for the second subheading **normal** and a further subheading **first,** which gives you the code Z34.0-.
Step 4   Find **Z34.0-** in the Tabular List. By Tabular List, you will see "**Encounter for Supervision of Normal First Pregnancy.**"
Step 5   Find **Z34.01** in the Tabular List, which indicates "**Encounter for Supervision of Normal First Pregnancy, First Trimester.**"

Example 5-43	

Z47.81   Encounter for orthopedic aftercare following surgical amputation
Instructional note: Use additional code to identify the limb amputated. (Z89.-)

Example 5-44	

Z85.3   Personal history of malignant neoplasm of breast

Example 5-45	

Z38.00   Single liveborn infant, delivered vaginally, born in hospital

2. When a person with a resolving disease or injury, such as a chronic, long-term condition that needs continuous care, seeks aftercare (Example 5-43).
3. When a circumstance influences an individual's health status but the illness is not current (Example 5-44).
4. When it is necessary to indicate the birth status of a newborn (Example 5-45).

These types of encounters are among the more common services for hospital outpatients and patients of private practitioners, health clinics, and others. Certain Z codes may appear only as a primary code and others only as secondary codes.

Some key words in patient care that indicate that a Z code might be necessary are *exposure, routine annual examination, admission, history of, encounter,* and *vaccination.* Z codes also are used when some circumstance or problem is present that influences the person's health status but is not in itself a current illness or injury, such as when the person is known to have an allergy to a specific drug. In this instance, the Z code cannot be used as a stand-alone code and should be used only as a supplementary code.

Example 5-46	Routine Annual Adult Physical Examination, without Abnormal Findings

Step 1   Look up **examination,** and notice **annual (adult)** as a subterm and the code **Z00.00.**
Step 2   Find **Z00.00** in the Tabular List and the wording "**Encounter for general adult medical examination without abnormal findings.**"

Additional code numbers are given for occupational health examinations and routine annual physical examinations; therefore select specific codes depending on the circumstances (Example 5-46).

Encounters for Reproductive Services

Z codes are used to report family planning, contraceptive or procreative management, and counseling. Codes from the category Z30 are used only when the encounter is for contraceptive management and must be specific to the type of contraceptive managed.

Z30.011   Encounter for initial prescription of contraceptive pills
Z30.012   Encounter for prescription of emergency contraception
Z30.013   Encounter for prescription of injectable contraceptive
Z30.014   Encounter for initial prescription of intrauterine contraceptive device
Z30.018   Encounter for initial prescription of other contraceptives
Z30.019   Encounter for initial prescription of unspecified contraceptive
Z30.02   Counseling and instruction in natural family planning to avoid pregnancy
Z30.09   Encounter for other general counseling and advice on contraception

Codes from the category Z30.4, encounter for surveillance of contraceptives, are available for reporting encounters for continued management. The codes from category Z30.4 are also specific to the type of contraceptive being used. When sterilization is performed for the major purpose of contraception rather than being an incidental result of the treatment of a disease, code Z30.2 is reported.

Diagnostic Coding and Reporting Guidelines for Outpatient Services

Section IV of the Official Guidelines contains a set of rules specific to reporting of outpatient services with which the insurance billing specialist should be familiar. The guidelines are approved for use for reporting hospital-based outpatient services and provider-based office visits.

The guidelines are used in conjunction with the general and disease-specific guidelines.

Outpatient Surgery

When patients present for outpatient surgery, the first-listed diagnosis should be the reason for the surgery. If the postoperative diagnosis is different and is confirmed, select the more specific postoperative diagnosis code.

Uncertain Diagnosis

When reporting hospital-based outpatient services and provider-based office visits, if the provider has documented a condition as "probable," "suspected," "questionable," "rule out," or "working diagnosis," do not code as if the patient has the condition. Instead, code for the symptom, sign, or reason for the visit. This guideline is different for medical record coders in the inpatient hospital setting.

Chronic Disease

Chronic diseases that are treated on an ongoing basis may be reported as long as evaluation and management of the condition are documented.

Code All Documented Conditions that Coexist

All conditions that coexist at the time of the visit that are evaluated and managed and affect patient care should be reported. If the condition was previously treated but no longer exists, it should be reported as a history code (Z80-Z87) if the condition has an impact on the current plan of care (Example 5-47).

Patients Receiving Diagnostic Services Only

Sequence first the diagnosis, condition, problem, or other reason for the visit for patients receiving diagnostic services. For routine laboratory or radiology testing in the absence of any signs or symptoms, assign Z01.89, encounter for other specified special examination (Example 5-48).

Example 5-47

A patient is seen by her primary care physician (PCP) for management of chronic hypertension. The physician also performed a completed skin assessment, based on the patient's history of malignant melanoma in situ, which was previously excised in full.	Hypertension: I10 Personal history of malignant neoplasm: Z85.820

Example 5-48

Patient seen in the emergency room for pain in the left leg is sent to x-ray. The x-ray is read and is negative.	Report as: Left leg pain M79.605

Example 5-49   Preoperative Examination

A patient to have surgery for gallstones is sent to a cardiologist for a preoperative examination to evaluate the patient's suspected cardiovascular disease.

Step 1   In the Alphabetic Index, look up **examination** and notice **preprocedural (preoperative)** and **cardiovascular** as subterms and the code **Z01.810.** Verify it in the Tabular List.

Step 2   Code the reason for the surgery—K80.20, cholelithiasis.

Preoperative Evaluations

Sometimes a patient receives a consultation for a preoperative medical evaluation as an inpatient or outpatient (Example 5-49) and the majority of the results are negative for chronic or current illness. A good-health diagnosis code will trigger a rejection by the third-party payer unless the insurance company allows or requires it. When reporting, sequence first a code from subcategory Z01.80, encounter for pre-procedural examination, to describe the preoperative consultation, followed by a code for the condition describing the reason for the surgery. Any additional findings related to the preoperative evaluation should also be reported.

General Medical Examinations with Abnormal Findings

General medical examinations are reported with the category of codes Z00.0-. Subcategories provide codes for examinations with and without abnormal findings. A general medical examination that results in an abnormal finding should be reported with the code for general medical examination with abnormal finding assigned as the first-listed diagnosis. A secondary code for the abnormal finding should also be reported.

Handy Hints for Diagnostic Coding

If your ICD-10-CM code books are not color-coded, identify important references with a colored highlighter pen. Also add tabs to main sections of the Alphabetic Index, Tabular List, and Drug and Chemical Table. Refer to the end of this chapter to learn how to locate and select diagnostic codes step by step.

Many times you will locate a diagnostic code in the Alphabetic Index only to find that the cross-referenced code is the same when verified in the Tabular List. In some situations you might indicate these codes in Volume 2 with a different-colored highlighter pen to remind you that this code is correct as described in the Alphabetic Index, which saves the time you would spend checking the Tabular List. However, keep in mind that the Tabular List has many instructional notes that are not indicated in the Alphabetic Index and must be followed for accurate coding.

Keep a list of diagnostic codes commonly encountered by your office. Some insurance companies publish lists of diagnostic codes that support medical necessity and are acceptable for specific procedures. Consult payer guidelines by calling the insurance company or managed care plan to determine whether certain procedures are a covered benefit for certain diagnoses and if not, have the patient sign a waiver. Reference books that show codes that link diagnostic and procedure codes are available. The American Medical Association (AMA) publishes a list of the most common diagnostic codes at the end of each of its mini-specialty code books.

In the past, some medical practices have developed an encounter form that is an all-encompassing billing document and reference page and that acts as a shortcut to locating diagnostic codes for conditions commonly seen by a physician specialist. Although these may have served a good purpose under the previous ICD-9 coding system, it is no longer recommended that these types of billing documents be used. Most often these types of documents are found to lack the specificity necessary to infer diagnosis details needed for accurate coding. Continuing their use in ICD-10-CM will only prevent reporting of the increased granularity.

Computer-Assisted Coding

Computer-assisted coding (CAC) is computer software that automatically generates a set of medical codes for review, validation, and use based on clinical documentation provided by health care practitioners. Many factors have pushed medical practices to adopt CAC. Some of these factors are as follows:
- Shortage of coders throughout the United States
- Financial need to reduce the cost of filing insurance claims
- Increased complexity of coding systems with implementation of the ICD-10-CM coding system
- Adoption of EHRs
- Advancement in natural language processing (NLP) technology
- Frequent changes in code numbers and coding rules and regulations
- Compliance liability for increased erroneous claims

CAC uses two technology options: structured input and NLP. In structured input, the physician inputs information on a data entry screen that has point-and-click fields, pull-down menus, structured templates, or macros. The system prompts the physician for detailed information. Words and phrases selected are linked to diagnostic and procedural codes that are automatically generated when all fields are completed. Input of the detailed information results in a completed document with the appropriate level of detail. Recommended diagnostic and procedural codes are then checked and edited by a coder.

The NLP system uses artificial medical intelligence. The physician dictates a report, handwrites a note, or inputs a picture file. The document is sent to an NLP engine that scans the health record; chooses important, relevant words; and converts them into suggested codes. A coder searches and validates the diagnostic and procedural codes and makes any changes, and then the codes are transmitted to billing. NLP systems must be updated regularly to address new medical terminology and conform to changes in coding guidelines.

Automated coding software uses a statistics-based method, rules-based method, or both methods to assign codes. In a statistics-based program, also called a *data-driven method*, the software predicts the code for a word or phrase based on statistics from the past. A rules-based or knowledge-driven method applies coding rules, such as those used in logic- or rules-based encoders, groupers, and imaged coding applications, to electronic clinical documents. The codes are processed through associated established rules for refinement and code assignment.

Another feature of CAC is the use of crosswalks or *data mapping*, which gives a coder the ability to input a discontinued code and find a new replacement code.

Sometimes professional coders disagree about which codes to apply to a specific case; thus checking and editing codes may be needed when using CAC. Usually, repetitive procedures are quick for coders to approve but complex procedures may need more time for validation. CAC technology helps coders to do their jobs faster and more efficiently and does not diminish the need for coders.

THE FUTURE OF DIAGNOSIS CODING

The ICD is constantly under revision to better reflect progress in health sciences and medical practices. Development of the next edition of ICD (ICD-11) for diagnosis coding began in April 2007 and included some very specific goals:
- To improve on the ability to function in an electronic environment

- To allow for collaborative web-based editing by interested parties while under peer review
- To incorporate international multilingual reference standards for scientific comparability

ICD-11 is alphanumeric, building on the structure of ICD-10, and will be similar in appearance. It will be a digital product that will link with terminologies (i.e., SNOMED CT) and support EHRs and information systems.

ICD-11 was scheduled for dissemination by 2012; however, the timeline was extended given the size of the task, the technical complexity of the system, and the limited funding and human resources for the project. The beta version of ICD-11 was produced in September 2013 and will undergo field trials and final review. According to the WHO, ICD-11 is expected to be unveiled to the world in May 2017.

PROCEDURE 5-1

Basic Steps in Selecting Diagnostic Codes from ICD-9-CM

OBJECTIVE: Accurately select and insert diagnostic codes for electronic transmission of an insurance claim

EQUIPMENT/SUPPLIES: ICD-9-CM diagnostic code book, medical dictionary, and pen or pencil

DIRECTIONS: Use a standard method and establish a routine for locating a code. Follow these recommended steps for coding the first diagnosis. There are no shortcuts. For each subsequent diagnosis in a patient's medical record, repeat these steps.

DIAGNOSIS: Refractory megaloblastic anemia with chronic alcoholic liver disease

1. Read the patient's medical record. Identify the main term or condition (not the anatomic site) in the Alphabetic Index (anemia). To locate the main term, ask what is wrong with the patient.
2. Refer to any notes under the main term (none shown).
3. Read any notes or terms enclosed in parentheses after the main term (nonessential modifiers) (none shown).
4. Look for appropriate subterm (megaloblastic). *Do not* skip over any subterms indented under the main term.
5. Look for appropriate subsubterm (refractory).

6. Follow any cross-reference instructions (none given).
7. Write down the code (281.3).
8. Verify the code number in the Tabular List.
9. Read and be guided by any instructional terms in the Tabular List. In this example, there are none given.
10. Read the complete description and then code to the highest specificity; that is, code to the highest number of digits (three, four, or five) in the classification (refractory megaloblastic anemia, 281.3). When a fourth or fifth digit is listed, its use is *not* optional. A three-digit code is considered a category unless no fourth or fifth digit appears after it. Fifth-digit codes appear either at the beginning of a chapter, section, or three-digit category or within the four-digit subcategory. To facilitate locating those codes that require a fourth or fifth digit, some publishers may insert a symbol (for example, *f*) in the code book. Do not arbitrarily use a zero as a filler character when listing a diagnostic code number. This may nullify the code or indicate a different disease. The code book includes decimal points but these are not required for transmission of insurance claims.
11. Assign the code.

PROCEDURE 5-2

Basic Steps in Selecting Diagnostic Codes from ICD-10-CM

OBJECTIVE: Accurately choose and insert diagnostic codes for electronic transmission of an insurance claim

EQUIPMENT/SUPPLIES: ICD-10-CM diagnostic code book, medical dictionary, and pen or pencil.

DIRECTIONS: Use a standard method and establish a routine for locating a code. Follow these steps for coding the first diagnosis. For each subsequent diagnosis in a patient's medical record, repeat these steps.

1. Read the patient's medical record to find the main term. To identify the main term, ask what is wrong with the patient.
2. Next, locate the main term (disease or condition), not the anatomic site, in the Alphabetic Index. The

Alphabetic Index is organized by main terms and has three sections:
- Section 1—Index to Diseases and Nature of Injury includes Neoplasm Table and Table of Drugs and Chemicals
- Section 2—Index to External Causes of Injury
- Section 3—Table of Drugs and Chemicals
3. Read any notes under the main term. Select and write down the code.
4. Next, go to the Tabular List, review how it is organized for the subclassification, read and be guided by any instructional terms, and then verify that the selected code gives the highest level of

Continued

PROCEDURE 5-2—cont'd

specificity (up to seven alphanumeric characters). Possible errors may occur when using the Tabular List and when coding diseases or conditions that begin with categories "O" and "I." These can look like the numbers "zero" and "one" (for example, I00 and O99 are correct—not 100 and 099). In these categories, special attention must be given. Always read the specific chapter guidelines and refer to the general guidelines in the code book for certain diagnoses and/or conditions in the classification before choosing a code.

5. Assign the code.

KEY POINTS

This is a brief chapter review, or summary, of the key issues presented. To further enhance your knowledge of the technical subject matter, review the key terms and key abbreviations for this chapter by locating the meaning for each in the Glossary at the end of this text, which appears in a section before the Index.

1. Accurate diagnostic coding can mean the financial success or failure of a medical practice.

2. Payment for outpatient services is related to procedure codes but must be supported and justified by the diagnosis.

3. Diagnostic coding was developed for the following reasons: (1) tracking of disease processes, (2) classification of causes of mortality, (3) medical research, and (4) evaluation of hospital service use.

4. When submitting insurance claims for patients seen in a physician's office or an outpatient hospital setting, the primary diagnosis, which is the main reason for the encounter, is listed first.

5. For services provided after October 1, 2015, always use the ICD-10-CM Alphabetic Index and then go to the Tabular (numerical) List before assigning a diagnostic code. For services provided prior to October 1, 2015, the same process is followed using ICD-9-CM.

6. Always code to the highest degree of specificity. The more digits a code has, the more specific the description is.

7. Always code the underlying disease, the etiology, or the cause first; subsequently list the secondary diagnosis.

8. Z codes in ICD-10-CM are used when a person who is not currently sick encounters health services for some specific purpose, such as to receive a vaccination.

9. External cause codes in ICD-10-CM are used to report the causes of injury rather than the nature of the injury or disease and to code adverse reactions to medications. In ICD-10-CM, these codes begin with V, W, X, and Y.

10. Always follow coding conventions because they assist in the selection of correct codes for the diagnoses encountered. These conventions are rules or principles for determining a diagnostic code when using diagnostic code books, such as each space, typefaces, indentations, punctuation marks, symbols, instructional notes, abbreviations, cross-reference notes, and specific usage of the words "and," "with," and "due to."

🖥 STUDENT ASSIGNMENT

✔ Study Chapter 5.
✔ Answer the fill-in-the-blank, multiple-choice, and true/false review questions in the *Workbook* to reinforce theory learned in this chapter and to help prepare for a future test.

✔ Complete the assignments in the *Workbook* to gain hands-on experience in diagnostic coding.
✔ Turn to the Glossary at the end of this text for a further understanding of the key terms and key abbreviations used in this chapter.

Marilyn Takahashi Fordney and Karen Levein

OBJECTIVES

After reading this chapter, you should be able to:

1. Explain the purpose and importance of coding for professional services.

2. Define terminology used in Current Procedural Terminology (CPT).

3. Demonstrate an understanding of CPT code conventions.

4. Describe various methods of payment by insurance companies and state and federal programs.

5. Describe the process to create a fee schedule using relative value studies conversion factors.

6. Discuss the format and content of the CPT code book, including category I, II, and III codes.

7. Interpret the meaning of CPT code book symbols.

8. Identify and discuss the complexity of evaluation and management (E/M) services codes.

9. Compare a surgical package and a Medicare global package.

10. Explain various types of code edits.

11. Explain how to choose accurate procedure codes for descriptions of services and procedures documented in a patient's medical record, including discussions on bundled codes, unbundling, downcoding, upcoding, and code monitoring.

12. Discuss helpful hints in coding.

13. Explain correct usage of modifiers in procedure coding.

KEY TERMS

alternative billing codes	global surgery policy	relative value unit
bilateral	Healthcare Common Procedure	resource-based relative value
bundled codes	Coding System	scale
comprehensive code	modifiers	surgical package
conversion factor	never event	technical component
Current Procedural Terminology	procedure code numbers	unbundling
customary fee	professional component	upcoding
downcoding	reasonable fee	usual, customary, and
fee schedule	relative value studies	reasonable

KEY ABBREVIATIONS

ABCS	ED	GPCIs	RVU
AHA	E/M service	HCPCS	TC
CF	EMTALA	NCCI edits	UCR
CPT	EOB	PC	
DME	FTC	RBRVS	
ECG	GAF	RVS	

UNDERSTANDING THE IMPORTANCE OF PROCEDURAL CODING SKILLS

Now that you have learned some terminology and the basics of diagnostic coding, the next step is to learn how to code procedures.

Procedure coding is the transformation of written descriptions of procedures and professional services to numeric designations (code numbers). The physician rendering medical care either writes or dictates this information in the patient's health record. Then the insurance billing specialist reads through the pertinent information and verifies this with the procedure codes marked on the encounter form. Routine office visits and procedures usually are listed with codes and brief descriptions on the encounter form. These services are documented in the record and circled or checked off on the encounter form by the physician when they are performed during the patient's visit.

With the implementation of computer technology and stricter adherence to federal regulations, more emphasis is being placed on correct procedural coding. Coding must be correct if claims are to be paid promptly and optimally. Every procedure or service must be assigned correct and complete code numbers. Because of the complexity of procedural coding, a working knowledge of medical terminology, including anatomy and physiology, is essential.

Procedure codes are a standardized method used to precisely describe the services provided by physicians and allied health care professionals, such as chiropractors and nurse practitioners. They allow claim forms to be optically scanned by insurance companies. The general acceptance of the codes by third-party payers and government agencies assures the physician who uses a standardized coding system that the services and procedures he or she performs can be objectively identified and priced. The American Hospital Association (AHA) and American Health Information Management Association (AHIMA) guidelines for outpatient services and procedure coding and reporting requirements for physician billing may be found by visiting their respective websites. The AHA Central Office is the official clearinghouse for information on proper use of ICD-9-CM and ICD-10-CM codes; Level I HCPCS codes (CPT-4 codes) for hospital providers; and certain Level II HCPCS codes for hospitals, physicians, and other health care professionals. In addition, CPT Assistant, published by the American Medical Association (AMA), gives guidelines for outpatient services and procedure coding.

The primary coding system used in physicians' offices for professional services and procedures is **Current Procedural Terminology (CPT),*** published and updated annually by the AMA. To obtain a current copy of CPT, visit the AMA's website. A relative value scale, called **relative value studies (RVS),** is also used for services and procedures; it is the system used by Medicare called **resource-based relative value scale (RBRVS).** RVS and RBRVS provide unit values for CPT codes that can then be converted into dollars by use of geographic and conversion factors.

Some managed care plans develop a few internal codes for use by the plan only. Sometimes the codes are used for tracking; other times, they are used to provide reimbursement for a service not defined within CPT on the basis of their benefit structure and internal needs.

Current Procedural Terminology

The first edition of *Physicians' Current Procedural Terminology* appeared in 1966 and it was subsequently revised in 1970, 1973, and 1977. Since 1984, *CPT,* Fourth Edition, has been updated and revised annually. Code numbers are added or deleted as new procedures are developed or existing procedures are modified. These changes are shown in each edition by the use of symbols, which are described and shown later in this chapter in Figure 6-4. The symbols with their meanings are located at the bottom of each page of code numbers in the CPT code book.

HIPAA Compliance Alert

CODING COMPLIANCE PLAN

Because the government is more involved in health care, each medical practice should construct and maintain a policy and procedure manual regarding coding guidelines so that it is in compliance with HIPAA. Establishing coding and billing policies and procedures helps physicians and their office staff to address potential risk areas for fraud and abuse. A plan should include the medical practice's basic ethical philosophy, outline policies, detail coding procedures, and create an environment of confidentiality. Billers and coders should sign a statement annually indicating that they have read, understood, and agreed with the medical practice's standards of conduct (see Figure 2-5). The plan should provide coders with the framework for correct coding and indicate that health record documentation must support the codes billed. An internal audit should be done on a regular basis, and action should be taken to correct the offense if noncompliance is discovered. Such plans must have a compliance officer or a committee that oversees the audits, monitors compliance issues, and trains employees in compliance issues.

---

*Available from Book and Pamphlet Fulfillment: OP-3416, American Medical Association, P.O. Box 10946, Chicago, IL 60610-0946, or visit CPT on the Internet at website www.ama-assn.org.

Example 6-1	Current Procedural Terminology Procedure Code Numbers

A 45-year-old woman is seen for an initial office visit for evaluation of recurrent right shoulder pain. The patient's condition warranted a detailed history and physical examination (D HX & PX) with low complexity medical decision making (LCMDM). The patient complains of pain radiating down her right arm. A complete radiographic study of the right shoulder is obtained in the office and read by the physician. A corticosteroid solution is injected into the shoulder joint.

CPT Code	Description of Services
99203	Office visit, new patient (**E/M service**)
73030	Radiologic examination, shoulder, two views (**Diagnostic service**)
20610	Arthrocentesis inj.; major joint, shoulder (**Therapeutic service**)

CPT uses a basic five-digit system for coding services rendered by physicians and two-digit add-on **modifiers** to indicate circumstances in which a procedure as performed differs in some way from that described in the code. **Procedure code numbers** represent diagnostic and therapeutic services on medical billing statements and insurance forms (Example 6-1).*

CPT emerged as the procedural coding of choice when the federal government developed the Health Care Financing Administration (HCFA) **Healthcare Common Procedure Coding System (HCPCS)** (pronounced "hick-picks") for the Medicare program. The HCFA then changed its acronym to CMS (Centers for Medicare and Medicaid Services). The Medicare HCPCS consists of the following two levels of coding:

- Level I: The AMA CPT codes and modifiers (national codes).
- Level II: The CMS-designated codes and alpha modifiers (national codes). Table 6-1 lists the Level II HCPCS national code content and code ranges with details of each alphanumeric code category. Several companies annually publish Level II HCPCS code books. Content, numbers of the appendices, color-coded coverage instructions, notes, and unlisted procedures vary between the editions. Notes or special instructions may appear in or following subsections or headings or as part of the description in a heading or code. Unlisted procedures may use one of the following terms: *unlisted*, *not otherwise classified (NOC)*, *unspecified*, *unclassified*, *other*, or *miscellaneous*. Examples of

Level II codes may be found in Table B-2 in Appendix B of the *Workbook*.

You may discover that one case can be coded in two coding levels. The CPT code should be used when both a CPT and Level II code have the same description. The Level II code should be used if the descriptions are not identical (for example, if the CPT code narrative is generic and the HCPCS Level II code is specific).

The guideline for selecting a code that most accurately identifies the service is as follows:
- *Level I HCPCS CPT codes* describes physician or provider service (PPS).
- *Level II HCPCS national codes* describes ambulance, medical and surgical supplies, enteral and parenteral therapy, outpatient PPS, dental procedures, durable medical equipment, procedures/professional services, alcohol and drug abuse treatment services, drugs administered other than oral method, orthotic procedures, prosthetic procedures, other medical services, pathology and laboratory services, casting and splinting supplies, diagnostic radiology services, temporary non-Medicare codes, T codes for state Medicaid agencies, and vision and hearing services.

Some private insurance companies may or may not accept certain Level II HCPCS codes and it is recommended to check the payer's provider manual or telephone the third-party payer before sending in a claim for services or equipment. It is also wise to check the payer's provider manual or telephone the third-party payer before submitting claims for medications and durable medical equipment. The HCPCS is updated each January 1, with periodic updates made throughout the year as needed. (See Chapter 12 for additional information on coding for Medicare cases.) In some states, the TRICARE and Medicaid programs accept HCPCS codes. Most commercial insurance companies have adopted the Level I (CPT) and Level II (HCPCS) code systems.

Procedure 6-1 at the end of this chapter gives step-by-step directions on how to use a HCPCS code book for billing purposes.

HIPAA Compliance Alert	**HIPAA DIAGNOSTIC AND PROCEDURAL CODE GUIDELINES**

Under HIPAA, providers and medical facilities are responsible for using ICD-9-CM diagnostic codes to document why patients are seen and CPT-4 and HCPCS codes for what is done to patients during their encounter. They are also responsible for implementing the updated codes in a timely manner, using the HIPAA-mandated transaction code set codes, and deleting old or obsolete codes.

---

*Examples shown in this chapter reflect wording pertinent to coding a specific procedure and may be missing complete chart entries; therefore, there may be a gap of information for the reader.

Table 6-1	Level II HCPCS National Code Content	
CODE CATEGORY	**CONTENTS**	**CODE RANGES**
Index	New/Revised/Deleted Codes and Modifiers. Alphabetically arranged. Table of Drugs. Level II National Modifiers.	
A codes	Transportation services, including ambulance (medical and surgical supplies, administrative, and miscellaneous and investigational services and supplies).	A0000-A9999
B codes	Enteral and parenteral therapy.	B4000-B9999
C codes	Temporary codes for hospital outpatient Prospective Payment System.	C1000-C9999
D codes	Dental procedures (diagnostic, preventive, restorative, endodontic, periodontic, prosthodontic, prosthetic, orthodontic, and surgical). These codes have been removed from the official HCPCS list but remain available from and are maintained by the American Dental Association.	D0000-D9999
E codes	Durable medical equipment (canes, crutches, walkers, commodes, decubitus care, bath and toilet aids, hospital beds, oxygen and related respiratory equipment, monitoring equipment, pacemakers, patient lifts, safety equipment, restraints, traction equipment, fracture frames, wheelchairs, and artificial kidney machines).	E0100-E9999
G codes	Procedures and professional services (temporary) under review before inclusion in the CPT code book.	G0000-G9999
H codes	Alcohol and drug abuse treatment services.	H0001-H9999
J codes	Drugs administered other than oral method (chemotherapy drugs, immunosuppressive drugs, inhalation solutions, and miscellaneous drugs and solutions).	J0100-J9999
K codes	Temporary codes (durable medical equipment and drugs). When these codes are approved for permanent inclusion in HCPCS, they become A, E, or J codes.	K0000-K9999
L codes	Orthotic procedures and devices (prosthetic devices, scoliosis equipment, orthopedic shoes, and prosthetic implants).	L0100-L4999
P codes	Pathology and laboratory services.	P0000-P9999
Q codes	Miscellaneous temporary codes.	Q0000-Q9999
R codes	Diagnostic radiology services codes.	R0000-R9999
S codes	Temporary national codes (non-Medicare) replaced many of the Level III (local) codes, which have been phased out.	S0009-S9999
T codes	National T codes established for state Medicaid agencies and not valid for Medicare.	T1000-T9999
V codes	Vision, hearing, and speech-language pathology services.	V0000-V2999

Contents in HCPCS books will vary by edition. It is a good idea to compare editions to see which one is best for your use. For example, the Professional Edition has appendices not included in the Standard Edition.
CPT, Current Procedural Terminology; *HCPCS*, Healthcare Common Procedure Coding System.

Alternative Billing Codes

Alternative billing codes (ABCs) were created and distributed by Alternative Link and approved for a pilot study. They are five-character alphabetic symbols with appended two-character practitioner modifiers that represent the practitioner type. These codes represent more than 4000 integrative health care products and services (Example 6-2). Integrative health care is care that incorporates the best approaches from conventional and complementary and alternative medicine.

The following areas of health care are represented by the ABCs and are within specialty areas:

Acupuncturist	Massage therapy
Ayurvedic medicine	Mental health care
Body work	Midwifery
Botanical medicine	Minority health care
Chiropractic	Naturopathic medicine
Clinical nutrition	Oriental medicine
Conventional nursing	Osteopathic medicine
Holistic dentists and physicians	Physical medicine
Homeopathy	Somatic educational
Indigenous medicine	Spiritual and prayer-based healing

As of October 16, 2006, Alternative Link discontinued its pilot study. Covered entities under the Health Insurance Portability and Accountability Act (HIPAA) may not use the codes in HIPAA transactions but may use them for non-HIPAA transactions, for research, management, and manual or paper-based commerce. Alternative Link continually refines the code set and has modeled the structure of the code set and **fee schedule** after systems that are already part of the transaction and code set regulations of HIPAA to ease their anticipated assimilation. This company established a **relative value unit (RVU)** scale similar to the reimbursement process

Example 6-2 Alternative Billing Code with Modifier

The following descriptions illustrate the coding hierarchy of ABCs with modifiers.

CODE: CEBAM-1G High-risk pregnancy identification, Antepartum, Midwifery, Practice specialties

Section	Subsection	Heading	Code	Practitioner Modifier
C	E	B	AM	-1G
↓	↓	↓	↓	↓
Practice Specialties	Midwifery	Prenatal	Intervention Management	Certified Nurse Midwife

CODE: BFBAJ-1H Weight management

Section	Subsection	Heading	Code	Practitioner Modifier
B	F	B	AJ	-1H
↓	↓	↓	↓	↓
Multispecialty	Nutrition Services	Management	Interventions Weight Management, group, each 15 min	Nurse Practitioner

of the Medicare physician fee schedule. It includes a conversion factor that is updated annually. For electronic commerce, which is a federally regulated use of code sets under HIPAA, ABCs may be used by any of more than 10,000 entities that secured rights to use the codes under section 4 5CFR162.940 of the Code of Federal Regulations and their contractual trading partners. Some coded procedures require additional certification or training and those codes may be used if a practitioner can supply the documentation.

ABCs may become mandatory. Sandia Health System in New Mexico has been paying ABC-coded claims since 1999. Numerous payers are in the process of implementing the ABCs for payment.

METHODS OF PAYMENT

Private insurance companies, as well as federal and state programs, adopt different methods for establishing payment rates for outpatient services: (1) fee schedules; (2) **usual, customary, and reasonable (UCR)**; and (3) relative value scales or schedules. Additional methods of payment for inpatient hospital claims are discussed in Chapter 17.

Fee Schedule

A fee schedule is simply a listing of accepted charges or established allowances for specific medical procedures. A medical practice can have more than one fee schedule unless specific state laws restrict this practice. Charges refer to the regular rates established by the provider for services rendered to both Medicare beneficiaries and other paying patients. Charges should be related consistently

to the cost of the services and uniformly applied to all patients whether inpatient or outpatient. The following situations can occur:

1. Providers *participating* in the Medicare program typically would be paid by the fiscal agent an amount from a fee schedule for Medicare patients.
2. Providers *not participating* in the Medicare program would be paid by the fiscal agent an amount based on limiting charges for each service set by the Medicare program.
3. Providers having a contractual arrangement with a managed care plan (for example, health maintenance organization, individual practice association, or preferred provider organization) would be paid on the basis of the fee schedule written into the negotiated contract.
4. Providers rendering services to those who have sustained industrial injuries use a separate workers' compensation fee schedule (see Chapter 15).

Section 1128(b) of the Social Security Act states that a physician may risk exclusion or suspension from the Medicare program if his or her Medicare charges are "substantially in excess of such individual's or entity's usual charges." An exception is charges negotiated for managed care contracts that are not considered the physician's usual charges. In those cases, it is possible that Medicare patients may be charged more than managed care patients. By implementing multiple fee schedules, a provider may risk charging federal or state health programs a fee that might be construed as more than the provider's "usual" charge for a given service. This could potentially result in a violation of the Social Security Act and managed care agreements.

To prevent a possible violation of Section 1128(b) of the Social Security Act, the provider should assign one fee for each procedure code when establishing a fee schedule. This fee should be billed to all third-party payers and to self-pay patients. The provider can establish fees on the basis of the amount that the payer reimburses, which is based on the contract with the insurance plan. By establishing one fee for each procedure instead of multiple fees for each procedure, the provider helps establish the usual and **customary fee** for his or her geographic area. By monitoring payments, it is possible to observe when third-party payers raise their allowable rates, which cannot be done if sending a claim on the basis of the payer's allowable. It is equally important to monitor third-party payer adjustments to determine how much revenue is lost because of poor contracts and to monitor employee theft.

The fees should be above the maximums paid by the third-party payers to whom the practice generally bills. Your physician employer may wish to evaluate the fee schedules annually to decide whether fees should be raised for certain procedures or services.

Because mistakes can be costly in terms of lost revenue and possible violations, one fee schedule for all patients, with provisions for financial hardship cases, is usually the safest course for health care providers. The physician may want to evaluate the fee schedule in use to annually increase fees caused by cost-of-living and cost-of-supply increases. Such a process is discussed below in the section titled "Developing a Fee Schedule Using Relative Value Studies Conversion Factors."

Usual, Customary, and Reasonable

Usual, customary, and reasonable (UCR) is a complex system in which three fees are considered in calculating payment. UCR is used mostly in reference to fee-for-service reimbursement. Figure 6-1 illustrates how a surgeon's payment is determined under this method. The usual fee is the fee that a physician usually charges (submitted fee) for a given service to a private patient. A fee is a customary fee if it is in the range of usual fees charged by providers of similar training and experience in a geographic area (for example, the history of charges for a given service). The **reasonable fee** is the fee that meets

PARTICIPATING SURGEON UCR CALCULATION

Four Example Cases

Surgeon's bill	Usual fee	compared to	Customary fee		Payment
1) $400	$350	→	$350 →	declared reasonable (extenuating circumstances)	$400
2) $400	$350	→	$350 →	declared customary (no unusual circumstances)	$350
3) $375	$350	→	$400 →	declared customary (does not exceed customary level)	$375
4) $350	$350	→	$400 →	declared customary (falls within customary range)	$350

Usual Fee—usual submitted fee for a given service to patient.

Customary Fee—in the range of usual fees charged by providers of similar training and experience in a geographical area (i.e., the history of charges for a given service).

Reasonable Fee—meets the aforementioned criteria or is, in the opinion of the medical review committee, justifiable considering the special circumstances of the case.

Payment—based on the lower of usual and customary fees.

FIGURE 6-1 Usual, customary, and reasonable (UCR) calculation for four participating surgeons' cases.

the aforementioned criteria or is, in the opinion of the medical review committee, justifiable considering the special circumstances of the case. Reimbursement is based on the lower of the two fees (usual and customary) and determines the approved or allowed amount. In a UCR system, payment can be extremely low for a rarely performed but highly complex procedure because there may be no history of billed charges from other physicians on which to base payment. Many private health insurance plans use this method and pay a physician's full charge if it does not exceed UCR charges. Depending on the policies of each insurance company, the UCR system is periodically updated. UCR is a method chosen by third-party payers and not the provider. If the physician has a UCR that is significantly lower than those of other practices in his or her area, document this and ask the third-party payer for a review and possible adjustment. Increasing numbers of plans are beginning to discontinue the UCR system and are adopting the Medicare RBRVS method for physician reimbursement. A description of this system is found in the "Relative Value Studies" section, which follows.

To be considered *customary* for Medicare reimbursement, a provider's charges for like services must be imposed on most patients regardless of the type of patient treated or the party responsible for payment of such services. Customary charges are those uniform charges listed in a provider's established charge schedule that is in effect and applied consistently to most patients and recognized for Medicare program reimbursement.

Relative Value Studies

In 1956 the California Medical Association Committee on Fees published the first edition of the *California Relative Value Studies* (CRVS).

CRVS was subsequently revised and published in 1957, 1960, 1964, 1969, and 1974. RVS, referred to as either relative value studies or scale, is a coded listing of procedure codes with unit values that indicate the relative value of the various services performed, taking into account the time, skill, and overhead cost necessary for each service (Example 6-3).

Example 6-3	Relative Value Scale	
Procedure		
Code	**Description**	**Units**
10060	Incision & drainage of cyst	**0.8**

Using a hypothetical figure of $153/unit, this procedure is valued at $122.40.

Math: $153.00 × 0.8 = $122.40

Units in RVS are based on the median charges of all physicians during the time period in which the RVS was published. A **conversion factor** is used to translate the abstract units in the scale to dollar fees for each service.

The RVS is a sophisticated system for coding and billing of professional services. After the successful use of the California RVS, many state and medical specialty associations adopted the CRVS method. In 1975 the Federal Trade Commission (FTC) challenged the legality of using the RVS as a fee schedule, stating that it could be interpreted as a form of price fixing in violation of antitrust laws. Since that time, many medical societies and medical specialty associations issued new publications that omitted unit values for the procedures listed but retained the procedure code portion of RVS.

Some states passed legislation mandating the use of RVS codes for procedures and the unit values as the schedule of fees for workers' compensation claims. In these states, the conversion factor to be used in applying the units is also stated in the law. The third-party payer pays a specific dollar amount for each unit listed for each procedure in the RVS code book.

An insurer or other third party could devise an RVS on the basis of its own data. This type of RVS would not be created by physicians in an effort to regulate fees and therefore would be acceptable on the basis of FTC guidelines. An example is *Optum's Relative Values for Physicians (RVP)*, which is based on survey data from Relative Value Studies, Inc. Additionally, a national RVS developed under a government contract may be acceptable and would not be in violation of antitrust laws.

Resource-Based Relative Value Scale

The RBRVS is an RVS developed for CMS by William Hsiao and associates at the Harvard School of Public Health. CMS used it to devise the Medicare fee schedule that was phased in from 1992 through 1996. This approach to fees was developed to redistribute Medicare dollars more equitably among physicians and to control escalating fees that were out of control using the UCR system. This became the basis for physicians' payments nationwide for a 5-year phase-in that began on January 1, 1992. This system consists of a fee schedule based on relative values. The formula for obtaining RVUs is somewhat complex and involves a bit of mathematics in computing three components: an RVU for the service, a geographic adjustment factor (GAF), and a monetary conversion factor (CF).

Relative Value Unit Formula

RVU × GAF × CF = Medicare $ per service

RVUs are based on the physician work RVU, the practice expense RVU, and the malpractice insurance RVU. To bring the fees in line for the region where the physician practices and to adjust for regional overhead and malpractice costs, each of the RVUs is adjusted for each Medicare local fiscal agent by geographic practice cost indices (GPCIs), pronounced "gypsies."

A CF is used to convert a geographically adjusted relative value into a payment amount. This CF is updated to a new amount each year. Figure 6-2 provides an example of calculating payment for one procedure code.

The figures to work out this formula in the chart for each service are published annually in the *Federal Register*.

RVUs help when determining cost accounting because they take into account the practice expense, malpractice expense, work effort, and cost of living. They are also helpful when negotiating the best contract available with managed care plans; therefore office managers or individuals assisting physicians should know and understand RBRVS data. A crosswalk is an effective way to see how the practice may be affected by an RBRVS contract (Table 6-2). To develop one, make several columns using spreadsheet software. In column A, list common

procedure codes used by the practice; in column B, list the code descriptions; and in column C, list the RBRVS RVUs. Leave column D blank to insert a conversion factor. In column E, put in the present fee-for-service rate (rounded-out figure). Divide the fee in column E by column C to get the conversion factor. Leave a blank for column F to insert a conversion factor for the contract. List the managed care contract payment in column G. Divide column G by column C to get the conversion factor for column F. Then divide the plan's contract fee by the physician's fee for column H to work out the percentage being paid at the contract rate.

Medicare Fee Schedule

Beginning in 1996, each local Medicare administrative contractor (MAC) annually sent each physician a Medicare fee schedule for his or her area or region number listing three columns of figures: participating amount, nonparticipating amount, and limiting charge for each procedure code number. Currently, fee schedules may be accessed online at your local MAC's website. To see an example of this, refer to the Mock Fee Schedule shown in Appendix A of the *Workbook*.

Developing a Fee Schedule Using Relative Value Studies Conversion Factors

A physician's fees can be adjusted if they are too high or too low but doing this can present a problem. It is legal to use an RVS guide for setting, realigning, or evaluating fees as long as the physician does not enter into any price-fixing agreements. Updating or establishing a fee schedule can be accomplished in a number of ways, ranging from easy to difficult. They are as follows:

1. Use the RBRVS fee profile sent to each physician's practice in the latter part of each year. This lists the codes most frequently used by the practice with their allowable charges and limiting charge amounts for the coming year. This is used for billing patients under the Medicare program. However, it can help you to update the office fee schedule but you must ensure that the charges are above the allowances on that schedule and above the allowances of the majority of the other third-party payers to whom the medical practice generally sends insurance claims.

HCPCS/CPT CODE	WORK RVUs	PRACTICE EXPENSE RVUs	MALPRACTICE RVUs
91000 RVUs	1.04	0.70	0.06
GPCI* ×1.028	+ ×1.258	+ ×1.370	= Total adjusted
1.07	0.88	0.08	RVUs, 2.03

For 2016, the conversion factor for nonsurgical care is
$36.1096 × 2.03 = Allowed amount $73.30

*The geographical practice cost indices (GPCI) for the medical practice whose location in the example is Oakland, California.

FIGURE 6-2 Formula used to calculate the fee for a specific procedure using the resource-based relative value scale (RBRVS) system.

Table 6-2	RBRVS Crosswalk						
A	B	C	D	E	F	G	H
CODE	CODE DESCRIPTION	RBRVS/RVU	CONVERSION FACTOR	FEE	CONTRACT CONVERSION FACTOR	CONTRACT FEE	% CONTRACT PAYMENT
99212	Office Visit	0.68	72.06	$49	64.71	$44.00	90%

RBRVS, Resource-based relative value scale; *RVU*, relative value unit.

2. Obtain the *Federal Register* with the printed relative values for most of the CPT code numbers and geographic cost indices for the region of service. Using a simple formula, calculate the actual Medicare reimbursement for the procedures the physician most frequently performs, making up a set of separate conversion factors for the Evaluation and Management (E/M), Anesthesia, Surgery, Radiology, Pathology, and Medicine sections. A fee schedule can be either updated or established from the calculations. Take into consideration that the fees should be above the maximums paid by the third-party payers to whom the practice generally bills. Procedure 6-2 at the end of this chapter is detailed, to assist you in gaining experience and skill if choosing to use this method.

3. A more time-consuming method is to review the medical practice's patient mix, that is, those patients with Medicare, the Blue Plans, Medicaid, managed care, private pay, workers' compensation, TRI-CARE, CHAMPVA, and so on. This may involve a detailed chart review of a large representative sampling of patients seen in the medical practice. Next, review the current fee schedule and current reimbursement amounts for the most commonly billed codes and the payments generated from each insurance plan in the study. A new fee schedule can be created from these data. The code books mentioned in this chapter can be obtained from various publishers and bookstores.

FORMAT AND CONTENT OF THE CPT CODE BOOK

The following explains content and procedures for the 2015 edition of the CPT published by the AMA. CPT code books published by other companies may contain differences; for example, the Index may appear at the beginning and not at the end of the book. CPT codes have three categories: I, II, and III. This code book is a systematic listing of five-digit code numbers with no decimals. CPT I is divided into six code sections with categories and subcategories. The CPT content is as follows:

Category I Codes	(99201 to 99607)
Evaluation and Management (E/M)	99201 to 99499
Anesthesia	00100 to 01999
Surgery	10021 to 69990
Radiology, Nuclear Medicine, and Diagnostic Ultrasound	70010 to 79999
Pathology and Laboratory	80047 to 89398
Medicine	90281 to 99607
Category II Codes	0001F to 7025F
Category III Codes	0019T to 0290T
Appendix A Modifiers	

Appendix B Summary of Additions, Deletions, and Revisions
Appendix C Clinical Examples
Appendix D Summary of CPT Add-on Codes
Appendix E Summary of CPT Codes Exempt from Modifier 51
Appendix F Summary of CPT Codes Exempt from Modifier 63
Appendix G Summary of CPT Codes That Include Moderate (Conscious) Sedation
Appendix H Alphabetical Clinical Topics Listing
Appendix I Genetic Testing Code Modifiers
Appendix J Electrodiagnostic Medicine Listing of Sensory, Motor, and Mixed Nerves
Appendix K Product Pending FDA Approval
Appendix L Vascular Families
Appendix M Renumbered CPT Codes-Citations Crosswalk
Appendix N Summary of Resequenced CPT Codes
Appendix O Multianalyte Assays with Algorithmic Analyses
Index

Each main section is divided into categories and subcategories according to anatomic body systems, procedure, condition, description, and specialty. Figure 6-3, *A*, illustrates the format of the Index, which is where you go to locate the CPT section, and Figure 6-3, *B*, illustrates the format of the CPT section.

Read through the clinical examples presented in Appendix C of the CPT. These examples will help you become familiar with some common case scenarios that might occur for the codes that appear in the E/M section of the CPT.

When on the job, you might want to make your CPT into a reference manual by customizing it. This can help you to find codes, modifiers, and rules, making your job easier. Break apart the manual into as many sections as needed on the basis of specialty, three-hole punch it, and place it in a binder. You may want to add indexes

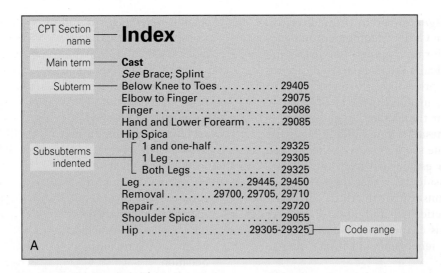

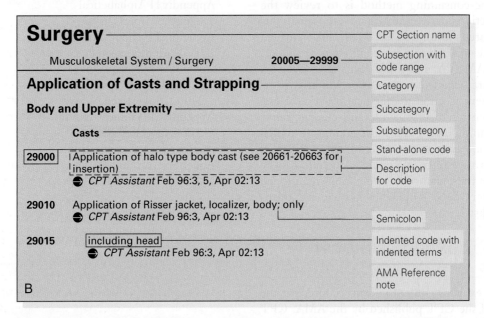

FIGURE 6-3 A, CPT format illustrating conventions of the Index and a section. **B,** CPT format illustrating conventions of the Index and a section.

with tabs to the frequently used sections. You can also add coding edits, Medicare updates, and notes at any place in the binder. Color-code any codes to which you usually add modifiers or that should not be used until you have reviewed certain data. For example, use red to highlight codes, descriptions, or entire sections to alert you or anyone using the reference to codes that are often denied. Use yellow to highlight a code that needs to be checked before using it in combination with other codes. Use a symbol (for example, * or ?) to identify services not covered under certain conditions. Appendix A of the CPT code book is a comprehensive list of the modifiers, so you might want to add any insurance plan bulletins pertinent to modifiers that affect the specialty you bill for to this section of the binder. Customizing

the CPT code book with a reference like this can save time and reduce coding errors.

Category I, II, and III Codes

To improve the existing CPT-4 code system, a CPT-5 Project was implemented. It is a revision of CPT-4 and includes two new code sets: category II codes, which are intended for performance measurement, and category III codes, which are intended for new and emerging technology. Existing CPT codes are considered category I.

Category II codes describe clinical components that typically may be included in E/M services or clinical services and do not have a relative value associated with them. They also describe results from clinical laboratory or radiology tests and other procedures, identified processes intended to address patient safety practices, or services reflecting compliance with state or federal laws.

Beginning with the CPT 2005 edition, Category II codes appear in a separate section located immediately after the Medicine section. They also have an alphanumeric identifier with a letter in the last field (for example, 0502F Subsequent prenatal care visit) to distinguish them from category I codes. Two modifiers are used to indicate that a service specified by a performance measure was considered but because of either medical or patient circumstance(s) documented in the medical record, the service was not provided. The modifiers are 1P, 2P, 3P, and 8P. Use of these codes is optional for correct coding.

Category III codes are a temporary set of tracking codes used to code emerging technologies that do not yet have any procedure code assignment in category I. They are intended to expedite data collection and assessment of new services and procedures to substantiate widespread use and clinical effectiveness. A category III code may become a category I code. When it is deleted from category III and adopted as a category I code, the CPT code book provides clear indication of this change by inserting a cross reference in place of the former category III code; for example, ▸(0024T has been deleted. To report use 93799)◂. The AMA website posts updates to this category in January and July of every year.

Code Book Symbols

With each new issuance of CPT, deletions and new codes and description changes are added. Become familiar with the new codes and any description changes or deleted codes related to codes that may exist on your medical practice's fee schedule. Figure 6-4 shows how to identify new codes and description changes by following the symbols that are used. The symbols placed below many codes throughout the code book indicate that the AMA has published reference material on those particular codes. The reference citation is also provided. When using a new code, marked with a bullet (•), it may take as long as 6 months before a third-party payer has a mandatory value assignment; therefore reimbursements are received in varying amounts during that time. An exception is in the Medicare program, which has a value assignment published annually each fall in the *Federal Register*. Revised codes or revised text, marked with a triangle (▴) or (▸ ◂), highlight what is new or deleted. This saves time in trying to figure out what was changed and prevents using these codes incorrectly. Appendix B in the CPT code book provides a summary of code additions, deletions, and revisions. Add-on codes, shown with a plus sign (+), means that the code can *only* be listed after the primary or parent code has been listed. Modifier -51 exempt

codes, shown with a symbol Ø, means that the modifier cannot be used with this code. More explanation about the add-on codes and modifier -51 appears at the end of this chapter. The symbol ⊙ is used to identify codes that include moderate (conscious) sedation; Appendix G in the CPT code book provides a complete list of these codes. The symbol is used to identify codes for vaccines that are pending Food and Drug Administration (FDA) approval. A complete list of these appears in Appendix K in the CPT code book. Resequenced codes that are not placed numerically are identified with the # symbol and a reference placed numerically (for example, "Code is out of numerical sequence. See …") is a navigational alert to direct the user to the location of the out-of-sequence code. A list appears in Appendix N. All of these symbols are located at the bottom of each page of codes in the CPT code book.

Evaluation and Management Section

The insurance billing specialist must become familiar with the terminology in the procedure code book to use it efficiently. Basic procedural code terminology is reviewed in Chapter 4 to give you a good foundation to begin coding. By now, you should know the difference between a new and an established patient, a consultation and a referral, and concurrent care versus continuity of care. This section familiarizes you with specific coding policies related to some of the terminology you have learned thus far.

The E/M section is divided into office visits, hospital visits, and consultations and these codes describe physician services involving the E/M of a patient's problem. Two subcategories of office visits exist: new patient and established patient. Hospital visits also have two bold-faced subcategories: initial and subsequent. Each subcategory has levels of E/M services identified by specific codes. This classification is based on the nature of the physician's work, such as type of service, place of service, and the patient's status.

In Chapter 4 you learned the CPT definitions for new patient and established patient. However, Medicare's revised definition of new patient is a "patient who has not received any professional services (that is, E/M service or other face-to-face service [for example, surgical procedure]) from the physician or physician group practice (same physician/same specialty) within the previous 3 years" (Example 6-4). This is referred to as the *3-year rule*. The CPT has a decision tree in the E/M services guidelines section for new versus established patients to help the provider.

The format for the levels of E/M service is as follows:
1. Under new patient or established patient, a code number is listed.
2. The place of service is listed.

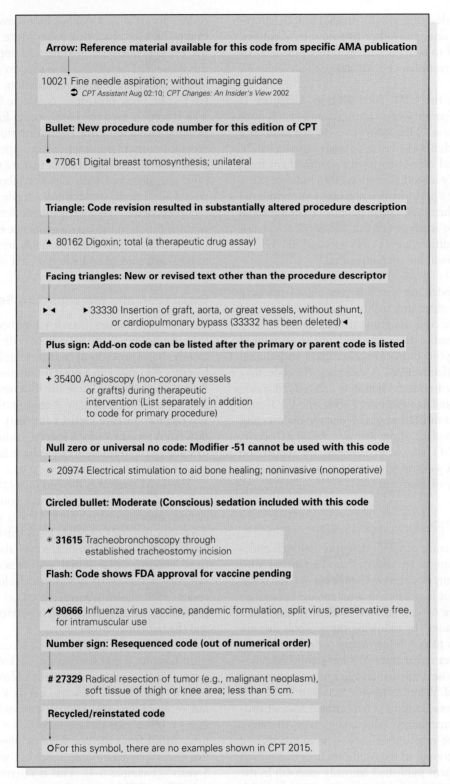

Arrow: Reference material available for this code from specific AMA publication

10021 Fine needle aspiration; without imaging guidance
    ⊃ *CPT Assistant* Aug 02:10; *CPT Changes: An Insider's View* 2002

Bullet: New procedure code number for this edition of CPT

● 77061 Digital breast tomosynthesis; unilateral

Triangle: Code revision resulted in substantially altered procedure description

▲ 80162 Digoxin; total (a therapeutic drug assay)

Facing triangles: New or revised text other than the procedure descriptor

►◄   ▶ 33330 Insertion of graft, aorta, or great vessels, without shunt,
                or cardiopulmonary bypass (33332 has been deleted) ◄

Plus sign: Add-on code can be listed after the primary or parent code is listed

+ 35400 Angioscopy (non-coronary vessels
        or grafts) during therapeutic
        intervention (List separately in addition
        to code for primary procedure)

Null zero or universal no code: Modifier -51 cannot be used with this code

⊘ 20974 Electrical stimulation to aid bone healing; noninvasive (nonoperative)

Circled bullet: Moderate (Conscious) sedation included with this code

⊙ **31615** Tracheobronchoscopy through
        established tracheostomy incision

Flash: Code shows FDA approval for vaccine pending

⚡ **90666** Influenza virus vaccine, pandemic formulation, split virus, preservative free,
        for intramuscular use

Number sign: Resequenced code (out of numerical order)

27329 Radical resection of tumor (e.g., malignant neoplasm),
        soft tissue of thigh or knee area; less than 5 cm.

Recycled/reinstated code

○For this symbol, there are no examples shown in CPT 2015.

FIGURE 6-4 Symbols that appear in the 2015 CPT code book and a brief explanation of what they tell the coder. These symbols and their meanings appear at the bottom of each page of codes in the CPT code book.

Example 6-4 Determination of a Medicare New Patient

On January 2, 20XX, Jason Emerson, new patient, is seen by Dr. Practon for an office visit. The service is billed using E/M code 99204.

On April 14, 20XX, Mr. Emerson returns to the office for an electrocardiogram and in-office laboratory test. Dr. Practon interprets the results of the test but does not perform an E/M service.

Note: In this case, the time interval to determine whether the patient is considered a new patient or established patient reverts to the January 2, 20XX, date and not the April 14, 20XX, date.

Example 6-5 Categories of Time

1. **Face-to-face:** Office and outpatient visits
   (Physician meets face-to-face with the patient or family.)
2. **Floor/unit time:** Hospital observation services, inpatient hospital care, initial and follow-up hospital consultations, and nursing facility services
   (Physician is present on the patient's hospital floor or unit providing bedside services to the patient, such as time with patient, time working on patient's chart, and discussing patient's care with nurses.)
3. **Non-face-to-face time:** Inpatient hospital pre-encounter and post-encounter time, obtaining records and test results, talking with other health care providers, and arranging for additional services
   (Physician does work related to the patient before or after face-to-face time or floor/unit time.)

3. The extent of the service is defined (for example, comprehensive history and comprehensive examination).
4. The nature of the presenting problem usually associated with the level is described.
5. The time typically needed to give the service is stated (Example 6-5).

You are allowed to use time to determine an E/M service level when counseling and/or coordinating care takes up more than 50% of the visit. Refer to Table 6-4, which appears later in this chapter and shows a summary of the E/M codes with these five components.

There are seven elements when selecting an E/M code to bill and providers consider them in the following order:
1. History
2. Examination
3. Medical decision making
4. Nature of presenting problem
5. Counseling
6. Coordination of care
7. Time

Hospital Inpatient Services

In the E/M section of the code book, the hospital inpatient service codes range from 99221 to 99239. If a patient is seen in the emergency department (ED) and is subsequently admitted to the hospital by the same physician on the same date of service as the ED visit, it is billed as initial hospital care. The physician includes the services related to the admission that he or she provided in the other hospital service departments as well as in the inpatient setting.

Consultation

As discussed in Chapter 4, a consultation includes services rendered by a physician whose opinion or advice is requested by another physician or agency in the evaluation or treatment of a patient's illness or a suspected problem. A referral is the transfer of the total or specific care of a patient from one physician to another for known problems.

Effective January 1, 2010, the CMS issued a policy that eliminated the use of all consultation codes (ranges 99241 through 99245 and 99251 through 99255) for inpatient and office or outpatient settings and for various places of service except for telehealth consultation (HCPCS G-codes). CMS indicates that the initial hospital care codes 99221 through 99223 should be used when billing a consultation on a hospital inpatient. The attending physician must append HCPCS Level II modifier AI (A-eye) *principal physician of record* to the code. If a transfer of care, codes 99201 through 99205 and 99211 through 99215 may be used.

The following information is for non-Medicare cases. Some insurance policies pay for only one consultation per patient per year and often require a written report to be generated.

A consulting physician must submit a written report containing his or her findings and opinions to the requesting physician. Codes for consultations are as follows:
- Office or other outpatient consultations (new or established patient): 99241 through 99245 (Example 6-6)
- Inpatient consultations (new or established patient): 99251 through 99255 (Example 6-7)

In the office setting, use the appropriate consultation code for the initial encounter; if a follow-up visit is required for additional diagnostic testing or examination, then use the appropriate established patient code. In a hospital setting, use the appropriate inpatient hospital consultation code; if a follow-up is required for additional services, then use subsequent hospital care codes. As discussed in Chapter 4, remember the four Rs: There must be a *requesting* physician and the consultant

---

Example 6-6   Outpatient Consultation

A 20-year-old female is seen for an office consultation for cystitis. She complains of burning on urination and urinary frequency. The patient's records from the referring physician were reviewed. Urine culture confirmed a urinary tract infection, which was reported to her primary care physician for treatment. Obtained problem-focused history and examination with straightforward medical decision making.

99241	Office consultation
87086	Urine culture, bacterial

Example 6-7   Inpatient Consultation

A 50-year-old male is seen for an initial inpatient consultation with a status post left hip fracture and a history of well-controlled type II diabetes mellitus. Consultation is requested for surgical clearance. Reviewed medical data on the unit. Obtained a detailed history and performed a detailed examination with low complexity medical decision making (LCMDM). Discussed diagnosis and treatment options with patient and completed medical record documentation. Will give ongoing consultation to referring physician.

99253	Inpatient consultation

---

must *render* an opinion and send a *report*. The requesting physician must document the *reason* on the medical record.

Critical Care

According to CPT guidelines, critical care is the direct delivery of medical care by a physician for a critically ill or injured patient. A critical illness or injury acutely impairs one or more vital organ systems and makes an imminent or life-threatening deterioration in the patient's condition highly probable. Critical care involves highly complex decision making to assess, manipulate, and support vital system functions to treat single or multiple vital organ system failure or prevent further life-threatening deterioration of the patient's condition. Examples of vital organ system failure include but are not limited to central nervous system failure; circulatory failure; shock; and renal, hepatic, metabolic, or respiratory failure.

Although critical care typically requires interpretation of multiple physiologic parameters or application of advanced technologies, it may be provided in life-threatening situations when these elements are not present. Critical care may be provided on multiple days, even if no changes are made in the treatment rendered to the patient, as long as the patient's condition continues to require the level of physician attention described in the preceding paragraph.

Providing medical care to a critically ill, injured, or postoperative patient qualifies as a critical care service only if both the illness or injury and the treatment being provided meet the preceding requirements. Critical care is usually but not always given in a critical care area, such as the coronary care unit, intensive care unit, pediatric intensive care unit, respiratory care unit, or emergency care facility. It could occur in the patient's room or in the ED.

Inpatient critical care services provided to neonates and infants 29 days through 24 months of age are reported with pediatric critical care codes 99468 through 99476. The pediatric critical care codes are reported as long as the infant or young child qualifies for critical care services during the hospital stay. Inpatient critical care services provided to neonates (28 days of age or younger) are reported with the neonatal critical care codes 99468 and 99469. The neonatal critical care codes are reported as long as the neonate qualifies for critical care services through the twenty-eighth postnatal day. The reporting of the pediatric and neonatal critical care services is not based on time or on the type of unit (for example, pediatric or neonatal critical care unit) nor is it dependent on the type of provider delivering the care. For additional instructions on reporting these services, see the section on Inpatient Neonatal and Pediatric Critical Care in the Evaluation and Management section of CPT.

Services for a patient who is not critically ill but is in a critical care or intensive care unit are reported by use of other appropriate in-hospital E/M codes.

Critical care and other E/M services may be provided to the same patient on the same date by the same physician.

Some services are included in critical care codes used to report critical care when performed during the critical period by the physician providing critical care. They are not coded in addition to critical care codes. These services are:
- Interpretation of cardiac output measurements (93561, 93562)
- Chest radiographs (71010, 71015, 71020)
- Pulse oximetry (94760, 94761, 94762)
- Blood gases and information data stored in computers (e.g., electrocardiograms, blood pressures, hematologic data [99090])
- Gastric intubation (43752, 43753)
- Temporary transcutaneous pacing (92953)
- Ventilator management (94002 through 94004, 94660, 94662)
- Vascular access procedures (36000, 36400, 36405, 36406, 36410, 36415, 36591, 36600)

Any services performed in excess of those listed earlier should be reported separately. Many third-party payers attempt to downcode claims by stating that the procedure is included with critical care. If denied, these claims should be appealed by attaching supporting documentation, such as a copy of the critical care guidelines. The payer may tell you that the codes are inclusive or that they are not a covered benefit.

Codes 99466 and 99467 should be reported for the physician's attendance during the transport of critically ill or injured pediatric patients younger than 24 months of age to or from a facility or hospital.

Critical care codes 99291 and 99292 are used to report the total duration of time spent by a physician providing critical care services to a critically ill or injured patient, even if the time spent by the physician on that date is not continuous. For any given period of time spent providing critical care services, the physician must devote his or her full attention to the patient and therefore cannot provide services to any other patient during the same period of time.

Time spent with the individual patient must be recorded in the patient's record. Time spent engaged in work directly related to the individual patient's care, whether that time was spent at the immediate bedside or elsewhere on the floor or unit even if not continuous, is reported as critical care. For example, time spent on the unit or at the nursing station on the floor reviewing test results or imaging studies, discussing the critically ill patient's care with other medical staff, or documenting critical care services in the medical record is reported as critical care, even though it does not occur at the bedside. Also, when the patient is unable or clinically incompetent to participate in discussions, time spent on the floor or unit with family members or surrogate decision makers obtaining a medical history, reviewing the patient's condition or prognosis, or discussing treatment or limitations of treatment may be reported as critical care, as long as the conversation bears directly on the management of the patient.

Time spent in activities that occur outside of the unit or off the floor (for example, telephone calls, whether taken at home, in the office, or elsewhere in the hospital) may not be reported as critical care because the physician is not immediately available to the patient.

Time spent in activities that do not directly contribute to the treatment of the patient may not be reported as critical care, even if they are performed in the critical care unit (for example, participation in administrative meetings or telephone calls to discuss other patients). Time spent performing separately reportable procedures or services should not be included in the time reported as critical care time.

Code 99291 is used to report the first 30 to 74 minutes of critical care on a given date. It should be used only once per date, even if the time spent by the physician is not continuous on that date. Critical care of less than 30 minutes total duration on a given date should be reported with the appropriate E/M code.

Code 99292 is used to report additional blocks of time, up to 30 minute each, beyond the first 74 minutes. This code has a plus sign (+) and is an "add-on" code. It is never used alone.

Pediatric and Neonatal Critical Care

According to CPT guidelines, the codes 99468 through 99476 are used to report inpatient services provided by a physician directing the care of a critically ill neonate or infant. The same definitions for critical care services apply for the adult, child, and neonate.

The initial day neonatal critical care code (99468) can be used in addition to codes 99360 Physician standby service, 99464 Attendance, or 99465 Newborn resuscitation, as appropriate, when the physician is present for the delivery and newborn resuscitation is necessary. Other procedures performed as a necessary part of the resuscitation (for example, endotracheal intubation) are also reported separately when performed as part of the preadmission delivery room care. They must be performed as a necessary component of the resuscitation and not done for convenience.

Codes 99468 and 99469 are used to report services provided by a physician directing the care of a critically ill neonate through the first 28 days of life. These codes describe care for the date of admission (99468) and subsequent days (99469) and should be reported only once per day per patient. Once the neonate is no longer considered critically ill, the Intensive Low Birth Weight Services codes for those with present body weight of less than 1500 grams (99478, 99479, and 99480) or the codes for Subsequent Hospital Care (99231 through 99233) for those with present body weight more than 5000 grams should be used.

Codes 99471 and 99472 are used to report services provided by a physician directing the care of a critically ill infant or young child from 29 days of postnatal age through 24 months of age. These codes represent care for the date of admission (99471) and subsequent days (99472) and should be reported by a single physician only once per day per patient in a given setting. The critically ill or injured child older than 2 years of age when admitted to an intensive care unit is reported with hourly critical care service codes (99291 and 99292). When an infant is no longer considered critically ill but continues to require intensive care, the Intensive Low Birth Weight Services code (99478) should be used to report services for infants with a body weight of less than 1500 grams. When the body weight of those infants exceeds 1500 grams, the Subsequent Intensive Care codes (99479 and 99480) should be used.

The pediatric and neonatal critical care codes include those procedures previously listed for the hourly critical care codes (99291 and 99292). In addition, the following procedures also are included (and are not separately reported by professionals but may be reported by facilities) in the pediatric and neonatal critical care service codes (99468-99472, 99475, 99476) and the intensive care services codes (99477-99480).

Any services performed that are not included in these listings may be reported separately. Facilities may report the included services separately.

Invasive or noninvasive electronic monitoring of vital signs

Vascular access procedures
- Peripheral vessel catheterization (36000)
- Other arterial catheters (36140, 36620)
- Umbilical venous catheters (36510)
- Central vessel catheterization (36555)
- Vascular access procedures (36400, 36405, 36406)
- Vascular punctures (36420, 36600)
- Umbilical arterial catheters (36660)

Airway and ventilation management
- Endotracheal intubation (31500)
- Ventilatory management (94002-94004)
- Bedside pulmonary function testing (94375)
- Surfactant administration (94610)
- Continuous positive airway pressure (CPAP) (94660)

Monitoring or interpretation of blood gases or oxygen saturation (94760-94762)

Car seat evaluation (94780-94781)

Transfusion of blood components (36430, 36440)

Oral or nasogastric tube placement (43752)

Suprapubic bladder aspiration (51100)

Bladder catheterization (51701, 51702)

Lumbar puncture (62270)

Any services performed that are not listed above may be reported separately.

When a neonate or infant is not critically ill but requires intensive observation, frequent interventions, and other intensive care services, the Continuing Intensive Care Services codes (99477-99480) should be used to report these services.

Emergency Department Services

Codes 99281 through 99285 describe various levels of emergency care provided in an ED. An *emergency department (ED)* is defined as an organized hospital-based facility for the provision of unscheduled episodic services to patients who present for immediate medical attention. However, some facilities must use the ED to accommodate after-hours patients and overflow clinic patients or to administer minor procedures in the absence of a clinic. When a patient is seen in the ED for a scheduled procedure, he or she must have a valid order for services. The patient should be registered as a clinic patient because his or her visit is not deemed an emergency. Medical necessity rules apply and the hospital should screen the procedure and diagnosis. As discussed in Chapter 4, medical necessity services are services provided that are consistent with the diagnosis. This type of patient falls under the regulations of the Emergency Medical Treatment and Active Labor Act (EMTALA). The facility may either perform an EMTALA screening for the patient or have the patient sign a document indicating that he or she is not in the ED for emergency services. In these cases, there is a charge for the scheduled service provided but it is usually inappropriate to charge an E/M visit in addition to the procedure charge.

Code 99288 is used when advanced life support is necessary during emergency care and the physician is located in a hospital emergency or critical care department and is in two-way voice communication with ambulance or rescue personnel outside the hospital.

If office services are provided on an emergency basis, code 99058 (office services provided on an emergency basis—found in the Medicine section) may be used when billing private insurance cases. CPT codes 99281 through 99285 should not to be used to report emergency care provided in an office setting. Medicare does not pay for code 99058 and other third-party payers also may deny this code. When a physician spends several hours attending to a patient, coding for prolonged services (99354 through 99357), in addition to an E/M service office visit, might be indicated.

If a patient comes into the office requiring emergency care for a wound trauma, you might bill for the office visit, suturing of the laceration, and the surgical tray. Most third-party payers only pay for suturing.

Example 6-8   Office Emergency

Incorrect Coding

99212	Office visit, level 2, established patient
12005	Simple repair of scalp laceration, 12.6 cm
99070	Surgical tray (itemized)

Correct Coding

99212	Office visit, level 2, established patient
99058	Office services provided on an emergency basis
12005	Simple repair of scalp laceration, 12.6 cm

Typically the payer will state that the office visit is included or bundled (codes grouped together that are related to a procedure) in the suture procedure. The payer will also typically state that surgical trays and supplies are included or bundled in the suture procedure. If you view the CMS National Correct Coding Initiative (NCCI) edits, you can see which codes are normally considered part of another procedure. If the NCCI edits do not show the codes as being inclusive, you should appeal the third-party payer's decision or bill the patient if allowed by federal or state law. This topic is explained in more detail below in the section titled "Coding Guidelines for Code Edits." However, if documentation supports coding the claim for office services provided on an emergency basis (99058), most payers will reimburse for the office visit in addition to the repair (Example 6-8). For example, if a patient has an extensive open wound of the arm, then a bill should be submitted only for the wound repair. If a patient has an extensive wound of the arm with abrasions of the shoulder, contusions of the ribs, and a sprained finger, then a bill should be submitted for the wound repair and an E/M code. The wound diagnosis would be associated with the wound repair and the diagnosis for the injuries would support the E/M visit. Ensure that the appropriate modifiers are appended to the CPT codes on the claim. For example, modifier -25 is used to report a significant and separately identifiable E/M service performed in addition to the procedure. A -25 modifier should be appended to the E/M in the previous example but the documentation in the chart must support the reasons for the codes.

Miscellaneous service codes 99050 through 99058 can be used depending on the hour at which the patient is seen as an emergency either in the physician's office or if taken to the ED of a hospital (24-hour facility). Most payers, including Medicare, do not pay for these codes. Some payers might pay for these codes and require documentation from the provider to support the code. Other codes under Miscellaneous Services in the Medicine section may be applicable for a patient receiving emergency care, so these should be scrutinized carefully.

Preventive Medicine

Preventive medicine is composed of services provided to prevent the occurrence of illness, injury, and disease, such as vaccine immunizations, antiseptic measures, regular exercise, routine physical examinations, and screening programs for detection of signs of disorders. Sometimes one aspect of preventive medicine is counseling, which is a discussion between the physician and a patient, family members, or both concerning the diagnosis, recommended studies or tests, treatment options, risks and benefits of treatment, patient and family education, and so on.

Codes 99381 through 99397 include counseling that is provided at the time of the initial or periodic comprehensive preventive medicine examination. Codes 99401 through 99412 should be used for reporting counseling given at an encounter separate from the preventive medicine examination.

Sometimes a Medicare patient may have an annual checkup but while having the examination, he or she tells the physician of experiencing pain. The physician provides both preventive and problem-focused services at the same time. You may bill Medicare only for covered screenings or services (for example, problem-focused E/M, Pap test, colon/rectal cancer screening, or prostate cancer screening) and must properly "carve out" the rest of the noncovered and/or preventive services (codes 99381 through 99397) to bill to the patient. *Carve out* refers to medical services not included as benefits. This term may also be seen in managed care billing and is discussed further in Chapter 11. For preventive medicine when billing a Medicare case, an Advance Beneficiary Notice of Noncoverage (ABN) is not required.

Categories and Subcategories

The E/M section of CPT has categories and subcategories that have from three to five levels for reporting purposes. These levels are based on key components, contributory factors, and face-to-face time with the patient or family. To begin the coding process, the provider of service must identify the category (for example, office, hospital inpatient or outpatient, or consultation) and then select the subcategory (for example, new patient or established patient). The description should be read thoroughly to note the key components (for example, history, examination, and medical decision making) and the contributory factors (for example, counseling, coordination of care, and nature of the presenting problem);

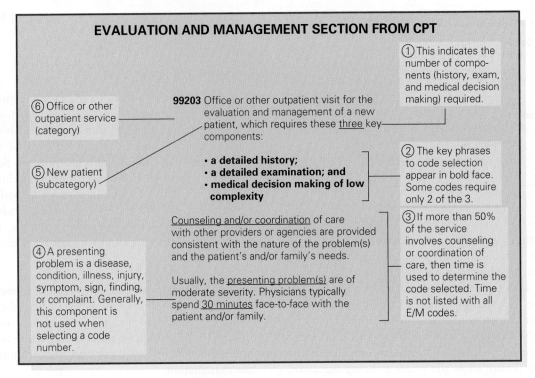

FIGURE 6-5 Evaluation and management (E/M) code 99203 defining the main words and phrases. This code is used for a new patient seen in the office or in an outpatient or ambulatory setting.

as well, face-to-face time of the service should be noted. Review the sample in Figure 6-5 illustrating an E/M code for a new patient seen in the office or in an outpatient or ambulatory setting.

Because key components are clinical in nature, the physician must document these factors in the patient's record. In a case in which counseling and coordination of care dominate (more than 50%) the face-to-face physician–patient encounter, time is considered the key component to qualify for a particular level of E/M services. Tables 6-3 and 6-4 give a concise view of the components for each code number.

Many physicians refer to the E/M codes as level 5 for the most complex to level 1 for the least complex. These levels coincide with the fifth or last digit of the CPT code, for example, 99205. It is common to hear a physician say, "Ted Brown was seen for a level 5 today." This terminology may appear on encounter forms with five-digit CPT code numbers and be referred to as levels 1 through 5 (Example 6-9).

Alternatively, this terminology may be seen abbreviated as L-1, L-2, and so on, but this usage is not preferred because it can be confused with the nomenclature for the sections of the lumbar vertebrae. The level also may be written out as level one, level two, and so on, depending on the complexity of the case.

A breakdown of the E/M levels with code numbers is shown in Table 6-5.

In some cases it is necessary to use a two-digit modifier to give a more accurate description of the services rendered. This is used in addition to the procedure code. Refer to the comprehensive list of modifiers at the end of this chapter (in Table 6-6) for more information.

Surgery Section
Coding from an Operative Report

It is best to obtain a copy of the patient's operative report from the hospital when coding surgery. A photocopy can be used so that you can make notes right on the document. When reviewing the report, use a ruler or highlighter pen. Use the ruler to read the report line by line. Highlight words that could indicate that the procedure performed may be altered by specific circumstances and to remind you that a code modifier may be necessary. Look up any unfamiliar terms using a medical dictionary or anatomic reference book and write the definitions in the margin.

Assign the code for the postoperative diagnosis shown at the beginning of the operative report. Also search for additional diagnoses in the body of the report that you can add as secondary diagnostic codes to support medical necessity, especially if the case is complex.

Table 6-3 Selection of Evaluation and Management Codes

CODE	HISTORY	EXAMINATION	MEDICAL DECISION MAKING	PROBLEM SEVERITY	COORDINATION OF CARE AND COUNSELING	TIME SPENT (AVG)
Office or Other Outpatient Services (Includes Hospital Observation Area)						
New Patient*						
99201	Problem focused	Problem focused	Straightforward	Minor or self-limited	Consistent with problem(s) and patient's needs	10 min face-to-face
99202	Expanded problem focused	Expanded problem focused	Straightforward	Low to moderate	Consistent with problem(s) and patient's needs	20 min face-to-face
99203	Detailed	Detailed	Low complexity	Moderate	Consistent with problem(s) and patient's needs	30 min face-to-face
99204	Comprehensive	Comprehensive	Moderate complexity	Moderate to high	Consistent with problem(s) and patient's needs	45 min face-to-face
99205	Comprehensive	Comprehensive	High complexity	Moderate to high	Consistent with problem(s) and patient's needs	60 min face-to-face
Established Patient*†						
99211	—	—	Physician supervision but presence not required	Minimal	Consistent with problem(s) and patient's needs	5 min face-to-face
99212	Problem focused	Problem focused	Straightforward	Minor or self-limited	Consistent with problem(s) and patient's needs	10 min face-to-face
99213	Expanded problem focused	Expanded problem	Low complexity	Low to moderate	Consistent with problem(s) and patient's needs	15 min face-to-face
99214	Detailed	Detailed	Moderate complexity	Moderate to high	Consistent with problem(s) and patient's needs	25 min face-to-face
99215	Comprehensive	Comprehensive	High complexity	Moderate to high	Consistent with problem(s) and patient's needs	40 min face-to-face
Hospital Observation Services						
99217	—	—	—	—	—	—
99218	Detailed or comprehensive	Detailed or comprehensive	Straightforward or low complexity	Low	Consistent with problem(s) and patient's needs	—
99219	Comprehensive	Comprehensive	Moderate complexity	Moderate	Consistent with problem(s) and patient's needs	—
99220	Comprehensive	Comprehensive	High complexity	High	—	—
Hospital Inpatient Services						
Initial Care‡						
99221	Detailed or comprehensive	Detailed or comprehensive	Straightforward or low complexity	Low	Consistent with problem(s) and patient's needs	30 min unit/floor
99222	Comprehensive	Comprehensive	Moderate complexity	Moderate	Consistent with problem(s) and patient's needs	50 min unit/floor
99223	Comprehensive	Comprehensive	High complexity	High	Consistent with problem(s) and patient's needs	70 min unit/floor
Subsequent Care‡§						
99231	Problem focused interval	Problem focused	Straightforward or low complexity	Stable, recovering or improving	Consistent with problem(s) and patient's needs	15 min unit/floor

Continued

Table 6-3 Selection of Evaluation and Management Codes—cont'd

CODE	HISTORY	EXAMINATION	MEDICAL DECISION MAKING	PROBLEM SEVERITY	COORDINATION OF CARE AND COUNSELING	TIME SPENT (AVG)
Hospital Inpatient Services						
99232	Expanded problem focused interval	Expanded problem focused	Moderate complexity	Inadequate response to treatment; minor complication	Consistent with problem(s) and patient's needs	25 min unit/floor
99233	Detailed interval	Detailed	High complexity	Unstable significant new problem(s) or complication(s)	Consistent with problem(s) and patient's needs	35 min unit/floor
99234	Detailed or comprehensive	Detailed or comprehensive	Straightforward or low complexity	Low	Consistent with problem(s) and patient's needs	—
99235	Comprehensive	Comprehensive	Moderate	Moderate	Consistent with problem(s) and patient's needs	—
99236	Comprehensive	Comprehensive	High	High	Consistent with problem(s) and patient's needs	—
99238	Hospital discharge day management	—	—	—	—	30 min or less
99239	Hospital discharge day management	—	—	—	—	More than 30 min

*Key component: For new patients for initial office and other outpatient services, all three components (history, physical examination, and medical decision making) are required in selecting the correct code. For established patients, at least two of these three components are required. Although average time spent is shown in the table, it is *not* a factor when billing but is shown to assist physicians in selecting the most appropriate level of evaluation and management service.

†Includes follow-up, periodic reevaluation, and management of new problems.

‡Key components: For initial care, all three components (history, physical examination, and medical decision making) are required in selecting the correct code. For subsequent care, at least two of these three components are required.

§All subsequent levels of service include a review of the medical record, diagnostic studies, and changes in the patient's status, such as history, physical condition, and response to treatment since the last assessment.

Table 6-4 Selection Criteria for Consultations

E/M CODE	HISTORY*	EXAMINATION	MEDICAL DECISION MAKING*	PROBLEM SEVERITY	COORDINATION OF CARE AND COUNSELING	TIMES (AVG)
Office or Other Outpatient						
99241	Problem focused	Problem focused	Straightforward	Minor or self-limited	Consistent with problem(s) and patient's needs	15 min face-to-face
99242	Expanded problem focused	Expanded problem focused	Straightforward	Low	Consistent with problem(s) and patient's needs	30 min face-to-face
99243	Detailed	Detailed	Low complexity	Moderate	Consistent with problem(s) and patient's needs	40 min face-to-face
99244	Comprehensive	Comprehensive	Moderate complexity	Moderate to high	Consistent with problem(s) and patient's needs	60 min face-to-face
99245	Comprehensive	Comprehensive	High complexity	Moderate to high	Consistent with problem(s) and patient's needs	80 min face-to-face
Initial Inpatient†						
99251	Problem focused	Problem focused	Straightforward	Minor or self-limited	Consistent with problem(s) and patient's needs	20 min unit/floor
99252	Expanded problem focused	Expanded problem focused	Straightforward	Low	Consistent with problem(s) and patient's needs	40 min unit/floor
99253	Detailed	Detailed	Low complexity	Moderate	Consistent with problem(s) and patient's needs	55 min unit/floor
99254	Comprehensive	Comprehensive	Moderate complexity	Moderate to high	Consistent with problem(s) and patient's needs	80 min unit/floor
99255	Comprehensive	Comprehensive	High complexity	Moderate to high	Consistent with problem(s) and patient's needs	110 min unit/floor

CPT codes, descriptions, and material are taken from *Current Procedural Terminology, CPT 2015, Professional Edition,* 2014, American Medical Association. All Rights Reserved.
*Key component: For office and initial inpatient consultations, all three components (history, physical examination, and medical decision making) are required for selecting the correct code.
†These codes also are used for residents of nursing facilities.

Example 6-9	Current Procedural Terminology Code Digit Analysis

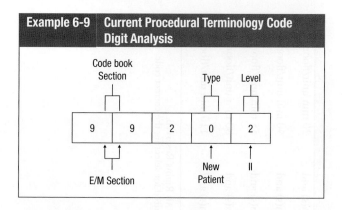

Table 6-5	Levels with Code Numbers			
	Office Visits		Consultations	
	NEW	**ESTABLISHED**	**OFFICE**	**HOSPITAL**
Level 1	99201	99211	99241	99251
Level 2	99202	99212	99242	99252
Level 3	99203	99213	99243	99253
Level 4	99204	99214	99244	99254
Level 5	99205	99215	99245	99255

Example 6-10	Integral Code

Partial and complete, which means the partial procedure is included in the complete procedure.
56620   Vulvectomy simple; partial
56625   complete
Partial and total, which means the partial procedure is included in the total procedure.
58940   Oophorectomy, partial or total, unilateral or bilateral
Unilateral and bilateral, which means the unilateral procedure is included in the bilateral procedure.
58900   Biopsy of ovary, unilateral or bilateral
Single and multiple, which means the single procedure is included in the multiple procedure.
49321   Laparoscopy, surgical, with biopsy (single or multiple)

If the complex surgical procedure is not accurately described in the procedure code nomenclature, include an operative report and list "Attachment" in Block 19 of the insurance claim form so that the claims adjuster clearly understands the case and generates maximum payment.

Code numbers that describe a part of the body treated render higher reimbursement, depending on their location (for example, suturing of a facial laceration pays a higher rate than suturing of an arm laceration).

Code only the procedures that actually were documented in the report. Check to make sure that they were neither a part of the main procedure nor bundled by NCCI edits, which is discussed later in this chapter.

Remember the rule: Not documented, not done.

Do not code using only the name of the procedure as it is given in the heading of the operative report. Read the report thoroughly before coding to see whether additional procedures were performed and whether they were part of the main procedure, performed independently, or unrelated. If the surgical position is noted, this can help you to identify the right approach code. You can also consult a good medical dictionary with illustrations of the various surgical positions. All codes include approach and closure except some skull base surgery codes. Information on how to code multiple procedures that are not inherent in a major procedure may be found in the "Modifier -51: Multiple Procedures" section at the end of this chapter.

Check to see how many surgeons were involved in the operative procedure and their roles (assistant surgeon, co-surgeon, team surgeon).

Reread the report to make certain that all procedural and diagnostic codes have been identified. Compare the content with the codes you are using. You cannot code circumstances that the physician relays to you verbally. Be sure that the words "extensive complications" are in the report if there are such complications.

Look for unusual details, such as special instruments used, unusually long or complex procedures, rare approach techniques, reoperation, or extensive scarring encountered. These conditions may need one or more modifiers appended to the code.

Surgical code descriptions may define a correct coding relationship wherein one code is part of another based on the language used in the description (Example 6-10). An explanation of how to read a description for stand-alone codes and indented codes can be found in Procedure 6-3 at the end of this chapter.

Confirm that the report findings agree with the procedure codes on the claim.

Surgical Package for Non-Medicare Cases

Surgical package is a phrase commonly encountered when billing. Generally, a surgical procedure includes the following:
- The operation
- Local infiltration; topical anesthesia or metacarpal, metatarsal, or digital block

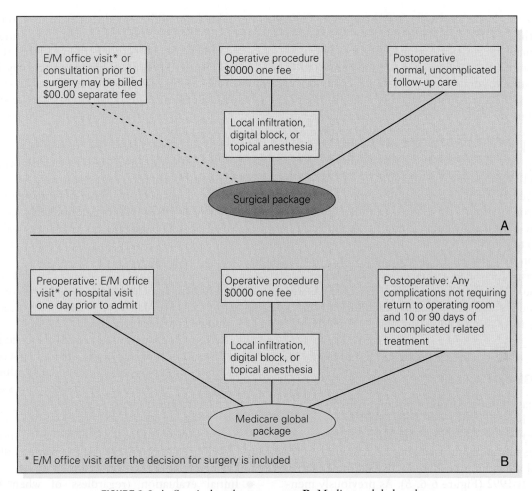

FIGURE 6-6 A, Surgical package concept. **B,** Medicare global package.

- After the decision for surgery is billed, the surgical package includes one related E/M encounter on the date immediately before or on the date of procedure (including history and physical). (See the section in this chapter titled "Modifier -57: Decision for Surgery.")
- Immediate postoperative care, including dictating operative notes and talking with the family and other physicians
- Writing orders
- Evaluating the patient in the postanesthesia recovery area
- Typical postoperative follow-up care (hospital visits, discharge, or follow-up office visits)

This is referred to as a "surgical package" for operative procedures and one fee covers the entire set of services (Figure 6-6, *A*). The majority of surgical procedures, including fracture care, are handled in this manner. Typical postoperative follow-up care includes only care that is usually a part of the surgical service. Complications, exacerbations, recurrence, or the presence of other diseases or injuries that require additional services should be

reported separately. The global period under CPT is not specifically stated, so from a CPT perspective the global surgical period extends from no more than 1 day before the day of the procedure to as long as is necessary for typical postoperative follow-up care to be completed. In essence, the postoperative period is open-ended. Medicare defines the postoperative global periods of 10 or 90 days and most third-party insurance companies apply the same criteria.

Visits not related to the original surgery and complications of the surgery (infection of the wound) are billable using modifier -24. Preoperative services, such as consultations, office visits, and initial hospital care, are often billed separately. An appropriate five-digit E/M code should be selected for these types of services. Payment of these services depends on third-party payment policy and the documentation—some are paid separately; some are not.

Insurance policies and managed care plans vary in what is included in the surgical package fee. Most follow Medicare guidelines; some do not. Plans may include all visits several weeks before surgery or they may include only visits that occur 1 day before the surgery. When a decision is made for surgery, a commonly asked question is whether a charge may be made for the consultation or office visit and admission if done on the same day. In most cases, the admission should be billed listing initial hospital care codes 99221 through 99223. However, the guidelines are different for surgeons. For example, surgical package rules apply if a patient is referred by his or her primary care physician for consultation by a surgeon and the surgeon recommends that the patient receive immediate transfer of care and admission for surgery. The consultation that resulted in the decision for surgery may be billed by adding modifier -57 (decision for surgery) to the consultation procedure code number. The surgeon may not charge for an admission because all E/M services provided within 24 hours of surgery are included (bundled) in the surgical fee. Most third-party reimbursement systems will not pay medical and surgical services to the same physician on the same date of service.

Medicare Global Package

Medicare has a **global surgery policy** for major operations that is similar to the surgical package concept. The Medicare global fee is a single fee for all necessary services normally furnished by the surgeon before, during, and after the procedure. This became effective on January 1, 1992 (Figure 6-6, *B*). As previously mentioned, CMS issued a policy that eliminated the use of all consultation codes (ranges 99241 through 99245 and 99251 through 99255) for inpatient and office/outpatient settings. Included in the global surgery package are the following:

● Preoperative visits (1 day before or day of surgery)
● Intraoperative services that are a usual and necessary part of the surgical procedure
● Complications after surgery that do not require additional trips to the operating room (medical and surgical services)
● Postoperative visits, including hospital visits, discharge, and office visits, for variable postoperative periods: 10 or 90 days
● Writing orders
● Evaluating the patient in the recovery area
● Normal postoperative pain management

Note: CMS proposes changes to the Medicare Global Package beginning in 2017 with the elimination of the 10-day follow-up period, followed by the elimination of the 90-day follow-up period in 2018. Be sure to check CMS updates.

Procedures shown in the *Federal Register* may show one of the three-digit or three-alpha codes in the global period column. These codes are not used on the claim form. They give information related to billing rules and regulations that indicate whether a global time period is part of a CPT code. This is particularly important when a patient comes in for a visit after surgery and helps in deciding whether the visit can be billed or is included in the surgical fee. These codes appear as follows:

000 No global period
010 For minor procedure with expected normal follow-up in a 10-day period
090 For major surgery with a 1-day preoperative period and a 90-day postoperative period included in the fee

MMM No global period. This is a service furnished in uncomplicated maternity cases, which includes prenatal care, delivery, and postnatal care.

XXX No global period. Visits, procedures, and follow-up services may be charged separately.

YYY The global period will be determined by the local Medicare fiscal agent because the code is for an unlisted procedure.

ZZZ The code is part of another service and falls within that service's global period.

Services provided for a Medicare patient not included in the global surgery package that may be billed are the following:

● Initial evaluation (regardless of when it occurs) (See the section titled "Modifier -57: Decision for Surgery.")
● Postoperative visits unrelated to the diagnosis for which the surgical procedure was performed (modifier -24 applies)
● Treatment necessary to stabilize a seriously ill patient before surgery
● Diagnostic tests and procedures
● Related procedure for postoperative complications that requires a return trip to the operating room (modifier -78 applies)
● Immunosuppressive therapy after transplant surgery

> **HIPAA Compliance Alert**
> ### HIPAA AND MEDICARE GLOBAL BILLING GUIDELINES
>
> Understanding which services are included, what constitutes the global surgical period, and how to code related or unrelated services in the global surgical package for Medicare patients is critical in ensuring correct payment and meeting compliance guidelines.

Never Event

Effective January 15, 2009, Medicare will not cover certain surgical never events and some insurance companies have stopped payment to hospitals for never events. A **never event** is an occurrence related to a surgical procedure that is performed on the wrong side, wrong site, wrong body part, or wrong person; retention of a foreign object in a patient after a procedure; patient death or disability associated with the use of contaminated drugs, devices, or biologics provided by the health care facility; patient death or serious disability associated with a medication error; stage 3 or 4 pressure ulcers acquired after admission to the health care facility; and patient death or disability associated with a fall while being cared for at the health care facility. Such occurrences should never happen in a medical practice and are usually preventable. Medicare will not cover hospitalization and other services related to these noncovered procedures. After discharge, reasonable and necessary services are covered whether they are or are not related to the surgical error.

Medically Unlikely Edits (MUEs)

Medically Unlikely Edits (MUEs) are frequency edits. These edits limit the number of units of a specific CPT code that a provider can bill for a single patient on 1 calendar day.

For example, code 10060, drainage of a skin abscess, can only be billed 1 unit but code 17003, destruction of premalignant lesions 2-14, can be billed up to 13 units.

Transfer to Another Facility

If a Medicare patient is discharged from one hospital facility and admitted to a different hospital or facility on the same day, a provider may get paid for both, depending on the circumstances of the case. A low-level admission code (for example, 99221) is used for the second hospital admission. A higher-level admission code may be used when the patient goes from a regular room status to a type of specialized hospital. Two separate revised CMS-1500 claim forms, one for the discharge and another for the admission, must be used because two different locations of service (hospital names) must appear on the claim forms.

Follow-Up (Postoperative) Days

The number of follow-up (postoperative) days that are included in the surgical package varies. The CPT code book does not specify how many days should be given, so an additional reference manual is necessary. Most states use an RVS for workers' compensation cases, which lists the follow-up days allowed for most surgical procedures.

Medicare lists a 90-day global period for all major procedures and 10 days for minor procedures. Some commercial third-party payers have a 45-day global period for all or some major procedures. A few commercial third-party payers treat major procedures like minor procedures in the surgical package by allowing 10 follow-up days instead of 90. However, most third-party insurance companies follow Medicare guidelines and adhere to the 10- and 90-day global periods. To obtain specific payer information, send the insurance company a list of the most common surgical procedures and ask for the surgical package rules and the number of global days that apply to each code. If this information is not available, it is wise to bill the private payer for the preoperative and all postoperative visits. When this information is received, a table should be created that shows global days on a payer-by-payer and procedure-by-procedure basis. On the chart of each patient scheduled for surgery, the type of surgery and how many days the insurance policy allows should be indicated. A bill should be submitted for all visits after the surgical package period expires.

For office visits by the physician during the postoperative period, use CPT code 99024 on the patient's financial account to indicate "No Charge." This code is located in the Medicine section under Special Services and Reports; Miscellaneous Services. It has no value, is unbundled with other codes, and is used for tracking purposes. Code 99024 on itemized billing statements lets the patient know how many office visits after surgery have been provided at no charge. There is no Medicare guideline for this code. It is not necessary to list this code when completing an insurance claim unless the third-party payer has specific instructions requesting that it be shown. If the patient has to be seen beyond the normal postoperative period, the reason must be documented in the patient's medical record and an applicable procedure code and fee for this service should be indicated on the claim form. A bill may be submitted for the office visit if the patient returns to the provider for treatment of an unrelated illness or injury during the postoperative (global) period. The diagnosis codes should support the reason for the visit. If the provider did not perform the surgery but is performing the postoperative care, the provider can charge for the visits but must use the appropriate modifier (-55) to explain the charge.

Repair of Lacerations

If multiple lacerations are repaired with the same technique and are in the same anatomic category, the insurance billing specialist should add up the total length of all lacerations and report one code to obtain maximum reimbursement. However, always read the notes and directives from the CPT manual when assigning these codes, as these sites and sums can be confusing. Anatomic

Example 6-11	Repair of Multiple Lacerations

Three lacerations of the face totaling 8.2 cm.

Incorrect Coding

12011	Repair 2.5-cm laceration of face
12013	Repair 2.7-cm laceration of face
12013	Repair 3-cm laceration of face

Correct Coding

12015	Repair 8.2-cm laceration of face

Example 6-12	Paring of Seven Corns

Incorrect Coding

11055	Paring; single lesion
11056-51	Two to four lesions
11057-51	More than four lesions
or	
11055 ×7	Paring; single lesion (× seven corns)

Correct Coding

11057	Paring; more than four lesions (seven corns)

categories are the scalp, neck, axillae, external genitalia, trunk, extremities (hands or feet), face, ears, eyelids, nose, lips, and mucous membranes. If the patient had three repairs and each was listed with a different code, the second and third codes are downcoded (coded down one level) by the third-party payer so that a smaller payment is generated. If a patient has lacerations on both sides of the face, the lengths of all lacerations should be combined because the anatomic region is the same, and a claim should be submitted for the total length. No modifier is used and the right and left sides of the face are not billed separately (Example 6-11).

Multiple Lesions

The descriptions for the surgical codes that relate to accessory structures (for example, scalp, arms, and legs) and lesions found in the integumentary system (pertaining to the skin) can cause confusion. Code descriptions, including indentations, should be read completely with attention paid to terms such as *complex, complicated, extensive,* and *multiple* (lesions). Lesion excision code selection is based on the lesion's clinical diameter plus margin before excision and the character of the lesion—benign or malignant. Measurements should be taken before excision because a specimen subject to pathology may shrink. Do not refer to a pathology report because the diameter of the mass may be measured after shrinkage or fragmentation of the specimen. Example 6-12 is a guide to obtain maximum reimbursement for the paring of seven corns.

MINOR OPERATING ROOM INSTRUMENT TRAY SUPPLY CHECKLIST

1 Adson Brown tissue forceps	_____
1 Adson tissue forceps with teeth	_____
1 long tissue forceps	_____
2 mosquito clamps	_____
1 Peck Joseph dissecting scissors	_____
1 Kahn dissecting scissors	_____
1 Reynolds dissecting scissors	_____
1 Stratte needle holder	_____
1 Webster needle holder	_____
4 small piercing towel clips	_____
2 double-skin hooks	_____
2 single-skin hooks	_____
1 knife handle	_____
1 #15 blade	_____
10 4 x 4s	_____
2 cotton-tipped applicators	_____
1 small basin	_____
3 sterile towels (drapes)	_____
1 Bovie pencil	_____
Sutures:_____ _____ _____	_____
Dressings: ½-inch Steri-strips	_____

A

OFFICE SURGERY MEDICAL RECORD CHECKLIST

Patient information sheet	_____
H and P or progress note	_____
Consent form	_____
Diagnostic studies	_____
Pathology report(s)	_____
Anesthesia record	_____
Circulating nurse's note	_____
Doctor's orders	_____
Discharge note	_____
Operative report	_____
Signature/operative report	_____

B

FIGURE 6-7 A, Checklist to document supplies used when billing for office surgery. This list can be kept with the patient's medical record. **B,** Checklist for identifying complete and incomplete medical records used for a patient receiving office surgery. As each item or document is completed, it is checked off so that the person reviewing the chart can see at a glance what needs to be finalized.

If possible, delay submission of the insurance claim for removal of a lesion or lesions until the pathology report is received. Usually a malignant lesion is reimbursed at a higher rate because of the more detailed nature of the procedure.

Supplies

When billing for office surgery and supplies used, checklists for the items used on the sterile tray (Figure 6-7, *A*) and for determining complete and incomplete records (see Figure 6-7, *B*) should be used. These items can be charged only if the surgery required the use of additional items not normally used for this type of surgery. Medicare pays for trays with some procedure codes but not with others.

Incident-To Services

According to federal Medicare billing guidelines, physicians can bill for services provided by allied health professionals who are members of their practice, such as physician assistants, therapists, nurses, and nurse practitioners, as long as the services relate to the professional services that the physician provides and direct supervision occurs. The physician does not need to be physically in the room with the ancillary provider but he or she must be available in the immediate office suite. Examples for using E/M code 99211 (established patient office visit) not requiring the presence of a physician include:

- Rechecking a patient for conjunctivitis
- Checking blood pressure of a patient who is being treated for high blood pressure
- Checking a wound beyond the global period
- Reading a tuberculin test result
- Recheck for issuing a return-to-work certificate

It is important that documentation includes the date of service, reason for the visit, medical necessity, patient encounter information, and signature of the practitioner. To verify that there was a supervising physician, add a place for the physician to countersign that he or she was available and directly supervised the visit.

Prolonged Services, Detention, or Standby

Codes 99354 through 99359 should be used to indicate prolonged services with direct face-to-face patient contact; for example, the physician has spent time beyond the usual amount allotted for the service (for example, 30 to 60 minutes). There are specific codes for services with face-to-face contact and without face-to-face contact. Prolonged service that is less than 30 minutes should not be billed using these codes because the time is included in the E/M code. Time should be documented in the health record to justify use of these codes. Reimbursement for prolonged attendance in the hospital is higher than payment for many other types of care and reimbursement for critical care is even higher.

Physician standby services over the first 30 minutes are billed using code 99360. Some insurance programs or plans (for example, Medicare) do not pay for physician standby services, so be sure to check before billing to see whether the commercial payer will pay. The charge for this type of service is based on what the physician believes to be the value of 1 hour of his or her time. An example of this might be when a pediatrician is on standby during a high-risk cesarean section performed on a pregnant woman.

Unlisted Procedures

When an unusual service is rendered, an unlisted code (Example 6-13) should be used rather than guessing or

Example 6-13	Unlisted Procedure Code
31599	Unlisted procedure, larynx

using an incorrect code. Supporting documentation (letter and copy of operative report) should be sent explaining the service.

Since the development of category III codes, it is important to double check that section of the CPT code book to verify whether a code exists before using an unlisted code. Unlisted codes may or may not end in -99 and are found at the end of each section or subsection. A comprehensive list of unlisted codes is found at the beginning of each section. Some MACs do not pay for any of the special -99 adjunct or unlisted codes. The following are guidelines for submitting a claim with an unlisted code to obtain maximum payment.

- Always send or transmit supporting documentation with the claim to clearly identify the procedure performed and the medical necessity. If detailed documentation cannot be submitted electronically or faxed to the third-party payer, send a paper claim with supporting documentation in a large envelope so that it is not folded. Do not use paper clips, staples, or tape to affix the attachments to the claim. Mark each attachment with the patient's name, insurance identification number, date of service, page number of the attachment, and total number of pages submitted (for example, page 2 of 3). This helps the claims processor to match the documentation to the claim in case they are separated. Do not use a highlighter to point out the pertinent operative note sections because highlighting may not show up when payers scan the claim. Instead, underline, star, or bracket the applicable sections for quick identification.
- File claims with unlisted procedure codes in a separate "tickler" file or in an electronic tracking system. Follow up the status of the claim if there is no response within 1 month.

Coding Guidelines for Code Edits

In 1996 the Medicare program implemented the NCCI. This initiative involves a code editing system consistent with Medicare policies to eliminate inappropriate reporting of CPT codes. *Code editing* is a computer software function that performs online checking of codes on an insurance claim to detect **unbundling,** splitting of codes, and other types of improper code submissions. Some coders refer to this process as *code screening*. NCCI edits are updated quarterly. Such software is used by private payers, federal programs, and state Medicaid programs. Some code pairs in the NCCI edits are followed by a

Example 6-14	Comprehensive and Component Codes	
Comprehensive code	93015	Cardiovascular stress test
Component codes	93016, 93017, 93018	
93015	Cardiovascular stress test using maximal or submaximal treadmill or bicycle exercise, continuous electrocardiographic monitoring, or pharmacologic stress; with physician supervision, with interpretation and report	
93016	Physician supervision only, without interpretation and report	
93017	Tracing only, without interpretation and report	
93018	Interpretation and report only	

Example 6-15	Separate Procedure
Separate procedure example: Inguinal hernia repair with lesion excised from spermatic cord **Comprehensive code:** 49505 Repair initial hernia age 5 years or older; reducible **Component code:** 55520 Excision of lesion of spermatic cord (separate procedure)	

Example 6-16	Mutually Exclusive	
47605	**Excision,** cholecystectomy; with cholangiography	
47563	**Laparoscopy,** surgical; cholecystectomy with cholangiography	

Note: Different methods of accomplishing the same procedure.

0 and others by a 1. If the superscript 0 appears with a code pair, it means that Medicare never allows a modifier to be used with the codes, so the code pair could never be reported together. The superscript 1 means that you may use a modifier under certain circumstances with appropriate documentation to have both codes reimbursed.

Because every medical practice has billing problems and questions unique to its specialty that arise because of denial or reduction in payment of claims, the billing specialist must become a detective and discover how to obtain maximum reimbursements in the appropriate specialty. The best way is to telephone the third-party payer to inquire about new coding options and to note improvements in reimbursement. Coding takes expertise. It is an art, not an exact science. The following explanations of various ways of coding claims assist in obtaining maximum reimbursement for each service rendered and avoiding denials, lowered reimbursement, and possible audit.

Comprehensive and Component Edits

A **comprehensive code** means a single code that describes or covers two or more component codes that are bundled together as one unit. A component code is a lesser procedure and is considered part of the major procedure. Each component code represents a portion of the service described in the comprehensive code and should be used only if a portion of the comprehensive service was performed (Example 6-14).

Under the Medicare program, NCCI component code edits involve procedures that meet any of the following criteria:
1. Code combinations that are specified as "separate procedures" by CPT

2. Codes that are included as part of a more extensive procedure
3. Code combinations that are restricted by the guidelines outlined in CPT
4. Component codes that are used incorrectly with the comprehensive code

If any one of these restricted code combinations is billed, Medicare allows payment for only the procedure with the highest relative value (Example 6-15).

For example, when performing an inguinal hernia repair, the surgeon makes an incision in the groin and dissects tissue to expose the hernia sac, internal oblique muscle, and spermatic cord. If a lesion is excised from the spermatic cord, it is considered a component of the comprehensive hernia repair procedure and is not separately billable. Medicare will deny code 55520 (lesion excision) as a component of procedure code 49505 (hernia repair) when performed during the same operative session.

Mutually Exclusive Code Edits

Mutually exclusive code edits (denials) relate to procedures that meet any of the following criteria:
1. Code combinations that are restricted by the guidelines outlined in CPT
2. Procedures that represent two methods of performing the same service
3. Procedures that cannot reasonably be done during the same session
4. Procedures that represent medically impossible or improbable code combinations

In Example 6-16, if one were to submit codes 47605 and 47563, both of these procedures are different

Example 6-17	Bundled Code	
Component code	19271	Excision of chest wall tumor involving ribs, with plastic reconstruction; without mediastinal lymphadenectomy
Comprehensive code	19272	with mediastinal lymphadenectomy

Example 6-18	Unbundled Code	
Incorrect Coding		
12011		Simple repair of superficial wounds of face, ears, eyelids, nose, lips and/or mucous membranes 2.5 cm or less.
12014		5.1 cm to 7.5 cm
Correct Coding		
12015		7.6 cm to 12.5 cm

methods of accomplishing the same result (removal of the gallbladder with cholangiography). They represent a duplication of effort and an overlap of services; therefore Medicare would deny code 47563 (laparoscopy) as mutually exclusive to code 47605 (the excision).

Bundled Codes

For insurance claim purposes, **bundled codes** means to group related codes together. To completely understand bundled codes, one must have a thorough knowledge of the service or procedure that is being provided or use an unbundling book as a reference guide.

Example 6-17 illustrates one type of bundling found in the CPT code book. Because code 19271 (excision of chest wall tumor without mediastinal lymphadenectomy) does not include mediastinal lymphadenectomy and code 19272 (with mediastinal lymphadenectomy) does include it, reporting both codes together would be a contradiction in the actual performance of the services at the same session. Hence when mediastinal lymphadenectomy is part of the procedure, submit code 19272 because code 19271 is bundled with it.

In the Medicare program, a number of services may be affected because CMS considers the services to be bundled. Because many commercial third-party payers may follow Medicare guidelines, an understanding of this bundling concept is necessary. When dealing with private insurance, an explanation of benefits (EOB) document may print out with the statement "Benefits have been combined," which means the same thing as bundling.

For example, when listing a sterile tray for an in-office surgical procedure, the tray is bundled with the procedure unless supplies are necessary in addition to those usually used. CPT code 99070 (supplies and materials) is not reimbursed by Medicare; however, HCPCS level II alphanumeric codes may be used in such cases. The cost of some services and supplies is bundled in E/M codes (for example, telephone services, reading of test results). However, Medicare pays for slings, splints, rib belts, cast supplies, Hexcelite and light casts, pneumatic ankle-control splints, and prosthetics but a supplier (provider) number is necessary to bill for take-home surgical supplies and durable medical equipment (DME). Medicare claims for supplies and DME go to one of four regional DME fiscal agents. Some coding reference books also include a comprehensive list of codes that CMS considers bundled for the Medicare program. When appealing a claim, a great deal of time may be spent on paperwork only to discover that the code is bundled and denial is imminent. When in doubt about whether or not services are combined, contact the third-party payer and ask.

Unbundling

Unbundling is coding and billing numerous CPT codes to identify procedures that usually are described by a single code. It is also known as *exploding* or *a la carte* medicine.

Some practices do this unwittingly but it is considered fraud if it is done intentionally to gain increased reimbursement. Unbundling can lead to downward payment adjustments and possible audit of claims.

Types of unbundling are as follows:
- Fragmenting one service into component parts and coding each component part as if it were a separate service (Example 6-18)
- Reporting separate codes for related services when one comprehensive code includes all related services (Example 6-19)
- Coding **bilateral** (both sides of the body) procedures as two codes when one code is proper (Example 6-20)
- Separating a surgical approach from a major surgical service that includes the same approach (Example 6-21)

Insurers use special software designed to detect unbundling. To avoid this problem, always use a current CPT code book. The use of outdated codes often inadvertently results in unbundling. A new technology or technique may have its own code when it is developed but may be bundled with another code as it becomes commonplace. If the practice uses a billing service, request in writing that the service's computer system include no unbundling programming.

Example 6-19   Unbundling (Comprehensive Code)

Unbundled Claim

58150	Total abdominal hysterectomy (corpus and cervix) with removal of tubes and with removal of ovary ($1200)
58700	Salpingectomy ($650)
58940	Oophorectomy ($685)
	Total Charge: $2535

Claim Coded Correctly

58150	Comprehensive code for all three services
	Total Charge: $1200

Example 6-20   Unbundling (Bilateral)

Incorrect Coding

77055-RT	Right mammography
77055-LT	Left mammography

Correct Coding

77056	Mammography, bilateral

Example 6-21   Bundling (Surgical Approach)

Incorrect Coding

49000	Exploratory laparotomy
44150	Colectomy, total, abdominal

Correct Coding

44150	Colectomy, total, abdominal (correct because it includes exploration of the surgical field)

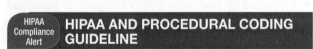

HIPAA AND PROCEDURAL CODING GUIDELINE

Always submit current CPT codes. If outdated codes are used, this could red flag a provider with Medicare as being in noncompliance.

Downcoding

Downcoding occurs when the coding system used on a claim submitted to a third-party payer does not match the coding system used by the company receiving the claim. The computer system converts the code submitted to the closest code in use, which is usually down one level from the submitted code. Therefore the payment that is generated is usually less. In many states, it is illegal for an insurance company to downcode a claim. Insurance commissioners have published bulletins warning payers to cease this claims adjudication practice. When a payer receives a claim, the payer is allowed to pay or deny the claim.

Example 6-22   Downcoding

Incorrect Coding

20010	Incision of abscess with suction irrigation

Correct Coding

20005	Incision of abscess, deep or complicated

(**Note:** 20010 has been deleted from CPT and would result in downcoding.)

If additional information is necessary to adjudicate the claim, it should be requested from the patient or provider. The payer is limited by the number of days it has to review the claim. At completion of the review, the payer must pay or deny the claim.

HIPAA Compliance Alert   **HIPAA DOCUMENTATION GUIDELINE**

Make sure that the documentation from the provider supports the code that is being submitted to prevent downcoding.

Use current CPT manuals. Review all Medicare updates for changes to HCPCS codes. Always monitor reimbursements and look for downcoding so that you become knowledgeable about which codes are affected (Example 6-22).

Downcoding also occurs when a claims examiner converts the CPT code submitted to a code in the RVS being used by the payer. This can occur in workers' compensation claims. When there is a choice between two or three somewhat similar codes, the claims examiner chooses the lowest-paying code. Any time the code that was submitted is changed, appeal the change immediately.

Downcoding also may occur when a claims examiner compares the code used with the written description of the procedure included in an attached document. If the two do not match, the payer will reimburse according to the lowest-paying code that fits the description given (Example 6-23). In this example the word "bone" is a clue to go to the musculoskeletal section of the code book and not the integumentary section. See Chapter 9 for additional information on and solutions to downcoding.

Upcoding

The term **upcoding** is used to describe deliberate manipulation of CPT codes for increased payment. This practice can be spotted by Medicare fiscal agents and third-party payers using prepayment and postpayment screens or "stop alerts," which are built into most computer coding software programs. An example of intentional upcoding might be a physician who selects one level of service code for all visits with the theory that the costs even out, such as always using code 99213. This opens the door to audits and in the end may cost the practice money. Upcoding may occur unintentionally if the coder is ill informed or does not keep current. Join a free list service (listserv) to keep current, make national coding contacts, and post questions to others who may know the answer to a current coding or billing dilemma.

Code Monitoring

Monitoring of CPT codes is done to maximize reimbursement from all third-party payers. First, determine which codes are used most often in the physician's practice. Many computer programs can generate a list of codes, ranking them according to frequency of use. If the practice does not have a computer, take a sampling of the charge slips to determine the prevalent codes. Once the high-volume codes are known, focus on coding strategies for the best possible reimbursement (Figure 6-8). Monitor every remittance advice (RA) and EOB that comes in directly or via patients. Every private insurance, Medicare, Medicaid, and TRICARE payment received should be checked for accuracy to see whether it is consistently the same or if

coding changes have occurred. Incorrect payments should be investigated and appealed. Examine all payments made for codes that do not match those submitted. Be sure to appeal every payment that is less than half of what the physician bills. An example of a code and payment tracking log to help monitor payments received is shown in Figure 6-8.

HELPFUL HINTS IN CODING

Office Visits

When an established patient is seen for an office visit and a clinical medical assistant incidentally takes the patient's blood pressure per the physician's standing order, the physician includes that service with the appropriate level of E/M code number (for example, 99213 or 99214). If the clinical medical assistant takes the blood pressure and the patient is not seen by the physician but the physician reviews the results, the appropriate E/M code number is 99211 (presence of physician not necessary). If more than one office visit is necessary per day, the requirements for use of modifiers -25 and -59 should be read before submitting a claim to determine whether one of them may be applicable.

Some insurance policies allow only two moderate- or high-complexity office visits per patient per year. Therefore contact the insurance company either online or by telephone to validate whether the patient is insured and also to learn if there are any limitations. A physician's practice should have a system in place to track this.

Drugs and Injections

When submitting claims for Medicare, Medicaid, and some private insurance carriers, insert the name of the drug, amount of dosage, strength, and how it was administered in Block 19 on the CMS-1500 claim form. This information must be documented in the patient's health record. If a drug is experimental or expensive, you need

---

Example 6-23   Downcoding

Document states: Excision of bone tumor from anterior tibial shaft.

Pathology report states: Tibia bone tumor; benign

Incorrect Coding

11400   Excision of benign lesion including margins except skin tag, trunk, arms or legs; excised diameter 0.5 cm or less

Correct Coding

27635   Excision of bone tumor of tibia, benign

CODE/PAYMENT TRACKING LOG					Date: 1-XX
CPT CODE	Practice fee	Medicare date and amount paid	Medicaid date and amount paid	TRICARE date and amount paid	Blue Shield date and amount paid
99201	$00.00	11-XX $00.00	8-XX $00.00	7-XX $00.00	4-XX $00.00
99202	$00.00	12-XX $00.00	9-XX $00.00	10-XX $00.00	6-XX $00.00
99211	$00.00	12-XX $00.00			11-XX $00.00
99212	$00.00				12-XX $00.00
99221	$00.00				
99231	$00.00				
99232	$00.00				
99241	$00.00				

FIGURE 6-8 Example of a code/payment tracking log.

to attach a copy of the invoice. CPT codes for immunization administration for vaccines are 90460 through 90474 and for therapeutic or diagnostic injections are 96372 to 96379. Separate codes are used to identify the product being administered, either immune globulin codes 90281 through 90399, vaccine/toxoid codes 90476 through 90749, or when billing a Medicare case, Level II HCPCS national alphanumeric codes A9500 or J0000. In Medicaid cases, it is permissible to bill for injectable medications. Separate codes are available for combination vaccines. See CPT codes 95004 through 95199 for allergy testing and codes 95115 through 95199 for allergen immunotherapy. If an anesthetic agent is being used, determine whether it is diagnostic, therapeutic, or prophylactic for pain. Medicare bills for immunosuppressive therapy are submitted to durable medical equipment fiscal agents, regional carriers (private companies) that contract with Medicare to process and pay insurance claims for medical equipment. *Immunosuppressive therapy* is treatment by administering an agent that significantly interferes with the ability of the body's immune system to respond to antigenic stimulation by inhibiting cellular and humoral immunity, such as preparing someone for a bone marrow transplant or to prevent rejection of donor tissue.

Some providers give mass immunizations to Medicare patients. A simplified process called *roster billing* was created that allows a provider to submit a vaccine roster with the CMS-1500 (02/12) claim form. The roster must include the Medicare patients' identification numbers, names, addresses, dates of birth, genders, and signatures when they received vaccinations for influenza and pneumococcal vaccines covered by Medicare. Paper or electronic claims may be submitted with the roster. Medicare annual Part B deductible and coinsurance amounts do not apply to these vaccines. HCPCS codes G0008, G0009, and G0010 are used with the appropriate vaccine product code and a V code from ICD-9-CM indicating the need for the immunization. For e-prescribing, a bonus is given to providers who electronically prescribe drugs. As of 2010, HCPCS code G8553 should be used for reporting.

Adjunct Codes

Adjunct codes are referred to in the Medicine section of the CPT as Special Services, Procedures and Reports and fall under the category of Miscellaneous Services. They are important to consider when billing because these codes provide the reporting physician with a means of identifying special services and reports that are provided in addition to the basic services provided. The circumstances that are covered under these codes (99000 through 99091) include handling of laboratory

---

Example 6-24	How to Report Modifier on Claim Form

Add a two-digit modifier to the five-digit code number.
Single line item:
12345-22 *OR* 1234522

---

specimens, telephone calls, seeing patients after hours, office emergency services, supplies and materials, special reports, travel, and educational services rendered to patients. Explain the circumstances on an attached document to justify the use of these codes when submitting an insurance claim. Some insurance companies pay for these services but others do not.

Basic Life or Disability Evaluation Services

Use code 99450 when reporting examinations done on patients for the purpose of trying to obtain life or disability insurance. Codes 99455 and 99456 may be used for work-related or medical disability examinations. Additional information about life or health insurance examinations is given in Chapter 4.

CODE MODIFIERS

The use of a CPT code's two-digit add-on modifier permits the physician to indicate circumstances in which a procedure as performed differs in some way from that described by its usual five-digit code (Example 6-24). It may be necessary when using a modifier to include an operative, pathology, x-ray, or special report to justify its use to a third-party payer. For each modifier listed at the end of this chapter in Table 6-6, there is a statement as to when it is appropriate to include a report. A modifier can indicate the following:

- A service or procedure has either a professional component (PC) or a technical component (TC).
- A service or procedure was performed by more than one physician or in more than one location.
- A service or procedure has been increased or reduced.
- A service or procedure was provided more than once.
- Only part of a service was performed.
- An adjunctive service was performed.
- A bilateral procedure was performed.
- Unusual events occurred.

Correct Use of Common CPT Modifiers

Any modifier that fits the situation being coded may be used, except when the modifier definition restricts the use of specific codes; for example, modifier -51, Multiple Procedures, states that -51 is to be appended for "multiple procedures, other than Evaluation and Management Services..." Discussion of the most commonly used modifiers follows.

Modifier -22: Increased Procedural Services

Modifier -22 is used when the service provided is substantially greater than that typically required for the listed procedure. If you add modifier -22, the documentation in the health record, such as operative reports and/or chart notes, must support the substantial additional work. Encourage your physician to use appropriate descriptions in the report and call these words to his or her attention. The reasons for use of this modifier are that the work encompasses increased intensity, time, technical difficulty of procedure, severity of the patient's condition, and physical and mental effort needed. This modifier may not be used with E/M services. Most third-party payers send an insurance claim to medical review before payment is made if modifier -22, indicating unusual services, appears on the claim. Because payments may be delayed, be cautious when using this modifier. An operative report should be submitted with the claim. If the third-party payer routinely denies the claim with modifier -22, an appeal for review should be made. See Chapter 9 for details on the Medicare redetermination (appeal) process.

Modifier -25: Significant, Separately Identifiable Evaluation and Management Service

In some cases, you may be confused whether to assign modifier -25 or -57. Modifier -25 is defined as "significant, separately identifiable evaluation and management service by the same physician on the same day of the procedure or other service." The industry standard is to use -25 when a diagnostic procedure or minor procedure is involved (for example, those with a 10-day follow-up period). Typically, E/M services that are modified with -25 are office visits performed on the day of a minor procedure for an established patient. However, the confusion results because the CPT book states: "This modifier is not used to report an E/M service that resulted in a decision to perform surgery. See modifier -57."

Modifier -26: Professional Component

Certain procedures are a combination of a **professional component (PC)** and a **technical component (TC)** and are considered a global service. Usually these involve radiology and pathology procedures. The professional (physician) component refers to a portion of a test or procedure that the physician does, such as interpreting an electrocardiogram (ECG), reading an x-ray film, or making an observation and determination using a microscope. The TC refers to the use of the equipment, the supplies, and the operator who performs the test or procedure, such as ECG machine and technician, radiography machine and technician, and microscope and technician. The TC is billed by the entity that owns the equipment. Do not modify procedures that are either 100% technical

Example 6-25	Professional and Technical Components	
73520-**26**	**Professional component** only for a radiograph of both hips. Use to bill physician's fee for interpretation of x-ray film.	$
73520-**TC** or **73525**	**Technical component** only for a radiograph of both hips. Use to bill fee for facility that owns equipment and employs technician. Modifier -TC is at carrier's discretion.	$
73520	**Global service:** Radiologic examination, hips, bilateral. Minimum of two views of each hip. Use to bill complete fee when physician owns equipment, employs technician, and interprets x-ray film.	$

or 100% professional or when the physician performs both the PC and the TC. Modifier -26 represents the PC only. Use of this modifier alerts the insurance company to expect a separate claim from another provider or facility for the TC.

In Example 6-25, the physician is performing only one of two services—he or she is interpreting the results of bilateral hip x-ray films.

The facility where the patient had the x-ray film taken bills only for the TC by using either 73525 or 73520 with modifier -TC. If the physician owns the equipment and reads the x-ray film, there is no need to modify the x-ray code (73520) because both the PC and the TC were done in the office. Modifier -TC is assigned at the carrier's discretion.

Modifier -51: Multiple Procedures

Multiple procedures are when more than one surgical service and/or related surgical service is performed on the same day or at the same surgical session by the same physician. In such cases, first report the primary service or procedure, which can be determined easily by the highest dollar value. Identify all additional services or procedures by appending codes with modifier -51 (Example 6-26).

The operative report should clearly state which procedures were done through separate incisions and which were done through the same incision. There are many circumstances when multiple procedures are performed. Modifier -51 may be used to identify the following:
- Multiple surgical procedures performed at the same session by the same provider
- Multiple related surgical procedures performed at the same session by the same provider

Example 6-26	Multiple Procedure Modifier -51

Excision of 2.0-cm benign lesion on the nose and at the same session a biopsy of the skin and subcutaneous tissue of the forearm.

Code	RVU	Description of Services
11442	$	Excision, other benign lesion including margins, face, ears, eyelids, nose, lips, mucous membrane; excised diameter 1.1 to 2.0 cm
11100-**51**		Biopsy of skin, subcutaneous tissue, or mucous membrane (including simple closure), unless otherwise listed; single lesion (**second; multiple procedure**)

- Surgical procedures performed in combination at the same session, whether through the same or another incision or involving the same or different anatomy
- A combination of medical and surgical procedures performed at the same session by the same provider

Usually, payment by third-party payers for the primary code is 100% of the allowable charge, for the second code is 50%, for the third code is 25%, and for the fourth and remaining codes is 10%. However, under NCCI guidelines, Medicare pays 100% of the allowable charge for the primary code, pays 50% for two to five secondary procedures, and does not require the assignment of modifier -51. Some computer systems can determine code order and automatically make the code adjustment for you. Many carriers no longer require modifier -51 because they process claims electronically and the software program recognizes when multiple procedures are performed and automatically makes the reduction in payment. Contact insurance carriers and ask which method is preferred when reporting multiple surgical procedures. Then note this for each payer's policy to refer to for future billings. Always bill the full amount and let the third-party payer make the payment adjustments for percentage considerations. For all third-party payers, it is recommended that you monitor the RA/EOB to ensure correct payment. A decision flow chart is provided for reference to help simplify the modifier decision process (Figure 6-9). As you read through the remainder of this chapter, follow the steps by answering the questions in Figure 6-9, *A*, as they apply to your billing scenario and refer to Figure 6-9, *B*, for key information and descriptions.

If multiple procedures are done as in-office procedures or services and you are using E/M codes, it may be possible to bill a higher-level E/M visit because the -51 modifier is not used with E/M services. Do not use the -51 modifier with add-on codes designated with a "+" (see Appendix D in CPT) or codes listed as exempt to modifier -51 (see Appendix E in CPT). Add-on codes are codes that cannot

Example 6-27	Add-On Code

Parent code	11000	Biopsy of skin … single lesion each separate/additional lesion (list separately in addition to code for primary procedure)
Add-on code	+11101	

Example 6-28	Decision for Surgery

A new patient is seen in the office complaining of a great deal of pain. Cholangiography is done and reveals blocked bile ducts. The patient is scheduled for surgery the next day.

8-1-20XX	99204-**57**	New patient office visit	$00.00
8-2-20XX	47600	Cholecystectomy	$000.00

stand alone. When billing with add-on codes, you must first list another code referred to as the "parent code" to give a full description for service billed (Example 6-27).

When making a decision about when to use an add-on code, look for a clue phrase that indicates additional procedures, such as "each additional," "list in addition to," and "second lesion."

Modifier -52: Reduced Services

Use of the modifier -52 indicates that under certain circumstances a service or procedure is partially reduced or eliminated at the physician's discretion. It is wise to provide an explanation of why the service was reduced. A cover letter or a copy of the operative report should not accompany these claims because usually they are not sent to medical review and attached documents may impede processing. Never use this modifier if the fee is reduced because of a patient's inability to pay.

Modifier -57: Decision for Surgery

The modifier -57 is used strictly to report an E/M service that resulted in the initial decision to perform a major surgical procedure within 24 hours of the office visit (for example, those with a 90-day follow-up period); see Examples 6-28 and 6-29. A -57 modifier may be used for inpatient or outpatient consultations, inpatient hospital visits, and new or established patient visits that occur the day of or the day before surgery. Do not attach modifier -57 to a hospital visit code for the day before surgery or the day of surgery when a decision for a major surgical procedure was made a week before surgery. Think of -57 as telling the insurance company that the office visit is not part of the global fee.

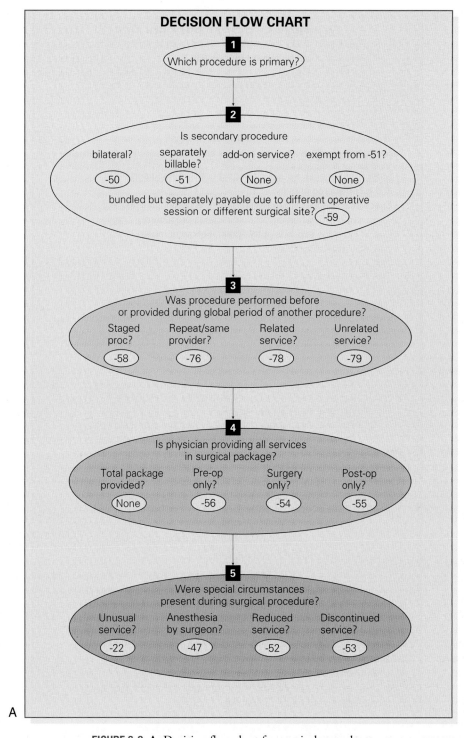

FIGURE 6-9 A, Decision flow chart for surgical procedures.

Continued

Consult Figure 6-10 when making the decision about which modifier to use for a surgical procedure that is performed within 24 hours of an office visit.

In Medicare cases, the CMS has published in the NCCI the specific codes for modifier -25 use after October 2000. Refer to the bulletin or newsletter pertinent to this update.

Modifier -58: Staged or Related Procedure

The modifier -58 is used to indicate that the performance of a procedure or service during the postoperative period was as follows:

- Planned (staged) at the time of the original procedure
- More extensive than the original procedure
- For therapy after a surgical procedure

MULTIPLE SURGICAL PROCEDURES

Multiple services must be related to:
- Same patient
- Same provider
- Same date of service

1

- List all procedures in order of reimbursement, highest to lowest.
- Most comprehensive service brings greatest reimbursement and is considered primary.
- Check all procedures to make sure there is no unbundling (i.e., using two codes when one code describes procedure).
- Decision making expands at this point. Follow numbered question to determine correct modifier usage.

2

-50 Bilateral procedure, not described by code
-51 Not bundled, separately billable
-59 Ordinarily bundled, separately payable due to special circumstance

3

- The term "primary procedure" can also refer to the first procedure initiating a global surgical period
-58 Current service was planned prospectively at time of first service
-76 Physician repeats procedure subsequent to original procedure
-78 Return to operating room for subsequent procedure, complication relating to original procedure
-79 Unrelated procedure performed during global period of previous surgery

4

- Surgical package means one fee covers the whole package, surgical procedure, and postoperative care.

5

-22 An extremely difficult procedure due to altered anatomy or unusual circumstances (add 10% to 30% reimbursement)
-47 When the surgeon administers regional or general anesthesia
-52 Procedure/service reduced or eliminated at the discretion of the physician
-53 Procedure is discontinued due to extenuating circumstances or because of threat to the patient

B

FIGURE 6-9, cont'd B, Guidelines and description of modifiers for multiple surgical procedures.

Such circumstances should be reported by adding modifier -58 to the staged or related procedure. The use of this modifier requires accurate documentation of events leading up to the initial surgery and any subsequent surgery. It is only possible to modify procedures if the coder has all of the relevant facts and circumstances. In Example 6-29, the fracture is considered surgery because it is in the surgery section of the CPT book. All fracture codes have 90-day postoperative periods.

Modifiers -62, -66, -80, -81, and -82: More Than One Surgeon

If more than one surgeon is involved, clarify for whom you are billing by using the appropriate two-digit modifier as follows:

- -62, Co-surgeon: Two surgeons work together as primary surgeons performing distinct parts of a procedure. Each physician reports his or her distinct operative work by adding this modifier.

Example 6-29 Decision for Surgery

A new patient comes to the office after sustaining a fall while in-line skating. She is in distress, complaining of right wrist pain and swelling of the joint. The injury is evaluated **(1)** with an x-ray film. **(2)** It is determined that the patient has a Smith fracture and manipulation is performed. A long-arm cast is applied **(3)** using fiberglass (Hexcelite) material **(4)**.

(1)	99203-57	Initial office evaluation (detailed) **with decision for surgery**
(2)	73100-RT	Radiologic examination, right wrist, antero-posterior (AP) and lateral (lat) views
(3)	25605	Closed treatment of distal radial fracture (for example, Colles or Smith type), with manipulation
(4)	99070	Supplies: Casting material (third-party payer) Medicine section code *or* Supplies: Hexcelite material (Medicare fiscal agent)
	A4590	HCPCS Level II code

The patient returns in 4 weeks for follow-up care **(1)**. The wrist is radiographed again **(2)**, the long-arm cast is removed **(3)**, and a short-arm cast is applied **(4)** using plaster material **(5)**.

(1)	No code	Follow-up care included in global fee
(2)	73100-RT	Radiologic examination, right wrist, AP and lat views
(3)	No code	Cast removal included in original fracture care (25605)
(4)	29075-**58**	Application, plaster, elbow to finger (short arm) **staged procedure**
(5)	99070	Supplies: Casting material (third-party payer) Medicine section code *or* Supplies: Plaster material (Medicare fiscal agent)
	A4580	HCPCS Level II code

- -66, Team surgery: A group of surgeons work together. Each participating physician adds this modifier to the basic procedure number for the service.
- -80, Assistant at surgery: Used when the surgery is not performed in a teaching hospital.
- -81, Minimum assistant surgeon.
- -82, Assistant surgeon: Used for surgeries performed in a teaching hospital when a qualified resident surgeon is not available to act as an assistant at surgery.

The assistant physician adds one of these modifiers to the usual procedure number (Examples 6-30 and 6-31).

Modifier -80 (assistant at surgery) is commonly used when billing for a physician who assists the primary physician in performing a surgical procedure (see Example 6-30).

The assisting doctor is paid a reduced fee of 16% to 30% of the allowed fee the primary surgeon receives for performing the surgery on the basis of the patient's contract. The assisting physician uses the same surgical code as the primary surgeon and adds the -80 modifier to it. The fee indicating a reduced percentage typically is listed as the fee on the claim form. However, some third-party payers may prefer having the full fee listed and making the reduction themselves. Under some insurance contracts, there may be some surgical procedures that restrict payment for an assistant surgeon.

Modifier -99: Multiple Modifiers

If a procedure requires more than one modifier code, use the two-digit modifier -99 after the usual five-digit CPT code number, all typed on one line; then list each modifier on a separate line (see Example 6-31). Some insurance

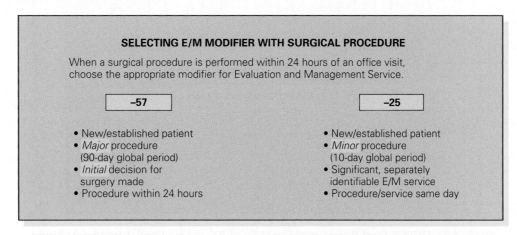

SELECTING E/M MODIFIER WITH SURGICAL PROCEDURE

When a surgical procedure is performed within 24 hours of an office visit, choose the appropriate modifier for Evaluation and Management Service.

–57	–25
• New/established patient	• New/established patient
• *Major* procedure (90-day global period)	• *Minor* procedure (10-day global period)
• *Initial* decision for surgery made	• Significant, separately identifiable E/M service
• Procedure within 24 hours	• Procedure/service same day

FIGURE 6-10 Two selections, with criteria to evaluate them, when choosing the appropriate code or modifier for evaluation and management (E/M) services when a surgical procedure is performed within 24 hours of an office visit.

companies require -99 with a separate note in Block 19 of the CMS-1500 claim form or in the freeform area of electronic submissions, indicating which two or more modifiers are being used.

Example 6-30   Assistant at Surgery

Closure of Intestinal Cutaneous Fistula

| Operating surgeon bills | 44640 | **No modifier** |
| Assistant surgeon bills | 44640-**80** | **With modifier** |

Example 6-31   Multiple Modifiers

A physician sees a patient who is grossly obese. The operative report documents that a bilateral sliding-type inguinal herniorrhaphy was performed and the procedure took 2 hours, 15 minutes.

49525-**99**	Bilateral repair sliding inguinal hernia requiring 2 hours 15 minutes
-**50**	
-**22**	

Example 6-32   HCPCS Modifiers

When taking x-ray films of both feet, the billing portion of the insurance claim appears as follows.

| 05/06/XX | 73620 **RT** | Radiologic examination, foot—right |
| 05/06/XX | 73620 **LT** | Radiologic examination, foot—left |

Healthcare Common Procedure Coding System

In addition to CPT modifiers, HCPCS Level II modifiers are used by Medicare and may be used by some commercial payers. HCPCS Level II modifiers may be two alpha digits (Example 6-32), two alphanumeric characters (Figure 6-11), or a single alpha digit used for reporting ambulance services or results of positron emission tomography scans. A brief list of these modifiers is found in Appendix A of the CPT code book. Modifiers also appear on the inside cover of the CPT code book. A comprehensive list may be found in an HCPCS national Level II code book. HCPCS reference books may be obtained from book stores, publishers, or online retailers.

Use the two-digit HCPCS modifiers whenever they are necessary. HCPCS modifiers further describe the services provided and can increase or decrease the physician's fee. If not used properly, they can drastically affect the physician's fee profile by reducing future payments to the physician.

Comprehensive List of Modifier Codes

Now that you have learned about some basic modifiers, read through the comprehensive list shown in Table 6-6 to gain information on additional modifiers and their use, illustrated by clinical examples.

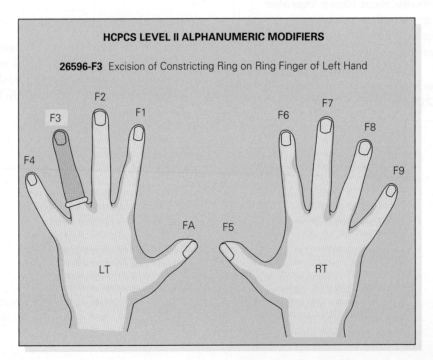

FIGURE 6-11 HCPCS Level II alpha modifiers (*LT* and *RT* used to identify left and right hands) and alphanumeric modifiers (*FA* through *F9*) used to identify digits (fingers) of left and right hands.

Table 6-6 CPT Modifier Codes

MODIFIER#	EXPLANATION	USE IN MAIN TEXT SECTIONS						
		E/M	ANESTHESIA	SURGERY	RADIOLOGY	PATHOLOGY	MEDICINE	TYPE
-22	**Increased Procedural Service:** When the work required to provide a service is substantially greater than typically required, it may be identified by adding modifier –22 to the usual procedure code. Documentation must support the substantial additional work and the reason for the additional work (that is, increased intensity, time, technical difficulty of procedure, severity of patient's condition, physical and mental effort required). **Note:** This modifier should not be appended to an E/M service.	Ø	Y	Y	Y	Y	Y	
-23	**Unusual Anesthesia:** Occasionally a procedure that usually requires either no anesthesia or local anesthesia must be done under general anesthesia because of unusual circumstances. This circumstance may be reported by adding the modifier –23 to the procedure code of the basic service.[†] **Examples:** A proctoscopy might require no anesthesia. A skin biopsy or excision of a subcutaneous tumor might require local anesthesia. If general anesthesia is necessary, append the procedure code with –23.	Ø	Y	Y	N	N	Ø	ANES
-24	**Unrelated E/M Service by the Same Physician during a Postoperative Period:** The physician may need to indicate that an evaluation and management service was performed during a postoperative period for a reason(s) unrelated to the original procedure. This circumstance may be reported by adding the modifier –24 to the appropriate level of E/M service.[†] **Example:** A patient seen for a postoperative visit after an appendectomy complains of a lump on the leg. The physician takes a history and examines the site and a biopsy is scheduled. The E/M code 99024 is used for the postsurgery examination and the modifier –24 is added for unrelated service rendered during a postoperative period. **Medicare Payment Rule:** No effect on payment; however, failure to use this modifier when appropriate may result in denial of the E/M service. CMS memo FQA-541 reads "a documented, separately identifiable related service is to be paid for. We would define 'related' as being caused or prompted by the same symptoms or conditions." Make sure to document that the E/M service was related to the procedure.	Y	Ø	Ø	Ø	Ø	Ø	GP E/M

Continued

Table 6-6 CPT Modifier Codes—cont'd

MODIFIER#	EXPLANATION	USE IN MAIN TEXT SECTIONS						TYPE
		E/M	ANESTHESIA	SURGERY	RADIOLOGY	PATHOLOGY	MEDICINE	
-25	**Significant, Separately Identifiable E/M Service by the Same Physician on the Same Day of the Procedure or Other Service:** It may be necessary to indicate that on the day a procedure or service identified by a CPT code was performed, the patient's condition required a significant, separately identifiable E/M service above and beyond the other service provided or beyond the usual preoperative and postoperative care associated with the procedure that was performed. A significant, separately identifiable E/M service is defined or substantiated by documentation that satisfies the relevant criteria for the respective E/M service to be reported (see CPT Evaluation and Management Services Guidelines for instructions on determining level of E/M service). The E/M service may be prompted by the symptom or condition for which the procedure and/or service was provided. As such, different diagnoses are not required for reporting of the E/M services on the same date. This circumstance may be reported by adding modifier –25 to the appropriate level of E/M service. **Note:** This modifier is not used to report an E/M service that resulted in a decision to perform surgery. See modifier –57. For significant, separately identifiable non-E/M services, see modifier –59. **Example:** A patient is seen for a diabetic follow-up and the physician discovers a suspicious mole on the patient's neck (0.4 cm), which is removed. The physician makes a minor adjustment of the oral diabetes medication. This case illustrates a significant E/M service provided on the same day as a procedure, so –25 is added to the E/M code. Code 11420 is used for removal of the benign lesion. **Note:** This modifier is not used to report an E/M service that resulted in a decision to perform surgery. See modifier –57.[†] **Medicare Payment Rule:** No effect on payment; however, failure to use this modifier when appropriate may result in denial of the E/M service.	Y	∅	∅	∅	∅	∅	BUN GP E/M

							BUN
-26	**Professional Component (PC):** Certain procedures are a combination of a professional physician component and a technical component (TC). When the professional (physician) component is reported separately, the service may be identified by adding the modifier -26 to the usual procedure number.* **Note:** The PC comprises only the professional services performed by the physician during radiologic, laboratory, and other diagnostic procedures. These services include a portion of a test or procedure that the physician does, such as interpretation of the results. The TC includes personnel, materials (including usual contrast media and drugs, film or xerograph, space, equipment, and other facilities) but excludes the cost of radioisotopes. When billing for the TC, use the usual five-digit procedure number with modifier -TC. **Example:** 70450-26 Computerized axial tomography, head or brain; without contrast material. *The modifier -26 indicates the physician interpreted this test only.* 70450-TC Computerized axial tomography, head or brain; without contrast material. *The modifier indicates the facility is billing only for the use of the equipment.*	N	N	N	Y	Y	Y
-27	**Multiple Outpatient Hospital E/M Encounters on the Same Date:** For hospital outpatient reporting purposes, use of hospital resources related to separate and distinct E/M encounters performed in multiple outpatient hospital settings on the same date may be reported by adding the modifier -27 to each appropriate level outpatient and/or emergency department (ED) E/M code(s). This modifier provides a means of reporting circumstances involving evaluation and management services provided by physician(s) in more than one (multiple) outpatient hospital settings (for example, hospital ED, clinic). Do not use this modifier for physician reporting ED or preventative medicine service codes. **Example:** Patient is seen in a hospital outpatient clinic. The patient falls in the treatment room and receives a cut on the right arm. The patient is taken to the ED for two stitches and a dressing. **Medicare Payment Rule:** Do not use modifier -27 for Medicare outpatients. Continue to use the -G0 (G-zero) modifier that CMS established to cover multiple procedures, same patient, same day.	Y	N	N	N	Y	Y

Continued

Table 6-6 CPT Modifier Codes—cont'd

MODIFIER#	EXPLANATION	USE IN MAIN TEXT SECTIONS						
		E/M	ANESTHESIA	SURGERY	RADIOLOGY	PATHOLOGY	MEDICINE	TYPE
-32	**Mandated Services:** Services related to mandated consultation and/or related services (for example, third-party payer, governmental, legislative, or regulatory requirement) may be identified by adding the modifier -32 to the basic procedure.‡ **Example:** A patient is referred to the physician by an insurance company for an unbiased opinion regarding permanent disability after 1 year of treatment following an accident. Add modifier -32 to the E/M code because the second opinion is mandated by the insurance company. **Medicare Payment Rule:** No effect on payment.	Y	Y	Y	Y	Y	Y	
-33	**Preventive Service:** When the primary purpose of the service is the delivery of an evidence-based service in accordance with a US Preventive Services Task Force A or B rating in effect and other preventive services identified in preventive services mandates (legislative or regulatory), the service may be identified by appending modifier -33, Preventive Service to the service. For separately reported services specifically identified as preventive, the modifier should not be used. *This modifier allows a provider to identify a service as preventive under the Patient Protection and Affordable Care Act and indicates that cost sharing does not apply.*	N	Y	Y	Y	N	N	
-47	**Anesthesia by Surgeon:** Regional or general anesthesia provided by the surgeon may be reported by adding the modifier -47 to the basic service; this does not include local anesthesia.† **Note:** Modifier -47 would not be used for anesthesia procedures 00100 through 01999. **Example:** A gastroenterologist performs an endoscopy for removal of esophageal polyps using the snare technique. The physician sedates the patient with Versed to perform the procedure. 43217 Esophagoscopy with removal of polyps by snare technique 43217-47 Administered Versed **Medicare Payment Rule:** Medicare will not reimburse the surgeon to administer anesthesia (any type).	Ø	Ø	Y	Ø	Ø	Ø	ANES
-50	**Bilateral Procedure:** Unless otherwise identified in the listings, bilateral procedures that are performed at the same session should be identified by adding modifier -50 to the appropriate 5-digit code. **Note:** It is important to read each surgical description carefully to look for the word "bilateral." A bilateral modifier on a unilateral procedure code indicates that the procedure was performed on both sides of a paired organ during the same operative session. **Example A:** 71060 Bronchography, bilateral (would be listed with no modifier) **Example B:** 19305 Mastectomy, radical 19305-50 Mastectomy, radical; bilateral **Medicare Payment Rule:** Payment is based on 150% (200% for x-rays) of the fee schedule amount.	N	N	Y	N	N	N	

Continued

Modifier						Description
-51	N	Y	Y	Ø	Y	**Multiple Procedures:** When multiple procedures, other than E/M services, physical medicine and rehabilitation services, or provision of supplies (for example, vaccines) are performed at the same session by the same provider, the primary procedure or service(s) may be identified by appending modifier -51 to the additional procedure or service code(s). **Note:** This modifier should not be appended to designated "add-on" codes (see Appendix D of CPT). Always list the procedure of highest dollar value first. **Example:** Patient had herniated disk in lower back with stabilization of the area where the disk was removed. 63030 Lumbar laminectomy with disk removal 22612-51 Arthrodesis (modifier used after the lesser of the two procedures) **Medicare Payment Rules:** Standard multiple surgery policy—100% of the fee schedule amount is allowed for the highest valued procedure, 50% for the second through fifth procedures, and "by report" for subsequent procedures.
-52	Y	N	Y	Y	Y	**Reduced Services:** Under certain circumstances a service or procedure is partially reduced or eliminated at the discretion of the physician or other qualified health care professional physician's election. Under these circumstances, the service provided can be identified by its usual procedure number and the addition of the modifier -52, signifying that the service is reduced. This provides a means of reporting reduced services without disturbing the identification of the basic service.§ **Note:** This means there will be no effect on the physician's fee profile in the computer data. It is not necessary to attach a report to the claim when using this modifier because it indicates a reduced fee. When a physician performs a procedure but does not charge for the service, such as a postoperative follow-up visit that is included in a global service, remember to use code 99024. Some physicians prefer to bill the insurance carrier the full amount and accept what the carrier pays as payment in full. In such cases, a modifier would not be used. **Example:** A patient is not able to participate or cooperate in a minimal psychiatric interview (90801) and the physician decides to attempt this at a later date. Modify the code with -52. **Medicare Payment Rule:** Payment is based on the extent of the procedure or service performed. Submit documentation with the claim.

Table 6-6 CPT Modifier Codes—cont'd

MODIFIER#	EXPLANATION	USE IN MAIN TEXT SECTIONS						TYPE
		E/M	ANESTHESIA	SURGERY	RADIOLOGY	PATHOLOGY	MEDICINE	
-53	**Discontinued Procedure:** Under certain circumstances, the physician may elect to terminate a surgical or diagnostic procedure. Due to extenuating circumstances or those that threaten the well-being of the patient, it may be necessary to indicate that a surgical or diagnostic procedure was started but discontinued. This circumstance may be reported by adding the modifier -53 to the code for the discontinued procedure. **Note:** This modifier is not used to report the elective cancellation of a procedure before the patient's anesthesia induction and/or surgical preparation in the operating suite. For outpatient hospital/ASC, see modifiers -73 and -74. **Example:** The physician is beginning a cholecystectomy on a patient. An earthquake of great magnitude occurs and the electricity is shut off. The backup generator comes on and electricity is restored; however, because of the disarray in the operative suite, the physician decides to discontinue the surgery. Code 47562 is used with -53 appended to it. **Medicare Payment Rule:** The carrier will determine the amount of payment "by report." Submit documentation with the claim identifying the extent of the procedure performed and the extenuating circumstances.	Ø	Y	Y	Y	Y	Y	
-54	**Surgical Care Only:** When one physician performs a surgical procedure and another provides preoperative and/or postoperative management, surgical services may be identified by adding the modifier -54 to the usual procedure number.* **Note:** Because many surgical procedures encompass a "package" concept that includes normal uncomplicated follow-up care, the surgeon will be paid a reduced fee when using this modifier. **Example:** A patient presents in the ED with severe abdominal pain. Dr. A, the on-call surgeon, examines the patient and performs an emergency appendectomy. Dr. A is leaving on vacation the next morning, so he calls his friend and colleague Dr. B. He asks him to visit the patient in the hospital the following day and take over the postoperative care. Dr. A bills using the appendectomy procedure code 44950 and modifies it with -54. **Medicare Payment Rule:** Payment is limited to the amount allotted for intraoperative services only.	N	N	Y	N	N	N	GP

-55	**Postoperative Management Only:** When one physician performs the postoperative management and another physician performs the surgical procedure, the postoperative component may be identified by adding the modifier -55 to the usual procedure number. **Note:** The fee to list would be approximately 30% of the surgeon's fee. **Example:** The Dunmires are relocating to Memphis, TN, when Mrs. Dunmire discovers a lump on her arm. She visits her family physician, Dr. A, who tells her it needs to be excised. She wants her physician (Dr. A) to do the surgery and Dr. A agrees if she promises to arrange for a physician in Memphis to follow up postoperatively. She makes arrangements with Dr. B in Memphis. Dr. B bills using the correct excision code that he obtained from Dr. A and modifies it with -55. **Medicare Payment Rule:** Payment will be limited to the amount allotted for postoperative services only. Payment to more than one physician for split surgical care of a patient will not exceed the amount paid for the total global surgical package.	N	N	Y	N	N	Y	GP
-56	**Preoperative Management Only:** When one physician performs the preoperative care and evaluation and another physician performs the surgical procedure, the preoperative component may be identified by adding the modifier -56 to the usual procedure number.[†] **Example:** Dr. A sees Mrs. Jones and determines that she needs to have a lung biopsy. He admits her to the hospital and Dr. A becomes ill. Dr. B is called in and performs the surgery. Dr. A bills for the preoperative care using the surgical code he obtained from Dr. B and modifies it with -56. **Medicare Payment Rule:** Payment for this component is included in the allowable amount for the surgery. If another physician performed the surgery, use an appropriate E/M code to bill for the preoperative service.	N	N	Y	N	N	Y	GP
-57	**Decision for Surgery:** An E/M service that resulted in the initial decision to perform the surgery may be identified by adding the modifier -57 to the appropriate level of E/M service.[‡] **Example:** A trauma patient is seen in the ED by an orthopedic surgeon for a consultation to determine whether surgery on a fractured femur is necessary. The surgeon subsequently performs surgery 24 hours later to provide time for the patient to clear his intestinal contents. The surgeon bills the E/M consultation code and adds the -57 modifier. By adding this modifier, the third-party payer is informed that the consultation is not part of the global surgical procedure. Medicare will pay if it is for major surgery that requires a 90-day postoperative follow-up but not for a minor surgical procedure (0- to 10-day postoperative follow-up). **Medicare Payment Rule:** Payment will be made for the E/M service in addition to the global surgery payment.	Y	N	N	N	N	Y	GP E/M

Continued

Table 6-6   CPT Modifier Codes—cont'd

MODIFIER#	EXPLANATION	USE IN MAIN TEXT SECTIONS						
		E/M	ANESTHESIA	SURGERY	RADIOLOGY	PATHOLOGY	MEDICINE	TYPE
-58	**Staged or Related Procedure or Service by the Same Physician during the Postoperative Period:** It may be necessary to indicate that the performance of a procedure or service during the postoperative period was (a) planned or anticipated (staged), (b) more extensive than the original procedure, or (c) for therapy after a surgical procedure. This circumstance may be reported by adding the modifier –58 to the staged or related procedure.‡ **Note:** For treatment of a problem that requires a return to the operating or procedure room (for example, unanticipated clinical condition), see modifier –78. **Example:** A patient has breast cancer and a surgeon performs a mastectomy. During the postoperative global period, the surgeon inserts a permanent prosthesis. The –58 modifier is added to the code for inserting the prosthesis, indicating that this service was planned at the time of the initial operation. If the modifier is not used, the insurance carrier may reject the claim because surgery occurred during the surgery's global period.	N	N	Y	Y	N	Y	GP BUN
-59	**Distinct Procedural Service:** Under certain circumstances, it may be necessary to indicate that a procedure or service was distinct or independent from other non-E/M services performed on the same day. Modifier –59 is used to identify procedures/services, other than E/M services, that are not normally reported together but are appropriate under the circumstances. Documentation must support a different session, different procedure or surgery, different site or organ system, separate incision/excision, separate lesion, or separate injury (or area of injury in extensive injuries) not ordinarily encountered or performed on the same day by the same individual. However, when another already established modifier is appropriate, it should be used rather than modifier –59. Modifier –59 should be used only if no more descriptive modifier is available and the use of modifier –59 best explains the circumstances. **Note:** Modifier –59 should not be appended to an E/M service. To report a separate and distinct E/M service with a non-E/M service performed on the same date, see modifier –25. **Example:** A patient is seen at a physician's office in the morning and the doctor orders a single view (71010) chest x-ray because the patient is complaining of a cough and chest congestion. The physician treats the patient for pneumonia. Later that same day, the patient is seen in the physician's office complaining of chest pain. The physician again orders a chest x-ray but this time a two-view x-ray (71020). Ordinarily, the single-view chest x-ray will be denied as a component of the two-view chest x-ray. However, because they were obtained at separate encounters, addition of the –59 modifier will indicate that these services are not combination components and should be paid for separately. **Medicare Payment Rule:** No effect on payment amount; however, failure to use modifier when appropriate may result in denial of payment for the services.	N	Y	Y	Y	Y	Y	BUN

	#	N	Ø	Y	Y	Ø
-62	Ø	Y	Y	Ø	N	#
-63	N	Y	Y	N	Y	
-66	Ø	Y	Y	Ø	N	#

-62 **Two Surgeons:** When two surgeons work together as primary surgeons performing distinct parts of a single reportable procedure, each surgeon should report his or her distinct operative work using the same procedure code and adding the modifier -62. If additional procedures (including add-on procedures) are performed during the same surgical session, separate codes may be reported without the modifier -62.
Note: If the co-surgeon acts as an assist in the performance of additional procedure(s) during the same surgical session, those services may be reported using separate procedure code(s) with modifier -80 or -81.
Example: A procedure for scoliosis is performed by a thoracic surgeon who does the anterior approach and an orthopedic surgeon who does the posterior approach and repair.
Medicare Payment Rule: Medicare allows 125% of the approved fee schedule amount for the -62 modifier if reported by both surgeons. That total fee is divided in half and dispersed to each surgeon at 62.5% of the approved amount.

-63 **Procedure Performed on Infants Less than 4 kg:** Procedures performed on neonates and infants up to a present body weight of 4 kg may involve significantly increased complexity and physician work commonly associated with these patients. This circumstance may be reported by adding the modifier -63 to the procedure number.
Note: Unless otherwise designated, this modifier may be appended only to procedures/services listed in the 20000-69999 code series. Modifier -63 should not be appended to any codes listed in the E/M services, Anesthesia, Radiology, Pathology/Laboratory, or Medicine sections.

-66 **Surgical Team:** Under some circumstances, highly complex procedures (requiring the concomitant services of several physicians, often of different specialties, plus other highly skilled, specially trained personnel and various types of complex equipment) are carried out under the "surgical team" concept. Such circumstances may be identified by each participating physician with the addition of the modifier -66 to the basic procedure number used for reporting services.*
Example: A kidney transplant, requiring use of a vascular surgeon, urologist, and nephrologist, with the assistance of anesthesiologist and pathologist, or open heart surgery using perfusion personnel, three cardiologists, and an anesthesiologist.
Medicare Payment Rule: Carrier medical staff will determine the payment amounts for team surgeries on a report basis. Submit supporting documentation with the claim.

Continued

Table 6-6 CPT Modifier Codes—cont'd

MODIFIER#	EXPLANATION	USE IN MAIN TEXT SECTIONS						TYPE
		E/M	ANESTHESIA	SURGERY	RADIOLOGY	PATHOLOGY	MEDICINE	
-73	**Discontinued Outpatient Hospital/ASC Procedure Before the Administration of Anesthesia:** Because of extenuating circumstances or those that threaten the well-being of the patient, the physician may cancel a surgical or diagnostic procedure subsequent to the patient's surgical preparation (including sedation when provided and being taken to the room where the procedure is to be performed) but prior to the administration of anesthesia (local, regional block[s], or general). Under these circumstances, the intended service that is prepared for but canceled can be reported by its usual procedure number and the addition of modifier -73. **Note:** The elective cancellation of a service before the administration of anesthesia and/or surgical preparation of the patient should not be reported. For physician reporting of a discontinued procedure, see modifier -53.	N	N	Y	N	N	N	
-74	**Discontinued Outpatient Hospital/ASC Procedure After Administration of Anesthesia:** Because of extenuating circumstances or those that threaten the well-being of the patient, the physician may terminate a surgical or diagnostic procedure after the administration of anesthesia (local, regional block[s], or general) or after the procedure was started (incision made, intubation started, or scope inserted). Under these circumstances, the procedure started but terminated can be reported by its usual procedure number and the addition of modifier -74. **Note:** The elective cancellation of a service before the administration of anesthesia and/or surgical preparation of the patient should not be reported. For physician reporting of a discontinued procedure, see modifier -53.	N	N	Y	N	N	N	
-76	**Repeat Procedure or Service by Same Physician or Other Qualified Health Care Professional:** It may be necessary to indicate that a procedure or service was repeated by the same physician or other qualified health care professional subsequent to the original procedure or service. This circumstance may be reported by adding modifier -76 to the repeated procedure or service. **Note:** This modifier should not be appended to an E/M service. **Example:** A patient is seen by his family physician in the morning for his regular appointment. At that time, his doctor orders an ECG (93000). The patient calls in to his doctor's office in the afternoon to state that he is having some odd chest pain. The physician may request that the patient return to the office for another ECG (93000). The second ECG should be billed with a -76 modifier. **Medicare Payment Rule:** Failure to use this modifier when appropriate (and to submit supporting documentation) may result in denial of the subsequent procedure.	N	N	Y	Y	N	Y	GP

-77	N	N	N	Y	Y	Y	GP
-78	N	N	N	Y	Y	Y	GP

-77 Repeat Procedure or Service by Another Physician or Other Qualified Health Care Professional: It may be necessary to indicate that a basic procedure or service was repeated by another physician or other qualified health care professional subsequent to the original procedure or service. This circumstance may be reported by adding modifier -77 to the repeated procedure or service.

Note: This modifier should not be appended to an E/M service.

Example: A femoral–popliteal bypass graft (35556) is performed in the morning and in the afternoon it becomes clotted. The original surgeon is not available and a different surgeon performs the repeat operation later in the day. The original surgeon reports 35556. The second surgeon reports 35556-77.

Medicare Payment Rule: Failure to use this modifier when appropriate (and to submit supporting documentation) may result in denial of the subsequent surgery.

-78 Unplanned Return to the Operating/Procedure Room by the Same Physician or Other Qualified Health Care Professional Following Initial Procedure for a Related Procedure during the Postoperative Period: It may be necessary to indicate that another procedure was performed during the postoperative period of the initial procedure (unplanned procedure following initial procedure). When the procedure is related to the first and requires the use of the operating or procedure room, it may be reported by adding the modifier -78 to the related procedure. (For repeat procedures, see modifier -76.)†

Example: A patient has an open reduction with fixation of a fracture of the elbow. While still hospitalized, the patient develops an infection and is returned to surgery for removal of the pin because it appears to be the cause of an allergic reaction. The original procedure would be billed for the open treatment of the fracture. The pin removal would be billed with modifier -78 because it is a related procedure.

Medicare Payment Rule: Medicare will pay the full value of the intra-operative portion of a given procedure. Documentation should be submitted with the claim to describe the clinical circumstances.

Continued

Table 6-6 CPT Modifier Codes—cont'd

MODIFIER#	EXPLANATION	USE IN MAIN TEXT SECTIONS						TYPE
		E/M	ANESTHESIA	SURGERY	RADIOLOGY	PATHOLOGY	MEDICINE	
-79	**Unrelated Procedure or Service by the Same Physician During the Postoperative Period:** The physician may need to indicate that the performance of a procedure or service during the postoperative period was unrelated to the original procedure. This circumstance may be reported by using the modifier -79. (For repeat procedures on the same day, see -76.)† **Example:** A patient in the hospital has colon resection surgery and is discharged home. After 7 days, the patient develops acute renal failure, is hospitalized, does not recover renal function, and hemodialysis is ordered. A nephrologist inserts a cannula for the dialysis. When billing for the nephrologist, the code for hemodialysis is shown with a -79 modifier, indicating that this is unrelated to the initial surgery. If modifier -79 is not used, the insurance carrier may not realize that the service is not related to the initial surgery and may reject the claim. **Medicare Payment Rule:** No effect on payment; however, failure to use this modifier when appropriate may result in denial of the subsequent surgery. Specific diagnostic codes will substantiate the medical necessity of the unrelated procedure. Documentation may be required to describe the clinical circumstances. A new global period begins for any procedure modified by -79.	N	N	Y	Y	N	Y	GP
-80	**Assistant Surgeon:** Surgical assistant services may be identified by adding the modifier -80 to the usual procedure number(s).* **Note:** Some insurance policies do not include payment for assistant surgeons, such as for 1-day surgery, but do pay for major or complex surgical assistance. In some instances, prior approval may be indicated owing to the patient's physiologic condition. Medicare will not pay assistant surgeons for operations that are not life threatening. Therefore Medigap (MG) insurance will not pay on this service because the service is not allowable. Assisting surgeons usually charge 16% to 30% of the primary surgeon's fee. **Example:** The primary surgeon performs a right ureterectomy, submitting code 50650-RT. The assistant surgeon would bill using the primary surgeon's code with modifier -80 (50650-80). **Medicare Payment Rule:** Payment is based on the billed amount or 16% of the global surgical fee, whichever is less, for procedures approved for assistant-at-surgery. Medicare will deny payment for an assistant-at-surgery for surgical procedures in which a physician is used as an assistant in less than 5% of the cases nationally.	Ø	N	Y	Y	N	N	#
-81	**Minimum Assistant Surgeon:** Minimum surgical assistant services are identified by adding the modifier -81 to the usual procedure number. **Note:** Payment is made to physicians but not to registered nurses or technicians who assist during surgery.* **Example:** A primary surgeon plans to perform a surgical procedure but during the operation circumstances arise that require the services of an assistant surgeon for a relatively short period. In this scenario, the second surgeon provides minimal assistance and may report using the procedure code with the -81 modifier appended.	Ø	N	Y	N	N	N	#

Modifier	Description						
-82	**Assistant Surgeon:** (When qualified resident surgeon is not available.) The unavailability of a qualified resident surgeon is a prerequisite for use of modifier -82 appended to the usual procedure code number(s).* **Note:** This modifier is usually used for services rendered at a teaching hospital. **Example:** A resident surgeon is scheduled to assist with an anorectal myomectomy (45108). Surgery is delayed due to the previous surgery, the shift rotation changes, and the resident is not available. A nonresident assists with the surgery and reports the procedure, appending it with modifier -82 (45108-82).	Ø	N	Y	N	N	#
-90	**Reference (Outside) Laboratory:** When laboratory procedures are performed by a party other than the treating or reporting physician, the procedure may be identified by adding the modifier -90 to the usual procedure number.† **Note:** Use this modifier when the physician bills the patient for the laboratory work and the laboratory is not doing its own billing. **Example:** Dr. Input examines the patient, performs venipuncture, and sends the specimen to an outside laboratory for a liver panel. The physician has an arrangement with the laboratory to bill for the test and in turn he bills the patient. Dr. Input bills for the examination (E/M code), venipuncture (36415 or for Medicare 0001), and acute hepatitis panel (80074), using modifier -90 (80074-90) to append to the hepatitis panel code.	N	Y	Y	Y	N	LAB
-91	**Repeat Clinical Diagnostic Laboratory Test:** In the course of treatment of the patient, it may be necessary to repeat the same laboratory test on the same day to obtain subsequent (multiple) test results. Under these circumstances, the laboratory test performed can be identified by its usual procedure number and the addition of modifier -91. **Note:** This modifier may not be used when tests are rerun to confirm initial results, due to testing problems with specimens or equipment, or for any other reason when a normal, one-time, reportable result is all that is required. This modifier may not be used when other code(s) describe a series of test results (for example, glucose tolerance tests, evocative/suppression testing). This modifier may be used only for laboratory test(s) performed more than once on the same day on the same patient. **Example:** A patient is scheduled for a nonobstetric dilation and curettage for dysfunctional uterine bleeding. When the patient arrives at the office, a routine hematocrit is obtained. During the procedure, the patient bleeds excessively. After the procedure, the physician orders a second hematocrit to check the patient for anemia due to blood loss. The first hematocrit is billed using CPT code 85013. The second hematocrit is billed using the same code appended with modifier -91 (85013-91).	N	Y	Y	Y	N	LAB

Continued

Table 6-6   CPT Modifier Codes—cont'd

MODIFIER#	EXPLANATION	USE IN MAIN TEXT SECTIONS						TYPE
		E/M	ANESTHESIA	SURGERY	RADIOLOGY	PATHOLOGY	MEDICINE	
-92	**Alternative Laboratory Platform Testing:** When laboratory testing is being performed using a kit or transportable instrument that wholly or in part consists of a single-use, disposable, analytic chamber, the service may be identified by adding modifier –92 to the usual laboratory procedure code (HIV testing 86701-86703). The test does not require permanent dedicated space; hence, by its design, it may be hand-carried or transported to the vicinity of the patient for immediate testing at that site, although location of the testing is not in itself determinative of the use of this modifier.	N	N	Y	Y	Y	Y	LAB
-99	**Multiple Modifiers:** Under certain circumstances, two or more modifiers may be necessary to delineate a service completely. In such situations modifier -99 should be added to the basic procedure and other applicable modifiers may be listed as part of the description of the service.‡ **Example:** An assistant surgeon helps to repair an enterocele where unusual circumstances appear because of extensive hemorrhaging. 57270-99 Repair of enterocele -22 Extensive hemorrhaging (unusual service) -80 Assistant surgeon **Medicare Payment Rule:** No effect on payment; however, the individual modifier payment policies apply, including any inherent effect they may have on payment.	N	N	Y	Y	N	Y	

Modified with permission from the *American Medical Association,* Chicago.

ANES, Modifier related to anesthesia; *ASC,* ambulatory surgery center; *BUN,* modifier related to bundling or Correct Coding Initiative; *CMS,* Centers for Medicare and Medicaid Services; *CPT,* Current Procedural Terminology; *ECG,* electrocardiogram; *ED,* emergency department; *E/M,* evaluation and management; *GP,* global package modifier; *HIV,* human immunodeficiency virus; *LAB,* modifier related to laboratory service; *N,* not usually used with the codes in that section of CPT; *PC,* professional component; *TC,* technical component; *Y,* yes, commonly used with the codes in that section of CPT; *#,* modifier related to number of surgeons; *Ø,* never used with the codes in that section of CPT.

*This modifier may affect reimbursement by third-party payer.

†This modifier may affect reimbursement, depending on the payer.

‡This modifier is informational in nature. Do not ask for an adjustment in reimbursement. Monitor reimbursement when using this modifier.

§This modifier affects reimbursement but not the physician's fee profile.

PROCEDURE 6-1

Locate Correct Level II HCPCS Codes for Professional Services

OBJECTIVE: Accurately locate and select Level II HCPCS codes for professional services

EQUIPMENT/SUPPLIES: HCPCS code book, medical dictionary, and pen or pencil

DIRECTIONS: Follow these step-by-step procedures, which include rationales, to practice this job skill.

1. Read the patient's medical record for items or services that might be covered under Level II HCPCS codes.
2. Go to the Index that is arranged alphabetically and locate the name of the supply, drug, or service. This will direct you to the proper code. Never code from the Index.

3. Turn to the code number in the section and verify that it is the proper code for the item or service the provider supplied to the patient.
4. Select the code.
5. Determine if a modifier is necessary to give a more accurate description of the service or item.
6. Enter the code number and modifier (if needed) to the proper field on the insurance claim form exactly as given for each service or item. Be careful not to transpose code numbers.

PROCEDURE 6-2

Determine Conversion Factors

OBJECTIVE: To determine the conversion factors for several procedure codes

EQUIPMENT/SUPPLIES: Current Procedural Terminology (CPT) code book, geographic practice cost indices (GPCIs) and relative value unit (RVU) pages from the *Federal Register,* calculator, and pen or pencil

DIRECTIONS: Follow these step-by-step procedures, which include rationales, to practice this job skill.

1. Choose 10 or more procedure codes commonly used in the medical practice and in the same section (E/M, Anesthesia, Surgery, Radiology, Pathology, or Medicine) and list the code numbers (at least 60).
2. Use the RVU formula: RVU × GAF × CF = Medicare $ per service, and use the GPCIs and RVU pages from the *Federal Register.* From the 60 or more codes that you have assembled, locate the first procedure code from the RVU pages of the *Federal Register.*
3. For the work amount, obtain the dollar amount from the work RVUs and multiply that by the GPCI of the locality name of where the medical practice is located.

4. For the overhead amount, obtain the dollar amount from the practice expense RVUs, and multiply that by the figure in the GPCI practice expense column.
5. For the malpractice amount, obtain the dollar amount from the malpractice RVUs and multiply that by the figure in the GPCI malpractice column.
6. Take the three results and add them together to obtain the total adjusted RVUs.
7. Use the current year Medicare conversion factor amount and multiply that by the total adjusted RVUs amount to get the allowed amount for the procedure code.
8. Repeat steps 2 through 7 for all additional procedure codes commonly used by the medical practice for each section of the CPT code book.
9. Look at all of the dollar figures you have determined for all of the procedure codes selected. For each section of the CPT code book, they should fall within the same general range. If they do not, reevaluate those fees that are too high or too low and readjust them depending on the service descriptions and market competition comparisons.

PROCEDURE 6-3

Choose Correct Procedural Codes for Professional Services

OBJECTIVE: Accurately locate and select procedural codes for professional services

EQUIPMENT/SUPPLIES: Current Procedural Terminology (CPT) code book, medical dictionary, and pen or pencil

DIRECTIONS: Follow these step-by-step procedures, which include rationales, to practice this job skill.

Figure 6-12 will help you in deciding how to search and choose correct CPT codes for a procedure, eponym, and acronym.

1. Read the patient's medical record and identify the main term by asking what is wrong with the patient.

Continued

PROCEDURE 6-3—cont'd

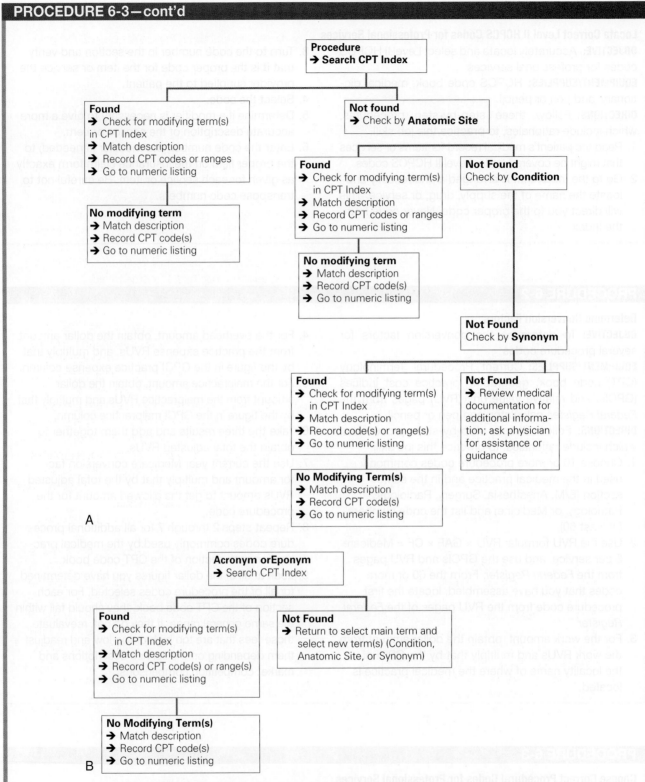

FIGURE 6-12 A, Decision tree when coding a medical procedure using the current edition of *Current Procedural Terminology (CPT)* published by the American Medical Association (AMA). **B,** Decision tree when coding a medical procedure using an acronym or eponym and using the current edition of *CPT* published by the AMA.

PROCEDURE 6-3—cont'd

2. Always read the Introduction section at the beginning of the code book, which may change annually with each edition.

3. Use the Index at the back of the book to locate a specific item by generalized code numbers, not by page numbers. Never code from the Index. Listings may be looked up according to names of procedures or services, organs, conditions, synonyms, eponyms, and abbreviations; for example, some primary entries might be as follows:

   a. Procedure or service
      Example: Anastomosis; Endoscopy; Splint
   b. Organ or other anatomic site
      Example: Salivary Gland; Tibia; Colon
   c. Condition
      Example: Abscess; Entropion; Tetralogy of Fallot
   d. Synonyms, eponyms, and abbreviations
      Example: EEG; Bricker operation; Clagett procedure

   If the procedure performed is not listed, check for the organ involved. If the procedure or organ is difficult to find, look up the condition. Key words, such as synonyms or eponyms, and abbreviations, will help you to find the appropriate code.

4. Locate the code number in the code section for the code range given in the Index.

5. Turn to the beginning of the section for the code range given in the Index and read the Guidelines at the beginning of the section. This gives general information and instructions on coding certain procedures within the section, defines commonly used terms, explains classifications within the section, and gives instructions specific to the section.

6. Turn to the correct section, subsection, category, or subcategory and read through the narrative description to locate the most appropriate code to apply to the patient's procedure. Look at the size of the title to find out the area you are in. Some code books have color-coded titles, making this determination easier. In the surgery section, each subsection is further divided into categories based on anatomic site. Within each category are subcategories listed by type of procedure (for example, excision, repair, destruction, graft) or condition (burn, fracture). Read the notes and special subsection information throughout the section.

7. Notice punctuation and indenting. Descriptions for stand-alone codes begin at the left margin and have a full description. No matter how many indented codes are listed, always go back to the stand-alone code to begin reading the description. A semicolon (;) separates common portions from subordinate designations; subterms are indented (Figure 6-13). Any terminology after the semicolon has a dependent status, as do the subsequent indented entries. In Figure 6-13, the procedure code number 11044 should read as follows: Debridement; skin, subcutaneous tissue, muscle, and bone. Figure 6-14 shows an insurance claim for a patient who has had six corns pared.

8. When trying to locate an E/M code, identify the place or type of service rendered. Then, identify whether the patient is new or established and locate the category or subcategory. Review any guidelines or instructions pertaining to the category or subcategory. Read the descriptors of the levels of E/M service. Identify the requirements necessary for code assignment. Ensure that the components necessary were performed by the physician and documented in the chart for the assigned E/M code. Commercial templates are available to aid in E/M code selection and help tremendously when verifying a code that has been selected by the physician.

9. For a code that has been assigned, note the following:

   • Parentheses ( ) further define the code and tell where other services are located (Figure 6-15).
   • Measurements throughout the code book are based on the metric system (Figure 6-16).
   • All anesthesia services are reported by use of the five-digit anesthesia code plus a physical status modifier. The use of other modifiers to explain a procedure further is optional. Example: Patient is a healthy 23-year-old Caucasian woman. Anesthesia is given for a vaginal delivery. The procedure code with modifier is 01960-P1.

11040	Debridement; skin, partial thickness
11041	skin, full thickness
11042	skin, and subcutaneous tissue
11043	skin, subcutaneous tissue, and muscle
11044	skin, subcutaneous tissue, muscle, and bone

FIGURE 6-13 Use of a semicolon.

Continued

PROCEDURE 6-3—cont'd

CODING FOR MULTIPLE LESIONS

Paring or Cutting

11055 Paring or cutting of benign hyperkeratotic lesion (e.g., corn or callus); single lesion

11056 two to four lesions

11057 more than four lesions

A

24. A. DATE(S) OF SERVICE From / To						B. PLACE OF SERVICE	C. EMG	D. PROCEDURES, SERVICES, OR SUPPLIES (Explain Unusual Circumstances) CPT/HCPCS | MODIFIER		E. DIAGNOSIS POINTER	F. $ CHARGES		G. DAYS OR UNITS	H. EPSDT Family Plan	I. ID. QUAL.	J. RENDERING PROVIDER ID. #
MM	DD	YY	MM	DD	YY											
05	11	20XX				11		99203		A	00	00	1		NPI	4627889700
05	11	20XX				11		11057		A	00	00	1		NPI	4627889700
															NPI	
															NPI	
															NPI	
															NPI	

B

FIGURE 6-14 A, Procedure codes from the Surgery section of the CPT code book. **B,** Blocks 24A through 24J of the revised CMS-1500 (02-12) insurance claim form showing placement of the code on Line 2.

BIOPSY

Defining further ⟶ **11100** Biopsy of skin, subcutaneous tissue and/or mucous membrane (including simple closure), unless otherwise listed (separate procedure); single lesion

11101 each separate/additional lesion

Location of other services ⟶ (For biopsy of conjunctiva, see 68100; eyelid, see 67810)

FIGURE 6-15 Use of parentheses in the Surgery section of the CPT code book.

13150 Repair, complex, eyelids, nose, ears, and/or lips; 1.0 cm or less (See also 40650–40654, 67961–67975)

13151 1.1 cm to 2.5 cm

13152 2.6 cm to 7.5 cm

FIGURE 6-16 Metric measurements in the Surgery section of the CPT code book.

PROCEDURE 6-3—cont'd

● The Surgery section is the largest segment of the code book. It has many subsections and subheadings. You must be able to break down a procedure and identify various terms that will direct you to the correct code. Blocks 24A through 24J of the revised CMS-1500 (02-12) insurance claim form show placement of the code on Line 2 (Example 6-33).

10. Determine if one or more modifiers are necessary to give a more accurate description of the services rendered or the circumstances in which they were performed.

11. Enter the five-digit code number and modifier to the proper field on the insurance claim form exactly as given for each procedure or service rendered. Be careful not to transpose code numbers.

Example 6-33   Blocks 24A through 24J of the CMS-1500 Claim Form

Closed Manipulative Treatment of a Clavicular Fracture

Section:	Surgery, Musculoskeletal System
Anatomic subheading:	Shoulder
Condition:	Fracture or Dislocation
Code:	23505

Thus when completing an insurance claim form for closed manipulative treatment, clavicular fracture, the billing portion appears as follows (Figure 6-17).

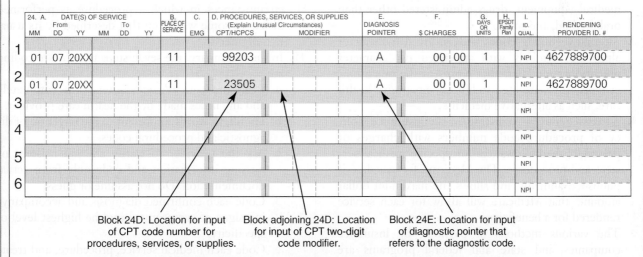

Block 24D: Location for input of CPT code number for procedures, services, or supplies.

Block adjoining 24D: Location for input of CPT two-digit code modifier.

Block 24E: Location for input of diagnostic pointer that refers to the diagnostic code.

FIGURE 6-17 The billing portion of a completed claim form for closed manipulation of a clavicular fracture.

KEY POINTS

This is a brief chapter review, or summary, of the key issues presented. To further enhance your knowledge of the technical subject matter, review the key terms and key abbreviations for this chapter by locating the meaning for each in the Glossary at the end of this text, which appears in a section before the Index.

1. CPT codes are a standardized five-digit numeric method used to precisely describe each service and procedure provided by physicians and allied health care professionals.

2. Medicare's Healthcare Common Procedure Coding System (HCPCS) has two levels: Level I—the American Medical Association's CPT codes and modifiers and Level II—Centers for Medicare and Medicaid Services (CMS) designated codes and alpha modifiers. HCPCS national codes are used to bill for ambulance, medical and surgical supplies, durable medical equipment, drugs administered other than oral method, and so on.

3. Alternative billing codes (ABCs) are five-character alphabetic symbols with appended two-character practitioner modifiers that represent the practitioner type. ABCs are used to bill for integrative health care, such as alternative medicine.

4. A fee schedule is a listing in an insurance policy of procedure code numbers with charges or pre-established allowances for specific medical services and procedures. The Medicare fee schedule is published annually and shows the maximum dollar amounts that Medicare will allow for each service rendered for a beneficiary.

5. The various methods of payment by insurance companies and state and federal programs are (1) fee schedules; (2) usual, customary, and reasonable (UCR); and (3) relative value studies or scale (RVS).

6. Each year when a new CPT code book is published, become familiar with code deletions, new codes, and description changes and observe the symbols and their interpretation in relation to the codes.

7. In CPT coding, *surgical package* is a term used to describe a surgical procedure code that includes the operation; local infiltration, digital block, or topical anesthesia; and normal, uncomplicated postoperative care all included in one fee. Under Medicare, a global surgery policy relates to surgical procedures in which preoperative and postoperative visits (24 hours before [major] and day of [minor]), usual intraoperative services, and complications not requiring an additional trip to the operating room are included in one fee.

8. Code edits are performed on submitted insurance claims to detect unbundling, splitting of codes, and other types of improper code submissions.

9. Ensure that the documentation from the provider supports the code submitted to prevent downcoding by the third-party payer.

10. Use two-digit add-on CPT modifiers to indicate circumstances in which a procedure as performed differs in some way from that described by its usual five-digit code.

11. In final summary, the seven steps to accurate coding are:

    a. Read the patient's encounter form completely and any notes made by the health care provider.

    b. Highlight words important to the selection of diagnostic and procedural codes.

    c. Ask the provider to clarify any inconsistent or missing information and code only from actual documentation. Do not assume or guess.

    d. Code each confirmed diagnosis and accompanying signs or symptoms using the highest level of specificity.

    e. Code each medical service, procedure, and treatment provided in the documentation.

    f. Verify medical necessity by associating each procedure code to the diagnostic code.

    g. Recheck the codes selected by rereading the code descriptions and match them with the provider's notes to confirm the codes assigned.

🖥 STUDENT ASSIGNMENT

✔ Study Chapter 6.
✔ Answer the fill-in-the-blank, multiple-choice, and true/false review questions in the *Workbook* to reinforce the theory learned in this chapter and help prepare for a future test.
✔ Complete the assignments in the *Workbook* to assist you in hands-on practical experience in procedural coding and learning medical abbreviations.

✔ Assignments related to the resource-based relative value scale (RBRVS) because of the complexity of that subject are presented later in the course when studying Chapter 12.
✔ Turn to the Glossary at the end of this text for a further understanding of the key terms and key abbreviations used in this chapter.

The Paper Claim CMS-1500 (02-12)

Linda Smith

OBJECTIVES

After reading this chapter, you should be able to:

1. Identify the circumstances in which paper claims continue to be used.
2. Discuss the history of the Health Insurance Claim Form (CMS-1500 [02-12]).
3. Define and discuss the two types of claims submission.
4. Explain the difference between clean, pending, rejected, incomplete, and invalid claims and discuss specific terms used to describe Medicare claims.
5. List the elements typically abstracted from the medical record that are included in a cover letter accompanying an insurance claim.
6. Describe basic guidelines for submitting insurance claims.
7. Explain how the diagnostic fields of the CMS-1500 (02-12) claim form would be completed.
8. Explain the difference between the PIN, UPIN, and NPI numbers.
9. Discuss claim signatures, the importance of proofreading every paper claim, and supporting documentation for claims.
10. Describe reasons why claims are rejected.
11. Identify claim submission errors and discuss the solutions to correct the errors.
12. Identify techniques required for submission of claims.
13. Demonstrate the ability to complete the CMS-1500 (02-12) claim form accurately for federal, state, and private payer insurance contracts using current basic guidelines.

KEY TERMS

clean claim
deleted claim
dirty claim
durable medical equipment number
electronic claim
employer identification number
facility provider number
group National Provider Identifier (group NPI)
Health Insurance Claim Form (CMS-1500 [02-12])
incomplete claim
intelligent character recognition
invalid claim
National Provider Identifier
optical character recognition
paper claim
pending claim
physically clean claim
rejected claim
Social Security number
state license number

KEY ABBREVIATIONS

ASCA	EIN	LMP	NUCC
CMS-1500	EMG	MSP	OCR
DME	EPSDT	NA, N/A	SOF
DNA	ICR	NPI	SSN

THE PAPER CLAIM CMS-1500 (02-12)

The CMS-1500 is the standard **paper claim** form used by health care professionals and suppliers to bill insurance carriers for services provided to patients.

The standard paper claim has gone through many transitions throughout the years. Paper claims were once used as our sole method of reporting health insurance claims but most health care providers and hospital facilities now send the majority of their claims to insurance carriers electronically, as a result of the Administrative Simplification Compliance Act (ASCA). ASCA was enacted by Congress to improve administration of the Medicare program by increasing efficiencies gained through **electronic claims** submission. ASCA required all claims sent to the Medicare program to be submitted electronically starting October 16, 2003. ASCA prohibits payment of services or supplies not submitted to Medicare electronically, with limited exceptions.

The paper claim continues to be an important part of the claims process that the insurance billing specialist must learn as a basic skill set. There are still circumstances under which the paper claim continues to be used, such as the following:

1. There are exceptions for which providers are not required to send claims to Medicare electronically under ASCA. ASCA provides an exception to the Medicare electronic claims submission requirements to "small providers." ASCA defines a small provider or supplier as a provider of services with fewer than 25 full-time equivalent employees or a physician, practitioner, facility, or supplier (other than a provider of services) with fewer than 10 full-time equivalent employees.
2. ASCA also allows an exemption to any health care provider who may be in an area that has disruptions in electricity and communication connections beyond control and expected to last more than 2 business days. Those health care providers may report claims to Medicare on paper.
3. ASCA does not preclude providers from submitting paper claims to other health plans. Other payers may allow or require submission of claims on paper.
4. There may be occasions whereby the practice's software program experiences technical downtime and the practice is unable to submit claims electronically for a period.
5. Paper claims often are used when reporting special services or require special processing due to unusual circumstances.
6. Paper claims are often used when resubmitting a claim for review following initial denial of the claim.
7. Paper claims can be provided to patients who have coverage with insurance with which the practice does not participate. The patient can then forward the paper claim to the insurance carrier for processing.
8. The paper claim may also be used to report patient encounter data to federal, state, and other public health agencies.

Essentially, the paper claim is the basis for electronic claim submission and many software and hardware systems depend on the existing CMS-1500 claim form in its current image. Because of this and because paper claims are still part of the claims process in many circumstances, it is essential for the insurance billing specialist to fully understand the basic guidelines for submitting paper claims and how to properly complete the claim form, whether they are filing electronic or paper claims.

National Uniform Claim Committee

The CMS-1500 claim form was developed by the National Uniform Claim Committee (NUCC). NUCC is a voluntary organization co-chaired by the American Medical Association (AMA) and Centers for Medicare and Medicaid Services (CMS). The committee is made up of health care industry stakeholders representing providers, payers, designated standards maintenance organizations, public health organizations, and vendors.

NUCC was formally named in the administrative simplification of the Health Insurance Portability and Accountability Act of 1996 (HIPAA) as the authoritative voice regarding national standard content. The committee is responsible for maintaining the integrity of the data sets and physical layout of the hard copy of the CMS-1500 claim form. It is further charged with the task of standardizing national instructions for completion of the claim form to be used by all payers, which may result in even more changes to the CMS-1500 claim form in the future.

History of the Paper Claim CMS-1500

The paper claim has origins as far back as 1958 when the Health Insurance Association of America (HIAA) and the AMA attempted to standardize the insurance claim form. Over the years, standardization has been the driving force to even further changes (Table 7-1). The current version of the claim form is referred to as the CMS-1500 (02-12).

Widespread use of the CMS-1500 (02-12) has saved time and simplified processing of claims for both physicians and carriers because it has eliminated the need to complete the many various insurance forms previously brought into the office by patients.

Table 7-1	History of the Paper Claim CMS-1500
YEAR	**DESCRIPTION**
1958	The Health Insurance Association of America (HIAA) and the American Medical Association (AMA) attempted to create a standardized insurance claim form that eventually became known as *COMB-1*, or *Attending Physician's Statement*.
1975	The AMA approved a "universal claim form," called the *Health Insurance Claim Form*, referred to as the *HCFA-1500*, which was an abbreviation for the *Health Care Financing Administration*. The AMA joined forces with the Centers for Medicare and Medicaid Services (CMS) and many other payer organizations, known as the *Uniform Claim Form Task Force*, to standardize and promote the use of their universal health claim form.
1990	The HCFA-1500 (12-90) was revised and printed in red ink, to allow optical scanning of claims. All services for Medicare patients from physicians and suppliers (except for ambulance services) reported after May 1, 1992, had to be billed on the scannable HCFA-1500 (12-90) form.
Mid-1990s	The Uniform Claim Form Task Force was replaced by the National Uniform Claim Committee (NUCC). The committee's goal was to develop the NUCC Data Set (NUCC-DS), a standardized data set for use in an electronic environment but applicable to and consistent with evolving paper claim form standards.
2001	The HCFA-1500 became known as the CMS-1500 when the Health Care Finance Administration was retitled the Centers for Medicare and Medicaid Services (CMS).
2005	It became necessary to change the CMS-1500 (12-90) so that it could accommodate reporting of the National Provider Identifier (NPI) for providers; this form was referred to as the CMS-1500 (08-05).
2009	NUCC began revision of the 1500 Claim Form to accommodate the updated Electronic Claims Submission (Version 5010 837P) changes and implementation of the new diagnosis coding system, ICD-10.
2012	NUCC released the revised version of the 1500 Health Insurance Claim Form (version 02-12), which accommodated changes needed for implementation of ICD-10.
January 6, 2014	Health plans, clearinghouses, and other information support vendors were required to handle and accept the newly revised (02-12) form effective January 6, 2014. Providers were allowed to use either the 08-05 or the revised (02-12) 1500 Claim Form until March 31, 2014.
April 1, 2014	The 1500 Claim Form (08-05) was discontinued and only revised claims (02-12) will be accepted for processing.

Insurance carriers with various computer programs and equipment may have instructions on completion of the form that vary by locality and program. Local representatives of insurance carriers should always be contacted to find out their specific claim form instructions for completion. Quantities of the CMS-1500 (02-12) can be purchased from many medical office supply companies or from the AMA by calling toll free to 800-621-8335. Medicare advised that the purchased red ink versions of the CMS-1500 (02-12) claim form cannot be duplicated by computer printer; therefore the claim forms must be originals and not photocopies or they will not be processed. This chapter focuses on the paper claim and Chapter 8 explains the intricacies of transmitting electronic claims as mandated by HIPAA.

TYPES OF SUBMITTED CLAIMS

A paper claim is one that is submitted on paper and converted to electronic form by insurance companies. Paper claims may be typed but are typically generated via computer.

An electronic claim is one that is submitted to the insurance carrier via dial-up modem (telephone line or computer modem), direct data entry, or over the internet by way of digital subscriber line (DSL) or file transfer protocol (FTP). Electronic claims are digital files that are not printed on paper claim forms when submitted to the payer.

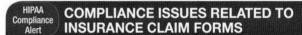

COMPLIANCE ISSUES RELATED TO INSURANCE CLAIM FORMS

HIPAA federal laws affect insurance claim submission. The provider rendering the service or procedure must be properly identified with the correct provider number. Claims must show only services rendered that have been properly documented and are medically necessary without evidence of fraud or abuse issues. HIPAA mandates use of electronic standards for automated transfer of certain health care data among health care payers, plans, and providers. The National Provider Identifier (NPI) system for health care providers became effective on May 27, 2007, in connection with the electronic transactions identified in HIPAA. Refer to Chapters 2 and 8 for a complete discussion about health care providers that are required to submit claims electronically.

Claim Status

Paper or electronic claims can be designated as clean, rejected, or pending (suspended).

A **clean claim** means that the claim was submitted within the program or policy time limit and contains all necessary information so that it can be processed and paid promptly. A **physically clean claim** is one that has no staples or highlighted areas and on which the bar code area has not been deformed.

A **rejected claim** means that the claim has not been processed or cannot be processed for various reasons (for example, the patient is not identified in the payer system, the provider of services is not active in the third-party payer records, or the claim was not submitted in a timely manner). A rejected claim is one that requires investigation, further clarification, and possibly answers to some questions. Such a claim should be resubmitted after proper corrections are made.

A **pending claim** is an insurance claim that is held in suspense for review or other reason by the third-party payer. The amount of time a claim is pended varies from carrier to carrier and from claim to claim. Some claims may take only an additional 9 to 10 days to process while others may take more time and may be dependent on additional information requests sent to the provider. The insurance billing specialist should handle all additional information requests promptly to eliminate long-term pending of claims. All pended claims should be monitored and followed up on if they are not promptly cleared for payment or denied.

Medicare Claim Status

In the Medicare program, specific terms are used to describe various claim processing situations. These terms may or may not be used by other insurance programs.

A *clean claim* means the following:
1. The claim has no deficiencies and passes all electronic edits.
2. The carrier does not need to investigate outside of the carrier's operation before paying the claim.
3. The claim is investigated on a postpayment basis, meaning that a claim is not delayed before payment and may be paid. After investigation, payments may be considered "not due" and a refund may be requested from the provider.
4. The claim is subject to medical review with attached information or forwarded simultaneously with electronic medical claim (EMC) records.

Further information on the many methods to ensure clean claims is given in the next chapter.

Medicare claims not considered "clean" claims, which require investigation or development on a prepayment basis (developed for Medicare Secondary Payer information), are known as *other claims.*

Participating provider electronic submissions are processed within approximately 14 days of receipt. Participating provider paper submissions and nonparticipating provider claims are not processed until at least 27 days after receipt.

An **incomplete claim** is any Medicare claim missing required information. It is identified to the provider so that it can be resubmitted as a new claim.

An **invalid claim** is any Medicare claim that contains complete, necessary information but is illogical or incorrect (for example, listing an incorrect provider number for a referring physician). An invalid claim is identified to the provider and may be resubmitted.

A **dirty claim** is a claim submitted with errors, one requiring manual processing for resolving problems, or one rejected for payment. Pending or suspense claims are placed in this category because something is holding the claim back from payment—perhaps review or some other problem.

A **deleted claim** is a claim canceled, deleted, or voided by a Medicare fiscal intermediary for the following reasons: CMS-1500 (02-12) or current CMS-1450 is not used, itemized charges are not provided, more than six line items are submitted on the CMS-1500 (02-12) claim form, patient's address is missing, internal clerical error was made, Certificate of Medical Necessity (CMN) for durable medical equipment (DME) was not with the Part B claim or was incomplete or invalid, and name of the store is not on the receipt that includes the price of the item.

The Omnibus Budget Reconciliation Act (OBRA) requires Medicare administrative contractors to pay the prompt payment interest rate on all clean claims not paid in a timely manner. The government updates the interest rate on January 1 and July 1 each year on the Treasury's Financial Management Service page.

ABSTRACTING FROM MEDICAL RECORDS

As discussed in Chapter 4, the insurance billing specialist must be skilled at abstracting information from medical records. Abstraction of technical information from patient records may be necessary for claims processing. Insurance carriers frequently request additional information to process the claim or to support medical necessity prior to payment of a claim (Figure 7-1).

Cover Letter Accompanying Insurance Claims

When requesting a review of a denied claim, the insurance billing specialist is required to send a cover letter with the claim. A letter accompanying insurance claims will generally require abstraction of information from the medical record and should include the patient's name; subscriber's name (if different from that of the patient); subscriber identification number; date and type of service; total amount of

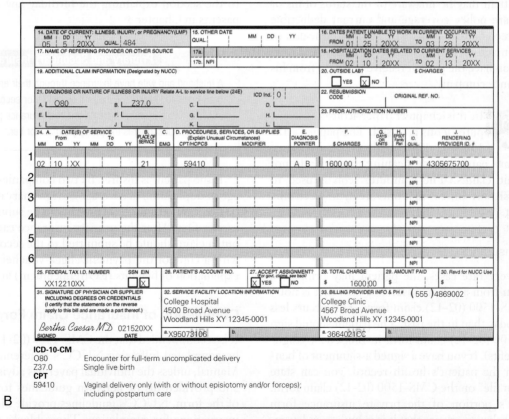

FIGURE 7-1 A, Example of a chart note illustrating important information to read through and abstract for insurance claim completion. **B,** The location of the abstracted information placed in the blocks on a CMS-1500 (02-12) insurance claim form in optical character recognition (OCR) format.

the claim; a short history; and a clear but concise explanation of the medical necessity, difficulty or complexity, or unusual circumstance (for example, emergency). The letter and insurance claim should be sent to the attention of the claims supervisor so that it may be directed to the appropriate person for processing.

HEALTH INSURANCE CLAIM FORM (CMS-1500 [02-12])

Basic Guidelines for Submitting a Claim

The **Health Insurance Claim Form (CMS-1500 [02-12]),** often known simply as the CMS-1500 claim form, is the form required when submitting Medicare claims and is accepted by nearly all state Medicaid programs and private third-party payers as well as by TRICARE and workers' compensation.

A claim form should be completed and submitted as required by payer rules on behalf of a patient who is covered by third-party insurance. If coverage is in question, the insurance carrier should be contacted about eligibility status. An official rejection from the insurance company is the best answer to present to the patient in this situation. The patient may be unaware of the status of his or her health care policy coverage and current deductible status. It is recommended that you submit an insurance claim and get paid for services rendered if there is coverage rather than have the patient receive payment from his or her insurance company.

 In this chapter, paper icons and computer icons are used. The paper CMS-1500 (02-12) icon identifies physicians' offices that are paper based, meaning that they do not file electronic claims. The computer icon is used to indicate physicians' offices that operate in an electronic environment.

Individual Insurance

In very rare cases, the patient may bring in a form from a private insurance plan that is not a CMS-1500 (02-12) claim form. This occurs less frequently today than in the past. The patient should sign the CMS-1500 (02-12) claim form in Block 13 (Assignment of Benefits). If you have a signed assignment of benefits form in the patient's health record, you can state "signature on file" on the CMS-1500 (02-12) claim form. The patient's portion of the private insurance form should be checked to ensure that it is complete and accurate. The forms should then be mailed together to the insurance carrier. Some companies allow staples and some do not. It is not recommended to let patients direct their own forms to insurance companies or employers.

Patients have been known to lose forms or alter data on documents before mailing, forget to send them, or mail them to an incorrect address.

Group Insurance

When a patient has group insurance through an employer, ensure that all information about the employer is complete and correct. If the employer's section is complete, both the CMS-1500 (02-12) and the group insurance forms should be sent directly to the insurance carrier after the physician's portion is completed.

Secondary Insurance

When two insurance policies are involved (sometimes called *dual coverage* or *duplication of coverage*), one is considered primary and the other secondary (Example 7-1). For billing purposes, generally the primary policy is the policy held by the patient when the patient and his or her spouse are both covered by employer-paid insurance. The patient's signature should always be acquired for assignment of benefits for both insurance companies. Regarding children, refer to the section explaining the birthday law and divorced parents in Chapter 3.

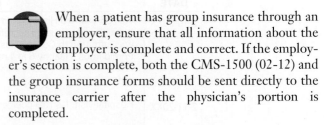

Example 7-1	Primary and Secondary Insurance Plans

A husband and wife have insurance through their employers and both have added the spouse to their plans for secondary coverage. If the wife is seen for treatment, the insurance plan to which she is the subscriber is the primary carrier for her.

If the patient is insured by two companies (dual coverage or duplication of coverage), the primary carrier should be determined and the claim should be submitted to that carrier first. After the primary insurance carrier has paid out, a claim should be submitted to the secondary carrier with a copy of the payment check voucher (or patient's explanation of benefits [EOB] document) attached.

Completion of Insurance Claim Forms

It is recommended that the CMS-1500 (02-12) claim form be completed following NUCC's Reference Instruction Manual, unless the individual payer has advised otherwise and provided his or her own guidelines for completion of the form. NUCC's guidelines provide block-by-block instructions for completion. Those blocks that are considered to be conditional will be noted in the instructions. If any questions are unanswerable, do not use the abbreviations DNA (Does Not Apply), NA (Not Applicable), or N/A (Not Applicable) but leave the space blank.

Diagnosis

In Block 21, diagnosis field of the CMS-1500 (02-12) claim form, all accurate diagnostic codes that affect the patient's condition should be inserted with the primary diagnosis code listed first followed by any secondary or tertiary diagnosis codes. The CMS-1500 (02-12) claim form has the ability to report 12 diagnostic codes. In Chapter 6, the sequence of diagnostic codes related to surgical procedures is explained in detail.

A diagnosis should never be submitted without supporting documentation in the medical record. The diagnosis must support the medical necessity of the treatment and services rendered. If there is no formal diagnosis at the conclusion of an encounter, the code(s) for the patient's symptom(s) should be submitted.

It is best to list only one illness or injury and its treatment per form, unless there are concurrent conditions to avoid confusing services with multiple medical conditions. A concurrent condition is a disorder that coexists with the primary condition, complicating the treatment and management of the primary disorder. It may alter the course of treatment required or lengthen the expected recovery time of the primary condition. It also is referred to as comorbidity or comorbidity condition.

Service Dates

Dates of service must be entered with no spaces using a 6-digit or 8-digit format; for example, January 2, 20XX, should appear as either 0102XX or 010220XX. The appropriate date of service format (6 digits or 8 digits) to be used is noted in NUCC's instructions section of each Item Number on the CMS-1500 (02-12) claim form. Do not use ditto marks (") to indicate repetition of dates for services performed on subsequent lines. Charges for services rendered in different years on the same claim form should not be submitted. This type of situation can occur when claims processing is affected by deductible and eligibility factors, thereby delaying reimbursement.

Consecutive Dates

Some carriers allow medical services or hospital or office visits to be grouped if each visit is consecutive, occurs in the same month, uses the same procedure

code, or results in the same fee. The total fee for the procedures should be listed in Block 24F and the number of times the procedure was performed or service supplied should be listed in Block 24G, as illustrated in the graphic at the bottom of this page (Example: $55.56 × 5 = $277.80). However, private insurance carriers should be contacted because some carriers require a single fee listed in Block 24F rather than the total fee for the procedures. If there is a difference in the procedure code or fee for several visits listed on the claim, each separately coded hospital or office visit must be itemized and each procedure or service code and charge entered on a separate line.

No Charge

Insurance claims should not be submitted for services that have no charge, such as global or surgical package postoperative visit, unless the patient requests that it be sent. These services should only appear documented in the patient's health and financial records.

Physicians' Identification Numbers

Insurance companies and federal and state programs require certain identification numbers on claim forms to be submitted from health care providers and facilities who provide and bill for services to patients. This can be confusing to the beginner, as well as to someone experienced in insurance billing procedures, because there are so many different numbers.

- *State license number.* To practice within a state, each physician must obtain a physician's **state license number.** Sometimes this number is requested on forms and is used as a provider number.
- *Employer identification number (EIN).* In a medical group or solo practice, each physician must have his or her own federal tax identification number, known as an **employer identification number (EIN)** or tax identification number (TIN). This is issued by the Internal Revenue Service for income tax purposes.

25. FEDERAL TAX I.D. NUMBER		SSN EIN
74 10640XX		☐ ☒

- *Social Security number.* In addition, each physician has a **Social Security number (SSN)** for other personal use and may have one or more EINs for financial reasons.

24. A.	DATE(S) OF SERVICE					B. PLACE OF SERVICE	C. EMG	D. PROCEDURES, SERVICES, OR SUPPLIES (Explain Unusual Circumstances)		E. DIAGNOSIS POINTER	F. $ CHARGES	G. DAYS OR UNITS	H. EPSDT Family Plan	I. ID. QUAL.	J. RENDERING PROVIDER ID. #
	From MM DD YY		To MM DD YY					CPT/HCPCS	MODIFIER						
1	10 04 XX		10 08 XX			21		99232		A	277 80	5		NPI	32783127XX
2														NPI	

A Social Security number is not typically used on the claim form unless the provider does not have an EIN, in which case the Social Security number may be required.

25. FEDERAL TAX I.D. NUMBER		SSN	EIN
082 XX 1707		X	

Provider Numbers. Claims may require several **National Provider Identifier (NPI)** numbers: one for the referring physician, one for the ordering physician, and one for the performing physician (billing entity). It is possible that the ordering physician and performing physician are the same. On rare occasions the number may be the same for all three but more frequently different numbers are required, depending on the circumstances of the case. For placement of the NPI number on the CMS-1500 (02-12) claim form, refer to the block-by-block instructions for Blocks 17a, 17b, and 24J. Keep in mind what role the physicians and their numbers represent in relation to the provider listed in Block 33. The following examples of blocks from the CMS-1500 (02-12) insurance claim form show where these numbers are commonly placed. Insurance billing manuals from major insurers give specific directions.

When a non-physician practitioner (NPP) bills incident-to a physician in the same group but that physician is out of the office on a day the NPP sees the patient, another physician in the same group can provide direct supervision to meet the incident-to requirements. Incident-to services are discussed in Chapter 6. When the ordering and supervising doctors are different individuals, the ordering doctor's name goes in Block 17 and his or her NPI goes in Block 17b. The NPI of the supervising doctor goes in Block 24J and the supervising physician signs the form in Block 31. The group's NPI goes in Block 33a.

To assist with claims completion, a reference list of provider numbers should be compiled for all ordering physicians and physicians who frequently refer patients. For Medicare claims, physicians' provider numbers can be obtained by calling their offices, contacting the Medicare carrier, or searching the NPI Registry on the internet. For license numbers, search the state licensing board on the internet. Refer to Appendix A in the *Workbook* for all physician provider numbers when completing *Workbook* assignments.

● *Provider identification number (PIN).* With the implementation of the NPI for compliance on May 23, 2007, PINs are no longer used.

● *Unique physician identification number (UPIN).* With the implementation of the NPI on May 23, 2007, UPINs are no longer used.

● **Group National Provider Identifier (group NPI).** The group NPI is used instead of the individual NPI for the performing provider who is a member of a group practice that submits claims to insurance companies under the group name.

33. BILLING PROVIDER INFO & PH #	(555) 4869002
College Clinic 4567 Broad Avenue Woodland Hills XY 12345-0001	
a. 3664021CC	b.

● *National Provider Identifier (NPI).* The NPI is a HIPAA administrative simplification standard. Covered health care providers and all health plans and health care clearinghouses must use the NPIs in the administrative and financial transactions adopted under HIPAA. Providers began using the NPI on May 23, 2007, except for small health plans whose compliance date was May 23, 2008. The NPI is a lifetime 10-digit number that replaces all other numbers assigned by various health plans. A health care provider is assigned only one NPI, which is retained for a lifetime even if he or she moves to another state. Under HIPAA, providers are required to share their NPIs with other providers, health plans, clearinghouses, and any entity that may need it for their own billing purposes.

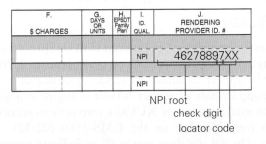

NPI root
check digit
locator code

● *Durable medical equipment (DME) number.* Medicare providers who charge patients a fee for supplies and equipment such as crutches, urinary catheters, ostomy supplies, surgical dressings, and so forth must bill Medicare using a **durable medical equipment (DME) number.** These claims are not sent to the regional fiscal intermediary but to another specific location.

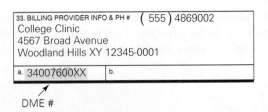

DME #

● *Facility provider number.* Each facility (for example, hospital, laboratory, radiology office, skilled nursing facility) is issued a **facility provider number** to be used by the performing physician to report services done at the location.

```
32. SERVICE FACILITY LOCATION INFORMATION
College Hospital
4500 Broad Avenue
Woodland Hills XY 12345-0001
a. X9507310XX          b.
```

- *Taxonomy code.* When applying for an NPI number, a health care provider must select the Health Care Provider Taxonomy code or code description that identifies the health care provider's type, classification, or specialization and report that in its NPI application. Some payers may either assign a provider identifier or prefer that the taxonomy code be inserted on CMS-1500 claim forms. Depending on issues of each case, provider taxonomy codes may or may not be required on the form. When needed, the blocks affected are Blocks 17a, 19, 24I, 24J, 32b, or 33b (Example 7-2).

Physician's Signature

The physician should sign the insurance claim form above or under the typed or preprinted physician's name. In the computerized office environment, the practice management system will generate a paper CMS-1500 (02-12) form. Generally, the participating contract with the third-party payer (including Medicare, Medicaid, and the Blue Plans) that is signed by the physician allows the physician's name to be printed in the signature block as it normally would be signed. This is an acceptable method for the provider's signature.

Insurance Billing Specialist's Initials

If more than one person is assigned to complete insurance paper claims, then the insurance billing specialist should place his or her initials in the bottom left or top right corner of the claim form. Placement of this reference should be consistent. The following are three good reasons to adopt this habit:
- To identify who in the office is responsible for the insurance form
- To decrease errors

- To avoid being accused of someone else's error, especially if another biller submitted a fraudulent claim

Proofread

Ideally, every paper claim should be proofread for transposition of numbers (group, policy, physician's ID, procedure, and diagnostic codes), misspelled name, missing date of birth, blanks, and attachments. Larger, more complex claims require special attention because they involve greater sums of money and may be more difficult to complete. Ensure that the bill is for the right patient by checking the address and date of birth to verify the correct individual. Review the encounter form to charge for the correct tests and number of tests so that the patient is not charged more than once for the same service. Review the bill for the correct number of units when reporting time-based services (for example, a patient seen for 16 minutes should show a billing for one 15-minute session). Check for any overcoding (for example, do not bill for a longer office visit that included paperwork time when only actual face-to-face time should have been charged). Double check to see if there are charges for items that can be included in the cost of something else, because unbundled charges are not allowed. Proofreading data prevents subsequent denials and avoids time-consuming responses to questions.

Supporting Documentation

Occasionally claims need supporting documents to further explain services billed and to obtain maximum reimbursement.

On any submitted supplemental document, the patient's name, subscriber's name (if different from that of the patient), date of service, and insurance identification number should be included in case the document becomes separated from the claim during processing. This same information should be placed on each page of the document, front and back if two-sided.

If a medication is expensive or experimental, a copy of the invoice received from the supply house or pharmacy should be sent.

When a procedure is complicated, takes additional time to perform, or falls outside of the manner in which

Example 7-2			
MEDICARE SPECIALTY CODE	MEDICARE PROVIDER/ SUPPLIER TYPE DESCRIPTION	PROVIDER TAXONOMY CODE	PROVIDER TAXONOMY DESCRIPTION: TYPE, CLASSIFICATION, SPECIALIZATION
33	Physician/Thoracic Surgery	208G00000X	Allopathic and Osteopathic Physicians/Thoracic Surgery
34	Physician/Urology	208800000X	Allopathic & Osteopathic Physicians/Urology
34	Physician/Urology	2088P0231X	Allopathic & Osteopathic Physicians/Urology, Pediatric Urology

the procedure is typically performed, it is reasonable for the provider to request additional reimbursement. In those cases, a copy of all pertinent reports (operative, radiology, laboratory, pathology, and discharge summary) should be included with the claim. For a treatment not listed in the procedure code book, a special detailed report should be sent that gives the nature, extent, and need for the services along with the time, effort, supplies, and equipment required. The correct code number should be used for unlisted services or procedures, which may or may not always end in "99" (Example 7-3).

Example 7-3	Unlisted Procedure
95199	Unlisted Allergy Testing Procedure

Office Pending File

As mentioned in Chapter 3, the office copy of the insurance form should be filed in a separate alpha (tickler) file for insurance claim copies unless the computer system maintains files. The tickler file should be reviewed for follow-up every 30 days.

 The practice management system will keep an accurate record of all patients and activity on their accounts.

COMMON REASONS WHY CLAIM FORMS ARE DELAYED OR REJECTED

It is wise to be aware of common billing errors and know how to correct them for quicker claim settlements and to reduce the number of appeals. This may help to avoid additional administrative burdens, such as telephone calls, resubmission of claims, and appeal letters. Also see Chapter 9 for information on solutions to denied or delayed claims as well as prevention measures. Table 7-2 contains some reasons why claims are rejected or delayed and suggested solutions when completing the CMS-1500 (02-12) insurance claim form blocks.

ADDITIONAL CLAIM SUBMISSION ERRORS

PROBLEM: Carolyn, the insurance billing specialist, telephoned the insurance company and discovered there was no record of the claim at the third-party payer.

SOLUTION: Always keep copies of paper claims. Send claims with large dollar amounts by certified mail with return receipt requested. Another option is to request that the customer service representative search the insurance carrier's imaging file for the period beginning on the date of service and ending on the date you are calling. Sometimes the claim was received and scanned but was never crossed over to the processing unit.

PROBLEM: Claire is in a hurry and submits a claim form that is illegible.

SOLUTION: Never handwrite a claim form. Check printer ink or toner and replace when necessary.

PROBLEM: Untimely or lack of response to claim development letters is discovered.

SOLUTION: Pay close attention to the due date shown in the letter and reply to development letters (third-party payer's request for additional information) as soon as possible. Send a copy of the claim with the letter and appropriate medical documentation listing the claim control number, if assigned.

PROBLEM: Phillip reviews the Medicare remittance advice and discovers a noncovered service that is deemed not a medical necessity.

SOLUTION: For Medicare claims, check the local coverage determination policies and national coverage determination policies for diagnosis requirements. For private claims, check the insurance policy for the service. Verify that the diagnosis billed indicates necessity for the medical procedure or service.

PROBLEM: Noncovered service occurs because a routine screening procedure is performed in conjunction with a routine examination.

SOLUTION: Determine if it is a diagnostic or preventive service and if the code is correct. Use the GY modifier when submitting a statutory-excluded service for payment by the secondary insurance carrier.

PROBLEM: Payment is adjusted because the care may be covered by another insurance plan per coordination of benefits.

SOLUTION: Annually check all Medicare patients' coverage. Verify eligibility on the Medicare interactive voice recognition system before transmitting the claim.

PROBLEM: Payment adjusted because the medical service is not paid separately because it is a global surgery or a National Correct Coding Initiative (NCCI) denial.

SOLUTION: Determine the global period for the surgical procedure. Use a modifier to report an unrelated or exception service within a global period. Check the NCCI edits to see if the code selected has been deleted or is a bundled service.

PROBLEM: Irene submits a claim with missing, incomplete, or invalid information regarding where the medical services were performed.

SOLUTION: Include the zip code of where the service was performed.

PROBLEM: In reviewing a Medicare remittance advice (RA) document, Anne notices that it indicates that Mrs. Bentley's medical expenses were incurred before insurance coverage.

Table 7-2	The Paper Claim: Problem Solving	
BLOCK NUMBER(S)	**PROBLEM**	**SOLUTION**
1	When submitting a paper claim, the wrong block is checked (that is, claim submitted to the secondary insurer instead of the primary insurer).	Obtain data from the patient during the first office visit as to which company is the primary insurer, depending on illness, injury, or accident. Submit the claim to the primary carrier and then send in a claim with a copy of the primary carrier's EOB to the secondary carrier.
1 to 13	Information missing on patient portion of the claim form.	Obtain a complete patient registration form from which information can be extracted. If patients are filling out their portion, educate patients on data requirements at the time of their first visit to the physician's office. Be sure to ask if there have been any changes on subsequent office visits.
1a	Patient's insurance number is incorrect or transposed (especially in Medicare and Medicaid cases).	Proofread numbers carefully from source documents. Always photocopy front and back sides of insurance identification cards.
2	Patient's name and insured's name are entered as the same when the patient is a dependent. A common error is that the patient is listed as the insured when he or she is not the insured (for example, spouse or child). Block 4 is used for listing the insured's name.	Verify the insured party and check for Sr, Jr, and correct birth date.
2	Patient name is missing, illegible, or incorrect.	Patient's name must be entered exactly as it appears on the patient's ID card.
3	Incorrect gender identification, resulting in a diagnosis or procedure code that is inconsistent with patient's gender.	Proofread the claim before mailing and review the patient's medical record to locate gender, especially if the patient's first name could be male or female.
5	Patient address is missing or illegible.	Enter the patient's complete address and telephone number. Do not puncture the address or phone number. When entering a 9-digit zip code, include the hyphen.
9a to 9d	Incomplete entry for other insurance coverage.	Accurately abstract data from the patient's registration form and input it to the computer database. Telephone the patient if information is incomplete.
10	Failure to indicate whether patient's condition is related to employment or an "other" type of accident.	Review patient's medical history to find out details of injury or illness and proofread claim before mailing. Telephone the employer to see if permission was given to treat the patient as a workers' compensation case.
14	Date of injury, date of LMP, or dates of onset of illness are omitted. This information is important for determining whether accident benefits apply, patient is eligible for maternity benefits, or there was a pre-existing condition.	Do not list unless dates are clearly documented in the patient's medical record. Read the patient's medical history and call the patient to obtain the date of accident or LMP. Compose an addendum to the record if necessary. Always proofread a paper claim before mailing in case data are missing.
17, 17a, 17b	Incorrect or missing name or NPI of referring physician on claim for consultation or other services requiring this information.	Check the patient registration form and the chart note for reference to the referring physician. Develop a list of NPI numbers for all physicians in the area.
19	Attachments (for example, prescription, operative report, manufacturer's invoice) or Medicaid verification (for example, labels, identification numbers) is missing.	Submit all information required for pricing or coverage on an 8.5- × 11-inch paper with the patient's name, subscriber name (if other than patient), and insurance identification number on each attachment (enclosure). Type the word "ATTACHMENT" in Block 19 or 10d. Never staple or clip documentation to a claim.
21	The diagnostic code is missing, incomplete, invalid, or not in standard nomenclature (for example, missing fourth or fifth digit); it includes a written description or does not correspond to the treatment (procedure code) rendered by the physician.	Verify and submit correct diagnostic codes by referring to an updated diagnostic code book and reviewing the patient record. Check with the physician if the diagnosis code listed does not go with the procedure code shown. Do not include decimal point.

Continued

Table 7-2 | **The Paper Claim: Problem Solving—cont'd**

BLOCK NUMBER(S)	PROBLEM	SOLUTION
24A	Omitted, incorrect, overlapping, or duplicate dates of service.	Verify against the encounter form or medical record that all dates of service are listed and accurate and appear on individual lines on paper claims. Date spans for multiple services must be adequate for the number and types of services provided. Each month should be on a separate line and each year should be on a separate claim.
24B	Missing or incorrect place of service code. If a physician sees a patient in a SNF that is in the same building as a domicile rest home or a hospice, it is possible to incorrectly document the SNF as the site for each patient.	Verify the place of service from the encounter form or medical record and list the correct code for place of service and submitted procedure.
24D	Procedure codes are incorrect, invalid, or missing.	Verify the coding system used by the third-party payer and submit correct procedure code(s) by referring to a current procedure code book. For Medicare patients and certain private insurance plans, check the HCPCS manual for CMS national and local procedure codes.
24D	Incorrect or missing modifier(s).	Verify usage of modifiers by referring to a current procedure code book and HCPCS manual. Submit valid modifiers with the correct procedure codes (see Chapter 6).
24E	Diagnosis Pointer is required.	Enter the associated diagnosis by referencing the pointers (A to L) listed in Block 21 that relate to the date of service and the procedures performed. Diagnosis codes must be valid ICD-9 or ICD-10 codes for the date of service.
24F	Omitted or incorrect amount billed.	Be certain that the fee column is filled in. Check the amounts charged with the appropriate fee schedule.
24G	Days/units are required on claim forms.	Enter quantity. Value entered must be greater than zero. (Field allows up to three digits.)
24G	Reasons for multiple visits made in 1 day are not stated on an attachment sheet.	Depending on insurance guidelines, submit documentation explaining reason for multiple visits. Use appropriate modifiers or upcode evaluation and management services to include all visits.
24G	Incorrect quantity billed.	Verify charge amounts. Ensure that the number of units listed is equal to the date span when more than one date of service is billed (for example, hospital visits).
24J	Provider's identification number is missing.	Verify and insert the required provider's number in this block.
24A to 24J, Line 6	More than six lines entered on a paper claim.	Insert service date and corresponding procedure on Lines 1 to 6 only. Complete an additional paper claim if more services should be billed.
27	Assignment acceptance must be indicated on the claim.	"Yes" or "No" must be checked.
28	Total amounts do not equal itemized charges.	Total charges for each claim and verify amounts with patient account. If number of units listed in Block 24G is more than one, multiply the units by the fee listed in Block 24F and add to all other charges listed.
31	Physician's signature is missing.	Have the physician or physician's representative sign the claim using a removable indicator "Sign Here" tag to indicate the correct location or key in "SOF" or "signature on file."
32	Information is not centered in block as required when submitting a paper claim.	Enter data centered in block.
33	Provider's address, NPI, or group number is missing.	The billing provider's name and address are required. A physical location must be entered; P.O. boxes are not acceptable. Obtain provider's data from a list that contains all physicians' professional information.

CMS, Centers for Medicare and Medicaid Services; *EOB*, explanation of benefits; *HCPCS*, Healthcare Common Procedure Coding System; *LMP*, last menstrual period; *NPI*, National Provider Identifier; *SNF*, skilled nursing facility.

SOLUTION: Annually verify all Medicare patients' coverage. Review the patient's Medicare card for entitlement and effective dates. Verify eligibility on the Medicare interactive voice recognition system before transmitting the claim. Verify that the claim is submitted with the correct Medicare number, including the alpha suffix.

CLAIM COMPLETION GUIDELINES*

Optical Character Recognition

The majority of paper claims are scanned using **optical character recognition (OCR),** also less commonly referred to as **intelligent character recognition (ICR)** or *image copy recognition (ICR),* devices (scanners). This technology has been used across the nation in processing insurance claims to enable greater speed and efficiency. A scanner can transfer printed or typed text and bar codes to the insurance company's computer memory. Scanners read at such a fast speed that they reduce data entry cost and decrease processing time.

More control is gained over data input using OCR. It improves accuracy thus reducing coding errors, because the claim is entered exactly as coded by the insurance billing specialist. Most insurance carriers have adopted the NUCC guidelines for completion of the CMS 1500 (02-12) claim form. It is recommended that claims be processed using NUCC guidelines unless carriers advise otherwise. NUCC guidelines provide instructions and examples that demonstrate how to enter the data in every field of the CMS 1500 (02-12) claim form.

Do's And Don'ts for Claim Completion

Basic do's and don'ts for completing claims follow.

Do: Use original claim forms printed in red ink; photocopies and forms generated from ink jet or laser printers cannot be scanned. Laser jet printing is preferable for computer-generated claims.

Do: Computer-generate or type all information in black ink.

Don't: Handwrite information on the document. Handwriting is accepted only for signatures. Handwritten claims require manual processing.

Do: Align the printer correctly so that characters appear exactly in the proper fields. Enter all information within designated fields.

Don't: Allow characters to touch lines.

Do: Keep characters within the borders of each field. Use 10-pitch Pica or Arial or 10-, 11-, or 12-point type.

Don't: Use script, slant, minifont, or italicized fonts or expanded, compressed, or bold print. Use fonts that have the same width for each character (proportional).

Don't: Strike over any errors when correcting or crowd preprinted numbers; OCR equipment does not read corrected characters on top of correction tape or correction fluid.

Do: Complete a new form for additional services if the case has more than six lines of service.

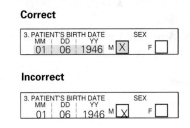

Don't: Use highlighter pens or colored ink on claims.

Don't: Use decimals in Block 21 or dollar signs ($) in the money column.

Correct

Incorrect

Don't: Use narrative descriptions of procedures, modifiers, or diagnoses; code numbers are sufficient.

Correct

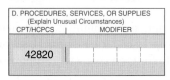

Incorrect

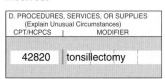

Don't: Use N/A or DNA when information is not applicable. Leave the space blank.

Correct

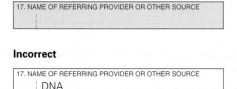

Incorrect

Don't: Use paper clips, cellophane tape, stickers, rubber stamps, or staples.

Do: Enter 6-digit or 8-digit date formats: 0601XX, 060120XX, or 06-01-20XX, depending on the block instructions.

Correct

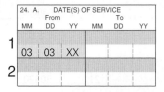

Correct

Do: Keep signature within signature block.

Correct

Incorrect

Do: Keep claim form clean and free from stains, tear-off pad glue, notations, circles or scribbles, strike-overs, crossed-out information, or white out.

Don't: Fold or spindle forms when mailing.

Don't: Send claim attachments smaller than 8½ × 11.

INSTRUCTIONS FOR COMPLETING THE HEALTH INSURANCE CLAIM FORM (CMS-1500 [02-12])

The NUCC has developed a general instruction guide for completing the CMS-1500 (02-12) claim form, which is referred to as *NUCC's Reference Instruction Manual.** Instructions align with the Health Care Claim Professional 837 and 5010. Updated versions of the instruction manual are released each July.

NUCC's Reference Instruction Manual is not specific to any applicable public or private payer. Refer to specific instructions issued by individual payers, clearinghouses, and vendors for further clarification of CMS-1500 (02-12) reporting requirements.

These instructions can be used to complete claims (see Figures 7-3 through 7-11). Blocks should be completed for all carriers as indicated in the "Instructions" unless a more specific guideline for the carrier is indicated.

_____

*Content from the NUCC's 1500 Health Insurance Claim Form Reference Instruction Manual is reprinted by permission of the American Medical Association.

HIPAA TRANSACTIONS AND CODE SETS STANDARDS

Question

Do the HIPAA transactions and code sets standards apply to paper claims and other nonelectronic transactions?

Answer

No. The HIPAA transactions and code sets standards only apply to electronic transactions conducted by covered entities. Other entities such as employers or casualty insurance plans may decide to use them voluntarily but are not required to do so.

For paper transactions, health plans are free to set their own data requirements. Other federal or state laws may require plans or providers to use specific code sets for certain paper transactions. However, all covered health plans and providers must be able to use the HIPAA standards for electronic transactions. Health plans may choose to require that paper claims include the same data elements, codes, and identifiers that are required by the HIPAA regulations for electronic transactions.

Block-By-Block Instructions for Completion of the CMS-1500 (02-12)

Carrier Block

The carrier block can be found in the upper right corner of the CMS-1500 (02-12) form.

DRAFT - NOT FOR OFFICIAL USE

HEALTH INSURANCE CLAIM FORM

APPROVED BY NATIONAL UNIFOR MCLAIM COMMITTEE (NUCC) 02/12

	PICA								PICA	

1. MEDICARE	MEDICAID	TRICARE	CHAMPVA	GROUP HEALTH PLAN	FECA BLK LUNG	OTHER	1a. INSURED'S I.D. NUMBER	(For Program in Item 1)
(Medicare#)	(Medicaid#)	(ID#DoD#)	(Member ID#)	X (ID#)	(ID#)	(ID#)	111704521	

2. PATIENT'S NAME (Last Name, First Name, Middle Initial)	3. PATIENT'S BIRTH DATE	SEX	4. INSURED'S NAME (Last Name, First Name, Middle Initial)
Forehand, Harry, N	MM 01 DD 06 YY 1946	M X F	Forehand, Harry, N

In the upper left corner of the form, a Quick Response (QR) code symbol and the date approved by the NUCC can be located. The payer is the carrier, health plan, third-party administrator, or other payer that will handle the claim. This information directs the claim to the appropriate payer. *Note:* Some carriers prefer that this area of the claim be left blank because identifying data are printed during the initial insurance claims processing stage.

Instructions: Enter in the white, open carrier area the name and address of the payer to whom the claim is being sent. Information should be entered in the following format:

1st line: Name of insurance carrier

2nd line: First line of address

3rd line: Second line of address (if necessary) (If address only has three lines, leave blank.)

4th line: City, state (two-character state code), and zip code (Examples 7-4 and 7-5)

Do not use punctuation (that is, commas and periods) or other symbols in the address (for example, 123 N Main Street 101 instead of 123 N. Main St, #101). When entering a 9-digit zip code, include the hyphen.

Example 7-4

Four-line address:

Worldwide Health Insurance Company

Suite 101

123 Main Street

Anytown IL 60605

Example 7-5

Three-line address:	123 Main Street
Worldwide Health Insurance Company	Anytown IL 60605

Block 1: Medicare, Medicaid, TRICARE, CHAMPVA, Group Health Plan, FECA, Black Lung, Other

This block is used to identify the insurance type to whom the claim is being submitted and may establish primary liability.

	PICA							PICA
1. MEDICARE	MEDICAID	TRICARE	CHAMPVA	GROUP HEALTH PLAN	FECA BLK LUNG	OTHER	1a. INSURED'S I.D. NUMBER	(For Program in Item 1)
(Medicare#)	(Medicaid#)	(ID#DoD#)	(Member ID#)	X (ID#)	(ID#)	(ID#)	111704521	
2. PATIENT'S NAME (Last Name, First Name, Middle Initial)			3. PATIENT'S BIRTH DATE MM DD YY	SEX			4. INSURED'S NAME (Last Name, First Name, Middle Initial)	
Forehand, Harry, N			01 06 1946	M X F			Forehand, Harry, N	

Instructions: Indicate the type of health insurance coverage applicable to this claim by placing an X in the appropriate box. Only one box can be marked. "Other" indicates health insurance including HMOs, commercial insurance, automobile accident, liability, or workers' compensation.

→*When completing the* Workbook *assignments for private payer cases or Medicare/Medigap cases, if the insured is employed, assume that the insurance is through the employer and is "group" insurance; otherwise, assume that it is an individual policy and enter "Other."*

Block 1a: Insured's ID Number

The "Insured's ID Number" is the identification number of the insured and identifies the insured to the payer.

	PICA							PICA
1. MEDICARE	MEDICAID	TRICARE	CHAMPVA	GROUP HEALTH PLAN	FECA BLK LUNG	OTHER	1a. INSURED'S I.D. NUMBER	(For Program in Item 1)
(Medicare#)	(Medicaid#)	(ID#DoD#)	(Member ID#)	X (ID#)	(ID#)	(ID#)	111704521	
2. PATIENT'S NAME (Last Name, First Name, Middle Initial)			3. PATIENT'S BIRTH DATE MM DD YY	SEX			4. INSURED'S NAME (Last Name, First Name, Middle Initial)	
Forehand, Harry, N			01 06 1946	M X F			Forehand, Harry, N	

Instructions: Enter the "Insured's ID Number" as shown on the insured's ID card for the payer to which the claim is being submitted. If the patient has a unique member identification number assigned by the payer, enter that number in this field.

 TRICARE Claims: Enter the sponsor's SSN or Department of Veterans Affairs (VA) file number.

 CHAMPVA Claims: Enter the sponsor's SSN or VA file number.

 Workers' Compensation Claims: Enter the employee ID or workers' compensation claim number. If none is assigned, enter the employer's policy number.

 Property and Casualty Claims: Enter the Federal Tax ID or SSN of the insured person or entity.

Block 2: Patient's Name

The "Patient's Name" is the name of the person who received the treatment or supplies.

PICA								PICA
1. MEDICARE (Medicare#)	MEDICAID (Medicaid#)	TRICARE (ID#DoD#)	CHAMPVA (Member ID#)	GROUP HEALTH PLAN ☒ (ID#)	FECA BLK LUNG (ID#)	OTHER (ID#)	1a. INSURED'S I.D. NUMBER (For Program in Item 1) 111704521	
2. PATIENT'S NAME (Last Name, First Name, Middle Initial) Forehand, Harry, N			3. PATIENT'S BIRTH DATE MM 01 DD 06 YY 1946		SEX M ☒ F ☐		4. INSURED'S NAME (Last Name, First Name, Middle Initial) Forehand, Harry, N	

Instructions: Enter the patient's full last name, first name, and middle initial. If the patient uses a last name suffix (for example, Jr, Sr), enter it after the last name and before the first name. Titles (for example, Sister, Capt, Dr) and professional suffixes (for example, PhD, MD, Esq) should not be included with the name.

Use commas to separate the last name, first name, and middle initial. A hyphen can be used for hyphenated names. Do not use periods within the name (Example 7-6).

Example 7-6   Surname Format

Hyphenated name: Smith-White = Smith-White

Prefixed name: MacIverson = MacIverson

Seniority name with numeric suffix: John R. Ellis, III = Ellis III, John, R

If the patient's name is the same as the insured's name (that is, the patient is the insured), it is not necessary to report the patient's name.

Block 3: Patient's Birth Date, Sex

The patient's birth date and sex (gender) is information that will identify the patient and it distinguishes persons with similar names.

PICA								PICA
1. MEDICARE (Medicare#)	MEDICAID (Medicaid#)	TRICARE (ID#DoD#)	CHAMPVA (Member ID#)	GROUP HEALTH PLAN ☒ (ID#)	FECA BLK LUNG (ID#)	OTHER (ID#)	1a. INSURED'S I.D. NUMBER (For Program in Item 1) 111704521	
2. PATIENT'S NAME (Last Name, First Name, Middle Initial) Forehand, Harry, N			3. PATIENT'S BIRTH DATE MM 01 DD 06 YY 1946		SEX M ☒ F ☐		4. INSURED'S NAME (Last Name, First Name, Middle Initial) Forehand, Harry, N	

Instructions: Enter the patient's 8-digit birth date (MM/DD/YYYY). Enter an X in the correct box to indicate sex of the patient. Only one box can be marked. If gender is unknown, leave blank. The patient's age must be as follows to correlate with the diagnosis in Block 21:
- Birth: Newborn diagnosis
- Birth to 17 years: Pediatric diagnosis
- 12 to 55 years: Maternity diagnosis
- 15 to 124 years: Adult diagnosis

Block 4: Insured's Name

The "Insured's Name" identifies the person who holds the policy, which would be the employee for employer-provided health insurance.

PICA								PICA
1. MEDICARE (Medicare#)	MEDICAID (Medicaid#)	TRICARE (ID#DoD#)	CHAMPVA (Member ID#)	GROUP HEALTH PLAN ☒ (ID#)	FECA BLK LUNG (ID#)	OTHER	1a. INSURED'S I.D. NUMBER (For Program in Item 1) 111704521	
2. PATIENT'S NAME (Last Name, First Name, Middle Initial) Forehand, Harry, N			3. PATIENT'S BIRTH DATE MM 01 DD 06 YY 1946		SEX M ☒ F ☐		4. INSURED'S NAME (Last Name, First Name, Middle Initial) Forehand, Harry, N	

Instructions: Enter the insured's full last name, first name, and middle initial. If the insured uses a last name suffix (for example, Jr, Sr), enter it after the last name and before the first name. Titles (for example, Sister, Capt, Dr) and professional suffixes (for example, PhD, MD, Esq) should not be included with the name.

Use commas to separate the last name, first name, and middle initial. A hyphen can be used for hyphenated names. Do not use periods within the name.

 Workers' Compensation Claims: Enter the name of the employer.

 Property and Casualty Claims: Enter the name of the insured person or entity.

Block 5: Patient's Address

The "Patient's Address" is the patient's permanent residence. A temporary address or school address should not be used.

5. PATIENT'S ADDRESS (No., Street)	6. PATIENT RELATIONSHIP TO INSURED	7. INSURED'S ADDRESS (No., Street)
1456 Main Street	Self [X] Spouse [ ] Child [ ] Other [ ]	1456 Main Street
CITY Woodland Hills	STATE XY	8. RESERVED FOR NUCC USE	CITY Woodland Hills	STATE XY
ZIP CODE 12345-0000	TELEPHONE (Include Area Code) (555) 4909876		ZIP CODE 12345-0000	TELEPHONE (Include Area Code) (555) 4909876

Instructions: Enter the patient's mailing address and telephone number. The first line is for the street address; the second line is for the city and two-character state code; the third line is for the zip code and phone number.

Do not use punctuation (that is, commas and periods) or other symbols in the address (for example, use 123 N Main Street 101 instead of 123 N. Main Street, #101). When entering a 9-digit zip code, include the hyphen.

If reporting a foreign address, contact payer for specific reporting instructions.

If the patient's address is the same as the insured's address, it is not necessary to report the patient's address.

"Patient's Telephone" does not exist in 5010A1. NUCC recommends that the phone number not be reported.

 Workers' Compensation Claims: If required by a payer to report a telephone number, do not use a hyphen or space as a separator within the telephone number.

 Property and Casualty Claims: If required by a payer to report a telephone number, do not use a hyphen or space as a separator within the telephone number.

 TRICARE Claims: An APO/FPO (Army Post Office/Fleet Post Office) address should not be used unless that person is residing overseas. Enter the patient's actual place of residence and not a post office box number.

 CHAMPVA Claims: An APO/FPO address should not be used unless that person is residing overseas. Enter the patient's actual place of residence and not a post office box number.

Block 6: Patient Relationship to Insured

The "Patient Relationship to Insured" indicates how the patient is related to the insured.

5. PATIENT'S ADDRESS (No., Street)		6. PATIENT RELATIONSHIP TO INSURED	7. INSURED'S ADDRESS (No., Street)	
1456 Main Street		Self [X] Spouse [ ] Child [ ] Other [ ]	1456 Main Street	
CITY	STATE	8. RESERVED FOR NUCC USE	CITY	STATE
Woodland Hills	XY		Woodland Hills	XY
ZIP CODE	TELEPHONE (Include Area Code)		ZIP CODE	TELEPHONE (Include Area Code)
12345-0000	(555) 4909876		12345-0000	(555) 4909876

"Self" would indicate that the insured is the patient. "Spouse" would indicate that the patient is the husband of the wife or qualified partner as defined by the insured's plan. "Child" would indicate that the patient is a minor dependent as defined by the insured's plan. "Other" would indicate that the patient is other than the self, spouse, or child, which may include employee, ward, or dependent as defined by the insured's plan.

Instructions: Enter an X in the correct box to indicate the patient's relationship to the insured when Block 4 is completed. Only one box should be marked.

 Workers' Compensation Claims: Check "Other."

Block 7: Insured's Address

The "Insured's Address" is the insured's permanent residence, which may be different from the patient's address in Block 5.

5. PATIENT'S ADDRESS (No., Street)		6. PATIENT RELATIONSHIP TO INSURED	7. INSURED'S ADDRESS (No., Street)	
1456 Main Street		Self [X] Spouse [ ] Child [ ] Other [ ]	1456 Main Street	
CITY	STATE	8. RESERVED FOR NUCC USE	CITY	STATE
Woodland Hills	XY		Woodland Hills	XY
ZIP CODE	TELEPHONE (Include Area Code)		ZIP CODE	TELEPHONE (Include Area Code)
12345-0000	(555) 4909876		12345-0000	(555) 4909876

Instructions: Enter the insured's address and telephone number. If Block 4 is completed, this field should be completed. The first line is for the street address; the second line is for the city and state; the third line is for the zip code and phone number.

Do not use punctuation (that is, commas and periods) or other symbols in the address (for example, use 123 N Main Street 101 instead of 123 N. Main Street, #101). When entering a 9-digit zip code, include the hyphen.

If reporting a foreign address, contact payer for specific reporting instructions.

"Insured's Telephone" does not exist in 5010A1. NUCC recommends that the phone number not be reported.

 Workers' Compensation Claims: Enter the employer's address. If required by a payer to report a telephone number, do not use a hyphen or space as a separator within the telephone number.

 Property and Casualty Claims: If required by a payer to report a telephone number, do not use a hyphen or space as a separator within the telephone number.

 TRICARE Claims: Enter sponsor's address (for example, an APO/FPO address, active duty sponsor's duty station, or the retiree's mailing address) if different from the patient's address.

CHAMPVA Claims: Enter sponsor's address (for example, an APO/FPO address, active duty sponsor's duty station, or the retiree's mailing address) if different from the patient's address.

Block 8: Reserved for NUCC Use

This field is reserved for NUCC use. NUCC will provide instructions for any use of this field.

5. PATIENT'S ADDRESS (No., Street)		6. PATIENT RELATIONSHIP TO INSURED		7. INSURED'S ADDRESS (No., Street)	
1456 Main Street		Self [X] Spouse [ ] Child [ ] Other [ ]		1456 Main Street	
CITY	STATE	8. RESERVED FOR NUCC USE		CITY	STATE
Woodland Hills	XY			Woodland Hills	XY
ZIP CODE	TELEPHONE (Include Area Code)			ZIP CODE	TELEPHONE (Include Area Code)
12345-0000	(555) 4909876			12345-0000	(555) 4909876

Instructions: This field was previously used to report "Patient Status." "Patient Status" does not exist in 5010A1, so this field has been eliminated.

Block 9: Other Insured's Name

The "Other Insured's Name" indicates that there is a holder of another policy that may cover the patient.

9. OTHER INSURED'S NAME (Last Name, First Name, Middle Initial)	10. IS PATIENT'S CONDITION RELATED TO:	11. INSURED'S POLICY GROUP OR FECA NUMBER
		A482
a. OTHER INSURED'S POLICY OR GROUP NUMBER	a. EMPLOYMENT? (Current or Previous) [ ] YES [X] NO	a. INSURED'S DATE OF BIRTH SEX MM DD YY 01 16 1946 M [X] F [ ]
b. RESERVED FOR NUCC USE	b. AUTO ACCIDENT? PLACE (State) [ ] YES [X] NO	b. OTHER CLAIM ID (Designated by NUCC)
c. RESERVED FOR NUCC USE	c. OTHER ACCIDENT? [ ] YES [X] NO	c. INSURANCE PLAN NAME OR PROGRAM NAME ABC Insurance Company
d. INSURANCE PLAN NAME OR PROGRAM NAME	10d. CLAIM CODES (Designated by NUCC)	d. IS THERE ANOTHER HEALTH BENEFIT PLAN? [ ] YES [X] NO *If yes,* complete items 9, 9a, and 9d.

Instructions: If Block 11d is marked YES, complete fields 9, 9a, and 9d; otherwise, leave fields 9, 9a, and 9d blank. When additional group health coverage exists, enter other insured's full last name, first name, and middle initial of the enrollee in another health plan if it is different from that shown in Block 2. If the insured uses a last name suffix (for example, Jr, Sr) enter it after the last name and before the first name. Titles (for example, Sister, Capt, Dr) and professional suffixes (for example, PhD, MD, Esq) should not be included with the name.

Use commas to separate the last name, first name, and middle initial. A hyphen can be used for hyphenated names. Do not use periods within the name.

 Workers' Compensation Claims: Leave blank. If the case is pending and not yet declared workers' compensation, insert "other insurance."

Block 9a: Other Insured's Policy or Group Number

The "Other Insured's Policy or Group Number" identifies the policy or group number for coverage of the insured as indicated in Block 9.

Instructions: Enter the policy or group number of the other or secondary insured.

Do not use a hyphen or space as a separator within the policy or group number.

Workers' Compensation Claims: Leave blank.

Block 9b: Reserved for NUCC Use

This field is reserved for NUCC use. NUCC will provide instructions for any use of this field.

Instructions: This field was previously used to report "Other Insured's Date of Birth, Sex." "Other Insured's Date of Birth, Sex" does not exist in 5010A1, so this field has been eliminated.

Block 9c: Reserved for NUCC Use

This field is reserved for NUCC use. NUCC will provide instructions for any use of this field.

Instructions: This field was previously used to report "Employer's Name or School Name." "Employer's Name or School Name" does not exist in 5010A1, so this field has been eliminated.

Block 9d: Insurance Plan Name or Program Name

The "Insurance Plan Name or Program Name" identifies the name of the plan or program of the other insured as indicated in Block 9.

Instructions: Enter the other or secondary insured's insurance plan or program name.

 Workers' Compensation Claims: Leave blank.

Block 10a to 10c: Is Patient's Condition Related To

This information indicates whether the patient's illness or injury is related to employment, auto accident, or other accident.

9. OTHER INSURED'S NAME (Last Name, First Name, Middle Initial)	10. IS PATIENT'S CONDITION RELATED TO:	11. INSURED'S POLICY GROUP OR FECA NUMBER A482
a. OTHER INSURED'S POLICY OR GROUP NUMBER	a. EMPLOYMENT? (Current or Previous) ☐ YES ☒ NO	a. INSURED'S DATE OF BIRTH MM | DD | YY 01 | 16 | 1946 SEX M ☒ F ☐
b. RESERVED FOR NUCC USE	b. AUTO ACCIDENT? PLACE (State) ☐ YES ☒ NO	b. OTHER CLAIM ID (Designated by NUCC)
c. RESERVED FOR NUCC USE	c. OTHER ACCIDENT? ☐ YES ☒ NO	c. INSURANCE PLAN NAME OR PROGRAM NAME ABC Insurance Company
d. INSURANCE PLAN NAME OR PROGRAM NAME	10d. CLAIM CODES (Designated by NUCC)	d. IS THERE ANOTHER HEALTH BENEFIT PLAN? ☐ YES ☒ NO *If yes*, complete items 9, 9a, and 9d.

"Employment (current or previous)" indicates that the condition is related to the patient's job or workplace. "Auto accident" indicates that the condition is the result of an automobile accident. "Other accident" indicates that the condition is the result of any other type of accident.

Instructions: When appropriate, enter an X in the correct box to indicate whether one or more of the services described in Block 24 are for a condition or injury that occurred on the job or as a result of an automobile or other accident. Only one box on each line should be marked.

The state postal code where the accident occurred must be reported if "YES" is marked in 10b for "Auto accident." Any item marked "YES" indicates there may be other applicable insurance coverage that would be primary, such as automobile liability insurance. Primary insurance information must then be shown in Block 11.

Block 10d: Claim Codes (Designated by NUCC)

The "Claim Codes" identify additional information about the patient's condition or the claim.

Instructions: When applicable, use the report "Claim Codes." Applicable claim codes are designated by NUCC. Refer to the most current instructions from the public or private payer regarding the need to report claim codes.

When required by payers to provide the subset of condition codes approved by NUCC, enter the "Condition Code" in this field. The condition codes approved for use on the 1500 Claim Form are available at www.nucc.org, under Code Sets.

Workers' Compensation Claims: A condition code is required when submitting a bill that is a duplicate (W2) or an appeal (W3 = Level 1, W4 = Level 2, W5 = Level 3). (The original reference number must be entered in Block 22 for these conditions.) *Note:* Do not use condition codes when submitting a revised or corrected bill.

➡ *When completing the* Workbook *assignments for Medicaid cases, enter the patient's Medicaid number preceded by "MCD," if Medicaid is the secondary payer. For all other cases, leave blank.*

Block 11: Insured's Policy, Group, or FECA Number

The "Insured's Policy, Group, or FECA Number" is the alphanumeric identifier for the health, auto, or other insurance plan coverage.

9. OTHER INSURED'S NAME (Last Name, First Name, Middle Initial)	10. IS PATIENT'S CONDITION RELATED TO:	11. INSURED'S POLICY GROUP OR FECA NUMBER A482
a. OTHER INSURED'S POLICY OR GROUP NUMBER	a. EMPLOYMENT? (Current or Previous) ☐ YES ☒ NO	a. INSURED'S DATE OF BIRTH MM DD YY 01 16 1946 SEX M ☒ F ☐
b. RESERVED FOR NUCC USE	b. AUTO ACCIDENT? PLACE (State) ☐ YES ☒ NO	b. OTHER CLAIM ID (Designated by NUCC)
c. RESERVED FOR NUCC USE	c. OTHER ACCIDENT? ☐ YES ☒ NO	c. INSURANCE PLAN NAME OR PROGRAM NAME ABC Insurance Company
d. INSURANCE PLAN NAME OR PROGRAM NAME	10d. CLAIM CODES (Designated by NUCC)	d. IS THERE ANOTHER HEALTH BENEFIT PLAN? ☐ YES ☒ NO *If yes*, complete items 9, 9a, and 9d.

The FECA number is the 9-digit alphanumeric identifier assigned to a patient claiming work-related condition(s) under the Federal Employees' Compensation Act 5 USC 8101.

Instructions: Enter the insured's policy or group number as it appears on the insured's health care identification card. If Block 4 is completed, this field should be completed.

Do not use a hyphen or space as a separator within the policy or group number.

TRICARE Claims: Leave blank.

CHAMPVA Claims: Enter the three-digit number of the VA station that issued the identification card.

Workers' Compensation Claims: Leave blank.

Block 11a: Insured's Date of Birth, Sex

The "Insured's Date of Birth, Sex" (gender) is the birth date and gender of the insured as indicated in Block 1a.

Instructions: Enter the 8-digit date of birth (MM/DD/YYYY) of the insured and an X to indicate the sex of the insured. Only one box should be marked. If gender is unknown, leave blank.

 TRICARE Claims: Enter sponsor's date of birth and gender if it is different from that listed in Block 3.

 CHAMPVA Claims: Enter sponsor's date of birth and gender if it is different from that listed in Block 3.

 Workers' Compensation Claims: Leave blank.

Block 11b: Other Claim ID (Designated by NUCC)

The "Other Claim ID" is another identifier applicable to the claim.

Instructions: Enter the "Other Claim ID." Applicable claim identifiers are designated by the NUCC.

The following qualifier and accompanying identifier has been designated for use:
Y4 Property Casualty Claim Number

Enter the qualifier to the left of the vertical, dotted line. Enter the identifier number to the right of the vertical, dotted line.

 Workers' Compensation Claims: Required if known. Enter the claim number assigned by the payer.

 Property and Casualty Claims: Required if known. Enter the claim number assigned by the payer.

 TRICARE Claims: Enter the sponsor's branch of service, using abbreviations (for example, United States Navy = USN).

 CHAMPVA Claims: Enter the sponsor's branch of service, using abbreviations (for example, United States Navy = USN).

Block 11c: Insurance Plan Name or Program Name

The "Insurance Plan Name or Program Name" is the name of the plan or program of the insured as indicated in Block 1a.

Instructions: Enter the "Insurance Plan Name or Program Name" of the insured. Some payers require an identification number of the primary insurer rather than the name in this field.

Workers' Compensation Claims: Leave blank.

Block 11d: Is There Another Health Benefit Plan?

This block indicates that the patient has insurance coverage other than the plan indicated in Block 1.

Instructions: When appropriate, enter an X in the correct box. If marked "YES," complete Blocks 9, 9a, and 9d. Only one box can be marked.

➡*When completing the* Workbook *assignments for Medicare, leave blank.*

Block 12: Patient's or Authorized Person's Signature

This block indicates that there is an authorization on file for the release of any medical or other information necessary to process and adjudicate the claim.

READ BACK OF FORM BEFORE COMPLETING & SIGNING THIS FORM.	13. INSURED'S OR AUTHORIZED PERSON'S SIGNATURE I authorize
12. PATIENT'S OR AUTHORIZED PERSON'S SIGNATURE I authorize the release of any medical or other information necessary to process this claim. I also request payment of government benefits either to myself or to the party who accepts assignment below.	payment of medical benefits to the undersigned physician or supplier for services described below.
SIGNED *Harry N. Forehand* DATE *March 3, 20XX*	SIGNED *Harry N. Forehand*

or

READ BACK OF FORM BEFORE COMPLETING & SIGNING THIS FORM.	13. INSURED'S OR AUTHORIZED PERSON'S SIGNATURE I authorize
12. PATIENT'S OR AUTHORIZED PERSON'S SIGNATURE I authorize the release of any medical or other information necessary to process this claim. I also request payment of government benefits either to myself or to the party who accepts assignment below.	payment of medical benefits to the undersigned physician or supplier for services described below.
SIGNED SIGNATURE ON FILE DATE	SIGNED SIGNATURE ON FILE

Instructions: Enter "Signature on File," "SOF," or legal signature. When legal signature is entered, enter the date signed in 6-digit (MMDDYY) or 8-digit (MMDDYYYY) format. If there is no signature on file, leave blank or enter "No Signature on File."

➡*When completing the* Workbook *assignments, enter "Signature on File," not "SOF," in this block.*

Block 13: Insured's or Authorized Person's Signature

This block indicates that there is a signature on file authorizing payment of medical benefits.

READ BACK OF FORM BEFORE COMPLETING & SIGNING THIS FORM.	13. INSURED'S OR AUTHORIZED PERSON'S SIGNATURE I authorize
12. PATIENT'S OR AUTHORIZED PERSON'S SIGNATURE I authorize the release of any medical or other information necessary to process this claim. I also request payment of government benefits either to myself or to the party who accepts assignment below.	payment of medical benefits to the undersigned physician or supplier for services described below.
SIGNED *Harry N. Forehand* DATE *March 3, 20XX*	SIGNED *Harry N. Forehand*

Or

READ BACK OF FORM BEFORE COMPLETING & SIGNING THIS FORM.	13. INSURED'S OR AUTHORIZED PERSON'S SIGNATURE I authorize
12. PATIENT'S OR AUTHORIZED PERSON'S SIGNATURE I authorize the release of any medical or other information necessary to process this claim. I also request payment of government benefits either to myself or to the party who accepts assignment below.	payment of medical benefits to the undersigned physician or supplier for services described below.
SIGNED SIGNATURE ON FILE DATE	SIGNED SIGNATURE ON FILE

Instructions: Enter "Signature on File," "SOF," or legal signature. If there is no signature on file, leave blank or enter "No Signature on File."

➡*When completing the* Workbook *assignments, enter "Signature on File," not "SOF," in this block.*

Block 14: Date of Current Illness, Injury, or Pregnancy (LMP)

This block identifies the first date of onset of illness, the actual date of injury, or the last menstrual period (LMP) for pregnancy.

14. DATE OF CURRENT: ILLNESS, INJURY, or PREGNANCY(LMP) MM DD YY 03 01 20XX QUAL. 431	15. OTHER DATE QUAL.	MM DD YY	16. DATES PATIENT UNABLE TO WORK IN CURRENT OCCUPATION MM DD YY MM DD YY FROM TO
17. NAME OF REFERRING PROVIDER OR OTHER SOURCE DN Perry Cardi MD	17a. 17b. NPI 67805027XX		18. HOSPITALIZATION DATES RELATED TO CURRENT SERVICES MM DD YY MM DD YY FROM TO
19. ADDITIONAL CLAIM INFORMATION (Designated by NUCC)			20. OUTSIDE LAB? $ CHARGES ☐ YES ☒ NO

Instructions: Enter the 6-digit (MMDDYY) or 8-digit (MMDDYYYY) date of the first date of the present illness, injury, or pregnancy. For pregnancy, use the date of the LMP as the first date.

Enter the applicable qualifier to identify which date is being reported:

431 Onset of Current Symptoms or Illness

484 Last Menstrual Period

Enter the qualifier to the right of the vertical, dotted line.

Block 15: Other Date

The "Other Date" identifies additional date information about the patient's condition or treatment.

14. DATE OF CURRENT: ILLNESS, INJURY, or PREGNANCY(LMP) MM DD YY 03 01 20XX QUAL. 431	15. OTHER DATE QUAL.	MM DD YY	16. DATES PATIENT UNABLE TO WORK IN CURRENT OCCUPATION MM DD YY MM DD YY FROM TO
17. NAME OF REFERRING PROVIDER OR OTHER SOURCE DN Perry Cardi MD	17a. 17b. NPI 67805027XX		18. HOSPITALIZATION DATES RELATED TO CURRENT SERVICES MM DD YY MM DD YY FROM TO
19. ADDITIONAL CLAIM INFORMATION (Designated by NUCC)			20. OUTSIDE LAB? $ CHARGES ☐ YES ☒ NO

Instructions: Enter an "Other Date" related to the patient's condition or treatment. Enter the date in the 6-digit (MMDDYY) or 8-digit (MMDDYYYY) format. Previous pregnancies are not a similar illness. Leave blank if unknown.

Enter the applicable qualifier between the vertical, dotted lines to identify which date is being reported.

454 Initial Treatment

304 Latest Visit or Consultation

453 Acute Manifestation of a Chronic Condition

439 Accident

455 Last X-ray

471 Prescription

090 Report Start

091 Report End

444 First Visit or Consultation

Block 16: Dates Patient Unable to Work in Current Occupation

Block 16 indicates the time span the patient is or was unable to work.

14. DATE OF CURRENT: ILLNESS, INJURY, or PREGNANCY(LMP) MM DD YY 03 01 20XX QUAL. 431	15. OTHER DATE QUAL.	MM DD YY	16. DATES PATIENT UNABLE TO WORK IN CURRENT OCCUPATION MM DD YY MM DD YY FROM TO
17. NAME OF REFERRING PROVIDER OR OTHER SOURCE DN Perry Cardi MD	17a. 17b. NPI 67805027XX		18. HOSPITALIZATION DATES RELATED TO CURRENT SERVICES MM DD YY MM DD YY FROM TO
19. ADDITIONAL CLAIM INFORMATION (Designated by NUCC)			20. OUTSIDE LAB? $ CHARGES ☐ YES ☒ NO

Instructions: If the patient is employed and is unable to work in current occupation, a 6-digit (MMDDYY) or 8-digit (MMDDYYYY) date must be shown for the "from–to" dates that the patient is unable to work. An entry in this field may indicate employment-related insurance coverage.

➡️*When completing the* Workbook *assignments, enter information when it is documented in the medical record.*

Block 17: Name of Referring Provider or Other Source

The name entered is the referring provider, ordering provider, or supervising provider who referred, ordered, or supervised the service(s) or supply(ies) on the claim. The qualifier indicates the role of the provider being reported.

14. DATE OF CURRENT: ILLNESS, INJURY, or PREGNANCY(LMP)	15. OTHER DATE	16. DATES PATIENT UNABLE TO WORK IN CURRENT OCCUPATION
MM 03	DD 01	YY 20XX QUAL. 431	QUAL.	MM	DD	YY	FROM	TO
17. NAME OF REFERRING PROVIDER OR OTHER SOURCE	17a.	18. HOSPITALIZATION DATES RELATED TO CURRENT SERVICES
DN Perry Cardi MD	17b. NPI 67805027XX	FROM	TO
19. ADDITIONAL CLAIM INFORMATION (Designated by NUCC)		20. OUTSIDE LAB? ☐ YES ☒ NO $ CHARGES

Instructions: Enter the name (first name, middle initial, last name) and credentials of the professional who referred, ordered, or supervised the service(s) or supply(ies) on the claim.

If multiple providers are involved, enter one provider using the following priority order:
1. Referring provider
2. Ordering provider
3. Supervising provider

Do not use periods or commas within the name. A hyphen can be used for hyphenated names.

Enter the applicable qualifier to the left of the vertical, dotted line to identify which provider is being reported.

DN Referring provider
DK Ordering provider
DQ Supervising provider

TRICARE Claims: If the patient is referred from a Military Treatment Facility (MTF), enter the name of the MTF and attach DD Form 2161 or SF 513, "Referral for Civilian Medical Care."

CHAMPVA Claims: If the patient is referred from an MTF, enter the name of the MTF and attach DD Form 2161 or SF 513, "Referral for Civilian Medical Care."

Block 17a: Other ID Number

The non-NPI ID number of the referring, ordering, or supervising provider is the unique identifier of the professional or provider designated taxonomy code.

14. DATE OF CURRENT: ILLNESS, INJURY, or PREGNANCY(LMP)	15. OTHER DATE	16. DATES PATIENT UNABLE TO WORK IN CURRENT OCCUPATION
MM 03	DD 01	YY 20XX QUAL. 431	QUAL.	MM	DD	YY	FROM	TO
17. NAME OF REFERRING PROVIDER OR OTHER SOURCE	17a.	18. HOSPITALIZATION DATES RELATED TO CURRENT SERVICES
DN Perry Cardi MD	17b. NPI 67805027XX	FROM	TO
19. ADDITIONAL CLAIM INFORMATION (Designated by NUCC)		20. OUTSIDE LAB? ☐ YES ☒ NO $ CHARGES

Instructions: The Other ID Number of the referring, ordering, or supervising provider is reported in 17a, the shaded area. The qualifier indicating what the number represents is reported in the qualifier field to the immediate right of 17a.

NUCC defines the following qualifiers used in 5010A1:

0B State License Number

1G Provider UPIN Number

G2 Provider Commercial Number

LU Location Number (This qualifier is used for Supervising Provider only.)

Block 17b: NPI

The NPI number refers to the HIPAA National Provider Identifier number.

Instructions: Enter the NPI number of the referring, ordering, or supervising provider in Block 17b.

Block 18: Hospitalization Dates Related to Current Services

Information in this field refers to an inpatient stay and indicates the admission and discharge dates associated with the service(s) on the claim.

14. DATE OF CURRENT: ILLNESS, INJURY, or PREGNANCY(LMP) MM DD YY 03 01 20XX QUAL. 431	15. OTHER DATE QUAL. MM DD YY	16. DATES PATIENT UNABLE TO WORK IN CURRENT OCCUPATION MM DD YY MM DD YY FROM TO
17. NAME OF REFERRING PROVIDER OR OTHER SOURCE DN Perry Cardi MD	17a. 17b. NPI 67805027XX	18. HOSPITALIZATION DATES RELATED TO CURRENT SERVICES MM DD YY MM DD YY FROM TO
19. ADDITIONAL CLAIM INFORMATION (Designated by NUCC)		20. OUTSIDE LAB? ☐ YES ☒ NO $ CHARGES

Instructions: Enter the inpatient 6-digit (MMDDYY) or 8-digit (MMDDYYYY) hospital admission date followed by the discharge date (if discharge has occurred). If not discharged, leave discharge date blank. This date is when a medical service is furnished as a result of or subsequent to a related hospitalization.

Block 19: Additional Claim Information (Designated by NUCC)

Block 19 identifies additional information about the patient's condition or the claim.

14. DATE OF CURRENT: ILLNESS, INJURY, or PREGNANCY(LMP) MM DD YY 03 01 20XX QUAL. 431	15. OTHER DATE QUAL. MM DD YY	16. DATES PATIENT UNABLE TO WORK IN CURRENT OCCUPATION MM DD YY MM DD YY FROM TO
17. NAME OF REFERRING PROVIDER OR OTHER SOURCE DN Perry Cardi MD	17a. 17b. NPI 67805027XX	18. HOSPITALIZATION DATES RELATED TO CURRENT SERVICES MM DD YY MM DD YY FROM TO
19. ADDITIONAL CLAIM INFORMATION (Designated by NUCC)		20. OUTSIDE LAB? ☐ YES ☒ NO $ CHARGES

Instructions: Refer to the most current instructions from the public or private payer regarding use of this field. Some payers ask for certain identifiers in this field. For example, when modifier 99 (multiple modifiers) is entered in Block 24D, an explanation of the modifiers might be inserted in Block 19. If identifiers are reported in this field, enter the appropriate qualifiers describing the identifier. Do not enter a space, hyphen, or other separator between the qualifier code and the number.

When reporting a second item of data, enter three blank spaces and then the next qualifier and number/code/information.

NUCC defines the following qualifiers, since they are the same as those used in 5010A1:

0B State License Number

1G Provider UPIN Number

G2 Provider Commercial Number

LU Location Number (This qualifier is used for Supervising Provider only.)

N5 Provider Plan Network Identification Number
SY Social Security Number (The SSN may not be used for Medicare.)
X5 State Industrial Accident Provider Number
ZZ Provider Taxonomy (The qualifier in the 5010A1 for Provider Taxonomy is PXC but ZZ will remain the qualifier for the 1500 Claim Form.)

The list above contains both provider identifiers and the provider taxonomy code. The provider identifiers are assigned to the provider either by a specific payer or by a third party in order to uniquely identify the provider. The taxonomy code is designated by the provider in order to identify his or her provider type, classification, and area of specialization. Both provider identifiers and provider taxonomy may be used in this field.

Workers' Compensation Claims: Additional claim information is required based on Jurisdictional Workers' Compensation Guidelines.

Supplemental Claims: For additional claim information, use the qualifier PWK for data followed by the appropriate report type code, the appropriate transmission type code, and then the attachment control number. Do not enter spaces between qualifiers and data. NUCC defines the following qualifiers, since they are the same as those used in 5010A1:

Report Type Code:

03	Report Justifying Treatment beyond Utilization
04	Drugs Administered
05	Treatment Diagnosis
06	Initial Assessment
07	Functional Goals
08	Plan of Treatment
09	Progress Report
10	Continued Treatment
11	Chemical Analysis
13	Certified Test Report
15	Justification for Admission
21	Recovery Plan
A3	Allergies/Sensitivities Document
A4	Autopsy Report
AM	Ambulance Certification
AS	Admission Summary
B2	Prescription
B3	Physician Order
B4	Referral Form
BR	Benchmark Testing Results
BS	Baseline
BT	Blanket Test Results
CB	Chiropractic Justification
CK	Consent Form(s)
CT	Certification
D2	Drug Profile Document
DA	Dental Models
DB	Durable Medical Equipment Prescription
DG	Diagnostic Report
DJ	Discharge Monitoring Report
DS	Discharge Summary
EB	Explanation of Benefits (Coordination of Benefits or Medicare Secondary Payer)

HC	Health Certificate
HR	Health Clinic Records
I5	Immunization Record
IR	State School Immunization Records
LA	Laboratory Results
M1	Medical Record Attachment
MT	Models
NN	Nursing Notes
OB	Operative Note
OC	Oxygen Content Averaging Report
OD	Orders and Treatments Document
OE	Objective Physical Examination (including vital signs) Document
OX	Oxygen Therapy Clarification
OZ	Support Data for Claim
P4	Pathology Report
P5	Patient Medical History Document
PE	Parenteral or Enteral Certification
PN	Physical Therapy Notes
PO	Prosthetics or Orthotic Certification
PQ	Paramedical Results
PY	Physician's Report
PZ	Physical Therapy Certification
RB	Radiology Films
RR	Radiology Reports
RT	Report of Tests and Analysis Report
RX	Renewable Oxygen Content Averaging Report
SG	Symptoms Document
V5	Death Notification
XP	Photographs

Transmission Type Code:

AA	Available on Request at Provider Site
BM	By Mail

Example: PWK03FX12363545465

Block 20: Outside Lab? $Charges

This block indicates that services have been rendered by an independent provider as indicated in Block 32 and the related costs.

14. DATE OF CURRENT: ILLNESS, INJURY, or PREGNANCY(LMP)	15. OTHER DATE	16. DATES PATIENT UNABLE TO WORK IN CURRENT OCCUPATION
MM DD YY	QUAL. MM DD YY	MM DD YY MM DD YY
03 01 20XX QUAL. 431		FROM TO
17. NAME OF REFERRING PROVIDER OR OTHER SOURCE	17a.	18. HOSPITALIZATION DATES RELATED TO CURRENT SERVICES
DN Perry Cardi MD	17b. NPI 67805027XX	MM DD YY MM DD YY FROM TO
19. ADDITIONAL CLAIM INFORMATION (Designated by NUCC)		20. OUTSIDE LAB? $ CHARGES
		☐ YES ☒ NO

Instructions: Complete this field when billing for purchased services by entering an X in "YES." If a "YES" is annotated, enter the purchase price under "$Charges" and complete Block 32. Each purchased service must be reported on a separate claim form because only one charge can be entered.

When entering the charge amount, enter the amount in the field to the left of the vertical line. The entered number should be right justified to the left of the vertical line. Enter 00 for cents if the amount is a whole number. Do not use dollar signs, commas, or a decimal point when reporting amounts. Negative dollar amounts are not allowed. Leave the right field blank.

Block 21: Diagnosis or Nature of Illness or Injury

The "ICD indicator" identifies the version of the International Classification of Diseases (ICD) code set being reported. The "Diagnosis or Nature of Illness or Injury" is the sign, symptom, complaint, or condition of the patient relating to the service(s) on the claim.

21. DIAGNOSIS OR NATURE OF ILLNESS OR INJURY Relate A-L to service line below (24E)			ICD Ind. 0	22. RESUBMISSION CODE	ORIGINAL REF. NO.
A. H66.009 B.	C.	D.			
E. F.	G.	H.		23. PRIOR AUTHORIZATION NUMBER	
I. J.	K.	L.			

24. A. DATE(S) OF SERVICE					B. PLACE OF SERVICE	C. EMG	D. PROCEDURES, SERVICES, OR SUPPLIES (Explain Unusual Circumstances) CPT/HCPCS MODIFIER	E. DIAGNOSIS POINTER	F. $ CHARGES	G. DAYS OR UNITS	H. EPSDT Family Plan	I. ID. QUAL.	J. RENDERING PROVIDER ID. #
From MM DD YY			To MM DD YY										
03 03 XX					11		99203	A	70 92	1		NPI	12458977XX

Instructions: Enter the applicable ICD indicator to identify which version of ICD codes is being reported.

9 ICD-9-CM

0 ICD-10-CM

Enter the indicator between the vertical, dotted lines.

Enter the patient's diagnosis and/or condition codes. List no more than 12 ICD-9-CM or ICD-10-CM diagnosis codes. Relate lines A to L to the lines of service in Block 24E by the letter of the line. Use the highest level of specificity. Do not provide narrative description in this field.

Block 22: Resubmission and/or Original Reference Number

"Resubmission" means the code and original reference number assigned by the destination payer or receiver to indicate a previously submitted claim or encounter.

21. DIAGNOSIS OR NATURE OF ILLNESS OR INJURY Relate A-L to service line below (24E)			ICD Ind. 0	22. RESUBMISSION CODE	ORIGINAL REF. NO.
A. H66.009 B.	C.	D.			
E. F.	G.	H.		23. PRIOR AUTHORIZATION NUMBER	
I. J.	K.	L.			

24. A. DATE(S) OF SERVICE					B. PLACE OF SERVICE	C. EMG	D. PROCEDURES, SERVICES, OR SUPPLIES (Explain Unusual Circumstances) CPT/HCPCS MODIFIER	E. DIAGNOSIS POINTER	F. $ CHARGES	G. DAYS OR UNITS	H. EPSDT Family Plan	I. ID. QUAL.	J. RENDERING PROVIDER ID. #
From MM DD YY			To MM DD YY										
03 03 XX					11		99203	A	70 92	1		NPI	12458977XX

Instructions: List the original reference number for resubmitted claims. Refer to the most current instructions from the public or private payer regarding use of this field (that is, code).

When resubmitting a claim, enter the appropriate bill frequency code left justified in the left side of the field.

7 Replacement of prior claim

8 Void/cancel of prior claim

This block is not intended for use of original claim submissions.

Block 23: Prior Authorization Number

This block identifies the payer assigned number authorizing the service(s).

21. DIAGNOSIS OR NATURE OF ILLNESS OR INJURY Relate A-L to service line below (24E)				ICD Ind. 0		22. RESUBMISSION CODE	ORIGINAL REF. NO.
A. H66.009	B.	C.	D.				
E.	F.	G.	H.			23. PRIOR AUTHORIZATION NUMBER	
I.	J.	K.	L.				

24. A. DATE(S) OF SERVICE From MM DD YY To MM DD YY	B. PLACE OF SERVICE	C. EMG	D. PROCEDURES, SERVICES, OR SUPPLIES (Explain Unusual Circumstances) CPT/HCPCS | MODIFIER	E. DIAGNOSIS POINTER	F. $ CHARGES	G. DAYS OR UNITS	H. EPSDT Family Plan	I. ID. QUAL.	J. RENDERING PROVIDER ID. #
03 03 XX	11		99203	A	70 92	1		NPI	12458977XX

Instructions: Enter any of the following: prior authorization number, referral number, mammography precertification number, or Clinical Laboratory Improvement Amendments (CLIA) number, as assigned by the payer for the current service.

Do not enter hyphens or spaces within the number.

Block 24A: Date(s) of Service (Lines 1 to 6)

Block 24A indicates the actual month, day, and year the service(s) was provided. Grouping services refers to a charge for a series of identical services without listing each date of service.

	24. A. DATE(S) OF SERVICE From MM DD YY To MM DD YY	B. PLACE OF SERVICE	C. EMG	D. PROCEDURES, SERVICES, OR SUPPLIES (Explain Unusual Circumstances) CPT/HCPCS | MODIFIER	E. DIAGNOSIS POINTER	F. $ CHARGES	G. DAYS OR UNITS	H. EPSDT Family Plan	I. ID. QUAL.	J. RENDERING PROVIDER ID. #
1	03 03 XX	11		99203	A	70 92	1		NPI	12458977XX
2									NPI	
3									NPI	
4									NPI	
5									NPI	
6									NPI	

25. FEDERAL TAX I.D. NUMBER	SSN EIN	26. PATIENT'S ACCOUNT NO.	27. ACCEPT ASSIGNMENT? (For govt. claims, see back)	28. TOTAL CHARGE	29. AMOUNT PAID	30. Rsvd for NUCC Use
XX12210XX	☐ ☒	010	☒ YES ☐ NO	$ 70 92	$	$

	24. A. DATE(S) OF SERVICE From MM DD YY To MM DD YY	B. PLACE OF SERVICE	C. EMG	D. PROCEDURES, SERVICES, OR SUPPLIES (Explain Unusual Circumstances) CPT/HCPCS | MODIFIER	E. DIAGNOSIS POINTER	F. $ CHARGES	G. DAYS OR UNITS	H. EPSDT Family Plan	I. ID. QUAL.	J. RENDERING PROVIDER ID. #
1	11 30 XX	21		99231	A	37 74	1		NPI	32783127XX
2	12 01 XX 12 03 XX	21		99231	A	37 74	3		NPI	32783127XX
3									NPI	
4									NPI	
5									NPI	
6									NPI	

25. FEDERAL TAX I.D. NUMBER	SSN EIN	26. PATIENT'S ACCOUNT NO.	27. ACCEPT ASSIGNMENT? (For govt. claims, see back)	28. TOTAL CHARGE	29. AMOUNT PAID	30. Rsvd for NUCC Use
XX12210XX	☐ ☒	102	☒ YES ☐ NO	$ 150 96	$	$

Instructions: Enter date(s) of service, both the "From" and "To" dates. If there is only one date of service, enter that date under "From." Leave "To" blank or re-enter the "From" date. If grouping services, the place of service, procedure code, charges, and individual provider for each line must be identical for that service. Grouping is allowed only for services on consecutive days. The number of days must correspond to the number of units in Block 24G.

When required by payers to provide additional anesthesia services information (for example, begin and end times), narrative description of an unspecified code, National Drug Code (NDC), Vendor Product Number–Health Industry Business Communications Council (VP–HIBCC) codes, Product Number Health Care Uniform Code Council–Global Trade Item Number (OZ-GTIN) codes, contract rate, or tooth numbers and areas of the oral cavity, enter the applicable qualifier and number/code/information starting with the first space in the shaded line of this field. Do not enter a space, hyphen, or other separator between the qualifier and the number/code/information. The information may extend to Block 24G.

Block 24B: Place of Service (Lines 1 to 6)

This block identifies the location where the service was rendered.

24. A. DATE(S) OF SERVICE			B. PLACE OF SERVICE	C. EMG	D. PROCEDURES, SERVICES, OR SUPPLIES (Explain Unusual Circumstances)		E. DIAGNOSIS POINTER	F. $ CHARGES	G. DAYS OR UNITS	H. EPSDT Family Plan	I. ID. QUAL.	J. RENDERING PROVIDER ID. #
From MM DD YY	To MM DD YY				CPT/HCPCS	MODIFIER						
1 03 03 XX			11		99203		A	70 92	1		NPI	12458977XX
2											NPI	
3											NPI	
4											NPI	
5											NPI	
6											NPI	

25. FEDERAL TAX I.D. NUMBER	SSN EIN	26. PATIENT'S ACCOUNT NO.	27. ACCEPT ASSIGNMENT? (For govt. claims, see back)	28. TOTAL CHARGE	29. AMOUNT PAID	30. Rsvd for NUCC Use
XX12210XX	☐ ☒	010	☒ YES ☐ NO	$ 70 92	$	$

Instructions: In Block 24B, enter the appropriate two-digit code from the Place of Service Code list for each item used or service performed. The Place of Service Codes can be referenced in Figure 7-2 and are available at www.cms.gov/physicianfeesched/downloads/Website_POS_database.pdf.

Block 24C: EMG (Lines 1 to 6)

"EMG" identifies whether the service was an emergency.

24. A. DATE(S) OF SERVICE			B. PLACE OF SERVICE	C. EMG	D. PROCEDURES, SERVICES, OR SUPPLIES (Explain Unusual Circumstances)		E. DIAGNOSIS POINTER	F. $ CHARGES	G. DAYS OR UNITS	H. EPSDT Family Plan	I. ID. QUAL.	J. RENDERING PROVIDER ID. #
From MM DD YY	To MM DD YY				CPT/HCPCS	MODIFIER						
1 03 03 XX			11		99203		A	70 92	1		NPI	12458977XX
2											NPI	
3											NPI	
4											NPI	
5											NPI	
6											NPI	

25. FEDERAL TAX I.D. NUMBER	SSN EIN	26. PATIENT'S ACCOUNT NO.	27. ACCEPT ASSIGNMENT? (For govt. claims, see back)	28. TOTAL CHARGE	29. AMOUNT PAID	30. Rsvd for NUCC Use
XX12210XX	☐ ☒	010	☒ YES ☐ NO	$ 70 92	$	$

**BLOCK 24B
PLACE OF SERVICE CODES**

01   Pharmacy
02   Unassigned
03   School
04   Homeless shelter
05   Indian health service free-standing facility
06   Indian health service provider-based facility
07   Tribal 638 free-standing facility
08   Tribal 638 provider-based facility
09   Prison/correctional facility
10   Unassigned
11   Doctor's office
12   Patient's home
13   Assisted living facility
14   Group home
15   Mobile unit
16   Temporary lodging
17-19   Unassigned
20   Urgent care facility
21   Inpatient hospital
22   Outpatient hospital or urgent care center
23   Emergency department—hospital
24   Ambulatory surgical center
25   Birthing center
26   Military treatment facility/uniformed service treatment facility
27-30   Unassigned
31   Skilled nursing facility (swing bed visits)
32   Nursing facility (intermediate/long-term care facilities)
33   Custodial care facility (domiciliary or rest home services)
34   Hospice (domiciliary or rest home services)
35-40   Unassigned
41   Ambulance—land
42   Ambulance—air or water
43-48   Unassigned
49   Independent clinic
50   Federally qualified health center
51   Inpatient psychiatric facility
52   Psychiatric facility—partial hospitalization
53   Community mental health care (outpatient, twenty-four-hours-a-day services, admission screening, consultation, and educational services)
54   Intermediate care facility/mentally retarded
55   Residential substance abuse treatment facility
56   Psychiatric residential treatment center
57   Non-residential substance abuse treatment facility
58-59   Unassigned
60   Mass immunization center
61   Comprehensive inpatient rehabilitation facility
62   Comprehensive outpatient rehabilitation facility
63-64   Unassigned
65   End-stage renal disease treatment facility
66-70   Unassigned
71   State or local public health clinic
72   Rural health clinic
73-80   Unassigned
81   Independent laboratory
82-98   Unassigned
99   Other place of service not identified above

FIGURE 7-2 Block 24B Place of Service Codes.

Instructions: Check with the payer to determine if this element is necessary. If required, enter Y for "YES," or leave blank if "NO," in the bottom, unshaded area of the field. The definition of an emergency would be defined by federal or state regulations or programs or payer contract, or would be as defined in 5010A1.

Block 24D: Procedures, Services, or Supplies (Lines 1 to 6)

This block identifies the medical services and procedures provided to the patient.

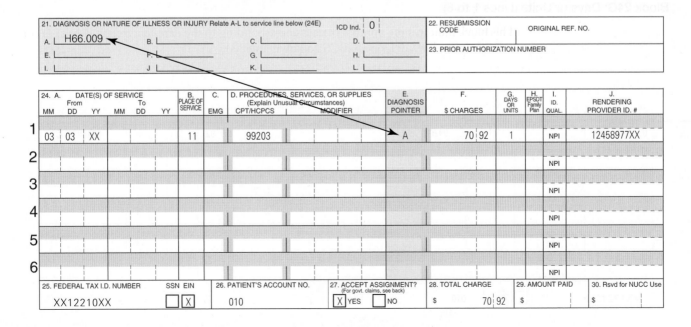

Instructions: Enter the Current Procedural Terminology (CPT) or Healthcare Common Procedure Coding System (HCPCS) code(s) and modifier(s) (if applicable) from the appropriate code set in effect on the date of service. This field accommodates the entry of up to four two-digit modifiers. The specific procedure code(s) must be shown without a narrative description.

Block 24E: Diagnosis Pointer (Lines 1 to 6)

The "Diagnosis Pointer" is the line letter from Block 21 that relates to the reason the service(s) was performed.

Instructions: In Block 24E, enter the diagnosis code reference letter (pointer) as shown in Block 21 to relate the date of service and the procedures performed to the primary diagnosis. When multiple services are performed, the primary reference number for each service should be listed first and other applicable services should follow. The reference letter(s) should be A to L or multiple letters as applicable. ICD-9-CM or ICD-10-CM diagnosis codes must be entered in Block 21 only. Do not enter them in Block 24E.

Enter numbers left justified in the field. Do not use commas between the numbers.

Block 24F: $Charges (Lines 1 to 6)

This block indicates the total billed amount for each service line.

24. A. DATE(S) OF SERVICE From MM DD YY To MM DD YY	B. PLACE OF SERVICE	C. EMG	D. PROCEDURES, SERVICES, OR SUPPLIES (Explain Unusual Circumstances) CPT/HCPCS | MODIFIER	E. DIAGNOSIS POINTER	F. $ CHARGES	G. DAYS OR UNITS	H. EPSDT Family Plan	I. ID. QUAL.	J. RENDERING PROVIDER ID. #
1 03 03 XX	11		99203	A	70 92	1		NPI	12458977XX
2								NPI	
3								NPI	
4								NPI	
5								NPI	
6								NPI	

25. FEDERAL TAX I.D. NUMBER	SSN EIN	26. PATIENT'S ACCOUNT NO.	27. ACCEPT ASSIGNMENT? (For govt. claims, see back)	28. TOTAL CHARGE	29. AMOUNT PAID	30. Rsvd for NUCC Use
XX12210XX	☐ ☒	010	☒ YES ☐ NO	$ 70 92	$	$

Instructions: Enter the charge for each listed service.

Enter numbers right justified in the dollar area of the field. Do not use commas when reporting dollar amounts. Negative dollar amounts are not allowed. Dollar signs should not be entered. Enter 00 in the cents area if the amount is a whole number.

➤ *When completing the* Workbook *insurance claim assignments, use the College Clinic Office Policies and Mock Fee Schedule at the back of the* Workbook. *For Medicare participating provider cases, use the Participating Provider Fee column. For nonparticipating provider cases, use the Limiting Charge column.*

Block 24G: Days or Units (Lines 1 to 6)

This block indicates the number of days corresponding to the dates entered in Block 24A or units as defined in CPT or HCPCS coding manual(s).

24. A. DATE(S) OF SERVICE From MM DD YY To MM DD YY	B. PLACE OF SERVICE	C. EMG	D. PROCEDURES, SERVICES, OR SUPPLIES (Explain Unusual Circumstances) CPT/HCPCS | MODIFIER	E. DIAGNOSIS POINTER	F. $ CHARGES	G. DAYS OR UNITS	H. EPSDT Family Plan	I. ID. QUAL.	J. RENDERING PROVIDER ID. #
1 03 03 XX	11		99203	A	70 92	1		NPI	12458977XX
2								NPI	
3								NPI	
4								NPI	
5								NPI	
6								NPI	

25. FEDERAL TAX I.D. NUMBER	SSN EIN	26. PATIENT'S ACCOUNT NO.	27. ACCEPT ASSIGNMENT? (For govt. claims, see back)	28. TOTAL CHARGE	29. AMOUNT PAID	30. Rsvd for NUCC Use
XX12210XX	☐ ☒	010	☒ YES ☐ NO	$ 70 92	$	$

Instructions: Enter the number of days or units. This block is most commonly used for multiple visits, units of supplies, anesthesia units or minutes, or oxygen volume. If only one service is performed, the numeral 1 must be entered.

Enter numbers left justified in this block. No leading zeros are required. If reporting a fraction of a unit, use the decimal point.

Anesthesia services must be reported as minutes. Units may only be reported for anesthesia services when the codes description includes a time period, such as "daily management."

Block 24H: EPSDT/Family Plan (Lines 1 to 6)

The "EPSDT/Family Plan" identifies certain services that may be covered under some state Medicaid plans.

24. A. DATE(S) OF SERVICE From MM DD YY	To MM DD YY	B. PLACE OF SERVICE	C. EMG	D. PROCEDURES, SERVICES, OR SUPPLIES (Explain Unusual Circumstances) CPT/HCPCS	MODIFIER	E. DIAGNOSIS POINTER	F. $ CHARGES	G. DAYS OR UNITS	H. EPSDT Family Plan	I. ID. QUAL.	J. RENDERING PROVIDER ID. #
1 03 03 XX		11		99203		A	70 92	1		NPI	12458977XX
2										NPI	
3										NPI	
4										NPI	
5										NPI	
6										NPI	

25. FEDERAL TAX I.D. NUMBER	SSN EIN	26. PATIENT'S ACCOUNT NO.	27. ACCEPT ASSIGNMENT? (For govt. claims, see back)	28. TOTAL CHARGE	29. AMOUNT PAID	30. Rsvd for NUCC Use
XX12210XX	☐ ☒	010	☒ YES ☐ NO	$ 70 92	$	$

Instructions: For Early and Periodic Screening, Diagnosis, and Treatment (EPSDT)–related services, enter the response in the shaded portion of the field as follows.

If there is a requirement to report a reason code for EPDST, enter the appropriate reason code as noted below. (A Y or N response is not entered with the code.) The two-character code is right justified in the shaded area of the field.

The following codes for EPSDT are used in 5010A1:

AV Available—Not Used (Patient refused referral.)

S2 Under Treatment (Patient is currently under treatment for referred diagnostic or corrective treatment or is scheduled for another appointment with screening provider for diagnostic or corrective treatment for at least one health problem identified during an initial or periodic screening service, not including dental referrals.)

NU Not Used (Used when no EPSDT patient referral was given.)

If the service is Family Planning, enter Y ("YES") or N ("NO") in the bottom, unshaded area of the field.

 Private Payers Claims: Leave blank.

 Medicare Claims: Leave blank.

 TRICARE Claims: Leave blank.

CHAMPVA Claims: Leave blank.

Workers' Compensation Claims: Leave blank.

Block 24I: ID Qualifier (Lines 1 to 6)

If the provider does not have an NPI number, enter the appropriate qualifier and identifying number in the shaded area.

24. A. DATE(S) OF SERVICE		B. PLACE OF SERVICE	C. EMG	D. PROCEDURES, SERVICES, OR SUPPLIES (Explain Unusual Circumstances) CPT/HCPCS | MODIFIER	E. DIAGNOSIS POINTER	F. $ CHARGES	G. DAYS OR UNITS	H. EPSDT Family Plan	I. ID. QUAL.	J. RENDERING PROVIDER ID. #
From MM DD YY	To MM DD YY									
1 03 03 XX		11		99203	A	70 92	1		NPI	12458977XX
2									NPI	
3									NPI	
4									NPI	
5									NPI	
6									NPI	

25. FEDERAL TAX I.D. NUMBER	SSN EIN	26. PATIENT'S ACCOUNT NO.	27. ACCEPT ASSIGNMENT? (For govt. claims, see back)	28. TOTAL CHARGE	29. AMOUNT PAID	30. Rsvd for NUCC Use
XX12210XX	☐ ☒X	010	☒ YES ☐ NO	$ 70 92	$	$

There will always be providers who do not have an NPI and will need to report non-NPI identifiers on their claim forms. The qualifiers will indicate the non-NPI number being reported.

Instructions: Enter in the shaded area of Block 24I the qualifier, identifying if the number is a non-NPI. The Other ID number of the rendering provider should be reported in Block 24J in the shaded area.

NUCC defines the following qualifiers used in 5010A1:

0B State License Number

1G Provider UPIN Number

G2 Provider Commercial Number

LU Location Number

ZZ Provider Taxonomy (The qualifier in the 5010A1 for Provider Taxonomy is PXC but ZZ remains the qualifier for the 1500 Claim Form.)

The list above contains both provider identifiers and the provider taxonomy code. The provider identifiers are assigned to the provider either by a specific payer or by a third party in order to uniquely identify the provider. The taxonomy code is designated by the provider in order to identify his or her provider type, classification, and area of specialization. Both provider identifiers and provider taxonomy may be used in this field.

The rendering provider is the person or company (laboratory or other facility) that rendered or supervised the care. In the case where a substitute provider (locum tenens) was used, enter that provider's information here. Report the identification number in Blocks 24I and 24J only when different from data recorded in Blocks 33a and 33b.

Block 24J: Rendering Provider ID. # (Lines 1 to 6)

The individual performing or rendering the service should be reported in Block 24J and the qualifier indicating if the number is a non-NPI goes in Block 24I. The non-NPI ID number of the rendering provider refers to the payer-assigned unique identifier of the professional.

24. A. DATE(S) OF SERVICE From			To			B. PLACE OF SERVICE	C. EMG	D. PROCEDURES, SERVICES, OR SUPPLIES (Explain Unusual Circumstances) CPT/HCPCS	MODIFIER	E. DIAGNOSIS POINTER	F. $ CHARGES		G. DAYS OR UNITS	H. EPSDT Family Plan	I. ID. QUAL.	J. RENDERING PROVIDER ID. #
MM	DD	YY	MM	DD	YY											
1 03	03	XX				11		99203		A	70	92	1		NPI	12458977XX
2															NPI	
3															NPI	
4															NPI	
5															NPI	
6															NPI	

25. FEDERAL TAX I.D. NUMBER	SSN	EIN	26. PATIENT'S ACCOUNT NO.	27. ACCEPT ASSIGNMENT? (For govt. claims, see back)	28. TOTAL CHARGE	29. AMOUNT PAID	30. Rsvd for NUCC Use
XX12210XX	☐	☒	010	☒ YES ☐ NO	$ 70 92	$	$

Instructions: The individual rendering the service should be reported in Block 24J. Enter the non-NPI ID number in the shaded area of the field. Enter the NPI number in the unshaded area of the field.

The rendering provider is the person or company (laboratory or other facility) that rendered or supervised the care. In the case where a substitute provider (locum tenens) was used, enter that provider's information here. Report the identification number in Blocks 24I and 24J only when different from data recorded in Blocks 33a and 33b.

Enter numbers left justified in the block.

Instructions and Examples of Supplemental Information in Block 24

The following are types of supplemental information that can be entered in the shaded areas of Block 24:

- Narrative descriptions of unspecified codes
- National Drug Codes (NDC) for drugs
- Vendor Product Number–Health Industry Business Communications Council (VP-HIBCC)
- Product Number Health Care Uniform Code Council–Global Trade Item Number (OZ-GTIN), formerly Universal Product Code (UPC) for products
- Contract rate
- Tooth numbers and areas of the oral cavity

The following qualifiers are to be used when reporting these services:

ZZ Narrative Description of Unspecified Code

N4 National Drug Codes (NDC)

VP Vendor Product Number–Health Industry Business Communications Council (HIBCC) Labeling Standard

OZ Product Number Health Care Uniform Code Council–Global Trade Item Number (GTIN)

CTR Contract Rate

JP Universal/National Tooth Designation System

JO ANSI/ADA/ISO Specification No. 3950-1984 Dentistry Designation System for Tooth and Areas of the Oral Cavity

If required to report other supplemental information not listed above, follow payer instructions for the use of a qualifier for the information being reported. When reporting a service that does not have a qualifier, enter two blank spaces before entering the information.

To enter supplemental information, begin at Block 24A by entering the qualifier and then the information. Do not enter a space between the qualifier and the number/code/information. Do not enter hyphens or spaces with the number/code.

More than one supplemental item can be reported in the shaded lines of Block 24. Enter the first qualifier and number/code/information at Block 24A. After the first item, enter three blank spaces and then the next qualifier and number/code/information.

When reporting dollar amounts in the shaded area, always enter the dollar amount, a decimal point, and cents. Use 00 for the cents if the amount is a whole number. Do not use commas. Do not enter dollar signs.

Additional Information for Reporting NDC. When entering supplemental information for NDC, add in the following order: qualifier, NDC code, one space, unit/basis of measurement qualifier, quantity. The number of digits for the quantity is limited to eight digits before the decimal and three digits after the decimal. If entering a whole number, do not use a decimal. Do not use commas.

When a dollar amount is being reported, enter the following after the quantity: one space, dollar amount. Do not enter a dollar sign.

The following qualifiers are to be used when reporting NDC unit/basis of measurement:
F2 International Unit
ML Milliliter
GR Gram
UN Unit

Additional Information for Reporting Tooth Numbers and Areas of the Oral Cavity. When reporting tooth numbers, add in the following order: qualifier, tooth number (for example, JP16). When reporting an area of the oral cavity, enter in the following order: qualifier, area of oral cavity code (for example, JO10).

When reporting multiple tooth numbers for one procedure, add in the following order: qualifier, tooth number, blank space, tooth number, blank space, tooth number, and so on (for example, JP1 16 17 32).

When reporting multiple tooth numbers for one procedure, the number of units reported in Block 24G is the number of teeth involved in the procedure.

When reporting multiple areas of the oral cavity for one procedure, add in the following order: qualifier, oral cavity code, blank space, oral cavity code, and so on (for example, JO10 20).

When reporting multiple areas of the oral cavity for one procedure, the number of units reported in Block 24G is the number of areas of the oral cavity involved in the procedure.

The following are the codes for tooth numbers, reported with the JP qualifier:
1-32 Permanent dentition
51-82 Permanent supernumerary dentition
A-T Primary dentition
AS-TS Primary supernumerary dentition

The following are the codes for areas of the oral cavity, reported with the JO qualifier:
00 Entire oral cavity
01 Maxillary arch
02 Mandibular arch
10 Upper right quadrant
20 Upper left quadrant
30 Lower left quadrant
40 Lower right quadrant

For further information on these codes, refer to the Current Dental Terminology (CDT) Manual available from the American Dental Association.

Block 25: Federal Tax ID Number

The "Federal Tax ID Number" is the unique identifier assigned by a federal or state agency.

25. FEDERAL TAX I.D. NUMBER SSN EIN	26. PATIENT'S ACCOUNT NO.	27. ACCEPT ASSIGNMENT?	28. TOTAL CHARGE	29. AMOUNT PAID	30. Rsvd for NUCC Use
XX12210XX ☐ ☒	010	☒ YES ☐ NO	$ 70 92	$	$

| 31. SIGNATURE OF PHYSICIAN OR SUPPLIER... Concha Antrum MD   030320XX SIGNED Concha Antrum MD DATE | 32. SERVICE FACILITY LOCATION INFORMATION a. NPI b. | 33. BILLING PROVIDER INFO & PH # (555) 4869002 College Clinic 4567 Broad Avenue Woodland Hills XY 12345-0001 a. 3664021CC b. |

Instructions: Enter the "Federal Tax ID Number" (EIN or SSN) of the billing provider identified in Block 33. This is the tax ID number intended to be used for 1099 reporting purposes. Enter an X in the appropriate box to indicate which number is being reported. Only one box can be marked.

Do not enter hyphens with numbers. Enter numbers left justified in the field.

→*When completing the* Workbook *assignments, enter the group's federal tax ID number and check the appropriate box except in Medicare/Medigap cases.*

Block 26: Patient's Account No

The "Patient's Account No." is the identifier assigned by the provider.

25. FEDERAL TAX I.D. NUMBER	SSN EIN	26. PATIENT'S ACCOUNT NO.	27. ACCEPT ASSIGNMENT? (For govt. claims, see back)	28. TOTAL CHARGE	29. AMOUNT PAID	30. Rsvd for NUCC Use
XX12210XX	☐ ☒	010	☒ YES ☐ NO	$ 70 ¦ 92	$	$

31. SIGNATURE OF PHYSICIAN OR SUPPLIER INCLUDING DEGREES OR CREDENTIALS (I certify that the statements on the reverse apply to this bill and are made a part thereof.)	32. SERVICE FACILITY LOCATION INFORMATION	33. BILLING PROVIDER INFO & PH # (555)4869002
Concha Antrum MD 030320XX		College Clinic 4567 Broad Avenue Woodland Hills XY 12345-0001
SIGNED *Concha Antrum MD* DATE	a. NPI b.	a. 3664021CC b.

Instructions: Enter the patient's account number assigned by the provider of service's or supplier's accounting system.

➡ *When completing the* Workbook *assignments, list the patient account number when provided.*

Block 27: Accept Assignment?

"Accept Assignment?" indicates that the provider agrees to accept assignment under the terms of the payer's program.

25. FEDERAL TAX I.D. NUMBER	SSN EIN	26. PATIENT'S ACCOUNT NO.	27. ACCEPT ASSIGNMENT? (For govt. claims, see back)	28. TOTAL CHARGE	29. AMOUNT PAID	30. Rsvd for NUCC Use
XX12210XX	☐ ☒	010	☒ YES ☐ NO	$ 70 ¦ 92	$	$

31. SIGNATURE OF PHYSICIAN OR SUPPLIER INCLUDING DEGREES OR CREDENTIALS (I certify that the statements on the reverse apply to this bill and are made a part thereof.)	32. SERVICE FACILITY LOCATION INFORMATION	33. BILLING PROVIDER INFO & PH # (555)4869002
Concha Antrum MD 030320XX		College Clinic 4567 Broad Avenue Woodland Hills XY 12345-0001
SIGNED *Concha Antrum MD* DATE	a. NPI b.	a. 3664021CC b.

Instructions: Enter an X in the correct box. Only one box can be marked.

➡ *When completing the* Workbook *assignments, check "Yes" if Medicare or Medicare with other insurance.*

Block 28: Total Charge

This block indicates the total billed amount for all services entered in Block 24F (Lines 1 to 6).

25. FEDERAL TAX I.D. NUMBER	SSN EIN	26. PATIENT'S ACCOUNT NO.	27. ACCEPT ASSIGNMENT? (For govt. claims, see back)	28. TOTAL CHARGE	29. AMOUNT PAID	30. Rsvd for NUCC Use
XX12210XX	☐ ☒	010	☒ YES ☐ NO	$ 70 ¦ 92	$	$

31. SIGNATURE OF PHYSICIAN OR SUPPLIER INCLUDING DEGREES OR CREDENTIALS (I certify that the statements on the reverse apply to this bill and are made a part thereof.)	32. SERVICE FACILITY LOCATION INFORMATION	33. BILLING PROVIDER INFO & PH # (555) 4869002
Concha Antrum MD 030320XX		College Clinic 4567 Broad Avenue Woodland Hills XY 12345-0001
SIGNED *Concha Antrum MD* DATE	a. NPI b.	a. 3664021CC b.

Instructions: Enter the total charges for the services (that is, total of all charges in Block 24F).

Block 29: Amount Paid

This block indicates payment received from the patient or other payers.

25. FEDERAL TAX I.D. NUMBER	SSN EIN	26. PATIENT'S ACCOUNT NO.	27. ACCEPT ASSIGNMENT? (For govt. claims, see back)	28. TOTAL CHARGE	29. AMOUNT PAID	30. Rsvd for NUCC Use
XX12210XX	☐ ☒	010	☒ YES ☐ NO	$ 70 ¦ 92	$	$

31. SIGNATURE OF PHYSICIAN OR SUPPLIER INCLUDING DEGREES OR CREDENTIALS (I certify that the statements on the reverse apply to this bill and are made a part thereof.)	32. SERVICE FACILITY LOCATION INFORMATION	33. BILLING PROVIDER INFO & PH # (555) 4869002
Concha Antrum MD 030320XX		College Clinic 4567 Broad Avenue Woodland Hills XY 12345-0001
SIGNED *Concha Antrum MD* DATE	a. NPI b.	a. 3664021CC b.

Instructions: Enter the total amount the patient and/or other payers paid on the covered services only.

Enter the number right justified in the dollar area of the field. Do not use commas when reporting dollar amounts. Negative dollar amounts are not allowed. Dollar signs should not be entered. Enter 00 in the cents area if the amount is a whole number.

Block 30: Reserved for NUCC Use

This field is reserved for NUCC use. NUCC will provide instructions for any use of this field.

25. FEDERAL TAX I.D. NUMBER SSN EIN	26. PATIENT'S ACCOUNT NO.	27. ACCEPT ASSIGNMENT? (For govt. claims, see back)	28. TOTAL CHARGE	29. AMOUNT PAID	30. Rsvd for NUCC Use
XX12210XX ☐ ☒	010	☒ YES ☐ NO	$ 70 ¦ 92	$ ¦	$ ¦
31. SIGNATURE OF PHYSICIAN OR SUPPLIER INCLUDING DEGREES OR CREDENTIALS (I certify that the statements on the reverse apply to this bill and are made a part thereof.) Concha Antrum MD 030320XX SIGNED *Concha Antrum MD* DATE	32. SERVICE FACILITY LOCATION INFORMATION a. NPI b.		33. BILLING PROVIDER INFO & PH # (555) 4869002 College Clinic 4567 Broad Avenue Woodland Hills XY 12345-0001 a. 3664021CC b.		

Instructions: This field was previously used to report "Balance Due." "Balance Due" does not exist in 5010A1, so this field has been eliminated.

Block 31: Signature of Physician or Supplier Including Degrees or Credentials

This block refers to the authorized or accountable person and the degree, credentials, or title.

25. FEDERAL TAX I.D. NUMBER SSN EIN	26. PATIENT'S ACCOUNT NO.	27. ACCEPT ASSIGNMENT? (For govt. claims, see back)	28. TOTAL CHARGE	29. AMOUNT PAID	30. Rsvd for NUCC Use
XX12210XX ☐ ☒	010	☒ YES ☐ NO	$ 70 ¦ 92	$ ¦	$ ¦
31. SIGNATURE OF PHYSICIAN OR SUPPLIER INCLUDING DEGREES OR CREDENTIALS (I certify that the statements on the reverse apply to this bill and are made a part thereof.) Concha Antrum MD 030320XX SIGNED *Concha Antrum MD* DATE	32. SERVICE FACILITY LOCATION INFORMATION a. NPI b.		33. BILLING PROVIDER INFO & PH # (555) 4869002 College Clinic 4567 Broad Avenue Woodland Hills XY 12345-0001 a. 3664021CC b.		

Instructions: Enter the legal signature of the practitioner or supplier, signature of the practitioner or supplier representative, "Signature on File," or "SOF." Enter either the 6-digit date (MM/DD/YY), 8-digit date (MM/DD/YYYY), or alphanumeric date (for example, January 1, 2003) on which the form was signed.

Block 32: Service Facility Location Information

The name and address of the facility where services were rendered identifies the site where services were provided.

25. FEDERAL TAX I.D. NUMBER SSN EIN	26. PATIENT'S ACCOUNT NO.	27. ACCEPT ASSIGNMENT? (For govt. claims, see back)	28. TOTAL CHARGE	29. AMOUNT PAID	30. Rsvd for NUCC Use
XX12210XX ☐ ☒	010	☒ YES ☐ NO	$ 70 ¦ 92	$ ¦	$ ¦
31. SIGNATURE OF PHYSICIAN OR SUPPLIER INCLUDING DEGREES OR CREDENTIALS (I certify that the statements on the reverse apply to this bill and are made a part thereof.) Concha Antrum MD 030320XX SIGNED *Concha Antrum MD* DATE	32. SERVICE FACILITY LOCATION INFORMATION a. NPI b.		33. BILLING PROVIDER INFO & PH # (555) 4869002 College Clinic 4567 Broad Avenue Woodland Hills XY 12345-0001 a. 3664021CC b.		

Instructions: Enter the name, address, city, state, and zip code of the location where the services were rendered. Providers of service (name of physician) must identify the supplier's name, address, zip code, and NPI number when billing for purchased diagnostic tests. When more than one supplier is used, a separate 1500 Claim Form should be used to bill for each supplier.

Enter the name and address information in the following format:

1st line: Name

2nd line: Address

3rd line: City, state, and zip code

Do not use punctuation (that is, commas and periods) or other symbols in the address (for example, use 123 N Main Street 101 instead of 123 N. Main Street, #101). Enter a space between the town name and state code; do not include a comma. When reporting a 9-digit zip code, include the hyphen.

If reporting a foreign address, contact payer for specific reporting instructions.

Block 32a: NPI#

The NPI number refers to the HIPAA National Provider Identifier number.

25. FEDERAL TAX I.D. NUMBER	SSN EIN	26. PATIENT'S ACCOUNT NO.	27. ACCEPT ASSIGNMENT? (For govt. claims, see back)	28. TOTAL CHARGE	29. AMOUNT PAID	30. Rsvd for NUCC Use
XX12210XX	☐ ☒	010	☒ YES ☐ NO	$ 70 | 92	$ |	$ |

31. SIGNATURE OF PHYSICIAN OR SUPPLIER INCLUDING DEGREES OR CREDENTIALS (I certify that the statements on the reverse apply to this bill and are made a part thereof.)	32. SERVICE FACILITY LOCATION INFORMATION	33. BILLING PROVIDER INFO & PH # (555) 4869002
Concha Antrum MD 030320XX SIGNED *Concha Antrum MD* DATE	a. NPI b.	College Clinic 4567 Broad Avenue Woodland Hills XY 12345-0001 a. 3664021CC b.

Instructions: If a service facility is entered in Block 32, enter the NPI number of the service facility location in Block 32a.

Block 32b: Other ID#

The non-NPI ID number of the service facility is the payer-assigned unique identifier of the facility.

25. FEDERAL TAX I.D. NUMBER	SSN EIN	26. PATIENT'S ACCOUNT NO.	27. ACCEPT ASSIGNMENT? (For govt. claims, see back)	28. TOTAL CHARGE	29. AMOUNT PAID	30. Rsvd for NUCC Use
XX12210XX	☐ ☒	010	☒ YES ☐ NO	$ 70 | 92	$ |	$ |

31. SIGNATURE OF PHYSICIAN OR SUPPLIER INCLUDING DEGREES OR CREDENTIALS (I certify that the statements on the reverse apply to this bill and are made a part thereof.)	32. SERVICE FACILITY LOCATION INFORMATION	33. BILLING PROVIDER INFO & PH # (555) 4869002
Concha Antrum MD 030320XX SIGNED *Concha Antrum MD* DATE	a. NPI b.	College Clinic 4567 Broad Avenue Woodland Hills XY 12345-0001 a. 3664021CC b.

Instructions: Enter the two-digit qualifier identifying the non-NPI number followed by the ID number. Do not enter a space, hyphen, or other separator between the qualifier and number.

NUCC defines the following qualifiers, since they are the same as those used in 5010A1:

0B State License Number

G2 Provider Commercial Number

LU Location Number

Block 33: Billing Provider Info & Ph#

The billing provider's or supplier's billing name, address, zip code, and phone number is the billing office location and telephone number of the provider and supplier.

25. FEDERAL TAX I.D. NUMBER	SSN EIN	26. PATIENT'S ACCOUNT NO.	27. ACCEPT ASSIGNMENT? (For govt. claims, see back)	28. TOTAL CHARGE	29. AMOUNT PAID	30. Rsvd for NUCC Use
XX12210XX	☐ ☒	010	☒ YES ☐ NO	$ 70 | 92	$ |	$ |

31. SIGNATURE OF PHYSICIAN OR SUPPLIER INCLUDING DEGREES OR CREDENTIALS (I certify that the statements on the reverse apply to this bill and are made a part thereof.)	32. SERVICE FACILITY LOCATION INFORMATION	33. BILLING PROVIDER INFO & PH # (555) 4869002
Concha Antrum MD 030320XX SIGNED *Concha Antrum MD* DATE	a. NPI b.	College Clinic 4567 Broad Avenue Woodland Hills XY 12345-0001 a. 3664021CC b.

Instructions: Enter the provider's or supplier's billing name, address, zip code, and phone number. The phone number is entered in the area to the right of the field title. Enter the name and address information in the following format:

1st line: Name

2nd line: Address

3rd line: City, state, and zip code

Block 33 identifies the provider that is requesting to be paid for the service rendered and should always be completed. Do not use punctuation (that is, commas and periods) or other symbols in the address (for example, use 123 N Main Street 101 instead of 123 N. Main Street, #101). Enter a space between the town name and two-character state code; do not include a comma. When reporting a 9-digit zip code, include the hyphen. Do not use a hyphen or space as a separator within the telephone number.

If reporting a foreign address, contact the payer for specific reporting instructions.

5010A1 requires the "Billing Provider Address" to be a street address or physical location. NUCC recommends that the same requirements be applied here.

Block 33a: NPI#

The NPI number refers to the HIPAA National Provider Identifier number.

25. FEDERAL TAX I.D. NUMBER SSN EIN	26. PATIENT'S ACCOUNT NO.	27. ACCEPT ASSIGNMENT? (For govt. claims, see back)	28. TOTAL CHARGE	29. AMOUNT PAID	30. Rsvd for NUCC Use
XX12210XX ☐ ☒	010	☒ YES ☐ NO	$ 70 ¦ 92	$	$
31. SIGNATURE OF PHYSICIAN OR SUPPLIER INCLUDING DEGREES OR CREDENTIALS (I certify that the statements on the reverse apply to this bill and are made a part thereof.) Concha Antrum MD 030320XX SIGNED *Concha Antrum MD* DATE	32. SERVICE FACILITY LOCATION INFORMATION a. NPI b.		33. BILLING PROVIDER INFO & PH # (555) 4869002 College Clinic 4567 Broad Avenue Woodland Hills XY 12345-0001 a. 3664021CC b.		

Instructions: Enter the NPI number of the billing provider in Block 33a.

Block 33b: Other ID#

The non-NPI number of the billing provider refers to the payer-assigned unique identifier of the professional.

25. FEDERAL TAX I.D. NUMBER SSN EIN	26. PATIENT'S ACCOUNT NO.	27. ACCEPT ASSIGNMENT? (For govt. claims, see back)	28. TOTAL CHARGE	29. AMOUNT PAID	30. Rsvd for NUCC Use
XX12210XX ☐ ☒	010	☒ YES ☐ NO	$ 70 ¦ 92	$	$
31. SIGNATURE OF PHYSICIAN OR SUPPLIER INCLUDING DEGREES OR CREDENTIALS (I certify that the statements on the reverse apply to this bill and are made a part thereof.) Concha Antrum MD 030320XX SIGNED *Concha Antrum MD* DATE	32. SERVICE FACILITY LOCATION INFORMATION a. NPI b.		33. BILLING PROVIDER INFO & PH # (555) 489002 College Clinic 4567 Broad Avenue Woodland Hills XY 12345-0001 a. 3664021CC b.		

Instructions: Enter the two-digit qualifier identifying the non-NPI number followed by the ID number. Do not enter a space, hyphen, or other separator between the qualifier and number. NUCC defines the following qualifiers used in 5010A1:

0B State License Number

G2 Provider Commercial Number

ZZ Provider Taxonomy (The qualifier in the 5010A1 for provider taxonomy is PXC but ZZ remains the qualifier for the 1500 claim form.)

The list above contains both provider identifiers and the provider taxonomy code. The provider identifiers are assigned to the provider either by a specific payer or by a third party in order to uniquely identify the provider. The taxonomy code is designated by the provider in order to identify his or her provider type, classification, and area of specialization. Both provider identifiers and provider taxonomy may be used in this field.

INSURANCE PROGRAM TEMPLATES

The following pages show the completed CMS-1500 (02-12) insurance claim forms and templates for the most common insurance programs encountered in a medical practice. Add a tab at the page margin for ease in flipping to this reference section when completing the *Workbook* assignments. The following examples illustrate entries for basic cases:

PRIVATE PAYER
NO SECONDARY COVERAGE

DRAFT - NOT FOR OFFICIAL USE

HEALTH INSURANCE CLAIM FORM

APPROVED BY NATIONAL UNIFOR MCLAIM COMMITTEE (NUCC) 02/12

CARRIER

| | PICA | | | | | | | | PICA | |

1. MEDICARE (Medicare#) MEDICAID (Medicaid#) TRICARE (ID#DoD#) CHAMPVA (Member ID#) GROUP HEALTH PLAN [X] (ID#) FECA BLK LUNG (ID#) OTHER (ID#)

1a. INSURED'S I.D. NUMBER (For Program in Item 1)
111704521

2. PATIENT'S NAME (Last Name, First Name, Middle Initial)
Forehand, Harry, N

3. PATIENT'S BIRTH DATE MM 01 DD 06 YY 1946 SEX M [X] F

4. INSURED'S NAME (Last Name, First Name, Middle Initial)
Forehand, Harry, N

5. PATIENT'S ADDRESS (No., Street)
1456 Main Street

6. PATIENT RELATIONSHIP TO INSURED
Self [X] Spouse Child Other

7. INSURED'S ADDRESS (No., Street)
1456 Main Street

CITY Woodland Hills   STATE XY

8. RESERVED FOR NUCC USE

CITY Woodland Hills   STATE XY

ZIP CODE 12345-0000   TELEPHONE (Include Area Code) (555) 4909876

ZIP CODE 12345-0000   TELEPHONE (Include Area Code) (555) 4909876

9. OTHER INSURED'S NAME (Last Name, First Name, Middle Initial)

10. IS PATIENT'S CONDITION RELATED TO:

11. INSURED'S POLICY GROUP OR FECA NUMBER
A482

a. OTHER INSURED'S POLICY OR GROUP NUMBER

a. EMPLOYMENT? (Current or Previous) YES [X] NO

a. INSURED'S DATE OF BIRTH MM 01 DD 06 YY 1946 SEX M [X] F

b. RESERVED FOR NUCC USE

b. AUTO ACCIDENT? PLACE (State) YES [X] NO

b. OTHER CLAIM ID (Designated by NUCC)

c. RESERVED FOR NUCC USE

c. OTHER ACCIDENT? YES [X] NO

c. INSURANCE PLAN NAME OR PROGRAM NAME
ABC Insurance Company

d. INSURANCE PLAN NAME OR PROGRAM NAME

10d. CLAIM CODES (Designated by NUCC)

d. IS THERE ANOTHER HEALTH BENEFIT PLAN? YES [X] NO *If yes*, complete items 9, 9a, and 9d.

READ BACK OF FORM BEFORE COMPLETING & SIGNING THIS FORM.

12. PATIENT'S OR AUTHORIZED PERSON'S SIGNATURE I authorize the release of any medical or other information necessary to process this claim. I also request payment of government benefits either to myself or to the party who accepts assignment below.

SIGNED *Harry N. Forehand*   DATE *March 3, 20XX*

13. INSURED'S OR AUTHORIZED PERSON'S SIGNATURE I authorize payment of medical benefits to the undersigned physician or supplier for services described below.

SIGNED *Harry N. Forehand*

PATIENT AND INSURED INFORMATION

14. DATE OF CURRENT: ILLNESS, INJURY, or PREGNANCY(LMP) MM 03 DD 01 YY 20XX QUAL. 431

15. OTHER DATE QUAL. MM DD YY

16. DATES PATIENT UNABLE TO WORK IN CURRENT OCCUPATION FROM MM DD YY TO MM DD YY

17. NAME OF REFERRING PROVIDER OR OTHER SOURCE
DN Perry Cardi MD

17a.
17b. NPI 67805027XX

18. HOSPITALIZATION DATES RELATED TO CURRENT SERVICES FROM MM DD YY TO MM DD YY

19. ADDITIONAL CLAIM INFORMATION (Designated by NUCC)

20. OUTSIDE LAB? YES [X] NO $ CHARGES

21. DIAGNOSIS OR NATURE OF ILLNESS OR INJURY Relate A-L to service line below (24E)   ICD Ind. 0
A. H66.009 B. C. D.
E. F. G. H.
I. J. K. L.

22. RESUBMISSION CODE   ORIGINAL REF. NO.

23. PRIOR AUTHORIZATION NUMBER

24. A. DATE(S) OF SERVICE From MM DD YY To MM DD YY	B. PLACE OF SERVICE	C. EMG	D. PROCEDURES, SERVICES, OR SUPPLIES (Explain Unusual Circumstances) CPT/HCPCS	MODIFIER	E. DIAGNOSIS POINTER	F. $ CHARGES	G. DAYS OR UNITS	H. EPSDT Family Plan	I. ID. QUAL.	J. RENDERING PROVIDER ID. #
1	03 03 XX	11		99203		A	70 92	1		NPI	1245897700
2										NPI	
3										NPI	
4										NPI	
5										NPI	
6										NPI	

PHYSICIAN OR SUPPLIER INFORMATION

25. FEDERAL TAX I.D. NUMBER   SSN EIN [X]
XX12210XX

26. PATIENT'S ACCOUNT NO.
010

27. ACCEPT ASSIGNMENT? (For govt. claims, see back) [X] YES NO

28. TOTAL CHARGE $ 70 92

29. AMOUNT PAID $

30. Rsvd for NUCC Use $

31. SIGNATURE OF PHYSICIAN OR SUPPLIER INCLUDING DEGREES OR CREDENTIALS (I certify that the statements on the reverse apply to this bill and are made a part thereof.)
Concha Antrum MD   030320XX
SIGNED *Concha Antrum MD* DATE

32. SERVICE FACILITY LOCATION INFORMATION

a. NPI   b.

33. BILLING PROVIDER INFO & PH # (555) 4869002
College Clinic
4567 Broad Avenue
Woodland Hills XY 12345-0001

a. 3664021CC   b.

NUCC Instruction Manual available at: www.nucc.org   PLEASE PRINT OR TYPE   OMB APPROVAL PENDING

FIGURE 7-3 Front side of the scannable Health Insurance Claim Form approved by the American Medical Association's (AMA's) Council on Medical Service. This form is also known as the CMS-1500 (02-12) and is shown illustrating completion to a private third-party payer with no secondary coverage. Third-party payer, state, and local guidelines vary and may not always follow the visual guide presented here.

MEDICAID
NO SECONDARY COVERAGE →

DRAFT - NOT FOR OFFICIAL USE

HEALTH INSURANCE CLAIM FORM

APPROVED BY NATIONAL UNIFOR MCLAIM COMMITTEE (NUCC) 02/12

| | | PICA | | | | | | | | | PICA | | |

1. MEDICARE	MEDICAID	TRICARE	CHAMPVA	GROUP HEALTH PLAN	FECA BLK LUNG	OTHER	1a. INSURED'S I.D. NUMBER (For Program in Item 1)
☐ (Medicare#)	☒ (Medicaid#)	☐ (ID#/DoD#)	☐ (Member ID#)	☐ (ID#)	☐ (ID#)	☐ (ID#)	276835090

2. PATIENT'S NAME (Last Name, First Name, Middle Initial)	3. PATIENT'S BIRTH DATE / SEX	4. INSURED'S NAME (Last Name, First Name, Middle Initial)
Abramson, Adam	MM 02 DD 12 YY 1995 M ☒ F ☐	Abramson, Adam

5. PATIENT'S ADDRESS (No., Street)	6. PATIENT RELATIONSHIP TO INSURED	7. INSURED'S ADDRESS (No., Street)
760 Finch Street	Self ☒ Spouse ☐ Child ☐ Other ☐	760 Finch Street

CITY	STATE	8. RESERVED FOR NUCC USE	CITY	STATE
Woodland Hills	XY		Woodland Hills	XY

ZIP CODE	TELEPHONE (Include Area Code)	ZIP CODE	TELEPHONE (Include Area Code)
12345	(555) 4826789	12345	(555) 4826789

9. OTHER INSURED'S NAME (Last Name, First Name, Middle Initial)	10. IS PATIENT'S CONDITION RELATED TO:	11. INSURED'S POLICY GROUP OR FECA NUMBER

a. OTHER INSURED'S POLICY OR GROUP NUMBER	a. EMPLOYMENT? (Current or Previous) ☐ YES ☒ NO	a. INSURED'S DATE OF BIRTH MM 02 DD 12 YY 1995 M ☒ F ☐

b. RESERVED FOR NUCC USE	b. AUTO ACCIDENT? ☐ YES ☒ NO PLACE (State)	b. OTHER CLAIM ID (Designated by NUCC)

c. RESERVED FOR NUCC USE	c. OTHER ACCIDENT? ☒ YES ☐ NO	c. INSURANCE PLAN NAME OR PROGRAM NAME Medicaid

d. INSURANCE PLAN NAME OR PROGRAM NAME	10d. CLAIM CODES (Designated by NUCC)	d. IS THERE ANOTHER HEALTH BENEFIT PLAN? ☐ YES ☒ NO If yes, complete items 9, 9a, and 9d.

READ BACK OF FORM BEFORE COMPLETING & SIGNING THIS FORM.

12. PATIENT'S OR AUTHORIZED PERSON'S SIGNATURE I authorize the release of any medical or other information necessary to process this claim. I also request payment of government benefits either to myself or to the party who accepts assignment below.	13. INSURED'S OR AUTHORIZED PERSON'S SIGNATURE I authorize payment of medical benefits to the undersigned physician or supplier for services described below.
SIGNED *Adam Abramson* DATE 7/14/XX	SIGNED *Adam Abramson*

14. DATE OF CURRENT: ILLNESS, INJURY, or PREGNANCY(LMP) MM DD YY QUAL.	15. OTHER DATE QUAL. MM DD YY	16. DATES PATIENT UNABLE TO WORK IN CURRENT OCCUPATION FROM MM DD YY TO MM DD YY

17. NAME OF REFERRING PROVIDER OR OTHER SOURCE	17a.	18. HOSPITALIZATION DATES RELATED TO CURRENT SERVICES
	17b. NPI	FROM MM DD YY TO MM DD YY

19. ADDITIONAL CLAIM INFORMATION (Designated by NUCC)	20. OUTSIDE LAB? ☐ YES ☒ NO $ CHARGES

21. DIAGNOSIS OR NATURE OF ILLNESS OR INJURY Relate A-L to service line below (24E) ICD Ind. 0	22. RESUBMISSION CODE ORIGINAL REF. NO.
A. T16.9xxA B. ____ C. ____ D. ____ E. ____ F. ____ G. ____ H. ____ I. ____ J. ____ K. ____ L. ____	23. PRIOR AUTHORIZATION NUMBER

24. A. DATE(S) OF SERVICE		B. PLACE OF SERVICE	C. EMG	D. PROCEDURES, SERVICES, OR SUPPLIES (Explain Unusual Circumstances)		E. DIAGNOSIS POINTER	F. $ CHARGES	G. DAYS OR UNITS	H. EPSDT Family Plan	I. ID. QUAL.	J. RENDERING PROVIDER ID. #
From MM DD YY	To MM DD YY			CPT/HCPCS	MODIFIER						
07 14 XX		23	Y	99282	25	A	37 00	1		NPI	37640017XX
07 14 XX		23	Y	69200		A	49 00	1		NPI	37640017XX
										NPI	
										NPI	
										NPI	
										NPI	

25. FEDERAL TAX I.D. NUMBER SSN EIN	26. PATIENT'S ACCOUNT NO.	27. ACCEPT ASSIGNMENT? (For govt. claims, see back)	28. TOTAL CHARGE	29. AMOUNT PAID	30. Rsvd for NUCC Use
XX12210XX ☒ ☐	030	☒ YES ☐ NO	$ 86 00	$	$

31. SIGNATURE OF PHYSICIAN OR SUPPLIER INCLUDING DEGREES OR CREDENTIALS (I certify that the statements on the reverse apply to this bill and are made a part thereof.) Pedro Atrics MD 071420XX SIGNED *Pedro Atrics MD* DATE	32. SERVICE FACILITY LOCATION INFORMATION College Hospital 4500 Broad Avenue Woodland Hills XY 12345-0001	33. BILLING PROVIDER INFO & PH # (555) 4869002 College Clinic 4567 Broad Avenue Woodland Hills XY 12345-0001
	a. X950731067 b.	a. 3664021CC b.

NUCC Instruction Manual available at: www.nucc.org   *PLEASE PRINT OR TYPE*   OMB APPROVAL PENDING

FIGURE 7-4 A Medicaid case with no secondary coverage, emphasizing basic elements.

MEDICARE
NO SECONDARY COVERAGE →

DRAFT - NOT FOR OFFICIAL USE

HEALTH INSURANCE CLAIM FORM

APPROVED BY NATIONAL UNIFOR MCLAIM COMMITTEE (NUCC) 02/12

| | PICA | | | | PICA | |

1. MEDICARE	MEDICAID	TRICARE	CHAMPVA	GROUP HEALTH PLAN	FECA BLK LUNG	OTHER	1a. INSURED'S I.D. NUMBER (For Program in Item 1)
[X] (Medicare#)	[ ] (Medicaid#)	[ ] (ID#DoD#)	[ ] (Member ID#)	[ ] (ID#)	[ ] (ID#)	[ ] (ID#)	123 XX 6789A

2. PATIENT'S NAME (Last Name, First Name, Middle Initial)
Hutch, Bill

3. PATIENT'S BIRTH DATE   SEX
MM 05 DD 07 YY 1910   M [X]   F [ ]

4. INSURED'S NAME (Last Name, First Name, Middle Initial)
Hutch, Bill

5. PATIENT'S ADDRESS (No., Street)
8888 Main Street

6. PATIENT RELATIONSHIP TO INSURED
Self [X]   Spouse [ ]   Child [ ]   Other [ ]

7. INSURED'S ADDRESS (No., Street)
8888 Main Street

CITY Woodland Hills   STATE XY

8. RESERVED FOR NUCC USE

CITY Woodland Hills   STATE XY

ZIP CODE 12345   TELEPHONE (Include Area Code) (555) 7321544

ZIP CODE 12345   TELEPHONE (Include Area Code) (555) 7321544

9. OTHER INSURED'S NAME (Last Name, First Name, Middle Initial)

10. IS PATIENT'S CONDITION RELATED TO:

11. INSURED'S POLICY GROUP OR FECA NUMBER

a. OTHER INSURED'S POLICY OR GROUP NUMBER

a. EMPLOYMENT? (Current or Previous)
[ ] YES   [X] NO

a. INSURED'S DATE OF BIRTH   SEX
MM 05 DD 07 YY 1910   M [X]   F [ ]

b. RESERVED FOR NUCC USE

b. AUTO ACCIDENT?   PLACE (State)
[ ] YES   [X] NO

b. OTHER CLAIM ID (Designated by NUCC)

c. RESERVED FOR NUCC USE

c. OTHER ACCIDENT?
[ ] YES   [X] NO

c. INSURANCE PLAN NAME OR PROGRAM NAME
Medicare

d. INSURANCE PLAN NAME OR PROGRAM NAME

10d. CLAIM CODES (Designated by NUCC)

d. IS THERE ANOTHER HEALTH BENEFIT PLAN?
[ ] YES   [X] NO   *If yes*, complete items 9, 9a, and 9d.

READ BACK OF FORM BEFORE COMPLETING & SIGNING THIS FORM.
12. PATIENT'S OR AUTHORIZED PERSON'S SIGNATUREI authorize the release of any medical or other information necessary to process this claim. I also request payment of government benefits either to myself or to the party who accepts assignment below.

SIGNED   Signature on file   DATE

13. INSURED'S OR AUTHORIZED PERSON'S SIGNATURE I authorize payment of medical benefits to the undersigned physician or supplier for services described below.

SIGNED

14. DATE OF CURRENT: ILLNESS, INJURY, or PREGNANCY(LMP)
MM DD YY   QUAL.

15. OTHER DATE
QUAL.   MM DD YY

16. DATES PATIENT UNABLE TO WORK IN CURRENT OCCUPATION
FROM MM DD YY   TO MM DD YY

17. NAME OF REFERRING PROVIDER OR OTHER SOURCE
DN Gerald Practon MD

17a.
17b. NPI 46278897XX

18. HOSPITALIZATION DATES RELATED TO CURRENT SERVICES
FROM MM DD YY   TO MM DD YY

19. ADDITIONAL CLAIM INFORMATION (Designated by NUCC)

20. OUTSIDE LAB? $ CHARGES
[ ] YES   [X] NO

21. DIAGNOSIS OR NATURE OF ILLNESS OR INJURY Relate A-L to service line below (24E)   ICD Ind. 0

A. J12.9   B. ___   C. ___   D. ___
E. ___   F. ___   G. ___   H. ___
I. ___   J. ___   K. ___   L. ___

22. RESUBMISSION CODE   ORIGINAL REF. NO.

23. PRIOR AUTHORIZATION NUMBER

24. A. DATE(S) OF SERVICE						B. PLACE OF SERVICE	C. EMG	D. PROCEDURES, SERVICES, OR SUPPLIES (Explain Unusual Circumstances) CPT/HCPCS	MODIFIER	E. DIAGNOSIS POINTER	F. $ CHARGES	G. DAYS OR UNITS	H. EPSDT Family Plan	I. ID. QUAL.	J. RENDERING PROVIDER ID. #
From MM	DD	YY	To MM	DD	YY										
1	03	10	XX				11		99205		A	132 00	1		NPI	64211067XX
2															NPI	
3															NPI	
4															NPI	
5															NPI	
6															NPI	

25. FEDERAL TAX I.D. NUMBER   SSN EIN
XX12210XX   [X]

26. PATIENT'S ACCOUNT NO.
040

27. ACCEPT ASSIGNMENT? (For govt. claims, see back)
[X] YES   [ ] NO

28. TOTAL CHARGE
$ 132 00

29. AMOUNT PAID
$

30. Rsvd for NUCC Use
$

31. SIGNATURE OF PHYSICIAN OR SUPPLIER INCLUDING DEGREES OR CREDENTIALS (I certify that the statements on the reverse apply to this bill and are made a part thereof.)
Brady Coccidioides   031020XX
SIGNED *Brady Coccidioides MD* DATE

32. SERVICE FACILITY LOCATION INFORMATION

a. NPI   b.

33. BILLING PROVIDER INFO & PH # (555) 4869002
College Clinic
4567 Broad Avenue
Woodland Hills XY 12345-0001

a. 3664021CC   b.

NUCC Instruction Manual available at: www.nucc.org   PLEASE PRINT OR TYPE   OMB APPROVAL PENDING

CARRIER · PATIENT AND INSURED INFORMATION · PHYSICIAN OR SUPPLIER INFORMATION

FIGURE 7-5 Example of a completed CMS-1500 (02-12) Health Insurance Claim Form for a basic Medicare case with no other insurance coverage. The physician has accepted assignment. Screened blocks should not be completed for a Medicare case with no other insurance.

MEDICARE/MEDICAID
(primary)   (secondary)
CROSSOVER CLAIM

DRAFT - NOT FOR OFFICIAL USE

HEALTH INSURANCE CLAIM FORM

APPROVED BY NATIONAL UNIFOR MCLAIM COMMITTEE (NUCC) 02/12

| | PICA | | | | | | PICA | |

1. MEDICARE [X] (Medicare#) **MEDICAID** [X] (Medicaid#) **TRICARE** (ID#DoD#) **CHAMPVA** (Member ID#) **GROUP HEALTH PLAN** (ID#) **FECA BLK LUNG** (ID#) **OTHER** (ID#)

1a. INSURED'S I.D. NUMBER (For Program in Item 1)
660 XX 2715A

2. PATIENT'S NAME (Last Name, First Name, Middle Initial)
Johnson, Kathryn

3. PATIENT'S BIRTH DATE MM 09 DD 07 YY 1937 **SEX** M □ F [X]

4. INSURED'S NAME (Last Name, First Name, Middle Initial)
Johnson, Kathryn

5. PATIENT'S ADDRESS (No., Street)
218 Vega Drive

6. PATIENT RELATIONSHIP TO INSURED
Self [X] Spouse □ Child □ Other □

7. INSURED'S ADDRESS (No., Street)
218 Vega Drive

CITY Woodland Hills **STATE** XY

8. RESERVED FOR NUCC USE

CITY Woodland Hills **STATE** XY

ZIP CODE 12345-0000 **TELEPHONE** (Include Area Code) (555) 4829112

ZIP CODE 12345-0000 **TELEPHONE** (Include Area Code) (555) 4829112

9. OTHER INSURED'S NAME (Last Name, First Name, Middle Initial)
Johnson, Kathryn

10. IS PATIENT'S CONDITION RELATED TO:

11. INSURED'S POLICY GROUP OR FECA NUMBER

a. OTHER INSURED'S POLICY OR GROUP NUMBER
MCD016745289

a. EMPLOYMENT? (Current or Previous) □ YES [X] NO

a. INSURED'S DATE OF BIRTH MM 09 DD 07 YY 1937 **SEX** M □ F [X]

b. RESERVED FOR NUCC USE

b. AUTO ACCIDENT? □ YES [X] NO **PLACE (State)**

b. OTHER CLAIM ID (Designated by NUCC)

c. RESERVED FOR NUCC USE

c. OTHER ACCIDENT? □ YES [X] NO

c. INSURANCE PLAN NAME OR PROGRAM NAME
Medicare

d. INSURANCE PLAN NAME OR PROGRAM NAME
Medicaid

10d. CLAIM CODES (Designated by NUCC)

d. IS THERE ANOTHER HEALTH BENEFIT PLAN?
[X] YES □ NO **If yes**, complete items 9, 9a, and 9d.

READ BACK OF FORM BEFORE COMPLETING & SIGNING THIS FORM.
12. PATIENT'S OR AUTHORIZED PERSON'S SIGNATURE I authorize the release of any medical or other information necessary to process this claim. I also request payment of government benefits either to myself or to the party who accepts assignment below.

SIGNED _Kathryn Johnson_ DATE _10/1/XX_

13. INSURED'S OR AUTHORIZED PERSON'S SIGNATURE I authorize payment of medical benefits to the undersigned physician or supplier for services described below.

SIGNED _Kathryn Johnson_

14. DATE OF CURRENT: ILLNESS, INJURY, or PREGNANCY(LMP) MM DD YY QUAL.

15. OTHER DATE QUAL. MM DD YY

16. DATES PATIENT UNABLE TO WORK IN CURRENT OCCUPATION FROM MM DD YY TO MM DD YY

17. NAME OF REFERRING PROVIDER OR OTHER SOURCE
DN Brady Coccidioides MD

17a.
17b. NPI 64211067XX

18. HOSPITALIZATION DATES RELATED TO CURRENT SERVICES FROM MM DD YY TO MM DD YY

19. ADDITIONAL CLAIM INFORMATION (Designated by NUCC)

20. OUTSIDE LAB? □ YES [X] NO **$ CHARGES**

21. DIAGNOSIS OR NATURE OF ILLNESS OR INJURY Relate A-L to service line below (24E) **ICD Ind.** 0
A. C43.70 B. C. D.
E. F. G. H.
I. J. K. L.

22. RESUBMISSION CODE **ORIGINAL REF. NO.**

23. PRIOR AUTHORIZATION NUMBER
7680560012

24. A. DATE(S) OF SERVICE			B. PLACE OF SERVICE	C. EMG	D. PROCEDURES, SERVICES, OR SUPPLIES (Explain Unusual Circumstances)		E. DIAGNOSIS POINTER	F. $ CHARGES	G. DAYS OR UNITS	H. EPSDT Family Plan	I. ID. QUAL.	J. RENDERING PROVIDER ID. #
From MM DD YY	To MM DD YY				CPT/HCPCS	MODIFIER						
1	10 01 XX		24		11600		A	195 00	1		NPI	50307117XX
2											NPI	
3											NPI	
4											NPI	
5											NPI	
6											NPI	

25. FEDERAL TAX I.D. NUMBER XX12210XX **SSN** □ **EIN** [X]

26. PATIENT'S ACCOUNT NO. 050

27. ACCEPT ASSIGNMENT? (For govt. claims, see back) [X] YES □ NO

28. TOTAL CHARGE $ 195 00

29. AMOUNT PAID $

30. Rsvd for NUCC Use $

31. SIGNATURE OF PHYSICIAN OR SUPPLIER INCLUDING DEGREES OR CREDENTIALS (I certify that the statements on the reverse apply to this bill and are made a part thereof.)
Cosmo Graff MD
SIGNED _Cosmo Graff, MD_ DATE 100320XX

32. SERVICE FACILITY LOCATION INFORMATION
Woodland Hills Ambulatory Center
1229 Center Street
Woodland Hills XY 12345-0001
a. X950513700 b.

33. BILLING PROVIDER INFO & PH # (555) 4869002
College Clinic
4567 Broad Avenue
Woodland Hills XY 12345-0001
a. 3664021CC b.

NUCC Instruction Manual available at: www.nucc.org **PLEASE PRINT OR TYPE** OMB APPROVAL PENDING

CARRIER — PATIENT AND INSURED INFORMATION — PHYSICIAN OR SUPPLIER INFORMATION

FIGURE 7-6 Example of a Medicare/Medicaid crossover claim. The CMS-1500 (02-12) claim form is sent to Medicare (primary payer) and then processed automatically by Medicaid (secondary payer).

MEDICARE/MEDIGAP
(primary)   (secondary)
CROSSOVER CLAIM

CARRIER

DRAFT - NOT FOR OFFICIAL USE

HEALTH INSURANCE CLAIM FORM
APPROVED BY NATIONAL UNIFOR MCLAIM COMMITTEE (NUCC) 02/12

| PICA | | PICA |

1. MEDICARE MEDICAID TRICARE CHAMPVA GROUP HEALTH PLAN FECA BLK LUNG OTHER	1a. INSURED'S I.D. NUMBER (For Program in Item 1)
[X] (Medicare#) (Medicaid#) (ID#/DoD#) (Member ID#) [X] (ID#) (ID#) (ID#)	419 XX 7272A

2. PATIENT'S NAME (Last Name, First Name, Middle Initial)	3. PATIENT'S BIRTH DATE SEX	4. INSURED'S NAME (Last Name, First Name, Middle Initial)
Barnes, Agusta, E	MM 08 DD 29 YY 1917 M [X] F [ ]	Barnes, Agusta, E

5. PATIENT'S ADDRESS (No., Street)	6. PATIENT RELATIONSHIP TO INSURED	7. INSURED'S ADDRESS (No., Street)
356 Encina Avenue	Self [X] Spouse [ ] Child [ ] Other [ ]	356 Encina Avenue

CITY	STATE	8. RESERVED FOR NUCC USE	CITY	STATE
Woodland Hills	XY		Woodland Hills	XY

ZIP CODE	TELEPHONE (Include Area Code)	ZIP CODE	TELEPHONE (Include Area Code)
12345-0000	(555) 4672646	12345-0000	(555) 4672646

9. OTHER INSURED'S NAME (Last Name, First Name, Middle Initial)	10. IS PATIENT'S CONDITION RELATED TO:	11. INSURED'S POLICY GROUP OR FECA NUMBER
Barnes, Agusta, E		A4612

a. OTHER INSURED'S POLICY OR GROUP NUMBER	a. EMPLOYMENT? (Current or Previous)	a. INSURED'S DATE OF BIRTH SEX
MEDIGAP 419167272	[ ] YES [X] NO	MM 08 DD 29 YY 1917 M [X] F [ ]

b. RESERVED FOR NUCC USE	b. AUTO ACCIDENT? PLACE (State)	b. OTHER CLAIM ID (Designated by NUCC)
	[ ] YES [X] NO	

c. RESERVED FOR NUCC USE	c. OTHER ACCIDENT?	c. INSURANCE PLAN NAME OR PROGRAM NAME
	[ ] YES [X] NO	ABC Insurance Company

d. INSURANCE PLAN NAME OR PROGRAM NAME	10d. CLAIM CODES (Designated by NUCC)	d. IS THERE ANOTHER HEALTH BENEFIT PLAN?
CALFCA002		[X] YES [ ] NO If yes, complete items 9, 9a, and 9d.

READ BACK OF FORM BEFORE COMPLETING & SIGNING THIS FORM.

12. PATIENT'S OR AUTHORIZED PERSON'S SIGNATURE I authorize the release of any medical or other information necessary to process this claim. I also request payment of government benefits either to myself or to the party who accepts assignment below.

SIGNED _Agusta E. Barnes_   DATE _11/21/XX_

13. INSURED'S OR AUTHORIZED PERSON'S SIGNATURE I authorize payment of medical benefits to the undersigned physician or supplier for services described below.

SIGNED _Agusta E. Barnes_

14. DATE OF CURRENT: ILLNESS, INJURY, or PREGNANCY(LMP) MM DD YY QUAL.	15. OTHER DATE QUAL. MM DD YY	16. DATES PATIENT UNABLE TO WORK IN CURRENT OCCUPATION FROM MM DD YY TO MM DD YY

17. NAME OF REFERRING PROVIDER OR OTHER SOURCE	17a.	18. HOSPITALIZATION DATES RELATED TO CURRENT SERVICES
DN Gaston Input MD	17b. NPI 32783127XX	FROM MM DD YY TO MM DD YY

19. ADDITIONAL CLAIM INFORMATION (Designated by NUCC)	20. OUTSIDE LAB? $ CHARGES
	[ ] YES [X] NO

21. DIAGNOSIS OR NATURE OF ILLNESS OR INJURY Relate A-L to service line below (24E)   ICD Ind. 0

A. R07.89   B. ___   C. ___   D. ___
E. ___   F. ___   G. ___   H. ___
I. ___   J. ___   K. ___   L. ___

22. RESUBMISSION CODE   ORIGINAL REF. NO.
23. PRIOR AUTHORIZATION NUMBER

24. A. DATE(S) OF SERVICE From To	B. PLACE OF SERVICE	C. EMG	D. PROCEDURES, SERVICES, OR SUPPLIES (Explain Unusual Circumstances) CPT/HCPCS MODIFIER	E. DIAGNOSIS POINTER	F. $ CHARGES	G. DAYS OR UNITS	H. EPSDT Family Plan	I. ID. QUAL.	J. RENDERING PROVIDER ID. #
1 11 21 XX	11		93350	A	183 00	1		NPI	67805027XX
2 11 21 XX	11		93017	A	68 00	1		NPI	67805027XX
3								NPI	
4								NPI	
5								NPI	
6								NPI	

25. FEDERAL TAX I.D. NUMBER SSN EIN	26. PATIENT'S ACCOUNT NO.	27. ACCEPT ASSIGNMENT? (For govt. claims, see back)	28. TOTAL CHARGE	29. AMOUNT PAID	30. Rsvd for NUCC Use
[ ][ ]	060	[X] YES [ ] NO	$ 251 00	$	$

31. SIGNATURE OF PHYSICIAN OR SUPPLIER INCLUDING DEGREES OR CREDENTIALS (I certify that the statements on the reverse apply to this bill and are made a part thereof.) Perry Cardi MD 112220XX SIGNED _Perry Cardi, MD_ DATE	32. SERVICE FACILITY LOCATION INFORMATION a. NPI b.	33. BILLING PROVIDER INFO & PH # (555) 4869002 College Clinic 4567 Broad Avenue Woodland Hills XY 12345-0001 a. 3664021CC b.

NUCC Instruction Manual available at: www.nucc.org   PLEASE PRINT OR TYPE   OMB APPROVAL PENDING

FIGURE 7-7 Example of a completed CMS-1500 (02-12) Health Insurance Claim Form for a Medicare (primary) and Medigap (secondary) crossover claim.

OTHER INSURANCE/MEDICARE-MSP
(primary)   (secondary)

DRAFT - NOT FOR OFFICIAL USE

HEALTH INSURANCE CLAIM FORM

APPROVED BY NATIONAL UNIFOR MCLAIM COMMITTEE (NUCC) 02/12

| | PICA | | | | | | PICA | |

1. MEDICARE [X] (Medicare#) MEDICAID [ ] (Medicaid#) TRICARE [ ] (ID#DoD#) CHAMPVA [ ] (Member ID#) GROUP HEALTH PLAN [X] (ID#) FECA BLK LUNG [ ] (ID#) OTHER [ ] (ID#)

1a. INSURED'S I.D. NUMBER (For Program in Item 1)
609 XX 5523A

2. PATIENT'S NAME (Last Name, First Name, Middle Initial)
Blair, Gwendolyn

3. PATIENT'S BIRTH DATE MM 09 DD 01 YY 1931 SEX M [ ] F [X]

4. INSURED'S NAME (Last Name, First Name, Middle Initial)
Blair, Gwendolyn

5. PATIENT'S ADDRESS (No., Street)
416 Richmond Street

6. PATIENT RELATIONSHIP TO INSURED
Self [X] Spouse [ ] Child [ ] Other [ ]

7. INSURED'S ADDRESS (No., Street)
416 Richmond Street

CITY Woodland Hills   **STATE** XY

8. RESERVED FOR NUCC USE

CITY Woodland Hills   **STATE** XY

ZIP CODE 12345-0000   **TELEPHONE** (Include Area Code) (555) 4591519

ZIP CODE 12345-0000   **TELEPHONE** (Include Area Code) (555) 4591519

9. OTHER INSURED'S NAME (Last Name, First Name, Middle Initial)
Blair, Gwendolyn

10. IS PATIENT'S CONDITION RELATED TO:

11. INSURED'S POLICY GROUP OR FECA NUMBER
7845931Q

a. OTHER INSURED'S POLICY OR GROUP NUMBER
609 XX 5523A

a. EMPLOYMENT? (Current or Previous) [ ] YES [X] NO

a. INSURED'S DATE OF BIRTH MM 09 DD 01 YY 1931 SEX M [ ] F [X]

b. RESERVED FOR NUCC USE

b. AUTO ACCIDENT? [ ] YES [X] NO PLACE (State)

b. OTHER CLAIM ID (Designated by NUCC)

c. RESERVED FOR NUCC USE

c. OTHER ACCIDENT? [ ] YES [X] NO

c. INSURANCE PLAN NAME OR PROGRAM NAME
ABC Insurance Company

d. INSURANCE PLAN NAME OR PROGRAM NAME
Medicare

10d. CLAIM CODES (Designated by NUCC)

d. IS THERE ANOTHER HEALTH BENEFIT PLAN?
[X] YES [ ] NO   *If yes,* complete items 9, 9a, and 9d.

READ BACK OF FORM BEFORE COMPLETING & SIGNING THIS FORM.
12. PATIENT'S OR AUTHORIZED PERSON'S SIGNATURE I authorize the release of any medical or other information necessary to process this claim. I also request payment of government benefits either to myself or to the party who accepts assignment below.

SIGNED Signature on file   DATE

13. INSURED'S OR AUTHORIZED PERSON'S SIGNATURE I authorize payment of medical benefits to the undersigned physician or supplier for services described below.

SIGNED Signature on file

14. DATE OF CURRENT: ILLNESS, INJURY, or PREGNANCY(LMP) MM DD YY QUAL.

15. OTHER DATE QUAL. MM DD YY

16. DATES PATIENT UNABLE TO WORK IN CURRENT OCCUPATION
FROM MM DD YY TO MM DD YY

17. NAME OF REFERRING PROVIDER OR OTHER SOURCE
DN Gerald Practon MD

17a.
17b. NPI 46278897XX

18. HOSPITALIZATION DATES RELATED TO CURRENT SERVICES
FROM MM DD YY TO MM DD YY

19. ADDITIONAL CLAIM INFORMATION (Designated by NUCC)

20. OUTSIDE LAB? [ ] YES [X] NO $ CHARGES

21. DIAGNOSIS OR NATURE OF ILLNESS OR INJURY Relate A-L to service line below (24E)   ICD Ind. 0

A. B35.1   B. ___   C. ___   D. ___
E. ___   F. ___   G. ___   H. ___
I. ___   J. ___   K. ___   L. ___

22. RESUBMISSION CODE   ORIGINAL REF. NO.

23. PRIOR AUTHORIZATION NUMBER

24. A. DATE(S) OF SERVICE From MM DD YY	To MM DD YY	B. PLACE OF SERVICE	C. EMG	D. PROCEDURES, SERVICES, OR SUPPLIES (Explain Unusual Circumstances) CPT/HCPCS	MODIFIER	E. DIAGNOSIS POINTER	F. $ CHARGES	G. DAYS OR UNITS	H. EPSDT Family Plan	I. ID. QUAL.	J. RENDERING PROVIDER ID. #
1 03 15 XX		11		99243	25	A	103 00	1		NPI	54022287XX
2 03 15 XX		11		11750		A	193 00	1		NPI	54022287XX
3										NPI	
4										NPI	
5										NPI	
6										NPI	

25. FEDERAL TAX I.D. NUMBER XX12210XX   SSN [ ] EIN [X]

26. PATIENT'S ACCOUNT NO. 070

27. ACCEPT ASSIGNMENT? (For govt. claims, see back) [X] YES [ ] NO

28. TOTAL CHARGE $ 296 00

29. AMOUNT PAID $ 100 00

30. Rsvd for NUCC Use $

31. SIGNATURE OF PHYSICIAN OR SUPPLIER INCLUDING DEGREES OR CREDENTIALS (I certify that the statements on the reverse apply to this bill and are made a part thereof.)
Nick Pedro DPM   031620XX
SIGNED *Nick Pedro, DPM* DATE

32. SERVICE FACILITY LOCATION INFORMATION

a. NPI   b.

33. BILLING PROVIDER INFO & PH # (555) 4869002
College Clinic
4567 Broad Avenue
Woodland Hills XY 12345-0001

a. 3664021CC   b.

NUCC Instruction Manual available at: www.nucc.org   *PLEASE PRINT OR TYPE*   OMB APPROVAL PENDING

FIGURE 7-8 Template for a case in which another insurance carrier is the primary payer and Medicare is the secondary payer (MSP).

TRICARE
NO SECONDARY COVERAGE

← CARRIER

HEALTH INSURANCE CLAIM FORM

APPROVED BY NATIONAL UNIFOR MCLAIM COMMITTEE (NUCC) 02/12

| | PICA | | | | | | PICA | |

1. MEDICARE	MEDICAID	TRICARE	CHAMPVA	GROUP HEALTH PLAN	FECA BLK LUNG	OTHER	1a. INSURED'S I.D. NUMBER (For Program in Item 1)
(Medicare#)	(Medicaid#)	X (ID#DoD#)	(Member ID#)	(ID#)	(ID#)	(ID#)	581147211

2. PATIENT'S NAME (Last Name, First Name, Middle Initial)
Smith, Susan, J

3. PATIENT'S BIRTH DATE   SEX
MM 03 | DD 16 | YY 1976   M☐ F☒

4. INSURED'S NAME (Last Name, First Name, Middle Initial)
Smith, William D

5. PATIENT'S ADDRESS (No., Street)
420 Maple Street

6. PATIENT RELATIONSHIP TO INSURED
Self☐ Spouse☒ Child☐ Other☐

7. INSURED'S ADDRESS (No., Street)
420 Maple Street

CITY
Woodland Hills
STATE XY

8. RESERVED FOR NUCC USE

CITY
Woodland Hills
STATE XY

ZIP CODE 12345-0000
TELEPHONE (Include Area Code) (555) 7899898

ZIP CODE 12345-0000
TELEPHONE (Include Area Code) (555) 7899898

9. OTHER INSURED'S NAME (Last Name, First Name, Middle Initial)

10. IS PATIENT'S CONDITION RELATED TO:

11. INSURED'S POLICY GROUP OR FECA NUMBER

a. OTHER INSURED'S POLICY OR GROUP NUMBER

a. EMPLOYMENT? (Current or Previous)
☐ YES ☒ NO

a. INSURED'S DATE OF BIRTH   SEX
MM 06 | DD 12 | YY 1974   M☒ F☐

b. RESERVED FOR NUCC USE

b. AUTO ACCIDENT?
☐ YES ☒ NO   PLACE (State)

b. OTHER CLAIM ID (Designated by NUCC)

c. RESERVED FOR NUCC USE

c. OTHER ACCIDENT?
☐ YES ☒ NO

c. INSURANCE PLAN NAME OR PROGRAM NAME
TRICARE

d. INSURANCE PLAN NAME OR PROGRAM NAME

10d. CLAIM CODES (Designated by NUCC)

d. IS THERE ANOTHER HEALTH BENEFIT PLAN?
☐ YES ☒ NO If yes, complete items 9, 9a, and 9d.

READ BACK OF FORM BEFORE COMPLETING & SIGNING THIS FORM.
12. PATIENT'S OR AUTHORIZED PERSON'S SIGNATURE I authorize the release of any medical or other information necessary to process this claim. I also request payment of government benefits either to myself or to the party who accepts assignment below.

SIGNED Signature on file   DATE

13. INSURED'S OR AUTHORIZED PERSON'S SIGNATURE I authorize payment of medical benefits to the undersigned physician or supplier for services described below.

SIGNED Signature on file

14. DATE OF CURRENT: ILLNESS, INJURY, or PREGNANCY(LMP)
MM 10 | DD 28 | YY 20XX   QUAL. 484

15. OTHER DATE
QUAL.   MM | DD | YY

16. DATES PATIENT UNABLE TO WORK IN CURRENT OCCUPATION
FROM 07 21 20XX TO 09 17 20XX

17. NAME OF REFERRING PROVIDER OR OTHER SOURCE
DN Adam Langerhans MD

17a.
17b. NPI 47680657XX

18. HOSPITALIZATION DATES RELATED TO CURRENT SERVICES
FROM 08 06 20XX TO 08 08 20XX

19. ADDITIONAL CLAIM INFORMATION (Designated by NUCC)

20. OUTSIDE LAB? ☐ YES ☒ NO $ CHARGES

21. DIAGNOSIS OR NATURE OF ILLNESS OR INJURY Relate A-L to service line below (24E)   ICD Ind. 0

A. O80   B. ____   C. ____   D. ____
E. ____   F. ____   G. ____   H. ____
I. ____   J. ____   K. ____   L. ____

22. RESUBMISSION CODE   ORIGINAL REF. NO.

23. PRIOR AUTHORIZATION NUMBER

24. A. DATE(S) OF SERVICE From / To	B. PLACE OF SERVICE	C. EMG	D. PROCEDURES, SERVICES, OR SUPPLIES (Explain Unusual Circumstances) CPT/HCPCS	MODIFIER	E. DIAGNOSIS POINTER	F. $ CHARGES	G. DAYS OR UNITS	H. EPSDT Family Plan	I. ID. QUAL.	J. RENDERING PROVIDER ID. #
1	08 06 XX	21		59400		A	1864 00	1		NPI	43056757XX
2										NPI	
3										NPI	
4										NPI	
5										NPI	
6										NPI	

25. FEDERAL TAX I.D. NUMBER   SSN EIN
XX12210XX   ☐ ☒

26. PATIENT'S ACCOUNT NO.
080

27. ACCEPT ASSIGNMENT? (For govt. claims, see back)
☒ YES ☐ NO

28. TOTAL CHARGE
$ 1864 00

29. AMOUNT PAID
$

30. Rsvd for NUCC Use
$

31. SIGNATURE OF PHYSICIAN OR SUPPLIER INCLUDING DEGREES OR CREDENTIALS (I certify that the statements on the reverse apply to this bill and are made a part thereof.)
Bertha Caesar MD   081020XX
SIGNED Bertha Caesar, M.D. DATE

32. SERVICE FACILITY LOCATION INFORMATION
College Hospital
4500 Broad Avenue
Woodland Hills XY 12345-0001
a. X950731067   b.

33. BILLING PROVIDER INFO & PH # (555) 4869002
College Clinic
4567 Broad Avenue
Woodland Hills XY 12345-0001
a. 3664021CC   b.

NUCC Instruction Manual available at: www.nucc.org   PLEASE PRINT OR TYPE   OMB APPROVAL PENDING

FIGURE 7-9 Example of a completed CMS-1500 (02-12) claim form used when billing for professional services rendered in a TRICARE standard case.

CHAMPVA
NO SECONDARY COVERAGE →

HEALTH INSURANCE CLAIM FORM

APPROVED BY NATIONAL UNIFOR MCLAIM COMMITTEE (NUCC) 02/12

| | PICA | | | | | | | | PICA | |

1. MEDICARE	MEDICAID	TRICARE	CHAMPVA	GROUP HEALTH PLAN	FECA BLK LUNG	OTHER	1a. INSURED'S I.D. NUMBER (For Program in Item 1)
(Medicare#)	(Medicaid#)	(ID#DoD#)	[X] (Member ID#)	(ID#)	(ID#)	(ID#)	560 XX 4444

2. PATIENT'S NAME (Last Name, First Name, Middle Initial)	3. PATIENT'S BIRTH DATE / SEX	4. INSURED'S NAME (Last Name, First Name, Middle Initial)
Dexter, Bruce, R	MM 03 DD 13 YY 1934 M [X] F [ ]	Dexter, Bruce, R

5. PATIENT'S ADDRESS (No., Street)	6. PATIENT RELATIONSHIP TO INSURED	7. INSURED'S ADDRESS (No., Street)
226 Irwin Road	Self [X] Spouse [ ] Child [ ] Other [ ]	226 Irwin Road

CITY	STATE	8. RESERVED FOR NUCC USE	CITY	STATE
Woodland Hills	XY		Woodland Hills	XY

ZIP CODE	TELEPHONE (Include Area Code)	ZIP CODE	TELEPHONE (Include Area Code)
12345-0000	(555) 4971338	12345-0000	(555) 4971338

9. OTHER INSURED'S NAME (Last Name, First Name, Middle Initial)	10. IS PATIENT'S CONDITION RELATED TO:	11. INSURED'S POLICY GROUP OR FECA NUMBER
		023

a. OTHER INSURED'S POLICY OR GROUP NUMBER	a. EMPLOYMENT? (Current or Previous) [X] YES [ ] NO	a. INSURED'S DATE OF BIRTH MM 03 DD 13 YY 1934 SEX M [X] F [ ]

b. RESERVED FOR NUCC USE	b. AUTO ACCIDENT? [ ] YES [X] NO PLACE (State)	b. OTHER CLAIM ID (Designated by NUCC)

c. RESERVED FOR NUCC USE	c. OTHER ACCIDENT? [ ] YES [X] NO	c. INSURANCE PLAN NAME OR PROGRAM NAME CHAMPVA

d. INSURANCE PLAN NAME OR PROGRAM NAME	10d. CLAIM CODES (Designated by NUCC)	d. IS THERE ANOTHER HEALTH BENEFIT PLAN? [ ] YES [X] NO *If yes*, complete items 9, 9a, and 9d.

READ BACK OF FORM BEFORE COMPLETING & SIGNING THIS FORM.

12. PATIENT'S OR AUTHORIZED PERSON'S SIGNATURE I authorize the release of any medical or other information necessary to process this claim. I also request payment of government benefits either to myself or to the party who accepts assignment below.

SIGNED Signature on file   DATE

13. INSURED'S OR AUTHORIZED PERSON'S SIGNATURE I authorize payment of medical benefits to the undersigned physician or supplier for services described below.

SIGNED Signature on file

14. DATE OF CURRENT: ILLNESS, INJURY, or PREGNANCY(LMP) MM DD YY QUAL.	15. OTHER DATE QUAL. MM DD YY	16. DATES PATIENT UNABLE TO WORK IN CURRENT OCCUPATION FROM MM DD YY TO MM DD YY

17. NAME OF REFERRING PROVIDER OR OTHER SOURCE DN Gerald Practon MD	17a.	18. HOSPITALIZATION DATES RELATED TO CURRENT SERVICES FROM MM 07 DD 29 YY 20XX TO MM 07 DD 31 YY 20XX
	17b. NPI 46278897XX	

19. ADDITIONAL CLAIM INFORMATION (Designated by NUCC)	20. OUTSIDE LAB? [ ] YES [X] NO $ CHARGES

21. DIAGNOSIS OR NATURE OF ILLNESS OR INJURY Relate A-L to service line below (24E)   ICD Ind. 0

A. N40.0   B.   C.   D.

E.   F.   G.   H.

I.   J.   K.   L.

22. RESUBMISSION CODE   ORIGINAL REF. NO.

23. PRIOR AUTHORIZATION NUMBER

24. A. DATE(S) OF SERVICE From MM DD YY To MM DD YY	B. PLACE OF SERVICE	C. EMG	D. PROCEDURES, SERVICES, OR SUPPLIES (Explain Unusual Circumstances) CPT/HCPCS MODIFIER	E. DIAGNOSIS POINTER	F. $ CHARGES	G. DAYS OR UNITS	H. EPSDT Family Plan	I. ID. QUAL.	J. RENDERING PROVIDER ID. #
1 07 29 XX	21		52601	A	1193 00	1		NPI	25678831XX
2								NPI	
3								NPI	
4								NPI	
5								NPI	
6								NPI	

25. FEDERAL TAX I.D. NUMBER SSN EIN	26. PATIENT'S ACCOUNT NO.	27. ACCEPT ASSIGNMENT? (For govt. claims, see back)	28. TOTAL CHARGE	29. AMOUNT PAID	30. Rsvd for NUCC Use
XX12210XX [ ] [X]	090	[X] YES [ ] NO	$ 1193 00	$	$

31. SIGNATURE OF PHYSICIAN OR SUPPLIER INCLUDING DEGREES OR CREDENTIALS (I certify that the statements on the reverse apply to this bill and are made a part thereof.) Gene Ulibarri MD 073020XX SIGNED *Gene Ulibarri MD* DATE	32. SERVICE FACILITY LOCATION INFORMATION College Hospital 4500 Broad Avenue Woodland Hills XY 12345-0001	33. BILLING PROVIDER INFO & PH # (555) 4869002 College Clinic 4567 Broad Avenue Woodland Hills XY 12345-0001
	a. X950731067 b.	a. 3664021CC b.

NUCC Instruction Manual available at: www.nucc.org   PLEASE PRINT OR TYPE   OMB APPROVAL PENDING

FIGURE 7-10 An example of a completed CMS-1500 (02-12) Health Insurance Claim Form for a CHAMPVA case with no secondary coverage.

WORKERS' COMPENSATION

DRAFT - NOT FOR OFFICIAL USE

HEALTH INSURANCE CLAIM FORM

APPROVED BY NATIONAL UNIFOR MCLAIM COMMITTEE (NUCC) 02/12

| | PICA | | | | | | | | | | PICA | | |

1. MEDICARE ☐ (Medicare#)	MEDICAID ☐ (Medicaid#)	TRICARE ☐ (ID#DoD#)	CHAMPVA ☐ (Member ID#)	GROUP HEALTH PLAN ☐ (ID#)	FECA BLK LUNG ☐ (ID#)	OTHER ☒ (ID#)	1a. INSURED'S I.D. NUMBER (For Program in Item 1)
							667289

2. PATIENT'S NAME (Last Name, First Name, Middle Initial)	3. PATIENT'S BIRTH DATE	4. INSURED'S NAME (Last Name, First Name, Middle Initial)
Barton, Peter, A	MM 11 DD 14 YY 1976 SEX M ☒ F ☐	D F Construction

5. PATIENT'S ADDRESS (No., Street)	6. PATIENT RELATIONSHIP TO INSURED	7. INSURED'S ADDRESS (No., Street)
14890 Daisy Avenue	Self ☐ Spouse ☐ Child ☐ Other ☒	1212 Hardrock Place
CITY Woodland Hills	STATE XY	8. RESERVED FOR NUCC USE	CITY Woodland Hills	STATE XY
ZIP CODE 12345-0000	TELEPHONE (Include Area Code) (555) 4277698		ZIP CODE 12345-0000	TELEPHONE (Include Area Code) (555) 4278200

9. OTHER INSURED'S NAME (Last Name, First Name, Middle Initial)	10. IS PATIENT'S CONDITION RELATED TO:	11. INSURED'S POLICY GROUP OR FECA NUMBER
a. OTHER INSURED'S POLICY OR GROUP NUMBER	a. EMPLOYMENT? (Current or Previous) ☒ YES ☐ NO	a. INSURED'S DATE OF BIRTH MM DD YY SEX M ☐ F ☐
b. RESERVED FOR NUCC USE	b. AUTO ACCIDENT? ☐ YES ☒ NO PLACE (State)	b. OTHER CLAIM ID (Designated by NUCC)
c. RESERVED FOR NUCC USE	c. OTHER ACCIDENT? ☐ YES ☒ NO	c. INSURANCE PLAN NAME OR PROGRAM NAME
d. INSURANCE PLAN NAME OR PROGRAM NAME	10d. CLAIM CODES (Designated by NUCC)	d. IS THERE ANOTHER HEALTH BENEFIT PLAN? ☐ YES ☐ NO If yes, complete items 9, 9a, and 9d.

READ BACK OF FORM BEFORE COMPLETING & SIGNING THIS FORM.

12. PATIENT'S OR AUTHORIZED PERSON'S SIGNATUREI authorize the release of any medical or other information necessary to process this claim. I also request payment of government benefits either to myself or to the party who accepts assignment below.

SIGNED _Signature on file_ DATE _____

13. INSURED'S OR AUTHORIZED PERSON'S SIGNATURE I authorize payment of medical benefits to the undersigned physician or supplier for services described below.

SIGNED _____

14. DATE OF CURRENT: ILLNESS, INJURY, or PREGNANCY(LMP) MM 01 DD 04 YY 20XX QUAL. 431	15. OTHER DATE QUAL. MM DD YY	16. DATES PATIENT UNABLE TO WORK IN CURRENT OCCUPATION FROM MM 01 DD 04 YY 20XX TO MM 03 DD 27 YY 20XX
17. NAME OF REFERRING PROVIDER OR OTHER SOURCE	17a. 17b. NPI	18. HOSPITALIZATION DATES RELATED TO CURRENT SERVICES FROM MM DD YY TO MM DD YY
19. ADDITIONAL CLAIM INFORMATION (Designated by NUCC)		20. OUTSIDE LAB? ☐ YES ☐ NO $ CHARGES

21. DIAGNOSIS OR NATURE OF ILLNESS OR INJURY Relate A-L to service line below (24E) ICD Ind. 0

A. M24.419   B. _____   C. _____   D. _____
E. _____   F. _____   G. _____   H. _____
I. _____   J. _____   K. _____   L. _____

22. RESUBMISSION CODE _____ ORIGINAL REF. NO. _____

23. PRIOR AUTHORIZATION NUMBER

24. A. DATE(S) OF SERVICE From MM DD YY	To MM DD YY	B. PLACE OF SERVICE	C. EMG	D. PROCEDURES, SERVICES, OR SUPPLIES (Explain Unusual Circumstances) CPT/HCPCS	MODIFIER	E. DIAGNOSIS POINTER	F. $ CHARGES	G. DAYS OR UNITS	H. EPSDT Family Plan	I. ID. QUAL.	J. RENDERING PROVIDER ID. #
1	02 27 XX		11		29055		A	150 00	1		NPI	12678547XX
2											NPI	
3											NPI	
4											NPI	
5											NPI	
6											NPI	

25. FEDERAL TAX I.D. NUMBER SSN EIN XX12210XX ☐ ☒	26. PATIENT'S ACCOUNT NO. 100	27. ACCEPT ASSIGNMENT? (For govt. claims, see back) ☐ YES ☐ NO	28. TOTAL CHARGE $ 150 00	29. AMOUNT PAID $	30. Rsvd for NUCC Use $

31. SIGNATURE OF PHYSICIAN OR SUPPLIER INCLUDING DEGREES OR CREDENTIALS (I certify that the statements on the reverse apply to this bill and are made a part thereof.) Raymond Skelton MD 022820XX SIGNED _Raymond Skelton, MD_ DATE	32. SERVICE FACILITY LOCATION INFORMATION a. NPI b.	33. BILLING PROVIDER INFO & PH # (555) 4869002 College Clinic 4567 Broad Avenue Woodland Hills XY 12345-0001 a. 3664021CC b.

NUCC Instruction Manual available at: www.nucc.org   PLEASE PRINT OR TYPE   OMB APPROVAL PENDING

PATIENT AND INSURED INFORMATION   *CARRIER*   *PHYSICIAN OR SUPPLIER INFORMATION*

FIGURE 7-11 An example of a completed CMS-1500 (02-12) Health Insurance Claim Form for a workers' compensation case.

KEY POINTS

This is a brief chapter review, or summary, of the key issues presented. To further enhance your knowledge of the technical subject matter, review the key terms and key abbreviations for this chapter by locating the meaning for each in the Glossary at the end of this book, which appears in a section before the Index.

1. There are two types of claims submitted to insurance companies for payment: *paper claims* and *electronic claims.*

2. A *clean claim* is one that was submitted to the third-party payer within the time limit, had the necessary information for processing, and was paid promptly. Under the Medicare program, a clean claim is one that has passed all electronic edits and is routed for payment.

3. Other types of claims are called *dirty* when a claim is submitted with errors; *incomplete* when missing required information; *invalid* when illogical or incorrect; *pending* when held in suspense for review; *rejected* when the claim needs investigation and answers to some questions; or *deleted* when the Medicare fiscal intermediary cancels, deletes, or voids a claim.

4. When two insurance policies are involved (*dual coverage* or *duplication of coverage*), one is considered primary and the other secondary. First, an insurance claim is submitted to the primary plan; after payment, the secondary carrier is billed with a copy of the explanation of benefits (EOB) from the primary carrier.

5. A diagnosis should never be submitted on an insurance claim without supporting documentation in the medical record.

6. Every insurance claim should be proofread for completeness and accuracy of content before it is submitted to the insurance carrier.

7. Be aware of common billing errors and learn how to correct them for quicker claim settlements and to reduce the number of appeals.

8. HIPAA transactions and code sets standards only apply to electronic transactions conducted by covered entities.

9. Copies of submitted insurance claim forms should be filed in a tickler file and reviewed for follow-up every 30 days unless the computer system maintains the files.

10. Ensure that the correct NPI is shown on the claim for the physician rendering the medical service to the patient.

STUDENT ASSIGNMENT

✔ Study Chapter 7.

✔ Answer the fill-in-the-blank, multiple-choice, and true/false questions in the *Workbook* to reinforce the theories learned in this chapter and to help prepare you for a future test.

✔ Complete the assignments in the *Workbook* to give you hands-on experience in abstracting information from case histories and financial accounting record cards as well as in completing insurance claim forms.

✔ Study the claim sample in the *Workbook* and try to locate as many errors as possible on the basis of the instructions you have been given in this chapter.

✔ Turn to the Glossary at the end of this text for a further understanding of the key terms and key abbreviations used in this chapter.

The Electronic Claim

Linda Smith

OBJECTIVES

After reading this chapter, you should be able to:

1. Define and discuss *electronic data interchange.*
2. Summarize the advantages of electronic claim submission.
3. Describe the clearinghouse process that follows after a claim is electronically received.
4. Identify the transactions and code sets to use for insurance claims transmission.
5. State which insurance claim data elements are required or situational for the 837P standard transaction format.
6. Define a claim attachment and discuss claim attachments standards.
7. Compare and contrast standard unique provider identifiers, health plan identifiers, and patient identifiers.
8. Describe necessary components when adopting a practice management system.
9. Describe the use of patient encounter forms and scannable encounter forms in electronic claim submission.
10. Name and discuss some methods of interactive computer transactions for transmitting insurance claims.
11. Discuss interactive transactions and relate the electronic funds transfer process and mandated requirements under the Affordable Care Act (ACA).
12. Define an electronic remittance advice and identify the ASC X12 Health Care Claim Payment/Advice (835).
13. List the six basic procedures for transmission of an electronic claim and discuss methods for sending claims.
14. Explain the difference between carrier-direct and clearinghouse electronically transmitted insurance claims.
15. List computer transmission problems that can occur.
16. List Health Insurance Portability and Accountability Act (HIPAA) administrative safeguards for electronic protected health information and discuss solutions to electronic processing problems.
17. State administrative, technical, and physical safeguards used to secure privacy of e-mail, internet, and instant messaging.
18. Explain handling of data storage and data disposal for good electronic records management.
19. Describe basic elements that should be considered when purchasing an in-office computer system.

KEY TERMS

Accredited Standards Committee X12
Accredited Standards Committee X12 Version 5010
application service provider
audit trail
back up
batch

business associate agreement
cable modem
claim attachments
clearinghouse
code sets
covered entity
data elements
digital subscriber line

direct data entry
electronic data interchange
electronic funds transfer
electronic remittance advice
encoder
encryption
HIPAA Transaction and Code Sets rule

National Standard Format	standard transactions	trading partner
password	T-1	trading partner agreement
real time	taxonomy codes	

KEY ABBREVIATIONS

ANSI	DHHS	EOMB	NDC
ASC X12	DSL	ePHI	NSF
ASET	EDI	ERA	PMS
ASP	EFT	HPID	TCS rule
ATM	EHR	IRS	UPS
DDE	EMC	MAC	

ELECTRONIC DATA INTERCHANGE

Electronic data interchange (EDI) is the exchange of data through computer systems (for example, health insurance claims are exchanged between health care providers and insurance carriers). This is a process by which understandable data are sent back and forth in a standardized format via computer linkages between entities, or **trading partners,** that function alternatively as sender and receiver. Technology and the use of EDI have made processing of transactions more efficient and reduced administrative overhead costs in health care and many other industries.

For security purposes, electronic transmissions are sent encrypted so that they cannot be opened and read if intercepted (received) by the wrong individual. **Encryption** is used to assign a "secret code" to represent data, which makes data unintelligible to unauthorized parties. In encrypted (encoded) versions, the data look like gibberish to unauthorized users and must be decoded to use or read. In electronically secure environments, the sending computer system encrypts or encodes the data being sent and the receiving computer decodes the data to make them understandable. Therefore both computers must speak the same "language." Standardizing transaction and **code sets** is required to use EDI effectively, so the industry has witnessed the implementation of standard formats, procedures, and data content through Health Insurance Portability and Accountability Act (HIPAA) regulations.

ELECTRONIC CLAIMS

An electronic claim, like a paper claim, is constructed from data that are used in the reimbursement process (the life cycle of a claim is discussed in Chapter 3). However, the method for submitting an electronic claim is EDI rather than the US Postal Service or paper fax transmission.

Since the 1960s and early 1970s, claims processing has transitioned from paper claims to electronic claims submission. As discussed in Chapter 7, the federal government has taken steps through the Administrative Simplification Compliance Act (ASCA) that require providers to submit claims electronically unless they have a waiver on file with their Medicare Administrative Contractor (MAC). Third-party payers have followed this lead, offering and encouraging electronic claims submission. Today, most health care providers submit electronic claims for reimbursement.

ADVANTAGES OF ELECTRONIC CLAIM SUBMISSION

Electronic claim submission offers many advantages to health care providers. Unlike paper claims, electronic transactions require no signature or stamp, no search for a third-party payer's address, no postage fees or trips to the post office, and no storage of claim forms in a file cabinet. Electronic transactions build an **audit trail,** which is a chronologic record of submitted data that can be traced to the source to determine the place of origin. Generally, cash flow is improved and less time is spent processing claims, thereby freeing staff for other duties. Information goes from one computer to another, which reduces overhead by decreasing labor costs and human error. After electronic submission of claims, payment can be received in 2 weeks or less. In comparison, when claims are completed manually and sent by mail, payment may take 4 to 6 weeks on average. With EDI, the audit trail offers proof of receipt and is generated by the carrier, thus eliminating the potential for insurance payers to make the excuse that the claim was never received and therefore not processed.

Another important advantage of electronic claims submission is the online error-edit process that may be incorporated in the software in the physician's office,

clearinghouse, or insurance company. This feature alerts the person processing the claim to any errors immediately so that a correction can be made before transmission of the claim. Information about problem claims can be telecommunicated immediately, allowing quicker submission of corrected or additional data.

Both paper and electronic claims begin with gathering data before, during, and after the service is rendered. You have learned that the information you need to obtain is crucial when submitting a paper claim for payment; therefore accurate information is key to successful electronic claim submission and timely reimbursement.

CLEARINGHOUSES

A clearinghouse is an entity that receives the electronic transmission of claims (EDI) from the health care provider's office and translates it to a standard format prescribed in HIPAA regulations. Once the clearinghouse receives a **batch** of claims, which is a group of claims for different patients sent at the same time from one facility, the clearinghouse's duties then include separating the claims by carrier, performing software edits on each claim to check for errors, and transmitting claims electronically to the correct insurance payer (Figure 8-1).

After receiving the claims transmission, a typical clearinghouse process is as follows:

- Claims are checked electronically (scrubbed) for missing or incorrect information using an elaborate editing process. Claims that do not meet all required data for further processing are rejected and not forwarded to the payer.
- Claims that are rejected during the editing process are sent back to the health care provider electronically along with a report that lists the needed corrections.
- Batches of claims that pass all edits are then sent to each separate insurance payer. Several claims can be submitted to various insurance payers in a single-batch electronic transmission.

Using a clearinghouse offers the following advantages:
- Translation of various formats to the HIPAA-compliant standard format
- Reduction in time of claims preparation
- Cost-effective method through loss prevention
- Fewer claim rejections
- Fewer delays in processing and quicker response time
- More accurate coding with claims edits
- Consistent reimbursement

Some medical practices choose not to use the services of a clearinghouse and have carrier-direct links to the insurance companies. For example, Centers for Medicare and Medicaid Services (CMS) allows claims to be submitted electronically to a MAC if they are using a computer with software that meets electronic filing requirements as established under HIPAA claim standards. Institutional

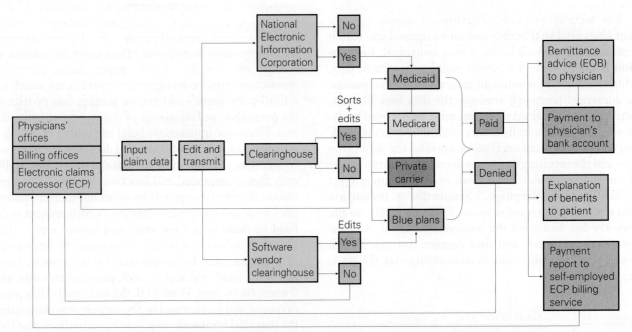

FIGURE 8-1 Flow sheet of electronic transmission systems showing path for claim payment via the National Electronic Information Corporation (NEIC), clearinghouse, and independent software vendor. This system also indicates when a payment is made to the physician and depicts where claims may not pass an edit or are denied. *EOB,* Explanation of benefits.

claims can be submitted to CMS MACs via direct data entry screens. The system called *electronic medical claims (EMCs)* is used for nearly all Medicare transactions, including claims submission, payment, direct deposit, online eligibility verification, coordination of benefits, and claims status.

TRANSACTION AND CODE SETS REGULATIONS: STREAMLINING ELECTRONIC DATA INTERCHANGE

Under HIPAA Title II Administrative Simplification, the Secretary of the United States Department of Health and Human Services (DHHS) is required to adopt standards to support the electronic exchange of health care transactions primarily between health care providers and plans. The purposes and objectives of this component of HIPAA were to achieve a higher quality of care and reduce administrative costs by streamlining the processing of routine administrative and financial transactions. As a result, the **HIPAA Transaction and Code Sets (TCS) rule** was developed to introduce efficiencies in the health care system. The DHHS estimated that by implementing TCS almost $30 billion over 10 years would be saved.

The intent of TCS requirements is to achieve a single standard. For example, in the pre-HIPAA environment, when submitting claims for payment, health care providers had been doing business with insurance payers who required the use of their own version of local code sets (for example, state Medicaid programs). A code set is any set of codes with their descriptions used to encode **data elements,** such as a table of terms, medical concepts, medical diagnostic codes, or medical procedure codes. Prior to HIPAA, there were more than 400 versions of a **National Standard Format (NSF)** that existed to submit a claim for payment. The TCS regulation required implementation of specific standards for transactions and code sets by October 16, 2003.

HIPAA standardization actions are similar to using a bank's automatic teller machine (ATM) or the grocery store's self-checkout. A magnetic strip on a bank card or the bar code on a grocery item can be swiped across a scanning device, allowing customers to process a transaction more quickly than with traditional methods. As these methods are adapted, there are benefits to both the end user and the business providing the technology (Table 8-1). Health care providers' offices benefit from less paperwork and standardizing data results in more accurate information and a more efficient organization.

As discussed in Chapter 2, HIPAA governs how a **covered entity** may handle health information. Whether a

Table 8-1	Recognized Benefits of Transaction and Code Sets and Electronic Data Interchange
BENEFIT	**RESULT**
More reliable and timely processing—quicker reimbursement from payer	Fast eligibility evaluation; reduced time in claim life cycle; industry averages for claim turnarounds are 9 to 15 days for electronic versus 30 to 45 days for paper claims, improving cash flow
Improved accuracy of data	Decreases processing time, increases data quality, and leads to better reporting
Easier and more efficient access to information	Improves patient support
Better tracking of transactions	Assists tracking of transactions (that is, when sent and received), allowing for monitoring (for example, prompt payments)
Reduction of data entry/manual labor	Electronic transactions assist automated processes (for example, automatic payment posting)
Reduction in office expenses	Lowers office supplies, postage, and telephone expenses

Data from HIPAAdocs Corporation, Columbia, Md.

provider transmits health information in electronic form in connection with a transaction covered by HIPAA will determine whether a provider is considered a covered entity (Figure 8-2). Under HIPAA, the following circumstances would likely make the provider a covered entity:

- If the provider submits electronic transactions to any payer, the provider is considered a covered entity.
- Large providers: If the provider submits paper claims to Medicare and has 10 or more employees, the provider is required to convert to electronic transactions no later than October 16, 2003. Therefore HIPAA compliance is required.

A provider is *not* considered a covered entity under HIPAA in the following circumstances:

- Small providers: If the provider has fewer than 10 employees and submits claims only on paper to Medicare (not electronically). The provider may continue to submit on paper and therefore is not required to comply with HIPAA guidelines (that is, not required to submit electronically).
- If the provider submitted only paper claims until and after April 14, 2003, and does not send claims to Medicare, the provider is not required to comply with sending electronic claims.

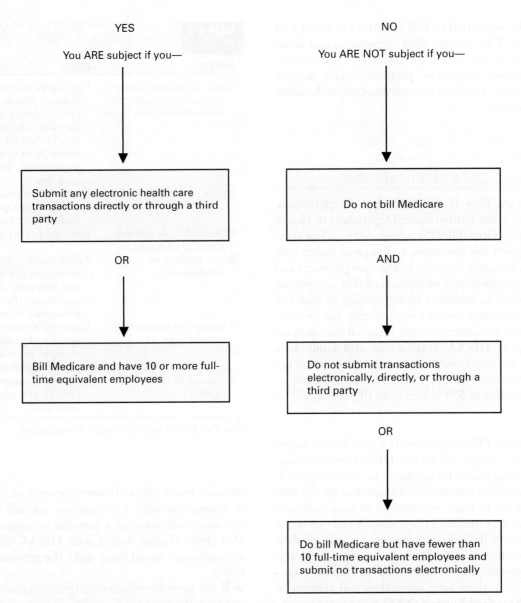

YES
You ARE subject if you—

Submit any electronic health care transactions directly or through a third party

OR

Bill Medicare and have 10 or more full-time equivalent employees

NO
You ARE NOT subject if you—

Do not bill Medicare

AND

Do not submit transactions electronically, directly, or through a third party

OR

Do bill Medicare but have fewer than 10 full-time equivalent employees and submit no transactions electronically

FIGURE 8-2 Decision flow chart of who is subject to the HIPAA Transaction and Code Sets (TCS) rule.

HIPAA Compliance Alert — PROVIDERS WHO MUST SUBMIT CLAIMS ELECTRONICALLY

According to CMS, "Providers who are **not** small providers (institutional organizations with fewer than 25 full-time employees or physicians with fewer than 10 full-time employees) **must** send all claims electronically in the HIPAA format."

Transaction and Code Sets Standards

TCS standards have been adopted for health care transactions. HIPAA **standard transactions** are the specific electronic file formats in which medical data are compiled to be used throughout the health care industry.

In general, code sets are the allowable sets of codes that anyone could use to enter into a specific space (field) on a form. All health care organizations using electronic transactions have to use and accept (either directly or through a clearinghouse) the code sets systems required under HIPAA that document specific health care data elements, including medical diagnoses and procedures, drugs, physician services, and medical suppliers. These codes have already been in common use throughout the industry and should have helped ease the transition to the new transaction requirements. What was a standard in the health care industry and recognized by most payers has now been *mandated* under HIPAA.

HIPAA standard codes are used in conjunction with the standard electronic transactions. This standardization

Table 8-2 | HIPAA Medical Code Sets and Elements

STANDARD CODE SETS	MEDICAL DATA ELEMENTS
Healthcare Common Procedure Coding System (HCPCS)	Items and supplies and non-physician services not covered by the American Medical Association's (AMA's) CPT-4 codes
Current Procedure Terminology (CPT) codes	Medical procedures and physicians services
International Classification of Diseases, Tenth revision, Clinical Modifications (ICD-10-CM)	Diseases, injuries, impairments, and other health-related problems and their manifestations
International Classification of Diseases, Tenth revision, Procedural Coding System (ICD-10-PCS)	Procedures or other actions taken for diseases, injuries, and impairments on hospital inpatients reported by hospitals, including prevention, diagnosis, treatment, and management
International Classification of Diseases, Ninth revision, Clinical Modifications, Volumes 1 and 2 (ICD-9-CM)	Diseases, injuries, impairments, and other health-related problems and their manifestations
International Classification of Diseases, Ninth revision, Clinical Modifications, Volume 3 (ICD-9-CM)	Procedures or other actions taken for diseases, injuries, and impairments on hospital inpatients reported by hospitals, including prevention, diagnosis, treatment, and management
National Drug Code (NDC)	Pharmaceuticals and biologics
Code on Dental Procedures and Nomenclature, Current Dental Terminology (CDT)	Dental services
Place of service (POS) codes	Indicates the setting in which services are provided

eliminates ambiguity when processing transactions. In turn, it improves the quality of data submitted for processing and improves the reimbursement cycle. *Medical code sets* are data elements used uniformly to document why patients are seen (that is, diagnosis, ICD-10-CM) and what is done to them during their encounter (that is, procedure, CPT-4, and HCPCS). Each covered entity organization is responsible for implementing the updated codes in a timely manner and deleting old or obsolete ones (Table 8-2). Because of this, medical practices may opt to subscribe to coding software or data files that have frequent updates and include new, updated, and deleted codes. Deleted codes become obsolete but are not removed because they have been used when billing past accounts.

Data Requirements

Your role as an insurance billing specialist will likely require you to understand which data elements are required to construct a HIPAA standard transaction compared to those essential for a paper CMS-1500 (02-12) form or an electronic claim.

The office's practice management software system produces the required HIPAA standard electronic formats. If the software is not capable of producing such formats, the continued use of clearinghouses eliminates much of the confusion by translating to the HIPAA standard format. You will be trained on the practice management software system as to where to insert or input additionally captured data that have not been collected on the CMS-1500 (02-12) or electronic claim.

HIPAA Compliance Alert — STANDARD TRANSACTION

When a patient comes to your office and is treated, his or her confidential health information is collected and put in the computerized practice management system (PMS). The services rendered are assigned a standard code from the HIPAA-required *code sets* (for example, CPT) and the diagnosis is selected from another code set (for example, ICD-10-CM). When claims are generated for electronic submission, all data collected are compiled and constructed into a HIPAA *standard transaction*. This electronic data interchange (EDI) is recognized across the health care sector in computers maintained by providers, clearinghouses, and insurance payers. The harmony among the covered entities results in a more efficient claim life cycle.

Required and Situational

In addition to the major code sets (ICD-10 and CPT/HCPCS), several *supporting code sets* encompass both medical and nonmedical data. When constructing a claim, the supporting code sets are made up of "Required" and "Situational" data elements, similar to those on the CMS-1500 (02-12) paper form. These supporting code sets are embedded in the data elements identified by the HIPAA standard electronic formats. You do not need to know all of these specific codes but it is helpful to know that they do exist, especially if you are active in the claims processing procedures. When reviewing reports from the clearinghouse or the insurance payer, you may have to correct claims that were rejected for not having correct data elements.

Required refers to data elements that must be used to be in compliance with a HIPAA standard transaction. Conversely, *situational* means that the item depends on the data content or context (Examples 8-1 and 8-2). For the required and situational status of data elements when electronically transmitting HIPAA-compliant electronic

Example 8-1	Required Data

Patient's birth date.
Patient's gender.

Example 8-2	Situational Data

Baby's birth weight when an infant is delivered.
Last menstrual period (LMP) when a woman is pregnant.

claim files (837P claims), refer to the extreme right column of Table 8-5, which appears later in this chapter.

Determining the required and situational data elements not currently collected for the CMS-1500 (02-12) claim or NSF electronic format can be complex; you will learn this process when you are in the office performing claims processing duties. As an insurance billing specialist, you are directly involved in the claims processing procedures and need to know the most important items to look for related to required and situational data to successfully construct a compliant and payable insurance claim.

In addition to other data elements required under HIPAA TCS standards, examples include the following:

Taxonomy Codes: Taxonomy is defined as the science of classification; thus these are numeric and alpha provider specialty codes (10 characters in length) that classify each health care provider. The taxonomy codes are self-selected by the provider, organized based on education and training, and used to define specialty, not specific services that are rendered. Common **taxonomy codes** include "general practice 208D0000X," "family practice 207Q00000X," and "nurse practitioner 363L00000X." Beginning January 2, 2007, CMS required providers submitting claims for their primary facility to include a taxonomy code. This code allows crosswalking to the Online Survey Certification and Reporting (OSCAR) system. Taxonomy codes are necessary because some institutional providers may choose not to apply for a unique national provider number for each of its subparts (for example, psychiatric unit or rehabilitation unit). Taxonomy codes are maintained by the National Uniform Claim Committee (NUCC).

Patient Account Number: To be assigned to every claim.

Relationship to Patient: Expanded to 25 different relationships, including indicators such as "grandson," "adopted child," "mother," and "life partner."

Facility Code Value: Facility-related element that identifies the place of service with at least 29 locations to choose from, including "office," "ambulance air or water," and "end-stage renal disease treatment facility."

ELECTRONIC STANDARD HIPAA 837P

The American National Standards Institute (ANSI) formed the **Accredited Standards Committee X12 (ASC X12),** which developed the US standards body for the cross-industry development, maintenance, and publication of electronic data exchange standards. In the health care industry, processing administrative functions can be costly and involve many paper forms and communications via telephone, fax, and postal services. Also, the security and privacy of an individual's health information may be jeopardized. To address the burden of these high overhead costs, the uniform adoption of HIPAA standards has brought forth electronic formats to complete the following health care–related transactions:

- Obtain authorization to refer to a specialist
- Submit a claim for reimbursement
- Request and respond to additional information needed to process a claim
- Health care claims or equivalent encounter information
- Health care payment and remittance advice
- Coordination of benefits
- Health care claim status
- Enrollment and disenrollment in a health plan
- Eligibility for a health insurance plan
- Health plan premium payments
- Referral certification and authorization
- First report of injury
- Health claims attachments
- Other transactions that DHHS may prescribe by regulation

Each of these standard transactions is identified by a three-digit number preceded by "ASC X12N" (Table 8-3). However, the transactions are referred to in the office simply by the three-digit number (for example, 837 or 837P [professional]). The 837P replaces the paper CMS-1500 (02-12) form and more than 400 versions of the electronic NSF.

Levels of Information for 837P Standard Transaction Format

Because the 837P is an electronic claims transmittal format, data collected to construct and submit a claim are grouped by levels. It is important for claims processing staff to know the language when following up on claims. You do not need to know exactly how these are grouped. However, if the clearinghouse or payer states that you have

Table 8-3	HIPAA Transaction Functions and Formats
STANDARD TRANSACTION FUNCTION	**INDUSTRY FORMAT NAME**
Official Title: Health Care Eligibility Benefit Inquiry and Response **Purpose:** Eligibility verification/response • When obtaining issues regarding benefits and coverage, this standard is used from a health care provider to a health plan or between two health plans. • The 270 is the "inquiry for eligibility verification." • The 271 is the "response."	ASC X12N 270/271
Official Title: Health Care Claim Status Request and Response **Purpose:** Health claim status inquiry/response • The 276 is the "inquiry" to determine the status of a claim. • The 277 is the "response."	ASC X12N 276/277
Official Title: Health Care Services Review—Request for Review and Response **Purpose:** Referral certification and authorization for patient health care services	ASC X12N 278
Official Title: Payroll Deducted and Other Group Premium Payment for Insurance Products **Purpose:** Health plan premium payments, including payroll deductions	ASC X12N 820
Official Title: Benefit Enrollment and Maintenance **Purpose:** Transmission of subscriber enrollment information to a health plan to establish coverage or terminate the policy	ASC X12N 834
Official Title: Payment and Remittance Advice **Purpose:** Transmission indicating the explanation of benefits or remittance advice from a health plan payer to the health care provider • This also may be data sent from a health plan directly to the provider's financial institution (bank) and may include payment and information about the processing of the claim.	ASC X12N 835
Official Title: Health Care Claim or Equivalent Encounter **Purpose:** To obtain payment for the transmitted health services encounter information • The 837P (Professional) replaces the paper CMS-1500 form and the electronic National Standard Format (NSF). • The 837I (Institutional) replaces the paper UB-04 often used in hospitals. • The 837D (Dental) is used for dentistry. • Additionally, the coordination of benefits (COB) for claims and payment will be transmitted through the 837 format.	ASC X12N 837 includes: • 837P—Health Care Claim, Professional • 837I—Health Care Claim, Institutional • 837D—Health Care Claim, Dental
Proposed Official Title: First Report of Illness, Injury, or Incident **Potential Purpose:** This standard will be used to report information on a claim pertaining to factors such as date of onset of illness or date of accident.	PROPOSED ASC X12N 148
Proposed Official Title: Health Claims Attachment **Potential Purpose:** Transmit additional information to claim • This means no more photocopied attachments stapled to paper claims or additional information mailed after the claim is initially received.	PROPOSED ASC X12 275 and HL7

an invalid item at the "high level," you need to understand that it could be incomplete or erroneous information pertaining to the provider, subscriber, or payer (Table 8-4).

A "friendlier" way to understand this new stream-of-data format is to address a "crosswalk" between the legacy CMS-1500 (02-12) paper claim and the 837P (Table 8-5; note that dates on HIPAA transactions will be in the 8-digit YYYYMMDD (for example, 20090806) electronic claim format.

Accredited Standards Committee X12 (ASC X12) Version 5010

Just as computer software programs are upgraded from time to time, the programs for transmission of insurance claims data must be upgraded periodically due to the continual changes to policies and regulations for payment of claims. Implementation of ICD-10-CM/PCS in 2015 resulted in the need to upgrade to HIPAA transaction standard **ASC X12 Version 5010** for electronic claim submission. Providers, payers, and clearinghouses were required to implement and start using this standard on January 1, 2012. The 5010 Version allows providers and payers to transmit either ICD-9 or ICD-10 data. Version 5010 also requires health insurers to specify when they received the claim from a physician practice, which allows physician practices to calculate interest due on untimely payments. There are many additional system improvements, such as returning claims that need corrections to the provider sooner, assignment of claim numbers closer to the time received by the payer, and more consistency

Table 8-4	Data Grouping in 837P Standard Transaction Format
LEVEL	INFORMATION
High-level information: Applies to the entire claim and reflects data pertaining to the billing provider, subscriber, and patient	• Billing/pay to provider information • Subscriber/patient information • Payer information
Claim-level information: Applies to the entire claim and all service lines and is applicable to most claims	Claim information
Specialty claim–level information: Applies to specific claim types	Specialty
Service line–level information: Applies to specific procedure or service that is rendered and is applicable to most claims	Service line information
Specialty service line–level information: Applies to specific claim types; required data are required only for the specific claim type	Specialty service line information
Other information	• Coordination of benefits (COB) • Repriced claim/line • Credit/debit information • Clearinghouse/value added network tracking

Table 8-5	Comparison of CMS-1500 (02-12) and 837P v5010*			
	1500 Form Locator		ANSI 837P Version 5010	
ITEM NUMBER	TITLE	LOOP ID	SEGMENT/ DATA ELEMENT	NOTES
N/A	Carrier Block	2010BB	NM103 N301 N302 N401 N402 N403	
1	Medicare, Medicaid, TRICARE, CHAMPUS, CHAMPVA, Group Health Plan, FECA, Black Lung, Other	2000B	SBR09	Required: **Claim filing indicator code.** Must = MB for Medicare Part B claims.
1a	Insured's ID Number	2010BA	NM109	Required: **Subscriber Primary Identifier.** Enter the patient's Health Insurance Claim Number.
2	Patient's Name	2010BA	NM103 NM104N M105	Required: **Subscriber last, first and middle name.** Enter the patient's name as shown on their insurance card.
3	Patient's Birth Date, Sex	2010BA	DMG02 DMG03	Required: **Subscriber birth date and gender code.** Enter the patient's birth date and sex.
4	Insured's Name	2330A	NM103 NM104 NM105	Situational: **Other insured last name, first name, middle name.** If there is insurance primary to Medicare, either through the patient's or spouse's employment or any other source, list the name of the insurance here. Required: If any other payers are known to potentially be involved in paying the claim.
5	Patient's Address	2010BA	N301 N302 N401 N402 N403	Required: **Subscriber address, city, state and zip code.** Enter the patient's mailing address.
6	Patient Relationship to Insured	2000B 2320	SBR02	Situational: **Individual relationship code.** Required when subscriber is the same as the patient. Individual relationship code is required if any other payers are known to potentially be involved in paying this claim.
7	Insured's Address	2330A	N301 N302 N401 N402 N403	Situational: **Other subscriber address, city, state, zip code.** Enter the mailing address of the insured. Required if any other payers are known to potentially be involved in paying this claim and the information is available.
8	Reserved for NUCC use.	Leave blank.		

Table 8-5	Comparison of CMS-1500 (02-12) and 837P v5010—cont'd			
1500 Form Locator			**ANSI 837P Version 5010**	
ITEM NUMBER	TITLE	LOOP ID	SEGMENT/ DATA ELEMENT	NOTES
9	Other Insured's Name	2330A	NM103 NM104 NM105	Situational: **Other insured last name, first name and middle name.** Enter the last name, first name and middle name of the insured. Required if other payers are known to potentially be involved in paying this claim.
9a	Other Insured's Policy or Group Number	2320 2320A	NM109 SBR03	Situational: **Other insured identifier and insured group or policy number.** Enter the policy number of the insured. Required if other payers are known to potentially be involved in paying this claim. Enter the insured's group or plan number.
9b	Reserved for NUCC use.	Leave blank.		
9c	Reserved for NUCC use.	2330B	N401 N402 N403	Situational: **Other payer city name, state code, zip code.** Enter the city, state and zip code of the insurer. Required if any other payers are known to potentially be involved in paying this claim.
9d	Insurance Plan Name or Program Name	2330B	NM109 NM103	Situational: **Other payer primary identifier, other payer organization name.** Enter the insurer's unique identifier. Enter the name of the insured's other insurance.
10a 10b 10c	Is Patient's Condition Related to: Employment? Auto accident? Other accident?	2300	CLM11-1 CLM11-2 CLM11-4	Situational: **Employment related indicator, auto accident indictor, other accident indicator.** Required if date of accident (DTP01=439) is used and the service is employment related or the result of an accident. Situational: **Auto Accident State or Province Code.** Identify state where automobile accident occurred if auto accident.
10d	Claim Codes (Designated by NUCC)	Leave blank.		
11	Insured's Policy, Group, or FECA Number	2320	SBR03	Situational: **Insured group or policy number.** If there is insurance primary to Medicare, enter the insured's policy or group number. Required if other payers are known to potentially be involved in paying this claim.
11a	Insured's Date of Birth, Sex	Leave blank.		
11b	Other Claim ID (Designated by NUCC)	Leave blank.		
11c	Insurance Plan Name or Program Name	2320 2330B 2330B	SBR04 NM103 NM109	Situational: **Other insured group name, other payer organization name, other payer primary identifier.** Enter the complete insurance plan or program name. Enter the payer ID of the other insurer.
11d	Is there another Health Benefit Plan?	Leave blank.		
12	Patient's or Authorized Person's Signature	2300	CLM09	Required: **Release of information code.** This item authorizes release of medical information necessary to process the claim. It also authorizes payment of benefits to the provider of service or supplier when assignment is accepted on the claim.
13	Insured's or Authorized Person's Signature	2300	CLM08	Required: **Benefits assignment certification.** This item authorizes payment of medical benefits to the physician or supplier.
14	Date of Current Illness, Injury, Pregnancy	2300	DTP03	Situational: **Accident date, onset of current illness or injury, initial treatment date.** Required if CLM 11-1 or 2 = (AA) or (OA) and on all claims involving spinal manipulations.
15	Other Date	Leave blank.		
16	Dates Patient Unable to Work in Current Occupation	2300	DTP03	Situational: **Initial disability period start and end.** If the patient is employed and is unable to work in his/her current occupation, enter the date(s) when patient is unable to work.

Continued

Table 8-5   Comparison of CMS-1500 (02-12) and 837P v5010—cont'd

	1500 Form Locator		ANSI 837P Version 5010	
ITEM NUMBER	TITLE	LOOP ID	SEGMENT/ DATA ELEMENT	NOTES
17	Name of Referring Provider or Other Source	2310A 2420F 2420E 2310D 2420D	NM103 NM104 NM105	Situational: **Referring provider, ordering provider and/or supervising provider last name, first name and middle name.** Enter the name of the referring or ordering physician if the service or item was ordered or referred by a physician. All physicians who order service or refer Medicare beneficiaries must report this data. This is also used if Medicare policy requires you to report a supervising physician. When a claim involves multiple referring and/or ordering physicians, a separate claim should be submitted for each.
17a		Leave blank.		
17b	NPI#	2310A 2420F 2420E 2310D 2420D	NM109	Situational: **Referring provider ID, Ordering provider ID and/or supervising provider ID.** Enter "XX" in the NM108 data element to indicate an NPI is present in NM109. Enter the NPI of the referring, ordering, or supervising physician or non-physician practitioner listed in Item 17.
18	Hospitalization Dates Related to Current Services	2300	DTP03	Situational: **Related Hospitalization Admission and Discharge Dates.** Enter the date when a medical service is furnished as a result of, or subsequent to, a related hospitalization.
19	Additional Claim Information (Designated by NUCC)	2300 2400 2310D 2420D	DTP03 NM109	Situational: **Last seen date.** Enter the date patient was last seen and the NPI of his/her attending physician when a physician providing routine foot care submits claim. Situational: **Supervising provider ID.** Enter "XX" in the NM108 data element to indicate an NPI is present in NM 109. Enter the NPI of his/her attending physician when a physician providing routine foot care submits claim. Situational: **Test Results.** Enter R1 or R2 in the MEA02 to qualify the Hemoglobin or Hematocrit test results. Enter the test results in the MEA03. Situational: **Code Category, Certification Condition Indicator, Homebound Indicator.** Required when an independent lab renders an EKG tracing or obtains a specimen from a homebound or institutionalized patient. Situational: **Extra narrative data.** Enter all applicable modifiers when modifier -99 is entered on the service line. Enter the statement, "Testing for hearing aid" when billing services involving the testing of a hearing aid is used to obtain intentional denials when other payers are involved. When dental examinations are billed, enter the specific surgery for which the exam is performed. Situational: **Description.** Enter the drug's name and dosage when submitting a claim for Not Otherwise Classified drugs. Enter a concise description of an unlisted procedure code or a Not Otherwise Classified drug. Enter the specific name and dosage amount when low osmolar contract material is billed, but only if HCPCS codes do not cover them. Situational: **Demonstration Project Identifier.** Required on claim where a demonstration project is being billed. Situational: **Assumed and Relinquished care dates.** Enter the date for a global surgery claim when providers share post-operative care.

Table 8-5 Comparison of CMS-1500 (02-12) and 837P v5010—cont'd

ITEM NUMBER	TITLE	LOOP ID	SEGMENT/ DATA ELEMENT	NOTES
				Situational: **Purchases Service Provider Identifier.** Enter "XX" in the NM108 data element to indicate an NPI is present in NM109. Enter the NPI of the physician who is performing the technical or professional component of a diagnostic test that is subject to the anti-markup payment limitation. Subjective: **Last X-ray.** Enter the x-ray date for chiropractic services (if an x-ray, rather than a physical exam was the method used to demonstrate subluxation). Situational: **Benefits Assignment Certification Indicator.** When a patient refuses to assign benefits to the provider, enter code "W".
20	Outside Lab Charges	2400 2420B	PS101 PS102 NMI	Situational: **Purchases service provider identifier, charge amount and service provider.** Required when billing for diagnostic tests subject to the anti-markup payment limitations. Loop 2420B is required when a 2400/PS1 segment is present. When submitting a PS1 segment, you must also submit the facility information in either loop 2310C or 2420C.
21	Diagnosis or Nature of Illness or Injury	2300	HI01-02 H102-02 HI03-02 HI04-02 H105-02 H106-02 H107-02 H108-02 H109-02 H110-02 H111-02 H112-02	Required: **Principal diagnosis code.** Required on all claims. Do not transmit the decimal points in the diagnosis codes. The decimal point is assumed. Enter the patient's diagnosis/condition. All physician and non-physician specialties use diagnosis codes to the highest level of specificity for the date of service. Enter the diagnoses in priority order. Situational: **Secondary and tertiary diagnosis codes.**
22	Resubmission and/or Original Reference Number	Leave blank.		
23	Prior Authorization Number	2300 2400 2310E 2420G	REF02 NM101 N301 N401 NM101	Situational: **Prior authorization number.** Enter the Quality Improvement Organization (QIO) prior authorization number for those procedures requiring QIO prior approval. Situational: **Investigational device exemption number.** Enter the Investigational Device Exemption (IDE) number when an investigational device is used in an FDA-approved clinical trial. Post Market Approval number should also be placed here when applicable. When more than one IDE applies, they must be split into separate claims. Situational: **Care Plan Oversight Number.** For physicians performing care plan oversight services, enter the NI of the home health agency (HHA) or hospice when CPT code G0181 or G0182 is billed. Situational: **CLIA number.** Enter the 10-digit CLIA certification number for laboratory services billed by an entity performing CLIA covered procedures. Situational: **Referring CLIA number.** Required for any laboratory that referred tests to another laboratory covered by the CLIA Act that is billed. Situational: **Ambulance Pick-up location, pick-up address, city state/zip.** Required when billing for ambulance or non-emergency transportation services. If the location is in an area where there are no street addresses, enter a description of where the service was rendered.

Continued

Table 8-5	Comparison of CMS-1500 (02-12) and 837P v5010—cont'd				

1500 Form Locator			ANSI 837P Version 5010		
ITEM NUMBER	**TITLE**	**LOOP ID**	**SEGMENT/ DATA ELEMENT**	**NOTES**	
24A	Date(s) of Service	2400	DTP03	Required: **Service date.** Enter the service date for each procedure or supply.	
24B	Place of Service	2300 2400	CLM05-1 SV105	Required: **Place of Service Code.** Enter the appropriate place of service code. Identify the setting, using a place of service code, for each item used or service performed.	
24C	EMG	Leave blank.			
24D	Procedures, Services, or Supplies	2400	SV101-2 SV101-3 SV101-4 SV101-5 SV101-6	Required: **Procedure code.** In product's Service ID Qualifier (SV101-1) enter (HC) for HCPCS codes. Enter the procedures, services or supplies using the HCPCS coding system. Situational: **Procedure modifier.** When applicable, show the HCPCS modifiers with the HCPCS codes.	
24E	Diagnosis Pointer	2400	SV107-1 SV107-2 SV107-3 SV107-4	Required: **Diagnosis code pointer.** A submitter must point to the primary diagnosis for each service line. Use remaining diagnosis pointers in declining level of importance to service line.	
24F	$Charges	2400	SV102	Required: **Line item charge amount.** Enter the charge amount for each service.	
24G	Days or Units	2400	SV104	Required: **Service unit count.** Enter the number of days or units. For anesthesia, show the elapsed time. Convert hours into minutes and enter the total minutes required for the procedure.	
24H 24I Shaded Line	EPSDT/Family Plan ID Qualifier	Leave blank. No longer used due to full implementation of NPI.			
24J	Rendering Provider ID#	2310B 2420A	NM109	Situational: **Rendering provider identifier.** Enter "XX" in the NM 108 data element to indicate an NPI is present in NM109. Enter the rendering provider's NPI number. This is required when the information is different than that in 2010AA billing provider.	
25	Federal Tax ID Number	2010AA	REF01 REF02	Required: **Billing Provider Tax Identification Number/Social Security Number.** Enter the provider of services or supplier Federal Tax ID number or Social Security number.	
26	Patient's Account No.	2300	CLM01	Required: **Patient control number.** Enter the patient's account number assigned by the provider of service's or supplier's accounting system.	
27	Accept Assignment?	2300	CLM07	Required: **Assignment or Plan Participation Code.** A=Assigned B=Assignment accepted on Clinical Lab services only C=Not assigned	
28	Total Charge	2300	CLM02	Required: **Total claim charge amount.** Enter the total charges for the services.	
29	Amount Paid	2300	AMT02	Situational: **Patient amount paid.** Required if patient has paid any amount towards the claim for covered services only.	
30	Reserved for NUCC Use.	Leave blank.			
31	Signature of Physician or Supplier Including Degrees or Credentials	2300	CLM06	Required: **Provider or supplier signature indicator.** A "Y" value indicates the provider signature is on file, an "N" value indicates the provider signature is not on file.	

Table 8-5	Comparison of CMS-1500 (02-12) and 837P v5010—cont'd			
1500 Form Locator			**ANSI 837P Version 5010**	
ITEM NUMBER	**TITLE**	**LOOP ID**	**SEGMENT/ DATA ELEMENT**	**NOTES**
32	Service Facility Location Information	2310C	NM103 N301 N401 N402 N403	Situational: **Laboratory or Facility Name, Address, City/State/Zip.** Required when the location of service is different than that carried in Loop ID-2010AA. If a modifier is billed indicating the service was rendered in a Health Professional Shortage Area or Physician Scarcity Area, the physical location where the service was rendered shall be entered. If an independent laboratory is billing, enter the place where the test was performed outside a physician's office. Providers of service shall identify the supplier's name, address and NPI when billing for anti-markup tests. Situational: **Ambulance Pick-up and Drop-off Location, address, city, state and zip.** Required when billing for ambulance or non-emergency transportation services. Situational: **Mammography certification.** If the supplier is a certified mammography screening center, enter the FDA approved certification number.
32a		2310C 2420C	NM109	Situational: **Laboratory/Facility Primary Identifier.** Enter "XX" in the NM108 data element to indicate an NPI is present in NM109. Enter the NPI of the service facility.
32b	No longer used due to full implementation of NPI			
33	Billing Provider Info & Ph #	2010AA	NM103 NM104 NM105 N301 N302 N401 N402 N403 PER04	Required: **Provider last or organization name, provider first name, middle initial, address, city, state, zip code, phone number.** Enter the provider of service/supplier's billing name, address, zip code and telephone number.
33a	NPI#	2010AA	NM109	Required: **Billing provider Identifier.** Enter "XX" in the NM108 data element to indicate an NPI is present in NM109. Enter the NPI of the billing provider or group.
33b	No longer used			

Copyright 1995-2012. American Medical Association. All Rights Reserved.
CHAMPUS, Civilian Health and Medical Program of the Uniformed Services; *CHAMPVA,* Civilian Health and Medical Program of the Department of Veterans Affairs; *CLIA,* Clinical Laboratory Improvement Amendments; *EKG,* electrocardiogram; *EMG,* emergency; *EPSDT,* Early Periodic Screening, Diagnosis, and Treatment; *FDA,* Food and Drug Administration; *FECA,* Federal Employees' Compensation Act; *HCPCS,* Healthcare Common Procedure Coding System; *ID,* identification; *NPI,* National Provider Identifier; *NUCC,* National Uniform Claim Committee.
*This crosswalk relates to the CMS-1500 (08-05) claim form. When it becomes available, a crosswalk relating to the new CMS-1500 (02-12) will be placed on the Evolve website.

of claims editing and error handling. A new electronic transaction standard, the Version 6020 standard for electronic claims submission, is currently under development.

CLAIM ATTACHMENTS STANDARDS

Claim attachments are supplemental documents providing additional medical information to the claims processor that cannot be accommodated within the claim format. Common attachments are Certificates of Medical

Necessity (CMNs), discharge summaries, and operative reports. Currently, practice management and claims software include a data field that allows you to indicate that a paper claims attachment is included with the claim.

HIPAA identified a health claim attachment as one of the transactions for which electronic standards were to be adopted. However, the final rule was never adopted. The ACA mandates a compliance date of January 1, 2016, for this regulation.

STANDARD UNIQUE IDENTIFIERS

Standard Unique Identifiers are used to identify the specific entities associated with the electronic claims process.

Standard Unique Employer Identifier

The employer identification number (EIN) is assigned by the Internal Revenue Service (IRS) and used to identify employers for tax purposes. HIPAA requires that the EIN be used to identify employers rather than inputting the name of the company when submitting claims. Employers use their EINs to identify themselves in transactions involving premium payments to health plans on behalf of their employees or to identify themselves or other employers as the source or receiver of information about eligibility. Employers also will use EINs to identify themselves in transactions when enrolling or disenrolling employees in a health plan.

Standard Unique Health Care Provider Identifier

In the past, health insurance plans have assigned an identifying number to each provider with whom they conduct business, which has resulted in providers having many different identifier numbers when submitting claims to several different payers.

Under HIPAA, all providers were required to obtain a National Provider Identifier (NPI) that is assigned to each provider for use in transactions with all health plans. The NPI is all numeric and 10 characters in length and became a requirement on all claims effective May 23, 2007.

According to CMS, NPI is a lasting identifier that will not change with changes to a health care provider's name, address, ownership, membership in health plans, or Healthcare Provider Taxonomy classification (taxonomy identifies the specialty).

Standard Unique Health Plan Identifier

Currently, health plans are identified in electronic transactions with multiple identifiers that differ in length, format, and meaning. The current versions of the adopted standards (ASC X12N) allow health plans to use these various identifiers in standard transactions that result in inconsistent use of identifiers for health plans.

The ACA requires implementation of standard unique health plan identifiers (HPIDs). The standard unique HPID rule will assign a standard identifier to identify health plans that process and pay certain electronic health care transactions. On October 4, 2012, a corrected and final rule was posted in the *Federal Register*, which stated that health plans (with the exception of small health plans) were required to obtain an HPID by November 5, 2014. Small health plans must obtain an HPID by November 5, 2015. Covered entities will be required to use HPIDs in the standard transactions on or after November 7, 2016.

The adoption of the HPID will increase standardization within HIPAA standard transactions and provide a platform for other regulatory initiatives. The use of HPIDs will bring a higher level of automation to offices providing health care services as they process billing and perform other insurance-related tasks, such as verification of patient eligibility and processing of remittance advices.

Standard Unique Patient Identifier

In addition to standardization of a unique provider identifier and a unique HPID, both HIPAA and the ACA support the creation of a unique patient identifier system. However, privacy and security concerns have stalled the efforts to implement the proposal. The intention to create a standard for a uniform patient identifier has also prompted protest among public interest groups who consider a universal identifier to be a civil liberties threat. Therefore the issue of a universal patient identifier is "on hold."

PRACTICE MANAGEMENT SYSTEM

The most important function of a practice management system (PMS) is accounts receivable. Many offices use features such as scheduling, electronic health record (EHR), and word processing to run an efficient office. However, the goal of maximum value can be attained if the PMS is able to prepare, send, receive, and process HIPAA standard electronic transactions. For older PMS versions, a clearinghouse converts old formats to HIPAA standard transactions. Keep in mind that HIPAA does not apply to the format of stored data within the PMS databases. Computer systems are free to use any data format when storing data because HIPAA standards apply only to the format in which data are transmitted.

If your practice is in the market for a new PMS, it is important to find a vendor that understands HIPAA thoroughly—including the Privacy and Security Rules. A PMS can help with administrative burdens, such as tracking the receipt of the Notice of Privacy Practices (NPP), noting a patient's treatment consent or authorization, and mapping disclosures. A HIPAA-ready PMS may allow the following:

- Setting security access to patient files in the software
- Indicating date of receipt and signature of NPP

- Inserting date of patient's authorization
- Maintaining files of practice's authorization and notification forms
- Tracking requests for amendments, requests for restrictions on use and disclosure of protected health information (PHI), and indications of whether the physician agreed to or denied the request
- Tracking expiration dates

When assessing the PMS's functionality in accounts receivable management, consider the ability to perform the following:

- Set up all practice providers as individuals to bill using correct and appropriate identifiers for each and every health care provider.
- Key in all patient demographics and insurance information.
- Electronic claim batch submission, either direct to payer or through a clearinghouse. Note that some PMS vendors sell an "add-on" module to go directly to some carriers, such as Medicare, Medicaid, and Blue Cross Blue Shield.

BUILDING THE CLAIM

Encounter or Multipurpose Billing Forms

As mentioned in Chapter 3, an *encounter form* (also known as a *charge slip*, *multipurpose billing form*, *patient service slip*, *routing form*, *super bill*, or *transaction slip*) is a document used to record information about the service rendered to a patient. The style and format of the billing form varies because it is customized to meet the needs of each health care office, based on the medical practice's specialty. For easy reference, many billing forms include preprinted procedural and diagnostic codes. The provider circles the codes and the insurance billing specialist takes that information and enters it in the computer system.

Scannable Encounter Form

Some encounter forms are designed so that they may be scanned to input charges and diagnoses in the patient's computerized account. Time is saved and fewer errors occur because no keystrokes are involved (Figure 8-3).

Keying Insurance Data for Claim Transmission

When one is operating computer software, the encounter form may be used to obtain patient information (Figure 8-4). A prompt (question field) appears on the screen and the data are keyed in reply to the prompt. Reusable data are entered initially in a file and identified by a number. Each treating physician, referring physician, patient, and

third-party payer has an assigned computer code number. Notice in Figure 8-4, Figure 8-5, and Figure 8-6 that a patient, Charles Weber, is input as account number WEBCH000; Star Insurance is STA00; and the provider is keyed as DIW, the initials of the provider. This information is stored in the database and is the same as that necessary for completing a claim manually. It is automatically retrieved by the system when a computer code number is keyed in and used to generate a computerized claim or electronic claim. Because there are computer code numbers and prompts for each item, there is less chance of error or omitting mandatory information. The program checks that data are complete and in proper format. It is important to understand how your particular management system works.

Some entries are made using a "macro." This technique involves a series of menu selections, keystrokes, or commands that have been recorded in memory and assigned a name or key combination. When the macro name is keyed in, the steps or characters in the macro are executed from beginning to end, saving time and keystrokes. However, when using a macro, template, or other automated billing system, ensure that the provider accurately individualizes each record to reflect what occurred during the visit. The practice of cutting and pasting diagnosis and treatment language from one record to another can generate a false claim.

Some general do's and don'ts for keying in data and billing electronic claims follow.

Do: Use the patient account numbers to differentiate between patients with similar names.

Do: Use correct numeric locations of service code, current valid Current Procedural Terminology (CPT), or Healthcare Common Procedure Coding System (HCPCS) procedure codes.

Do: Print an insurance billing worksheet or perform a front-end edit (online error checking) to look for and correct all errors before the claim is transmitted to the third-party payer.

Do: Request electronic error reports from the third-party payer to make corrections to the system.

Do: Obtain and cross-check the electronic status report against all claims transmitted.

Don't: Bill codes using modifier -22 electronically unless the carrier receives documents (called *attachments*) to justify more payment.

After input is complete, the information is stored in memory and a claim may be transmitted individually or

CFR

PAT 4140.0

DOCTOR: 2 FRANK CHI, M.D.

APPT DATE: 05/27/XX

ROOM:	APPT TIME: 2:30 PM
APPTLOC:	APPT LEN: 10 min.
APPTCD:	DEPT/LOC: 0, n/a

( ) 985-6575 01/22/1936 F63
PRI: (Y) BLUE SHIELD ENVOY
201-XX-9969
SEC:

REASON: OX, F/U visit   DSET/PRT: 1, 12
LAST DX: 000.0 No diagnosis applicable   ACCT BAL: 75.00
SSN/STA: 201-XX-9969, 1 Active   PAT DUE: 0.00
OVERLAY: 1 INTERNAL MEDICINE   VOUCHER: 7887

NEW PT OFFICE VISITS
①②③④Ⓟ/Ⓛ 99203 NP LEVEL THREE
①②③④Ⓟ/Ⓛ 99204 NP LEVEL FOUR
①②③④Ⓟ/Ⓛ 99205 NP LEVEL FIVE
EST PT OFFICE VISIT
①②③④Ⓟ/Ⓛ 99211 EST PT LEVEL ONE
①②③④Ⓟ/Ⓛ 99212 EST PT LEVEL TWO
①②③④Ⓟ/Ⓛ 99213 EST PT LEVEL THREE
①②③④Ⓟ/Ⓛ 99214 EST PT LEVEL FOUR
①②③④Ⓟ/Ⓛ 99215 EST PT LEVEL FIVE
①②③④Ⓟ/Ⓛ 00003 GLOBAL VISIT

OTHER PROCEDURES
①②③④Ⓟ/Ⓛ 99000 COLL & PREP/PAP TEST
①②③④Ⓟ/Ⓛ 93000 EKG WITH INTERPRETATION
①②③④Ⓟ/Ⓛ 82270 HEMOCCULT
①②③④Ⓟ/Ⓛ 81000 URINALYSIS

INJECTIONS
①②③④Ⓟ/Ⓛ ~FLU, FLU INJ/ADMIN/MCR
①②③④Ⓟ/Ⓛ ~9065 FLU INJ/NON MCR
①②③④Ⓟ/Ⓛ ~PNEU PNEUMO/ADMIN/MCR
①②③④Ⓟ/Ⓛ ~9073 PNEUMO INJ NON MCR

UNLISTED PROCEDURES

STOP FOR VERIFICATION
BREASTS
①②③④Ⓟ/Ⓛ N60.29 FIBROADENOSIS, BREAST
①②③④Ⓟ/Ⓛ N63 LUMP OR MASS IN BREAST

CARDIOVASCULAR
①②③④Ⓟ/Ⓛ I71.4 ABDOM AORTIC ANEURYSM
①②③④Ⓟ/Ⓛ I20.9 ANGINA
①②③④Ⓟ/Ⓛ I74.11 AORTIC VALVE DISORDER
①②③④Ⓟ/Ⓛ I48.91 ATRIAL FIBRILLATION
①②③④Ⓟ/Ⓛ I48.92 ATRIAL FLUTTER
①②③④Ⓟ/Ⓛ I49.1 ATRIAL PREMATURE BEATS
①②③④Ⓟ/Ⓛ I44.0 ATRIOVENT BLOCK-1ST DE
①②③④Ⓟ/Ⓛ R01.1 CARDIAC MURMURS NEC
①②③④Ⓟ/Ⓛ I51.7 CARDIOMEGALY
①②③④Ⓟ/Ⓛ I50.9 CONGESTIVE HEART FAILU
①②③④Ⓟ/Ⓛ I42.1 HYPERTR OBSTR CARDIOMY
①②③④Ⓟ/Ⓛ I25.1Ø ISCHEMIC CHR HEART DIS
①②③④Ⓟ/Ⓛ R00.2 PALPITATIONS
①②③④Ⓟ/Ⓛ I47.1 PAROX ATRIAL TACHYCARD
①②③④Ⓟ/Ⓛ I47.2 PAROX VENTRIC TACHYCAR

CHEST
①②③④Ⓟ/Ⓛ J20.9 BRONCHITIS, ACUTE
①②③④Ⓟ/Ⓛ J41.0 BRONCHITIS, CHRONIC
①②③④Ⓟ/Ⓛ J44.9 CH OB ASTH W/O STAT AS
①②③④Ⓟ/Ⓛ J45.20 EXT ASTHMA W/O STAT AS

①②③④Ⓟ/Ⓛ J44.1 OBS CHR BRNC W ACT EXA
①②③④Ⓟ/Ⓛ J44.9 OBS CHR BRNC W/O ACT E

ENDOCRINE
①②③④Ⓟ/Ⓛ E10.40 DMI NEURO CMP CONTROLL
①②③④Ⓟ/Ⓛ E10.9 DMI WO CMP CONTROLLED
①②③④Ⓟ/Ⓛ E10.65 DMI UNCONTROLLED
①②③④Ⓟ/Ⓛ E11.40 DMII NEURO CMP CONTROL
①②③④Ⓟ/Ⓛ E11.9 DMII WO CMP CONTROLLED
①②③④Ⓟ/Ⓛ E11.65 DMII UNCONTROLLED
①②③④Ⓟ/Ⓛ E78.0 HYPERCHOLESTEROLEMIA
①②③④Ⓟ/Ⓛ E78.1 HYPERGLYCERIDEMIA
①②③④Ⓟ/Ⓛ E03.9 HYPOTHYROIDISM
①②③④Ⓟ/Ⓛ E66.01 MORBID OBESITY
①②③④Ⓟ/Ⓛ E04.1 THYROID NODULE

EXTREMITIES
①②③④Ⓟ/Ⓛ E60.9 EDEMA
①②③④Ⓟ/Ⓛ I74.3 LOWER EXT EMBOLISM
①②③④Ⓟ/Ⓛ I80.0- PHLEBITIS-LEG
①②③④Ⓟ/Ⓛ I70.219 PVD W/CLAUDICATION
①②③④Ⓟ/Ⓛ I83.90 VARICOSE VEIN OF LEG

GI
①②③④Ⓟ/Ⓛ R10.13 ABDMNAL PAIN EPIGASTRI
①②③④Ⓟ/Ⓛ R10.12 ABDMNAL PAIN LFT UP QU
①②③④Ⓟ/Ⓛ R10.32 ABDMNAL PAIN LT LWR QU
①②③④Ⓟ/Ⓛ R10.33 ABDMNAL PAIN PERIUMBIL
①②③④Ⓟ/Ⓛ R10.31 ABDMNAL PAIN RT LWR QU
①②③④Ⓟ/Ⓛ R10.11 ABDMNAL PAIN RT UPR QU
①②③④Ⓟ/Ⓛ K92.1 BLOOD IN STOOL
①②③④Ⓟ/Ⓛ K81.2 CHOLECYSTITIS, ACUTE
①②③④Ⓟ/Ⓛ K59.00 CONSTIPATION
①②③④Ⓟ/Ⓛ R19.7 DIARRHEA
①②③④Ⓟ/Ⓛ K57.32 DIVERTICULITIS
①②③④Ⓟ/Ⓛ K57.30 DIVERTICULOSIS
①②③④Ⓟ/Ⓛ K580.20 GALLSTONE(S), CHRONIC
①②③④Ⓟ/Ⓛ K29.00 GASTRITIS
①②③④Ⓟ/Ⓛ K51.9 GERD
①②③④Ⓟ/Ⓛ K64.4 HEMORRHOID, EXT W/O COM
①②③④Ⓟ/Ⓛ K64.8 HEMORRHOID, INT W/O COM
①②③④Ⓟ/Ⓛ K58.9 IRRITABLE COLON
①②③④Ⓟ/Ⓛ R11.2 NAUSEA WITH VOMITING
①②③④Ⓟ/Ⓛ K62.5 RECTAL & ANAL HEMORRHA
①②③④Ⓟ/Ⓛ K21.0 REFLUX ESOPHAGITIS
①②③④Ⓟ/Ⓛ Z12.12 SCREEN COLORECTAL

GU
①②③④Ⓟ/Ⓛ N41.0 ACUTE PROSTATITIS
①②③④Ⓟ/Ⓛ N40.0 BPH
①②③④Ⓟ/Ⓛ N20.0 CALCULUS OF KIDNEY
①②③④Ⓟ/Ⓛ N20.1 CALCULUS OF URETER
①②③④Ⓟ/Ⓛ N30.00 CYSTITIS, ACUTE
①②③④Ⓟ/Ⓛ N30.10 CYSTITIS, CHRONIC
①②③④Ⓟ/Ⓛ R31.9 HEMATURIA
①②③④Ⓟ/Ⓛ N52.9 IMPOTENCE, ORGANIC ORI
①②③④Ⓟ/Ⓛ R80.9 PROTEINURIA

HEENT
①②③④Ⓟ/Ⓛ H61.23 CERUMEN, IMPACTED
①②③④Ⓟ/Ⓛ H10.019 CONJUNCTIVITIS
①②③④Ⓟ/Ⓛ R04.0 EPISTAXIS
①②③④Ⓟ/Ⓛ R51 HEADACHE
①②③④Ⓟ/Ⓛ J04.0 LARYNGITIS/TRACHEITI
①②③④Ⓟ/Ⓛ J06.0 LARYNGOPHARYNGITIS, A
①②③④Ⓟ/Ⓛ R42 LIGHT-HEADEDNESS
①②③④Ⓟ/Ⓛ G43.109 MIGRAINE
①②③④Ⓟ/Ⓛ J00 NASOPHARYNGITIS, ACUT
①②③④Ⓟ/Ⓛ H65.00 OTITIS MEDIA
①②③④Ⓟ/Ⓛ J02.9 PHARYNGITIS, ACUTE
①②③④Ⓟ/Ⓛ J30.1 RHINITIS ALLERGIC
①②③④Ⓟ/Ⓛ J01.00 SINUSITIS, ACUTE
①②③④Ⓟ/Ⓛ R55 SYNCOPE/VERTIGO

HEMATOLOGIC
①②③④Ⓟ/Ⓛ D50.0 CHR BLOOD LOSS ANEMI
①②③④Ⓟ/Ⓛ D50.8 IRON DEF ANEMIA DIET
①②③④Ⓟ/Ⓛ D51.0 PERNICIOUS ANEMIA

HYPERTENSION
①②③④Ⓟ/Ⓛ I13.11 BEN HY HT/REN/CHF
①②③④Ⓟ/Ⓛ I12.9 BEN HTN REN W/O REN
①②③④Ⓟ/Ⓛ I12.0 BEN HYP WITH REN FAI
①②③④Ⓟ/Ⓛ I10 BENIGN HYPERTENSION
①②③④Ⓟ/Ⓛ I10 MALIGNANT HYPERTENSI
①②③④Ⓟ/Ⓛ I95.1 ORTHOSTATIC HYPOTENS

NEURO
①②③④Ⓟ/Ⓛ G40.309 GEN CNV EPIL W/O INT
①②③④Ⓟ/Ⓛ I82.3 TIA
①②③④Ⓟ/Ⓛ I65.29 CAROTID STENOSIS
①②③④Ⓟ/Ⓛ I67.2 CEREBRAL ATHEREOSCLER

OB GYN
①②③④Ⓟ/Ⓛ B37.3 CANDIDAL VULVOVAGINI
①②③④Ⓟ/Ⓛ N95.1 MENOPAUSAL SYMPTOMS
①②③④Ⓟ/Ⓛ Z12.4 SCREEN MAL NEOP-CERV

RHEUMATOLOGIC
①②③④Ⓟ/Ⓛ M54.2 CERVICAL PAIN
①②③④Ⓟ/Ⓛ M10.00 GOUT
①②③④Ⓟ/Ⓛ M54.5 LUMBAGO/BACK PAIN
①②③④Ⓟ/Ⓛ M79.609 PAIN IN LIMB
①②③④Ⓟ/Ⓛ M54.6 PAIN IN THORACIC SPI
①②③④Ⓟ/Ⓛ M06.9 RHEUMATOID ARTHRITIS
①②③④Ⓟ/Ⓛ M54.30 SCIATICA
①②③④Ⓟ/Ⓛ M32.10 SYST LUPUS ERYTHEMAT

MISC
①②③④Ⓟ/Ⓛ R50.9 FEVER UNKN ORGIN
①②③④Ⓟ/Ⓛ B00.9 HERPES SIMPLEX NOS
①②③④Ⓟ/Ⓛ R06.02 SHORTNESS OF BREATH

UNLISTED DIAGNOSIS
STOP FOR VERIFICATION

---

①②③④Ⓟ/Ⓛ **REFERRALS**   ①②③④Ⓟ/Ⓛ **LOCATIONS**   ①②③④Ⓟ/Ⓛ **DOCTORS**   ①②③④Ⓟ/Ⓛ **NEXT VISIT**
①②③④Ⓟ/Ⓛ   ①②③④Ⓟ/Ⓛ   ①②③④Ⓟ/Ⓛ   ①②③④Ⓟ/Ⓛ ____ DAYS
①②③④Ⓟ/Ⓛ   ①②③④Ⓟ/Ⓛ   ①②③④Ⓟ/Ⓛ   ①②③④Ⓟ/Ⓛ _1_ WEEKS
①②③④Ⓟ/Ⓛ   ①②③④Ⓟ/Ⓛ   ①②③④Ⓟ/Ⓛ F. CHI, MD   ①②③④Ⓟ/Ⓛ ____ MONTHS
①②③④Ⓟ/Ⓛ   ①②③④Ⓟ/Ⓛ   ①②③④Ⓟ/Ⓛ A. SWERD, MD   ①②③④Ⓟ/Ⓛ
  ①②③④Ⓟ/Ⓛ J. STEVEN, MD   ①②③④Ⓟ/Ⓛ

FIGURE 8-3 Scannable encounter form. Primary service or procedure is marked (with a No. 2 pencil) in the Number 1 location and linked to the primary diagnosis, which also is marked in the Number 1 location. The secondary procedures are marked in the Number 2 location, as is the secondary diagnosis. The primary linkage for all services and procedures is connected to the physician performing the service and the location in which it took place. Since there are five levels for both new and established patient office visits, an encounter form should include all levels. If information is missing, as shown in this example, an audit could be triggered because it appears to construe that this medical practice never bills any service lower than a Level 3, indicating fraud to an auditor. *(Form template from Pearson NCS, Inc., Bloomington, Minn. Form data are fictitious and not a part of the template.)*

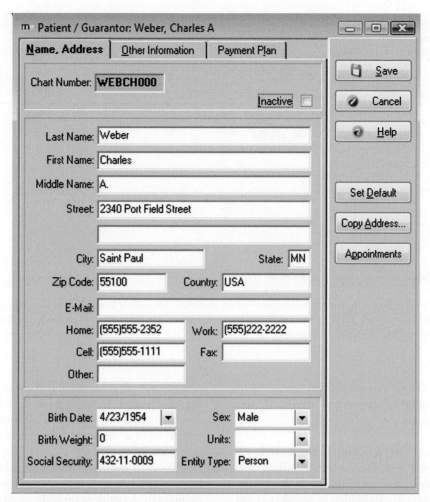

FIGURE 8-4 Patient entry screen using practice management software. *(Screenshot used by permission of MCKESSON Corporation. All Rights Reserved. ©MCKESSON Corporation 2012.)*

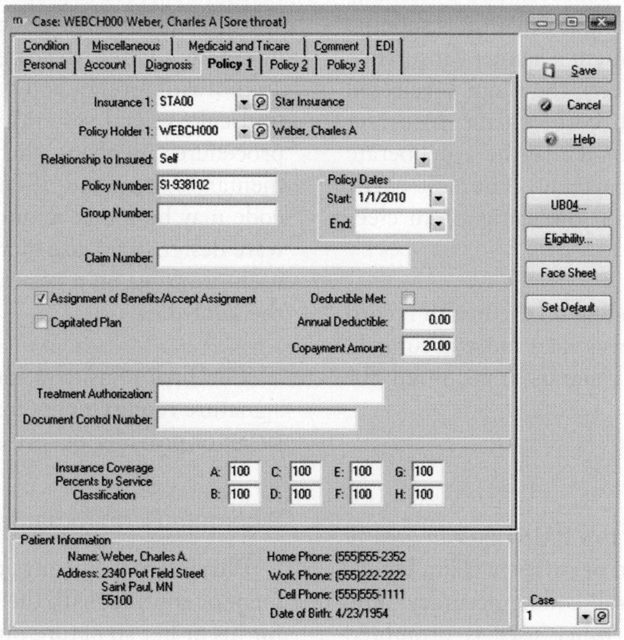

FIGURE 8-5 Insurance information using practice management software. Notice that the code for the payer is "STA00." *(Screenshot used by permission of MCKESSON Corporation. All Rights Reserved. ©MCKESSON Corporation 2012.)*

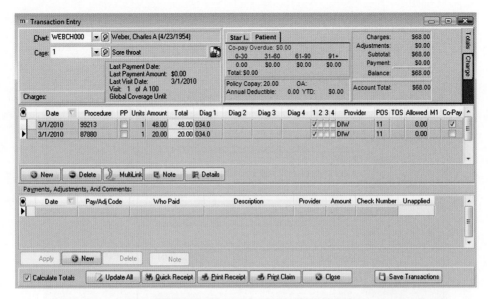

FIGURE 8-6 Entering patient information in an electronic encounter form. Notice that the provider's initials are DIW. *(Screenshot used by permission of MCKESSON Corporation. All Rights Reserved. ©MCKESSON Corporation 2012.)*

in batches. Batched claims can be divided according to insurance type or date(s) of service and are ideally sent during low-volume times.

Because the health care provider is responsible for submitting an accurate bill, the insurance billing specialist inputs the codes. Medicare and other third-party payer's claims examiners are forbidden to recode a claim. During the edit and error process, software code editors identify invalid codes, age conflicts, gender conflicts, procedural and diagnostic code conflicts, and other data before issuing payment. If certain information is submitted incorrectly (for example, patient's name or insurance identification number is incorrect), the claim is rejected and must be resubmitted with correct data. Incorrect coding may be keying errors or it may be a deliberate attempt to obtain fraudulent payment. The edit check allows immediate feedback about the status of an electronically transmitted claim.

The physician may revise coding on the health record and on the claim to reflect the services more accurately until the time at which the claim is transmitted for payment.

Encoder

An **encoder** is add-on software to a PMS that can greatly reduce the time it takes to build or review a claim before batching and can improve overall coding accuracy. The insurance billing specialist or other user is prompted with a series of questions or choices leading to or affecting a specific code assignment by displaying code-specific edits. Using an encoder can enhance a medical practice's compliance program when it comes to accuracy in its billing procedures. Used as an audit tool, the encoder can also be helpful in performance improvement by identifying problem areas in the billing process.

However, there are instances when an encoder does not accurately assign codes; therefore one must never be completely dependent on code-assist software. For example, if a patient has three thorns incised and extracted (removed), the CPT code 10120 "incision and removal of foreign body, subcutaneous tissue; simple (integumentary system)" might be generated by the encoder. However, if internally audited, the case may warrant CPT code 27372 "removal of foreign body, deep, thigh region in knee area (musculoskeletal system)." Thus one learns that not all procedures involving the skin are found in the integumentary system and, if deeper skin layers are affected, a code may be found in another system. A *grouper* is software designed for use in a network that serves a group of users working on a related project that allows access to the same data.

The final considerations in building a claim are the signature requirements for both the patient and the physician or provider of service.

Signature Requirements

Physician. The physician's signature on the agreement or contract with the third-party payer is a substitute for his or her signature on the claim form.

Patient. For assignment of benefits, each patient's signature must be obtained and retained in the office

PATIENT'S MEDICARE ELECTRONIC SIGNATURE MONTHLY AUTHORIZATION FORM

I authorize any holder of medical or other information about me to release to the Social Security Administration and Centers for Medicare and Medicaid Services or its intermediaries or carriers any information needed for this or a related Medicare claim. I permit a copy of this authorization to be used in place of the original, and request payment of medical insurance benefits either to myself or to the party who accepts assignment.

_____   _____
Signature of Patient   Date

A

PATIENT'S MEDICARE ELECTRONIC SIGNATURE ONE-TIME AUTHORIZATION FORM

I request that payment of authorized Medicare benefits be made either to me or on my behalf to _____ for services furnished me by that physician or supplier. I permit a copy of this authorization to be used in place of the original and authorize any holder of medical information about me to release to the Centers for Medicare and Medicaid Services or its agents any information needed to determine these benefits or the benefits payable for related services.

_____   _____
Signature of Patient   Date

B

FIGURE 8-7 Examples of patients' Medicare electronic signature authorization forms. **A,** Monthly form. **B,** One-time form.

records because there are no handwritten signatures on electronic claims (Figure 8-7). Office policy varies on obtaining the patient's signature for release of medical information. A clause on the patient registration form or an authorization and assignment release document may be designed specifically to obtain signatures for transmitting electronic claims and acceptance of financial responsibility by the patient. The CMS-1500 (02-12) Health Insurance Claim Form also may be used for this purpose and the patient should sign in Block 12 or 13 for a specific date of service. Most PMSs ask whether the patient's signature is on file and require a "yes" or "no" answer to complete the required field when the claim is submitted. When a physician sees a patient in the hospital who has never been to the office, the authorizations obtained by the hospital apply to that provider's filing of a claim (for example, as in a consultation process).

Clean Electronic Claims Submission

Clean claims are the key to a healthy revenue cycle, whereas a denied claim can delay payment for 30 to 100 days or more. By ensuring that clean claims are submitted initially, your chances of getting paid promptly are increased. According to industry experts, 90% of claim denials are preventable. The following is a review of some methods used to ensure clean electronic claims:

● Incorporate claim scrubber software (prebill/edit processing) to identify errors and correct them on initial submission
● Verify, file, and keep all transmission reports
● Track clearinghouse claims to ensure successful transmission
● Ensure that your computer software is consistent with the claims rules
● Verify that your software correctly prints the CMS-1500 claim form
● Use encoder software
● Use an electronic clearinghouse
● Perform single and batch claims review

PUTTING HIPAA STANDARD TRANSACTIONS TO WORK

Interactive Transactions

Interactive transactions involve back-and-forth communication between two computer systems. One requests information and the other provides information during what is referred to as *online real time*. **Real time** allows for instant information. An inquiry is made and an answer received within seconds. It can involve eligibility verification, deductible status, claim inquiries, status of claims, and other insurance claim data. Other information, such as fee schedules, allowables, procedure codes, and postoperative days for specific procedures, also may be accessed. Many insurance companies, such as Medicare fiscal intermediaries, provide access to information on assigned pending and paid claims. Additional information that may be determined includes whether the individual has other coverage and which third-party payer should be billed as primary.

Electronic Funds Transfer

Many third-party payers deposit payments in the physician's bank account automatically via **electronic funds transfer (EFT).** EFT is a paperless computerized system that enables funds to be debited, credited, or transferred and eliminates the need for personal handling of checks. A deposit-only bank account, sometimes called *zero-balance account (ZBA),* provides protection against cyber-thieves (identity or other theft). This account has blocks and filters so that it accepts only deposits. However, if the health plan's EFT agreement allows it to recoup overpayments from the provider's bank account, this restriction would have to be removed.

Under the ACA, the federal government has established a uniform procedure for electronically transferring funds as part of HIPAA Title II Administrative Simplification. Health care providers and others were required to comply with CMS's EFT rules by January 1, 2014. The benefits to a health care organization for using EFT include reduction in the amount of paper in the office, time savings for staff and avoiding the hassles associated with depositing checks at the bank, elimination of the risk of paper checks being lost or stolen in the mail, faster access to funds, and easier reconciliation of payments with bank statements.

ELECTRONIC REMITTANCE ADVICE

An **electronic remittance advice (ERA)** is a notice of payments and adjustments sent to providers, billers and suppliers. After a claim has been received and processed, the insurance carrier produces the ERA, which may serve as a companion to a claim payment or as an explanation when there is no payment. The ERA explains reimbursement decisions, including the reasons for payments and adjustments of processed claims. The ERA is similar to the remittance advice (RA) for paper claims, except that the ERA offers additional information and administrative efficiencies.

If the medical practice elects to set the software system to automatically post the information to patients' accounts, then data entry is not required. The computer tests the claims computer data against various guidelines or parameters known as *screens*. If the services billed on the claim exceed the screens, the claim is denied, returned to the physician for more information, or sent for review. If a claim is denied or rejected, the insurance billing specialist receives a printout stating the reason. The missing, miscoded, or incomplete information should be added or corrected and the claim resubmitted; this process is more efficient than remaining on a telephone, on hold, or resubmitting a claim via standard mail.

A Medicare ERA, formerly known as *explanation of Medicare benefits (EOMB* or *EOB)*, is based on the ANSI ASC X12 Health Care Claim Payment/Advice (835), or "ANSI 835." A subcommittee, X12N, has developed standards for a variety of electronic transactions between third-party payers and health care providers.

The use of ANSI 835 Version 5010 generates an electronic Medicare RA similar to the Standard Paper Remittance Advice (SPR) (Figure 8-8). To improve cash flow, ANSI 835 also allows EFT of Medicare payments to the physician's bank account, which is called *direct deposit*.

DRIVING THE DATA

Basic procedures for transmission of a claim electronically are as follows:
1. Set up the database.
2. Enter data.
3. Batch or compile a group of claims.
4. Connect the computerized database with the clearinghouse or direct to the payer.

5. Transmit the claims.
6. Review the clearinghouse reports.

METHODS FOR SENDING CLAIMS

The methods for getting claims submitted to either the payer or the clearinghouse vary according to the office system in place. Methods can include the following:
1. Data transmission via **cable modem, digital subscriber line (DSL),** or **T-1.**
   a. *Cable modem.* A modem used to connect a computer to a cable television system that offers online services.
   b. *DSL.* A high-speed connection through a telephone line jack and usually a means of accessing the internet.
   c. *T-1.* A T-carrier channel that can transmit voice or data channels quickly.
2. Data directly keyed into payer system: **Direct data entry (DDE)** via dial-up modem or internet
   a. *DDE.* Keying claim information directly into the payer system by accessing it over modem dial-up or DSL. This is a technology used to directly enter the information into the payer system via the access, whether it is dial-up or DSL.
3. *PMS.* An in-house shared system or **application service provider (ASP)**
   a. *ASP.* "Renting" a PMS available over the internet. All data are housed on the server of the ASP but the accounts are managed by the health care provider's staff. Claims are batched and submitted as though the software is stored on the desktop at the provider's office.

COMPUTER CLAIMS SYSTEMS

Payer or Carrier-Direct

For a better understanding of how insurance claims are transmitted, know the types of systems and how they work (for example, payer or carrier-direct and clearinghouse).

Fiscal agents for Medicaid, Medicare, TRICARE, and many private third-party payers use the carrier-direct system. With this system, the data are transmitted electronically directly to the payer's system. This eliminates the need for a clearinghouse.

It is necessary to have a signed agreement with each carrier with whom the physician wishes to submit electronic claims.

Once enrollment is complete, a submitter number may be assigned. Submitters must send a test file to the insurance carrier to ensure accurate file format, completeness, and validity. Any problems discovered during the test

No. 1 ABC INSURANCE COMPANY	5780 MAIN STREET	WOODLAND HILLS	XY	12345	TEL # 5557639836
No. 2 Prov #	No. 3 Prov Name	No. 4 Part B	No. 5	Paid Date:	No. 6 Remit # Page:

Claim information block

PATIENT NAME No. 7	PATIENT CNTRL NUMBER No. 12		
HIC NUMBER No. 8	ICN NUMBER No. 13		
FROM DT–THRU DT Nos. 9 / 10	NACHG Nos. 14	HICHG No. 15	TOB No. 16
CLM STATUS No. 11	COST Nos. 17	COVDY No. 18	NCOVDY No. 19

Charges / adjustments grid

RC No. 20	REM No. 21	DRG # No. 22	DRG OUT AMT No. 27	COINSURANCE No. 30	PAT REFUND No. 34	CONTRACT ADJ No. 38
RC No. 20	REM No. 21	OUTCD Nos. 23 / CAPCD 24	MSP PAYMT No. 28	COVD CHGS No. 31	ESRD NET ADJ No. 35	PER DIEM RTE No. 39
RC No. 20	REM No. 21	PROF COMP No. 25		NCOVD CHGS No. 32	INTEREST No. 36	PROC CD AMT No. 40
		DRG AMT No. 26	DEDUCTIBLES No. 29	DENIED CHGS No. 33	PRE PAY ADJ No. 37	NET REIMB No. 41

Detail / subtotal number rows

	COST	COVDY	NCOVDY	PROF COMP	DRG AMT	DRG OUT AMT	MSP PAYMT	DEDUCTIBLES	COINSURANCE	COVD CHGS	NCOVD CHGS	DENIED CHGS	PAT REFUND	ESRD NET ADJ	INTEREST	PRE PAY ADJ	CONTRACT ADJ	PER DIEM RTE	PROC CD AMT	NET REIMB
(claim line)	Nos. 17	No. 18	No. 19	No. 25	No. 26	No. 27	No. 28	No. 29	No. 30	No. 31	No. 32	No. 33	No. 34	No. 35	No. 36	No. 37	No. 38	No. 39	No. 40	No. 41
SUBTOTAL FISCAL YEAR	Nos. 17	No. 18	No. 19	No. 25	No. 26	No. 27	No. 28	No. 29	No. 30	No. 31	No. 32	No. 33	No. 34	No. 35	No. 36	No. 37	No. 38	No. 39	No. 40	No. 41
SUBTOTAL PART B	Nos. 17	No. 18	No. 19	No. 25	No. 26	No. 27	No. 28	No. 29	No. 30	No. 31	No. 32	No. 33	No. 34	No. 35	No. 36	No. 37	No. 38	No. 39	No. 40	No. 41

FIGURE 8-8 A, Example of a computer-generated Medicare Part B remittance advice (RA) document received by a provider from the payer or fiscal intermediary.

Continued

A

Medicare Standard Remittence Advice

Claim Adjustment Reason Codes (CARCs) provide financial information about claim decisions. CARCs communicate an adjustment, or why a claim (or service line) was paid differently than it was billed.

1	Deductible amount
2	Coinsurance amount
3	Copayment amount
4	The procedure code is inconsistent with the modifier used or a required modifier is missing.
5	The procedure code/bill type is inconsistent with the place of service.
6	The procedure/revenue code is inconsistent with the patient's age.

Remittance Advice Remark Codes (RARCs) are used in conjunction with CARCs on the Medicare remittance advice to further explain an adjustment or to indicate if and what appeal rights apply. RARCs are maintained by CMS, but may be used by any health care payer when appropriate.

M2	Not paid separately when the patient is an inpatient.
M19	Missing oxygen certification/recertification
M20	Missing/invalid HCPCS code

B

FIGURE 8-8, cont'd **B,** Medicare standard remittance advice.

period must be corrected and a new test submitted for review before final approval. Test submissions may be a cross-section of claim type data (from previously adjudicated claims) that might be expected in a production environment. The test file must consist of a minimum number of claims, dependent on the requirements of the insurance carrier, for each claim type to be billed. The test procedure must be completed for each claim type. A new test must be submitted when software is upgraded or the submission method changes. Test claims are not processed for payment. It is only after receiving written notification from the insurance carrier that claims may be transmitted electronically.

Clearinghouses

Clearinghouses may charge a flat fee per claim or a monthly fee. Some clearinghouses offer to file claims free of charge to the provider but they recoup the expense from the payer. Most often, a vendor agreement of sorts

will be in place between the clearinghouse and the provider submitting the claims. These contracts may be a **business associate agreement,** a **trading partner agreement,** or other contract.

TRANSMISSION REPORTS

Whether claims are submitted carrier-direct or through a clearinghouse, reports are generated and accessible to track each function of the claims process. Examples are as follows:

Send and Receive File Reports: Shows that a file is received by the clearinghouse and/or payer and also notifies the billing specialist when a file has been sent to the provider's account for review (Figure 8-9).

Batch Claim Report Billed Summary: Lists each patient's name, total charges for medical services, batch number, billing number, name of insurance company

```
                        Raw 837
                     ==========

              Electronic Technologies, Inc.
              ===========================


  ISA*00* *00*
  *ZZ*1234*ZZ*VB6786786*041110*0310*U*00401*123456789*0*P*:~GS*HC*12
  34*VB6786786*20041110*0310*123456789*X*004010X098A1~ST*837*0001~B
  HT*0019*00*1*20041110*0310*CH~REF*87*004010X098A1~NM1*41*2*GERI
  ATRIC ASSOCIATES LLC*****46*1234~PER*IC*JIM
  JONES*TE*8005551212~NM1*40*2*MASSACHUSETTS INS
  PLAN*****46*XYZ1~HL*1**20*1~NM1*85*2*ALABAMA MEDICAL
  ASSOC*****24*54-5555555~N3*PO BOX
  123456~N4*BOSTON*MA*12345~REF*1D*123456789~HL*2*1*22*0~SBR*P*1
  8*******MC~NM1*IL*1*JONES*DEBRA*K***MI*123456789123~N3*11
  JEFFERS POND
  ROAD~N4*BOSTON*MA*12345~DMG*D8*19640812*F~NM1*PR*2*VMAP
  FHSC FA*****PI*DMAS~N3*PO BOX
  123~N4*BOSTON*MA*12345~CLM*123456*150***11::1*Y*A*Y*Y*B~REF*X
  4*1242522DD~HI*BK:6110~NM1*DN*1*JACKSON*DONALD~REF*1D*12345
  6789~NM1*82*1*ROWLAND*DAVID****24*54-
  5555555~PRV*PE*ZZ*207ZP0102X~REF*1D*123456789~NM1*77*2*NORTH
  OFFICE*****24*54-5555555~N3*123 LIPPLE
  AVENUE~N4*BOSTON*MA*12345~LX*1~SV1*HC:88305:26*150*UN*1***1~
  DTP*472*D8*20041028~REF*6R*11265594~
          .
          .
          .
          .
          .

  SE*160*0001~GE*1*123456789~IEA*1*123456789~
```

A

```
                        Human-Readable 837
                        ==================
                   Electronic Technologies, Inc.
                        ==================
```

INTERCHANGE HEADER - Production File

Authorization: none	Password: none
SubmitterID: 1234	ReceiverID: VB6786786
Date: 11.10.2004	Time: 0310
Run #: 003	Control #: 123456789

Request Acknowledgement: No Sub-element Separator: :

FUNCTIONAL GROUP HEADER - HC

Submitter ID: 1234	ReceiverID: VB6786786
Date: 11.10.2004	Time: 0310 Control #: 123456789

ANSI X10 Version: 004010X098A1

TRANSACTION SET HEADER- 837

Control #: 0001

Structure Code: 0019	Purpose Code: 00
Reference ID: 1	Type: CH
Date: 11.10.2004	Time: 0310

Functional Category: 004010X098A1

Submitter - Non-Person

GERIATRIC ASSOCIATES LLC (Electronic Transmitter ID #,1234)
Contact: JIM JONES
Phone Number: 800.555.1212

Receiver - Non-Person

MASSACHUSETTS INS PLAN (Electronic Transmitter ID #,XYZ1)

BATCH #1

Billing Provider - Non-Person

ALABAMA MEDICAL ASSOC (Employer ID Number,54-5555555)
PO BOX 123456
BOSTON, MA 12345
Provider Number: 123456789

PATIENT #1

Primary Insurance

Patient Relationship: Self

Subscriber - Person

JONES, DEBRA K (Member ID Number,123456789123)
11 JEFFERS POND ROAD
BOSTON, MA 12345

Date of Birth: 19640812 Gender Code: F

Payer - Non-Person

VMAP FHSC FA (Payer ID Number,DMAS)
PO BOX 123
BOSTON, MA 12345

Account Number:	123456
Claim Amount:	$150
Facility:	Office
This Claim is	ORIGINAL
Provider Signature:	On File Assignment Code: Assigned
Assignment of Benefits Indicator:	Y
Release of Information:	Yes, Provider Has a Signed Statement
Permitting Release of Medical Billing	
Data Related to a Claim	
CLIA Number:	1242522DD
Principal Diagnosis Code:	6110

Referring Prov. - Person

JACKSON, DONALD
MA Provider Number: 123456789

Rendering Prov. - Person

ROWLAND, DAVID (Employer ID Number,54-5555555)
Provider Taxonomy Code: 207ZP0102X
MA Provider Number: 123456789

Service Location - Non-Person

NORTH OFFICE (Employer ID Number,54-5555555)
123 LIPPLE AVENUE
BOSTON, MA 12345

Service Line # 1

Service Code:	88305
Modifier:	26
Amount:	$150 Measurement: Unit Quantity: 1
Diagnosis Pointer:	1
Date of Service:	20041028
Prov. Control #:	11265594

PATIENT #2
          .
          .
          .

TRANSACTION SET TRAILER

Included Segments: 160
Control #: 0001

FUNCTIONAL GROUP TRAILER

Transaction Sets Included: 1
Group Control #: 123456789

INTERCHANGE TRAILER

Included Functional Groups: 1
Control #: 123456789

B

FIGURE 8-9 A, Raw 837 clearinghouse transmission report. If you print the 837 electronic claims transmission file, it looks similar to this; however, the report becomes readable after it comes back from the clearinghouse showing the patients' claims that were submitted. **B,** Readable 837 clearinghouse transmission report. *(Reports supplied by Electronic Technologies, Inc., Delmar, NY.)*

BATCH CLAIM REPORT Billed Summary					
Patient code	Total charges	Batch #	Billing #	Insurance co. billed	Date sent
BORTOLUSSI	465.00	2	1005	ABCI000001	05/25/2005
BLACKWOOD	16.07	3	1006	TRICARE	05/25/2005
HELMS	33.25	4	1007	MDCR	05/25/2005
JAMESON	41.07	5	1008	ROYAL	05/25/2005
KELSEY	66.23	8	1010	XYZI000001	06/09/2005
	621.62				

FIGURE 8-10 Batch Claim Report Billed Summary by chronologic date.

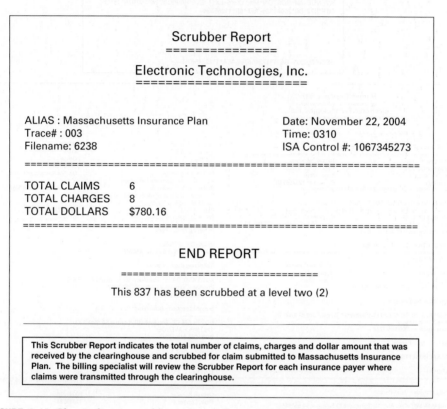

FIGURE 8-11 Clearinghouse scrubber report. *(Report supplied by Electronic Technologies, Inc., Delmar, NY.)*

billed, and chronologic date on which the claim was transmitted (Figure 8-10).

Scrubber Report: Indicates the total number of claims, charges, and dollar amounts that were received by the clearinghouse and scrubbed for claims submitted to Massachusetts Insurance Plan (Figure 8-11). The insurance billing specialist reviews the scrubber report for each insurance payer when claims have been transmitted through the clearinghouse.

Transaction Transmission Summary: Shows how many claims were originally received by the clearinghouse

and/or payer and how many claims were rejected automatically (not included for further processing) (Figure 8-12).

Rejection Analysis Report: Identifies the most common reasons that claims are rejected and indicates what claims were not included for processing (Figure 8-13). Corrections must be made by the insurance billing specialist and the claims need to be refiled.

Electronic Inquiry or Claims Status Review: Lists files received from the provider's office and indicates the progress of the claim. For example, if a claim is sent to

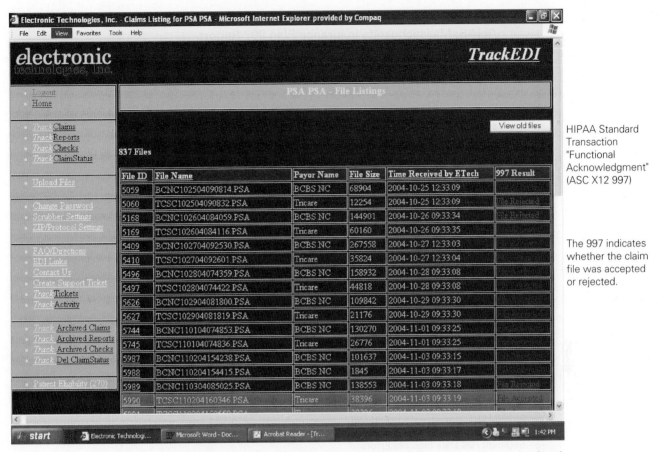

FIGURE 8-12 Clearinghouse 997 report that shows which 837 claim files were accepted and rejected. *(Report supplied by Electronic Technologies, Inc., Delmar, NY.)*

a clearinghouse and forwarded to a payer, the clearinghouse can indicate that the status is confirmed received by the payer.

Electronic Processing Problems

Some problems can occur in electronic claims submission. Usually a status report of claims is received electronically from the third-party payer. It consists of an acknowledgment report and indicates assigned and unassigned claims, crossed over and not crossed over claims, claims accepted with errors, and rejected claims (see Figure 8-13). Data transmission problems arise periodically because of hardware or software problems.

Changes to the standard electronic claims submission process can also result in errors. The upgrade to HIPAA transaction standard ASC X12 Version 5010 resulted in these common errors:

Billing Provider Address: The 5010 guidelines require providers to enter the physical address; post office boxes or lock box addresses cannot be used as a provider's address.

Zip Code: The 5010 guidelines require a nine-digit zip code when reporting billing provider and service facility locations.

Anesthesia Minutes: The 5010 guidelines require that anesthesia services be reported in actual minutes rather than units.

Primary Identification Code Qualifiers: The 5010 guidelines allow only an NPI as a primary identifier. EINs or Social Security numbers (SSNs) cannot be used as a primary identifier.

Billing Provider NPI Number: The 5010 guidelines require that a consistent NPI number be reported with all payers.

National Drug Code (NDC): The 5010 guidelines require that a drug quantity and unit of measure be reported on the claim form when an NDC is used.

Most billing software bundles claims into a batch and then claims are transmitted together. If one claim in the batch contains an error (for example, missing patient

ALIAS: Massachusetts Insurance Plan 997 Report
===
CLAIMS 997 ACKNOWLEDGMENT FILE

Trace#: 941   ID: 114120941
SUBMISSION DATE: 11.22.2004   997 DATE: 11.23.2004
TIME SUBMITTED: 0112   997 TIME: 111346
===============   ===

ERROR CODE	PATIENT ACCT #	LINE# / CHARGE#
251:NM1:9	628263478	2893

DESCRIPTION: Payer Name
Segment Has Data Element Errors
DETAIL: Subscriber Identifier - (Mandatory data element missing)
SUBMITTED:

ERROR CODE	PATIENT ACCT #	LINE# / CHARGE#
251:NM1:10	123456	5454545

DESCRIPTION: Payer Name
Segment Has Data Element Errors
DETAIL: (Invalid character in data element)
SUBMITTED:

ERROR CODE	PATIENT ACCT #	LINE# / CHARGE#
251:NM1:8	4515485	3157654

DESCRIPTION: Payer Name
Segment Has Data Element Errors
DETAIL: Identification Qualifier (Conditional required data element
missing)
SUBMITTED:

This transaction was :   Rejected
Rejection Reason :   One or More Segments in Error
This Functional Group was :   Rejected
Transaction Sets Included :   1
Transaction Sets Received :   1
Transaction Sets Accepted :   0

FIGURE 8-13 Clearinghouse 997 report showing the claims acknowledgment file. This report shows error codes and details the types of errors made. It also shows patient account numbers and names of the payers. *(Report supplied by Electronic Technologies, Inc., Delmar, NY.)*

name or missing diagnosis code), the third-party payer may reject the entire batch and return all claims to the provider. Some batches contain errors that occur in every transaction in the batch. These are called *syntax errors*. Syntax errors are inaccuracies that violate the HIPAA standard transaction format, such as incorrect sequence of patient information or incorrect batch header. Such errors make it difficult for the third-party payer's software to read the transactions in a batch. There are other errors in which only one transaction in the batch has a syntax error or one of the batch's transactions has a data content error. In these instances, it would be inappropriate for a third-party payer to reject the entire batch. Usually the payer returns any noncompliant claims and

processes the remaining claims in the batch. To avoid these types of rejections, it is important to use software that will separate out noncompliant transactions so that those can be removed from the batch and fixed before submission.

Solutions to Electronic Processing Problems

1. Review claims filed electronically by validating that you received confirmation that the claims were processed by the clearinghouse and received by the insurance carrier. Check for error messages from the clearinghouse and payer. Immediately respond to rejected claims.

Table 8-6	Daily, Weekly, and End-of-Month Guidelines and Protocols	
DAILY	**WEEKLY**	**END OF MONTH**
Post charges in practice management system.	Batch, scrub, edit, and transmit claims (daily or weekly).	Run month-end aging reports.
Post payments in practice management system.	Analyze previous week's rejected and resubmitted claims.	Review all claim rejection reports (clearinghouse and payer), ensuring all problems are resolved and claims accepted.
Batch, scrub, edit, and transmit claims (daily or weekly); retrieve transmission reports.	Note any problematic claims and resolve outstanding files.	Update practice management system with payer information, such as EIN and NPI.
Run daysheet.	Research unpaid claims.	Run patient statements in office or through clearinghouse.
Review clearinghouse/payer transmission confirmation reports.	Make follow-up calls to resolve reasons for rejections, such as incorrect NPI, missing patient ID, incomplete data elements, and wrong format.	
Audit claims batched and transmitted with confirmation reports.		
Correct rejections and resubmit claims.		

EIN, Employer identification number; *ID,* identification; *NPI,* National Provider Identifier.

2. Produce monthly aging of accounts and check the large amounts not paid in the 60-day aging column. Look at service dates of claims and the amounts. If there are many outstanding claims with the same service dates, it is possible that these claims did not reach the payer. Immediately confirm with the payer whether the claims were received and refile if appropriate.

3. File claims within the time limits because many payers have a 90-day filing deadline. Payers will not reimburse a time delinquent claim unless you can prove that the payer received the claim. Electronic confirmation that a claim reached the clearinghouse is not sufficient.

4. Double check that the correct code for place of service is shown, especially if your physician does procedures in different locations (office 11, hospital inpatient 21, ASC 24, or nursing home 12). The payment amount may be more or less, depending on the location.

5. Be accurate in linking the correct diagnosis codes to the procedure codes. Usually payers use the first diagnosis codes (primary and underlying) to process claims. Additional diagnostic codes may be used only for informational purposes or not considered at all.

Billing and Account Management Schedule

Maintaining a schedule will help with EDI transmissions, which will enable better cash flow. Table 8-6 suggests guidelines and procedures that can be tailored to the needs of your billing office.

Administrative Simplification Enforcement Tool

To address issues of noncompliance with the HIPAA TCS rule, the federal government has implemented the use of an electronic tool to assist health care providers, payers, clearinghouses, and others to submit complaints. This online tool, the *Administrative Simplification Enforcement Tool (ASET),* enables individuals or organizations to file a complaint online against an entity "whose actions impact the ability of a transaction to be accepted and/or efficiently processed."

The Security Rule: Administrative, Physical, and Technical Safeguards

Security measures encompass all administrative, physical, and technical safeguards in an information system. The Security Rule addresses only electronic protected health information (ePHI) but the concept of protecting PHI that will become ePHI puts emphasis on security for the entire office. The Security Rule is divided into the following three main sections:
- Administrative safeguards
- Technical safeguards
- Physical safeguards

Administrative safeguards prevent unauthorized use or disclosure of PHI through development, implementation, and maintenance of security measures to protect ePHI. These management controls guard data integrity, confidentiality, and availability and include the following:
- Information access controls authorize each employee's physical access to PHI. This is management of **passwords** and management of access for each individual employee that restricts access to records in accordance with the employee's responsibility in the health care organization. For example, usually the health information records clerk who has authorization to retrieve health records will

not have access to billing records located on the computer.

● Internal audits review who has had access to PHI to ensure that there is no intentional or accidental inappropriate access, in both the PMS system and the paper records or charges.

● Risk analysis and management is a process that assesses the privacy and security risks of various safeguards and the cost in losses if those safeguards are not in place. Each organization must evaluate its vulnerabilities and the associated risks and decide how to lessen those risks. Reasonable safeguards must be implemented to protect against known risks.

● Termination procedures should be formally documented in the office policies and procedures (P&P) manual and include terminating an employee's access to PHI. Other procedures include changing office security pass codes, deleting user access to computer systems, deleting terminated employees' e-mail accounts, and collecting any access cards or keys.

Technical safeguards are technologic controls in place to protect and control access to information on computers in the health care organization and include the following:

● Access controls through limitations created for each staff member based on job category (for example, receptionist, administrative medical assistant, clinical medical assistant, bookkeeper, or insurance billing specialist).

● Audit controls keep track of log-ins to the computer system, administrative activity, and changes to data. This includes changing passwords, deleting user accounts, and creating new user accounts.

● Automatic log-offs prevent unauthorized users from accessing a computer when it is left unattended. The computer system or software program should automatically log off after a predetermined period of inactivity. Each user should have a unique identifier or "user name" and an unshared, undisclosed password to log in to any computer with access to PHI. Identifying each unique user allows the functions of auditing and access controls to be implemented. Passwords for all users should be changed on a regular basis and should never be common names or words.

Physical safeguards also prevent unauthorized access to PHI. These physical measures and P&P protect a covered entity's electronic information systems and related buildings and equipment from natural and environmental hazards and unauthorized intrusion. Appropriate and reasonable physical safeguards should include the following:

● Media and equipment controls are documented in the office P&P manual regarding management of the PHI. Typical safeguard policies include how the office handles the retention, removal, and disposal of paper records as well as recycling computers and destroying obsolete data disks or software programs containing PHI.

● Physical access controls limit unauthorized access to areas in which equipment and medical charts are stored. Locks on doors are the most common type of control.

● Secure workstation locations minimize the possibility of unauthorized viewing of PHI. This includes ensuring that password-protected screen savers are in use on computers when unattended and that desk drawers are locked.

 COMPUTER CONFIDENTIALITY

Confidentiality Statement

Most information in patients' medical records and physicians' financial records is considered confidential and sensitive. Employees who have access to such computer data should have integrity and be well chosen because they have a high degree of responsibility and accountability. It is wise to have those handling sensitive computer documents sign an annual confidentiality statement, as recommended by the Alliance of Claims Assistance Professionals (ACAP) (Figure 8-14). This way, the statement can be updated when an individual's responsibilities increase or decrease. The statement should contain the following:

● Written or oral disclosure of information pertaining to patients is prohibited.

● Disclosure of information without consent of the patient results in serious penalty (for example, immediate dismissal).

An additional example of an employee confidentiality agreement that may be used by an employer when hiring an insurance biller is shown in Figure 2-5.

Prevention Measures

Employees can take a number of preventive measures to maintain computer security.

1. Obtain a software program that stores files in coded form.

2. Never leave disks or tapes unguarded on desks or anywhere else in sight.

3. Use a privacy filter over the computer monitor so that data may be read only when the user is directly in front of the computer.

4. Log off the computer terminal before leaving a workstation. Check and double check the credentials of any consultant hired.

5. Read the manuals for the equipment, especially the sections titled "Security Controls," and follow all directions.
6. Store confidential data on disks rather than only on the computer's hard drive. Disks should be stored in a locked, secure location, preferably one that is fireproof and away from magnetic fields.
7. Make sure the computer system has a firewall installed and proper antivirus/antispyware software. Hackers can also access digital copiers, laser printers, fax machines, and other electronic equipment with internal memories. Develop passwords for each user and access codes to protect the data. A password is a combination of letters, numbers, or symbols that an individual is assigned to access the system. Passwords should be changed at regular intervals and never written down. A good password is composed of more than eight characters and is case sensitive. *Case sensitive* means that the password must be entered exactly as stored using upper- or lower-case characters. Delete obsolete passwords from the system. Change any passwords known by an employee who is fired or resigns. Individuals with their own passwords allow the employer to distinguish work done by each employee. *If errors or* problems occur, focus may then be directed toward correcting the individual user.
8. A strong password:
   • Is at least eight characters long.
   • Does not contain your user name, real name, or company name.
   • Does not contain a complete word.
   • Is significantly different from a previous password.
   • Contains characters from these 4 categories: Upper case, Lower case, Numbers, Symbols.
     • Example: Iluv2pla2BA4$
9. Send only an account number (not the patient's name) when e-mailing a colleague with specific questions (for example, about coding).

RECORDS MANAGEMENT

Data Storage

A paperless office requires an organized and efficient system for keeping files that have been saved to the hard drive protected from accidental destruction. Keep financial records on computer disks or tapes and store them in an area that does not have temperature extremes or magnetic fields.

When data are keyboarded, it is wise to **back up** (save data) frequently, preferably daily. Automated backup is possible and the computer regularly initiates the process. Most financial software programs display a screen prompt instructing the operator to back up before quitting the program. If there is no automated backup, always back up files at the end of the day or several times a week so that information is not lost during a power outage (for example, surge, spike, blackout, brownout, lightning strike), computer breakdown, or head crash. Head crash occurs when the read-write head on a disk drive strikes the surface of the disk, causing damage at the point of impact.

About once a week, a verification process should be done that compares the original records with the copies. This can take 20% to 30% longer than ordinary backup but if a comparison is not made, there is no way to ensure that the data have been backed up. Store backup copies away from the office in case of fire, flood, or theft.

Maintain a notebook (log) of the documents on computer disks or CDs with an index located at the front of the book. The log enables you to keep track of files and should list when the files were backed up last so that they can be located quickly. Be sure that another employee knows where this notebook is kept and is familiar with how to track down files through this system. Note the code for accessing these documents and date revisions when updating old documents. Do not put anything related to PHI in this log (for example, 31403.DOC, Mrs. Private Patient Positive HIV Report).

Data Disposal

Another HIPAA security rule is the establishment of policies and procedures for final disposal of ePHI and the hardware or electronic media on which it is stored. It is easy to recover ePHI from hard drives, CD-ROMs, and other media storage devices if it is not properly erased or destroyed. Simply deleting files or formatting drives is not sufficient to keep ePHI from being accessed. Covered entities must implement reasonable safeguards when disposing of information. Some acceptable methods are as follows:

● Reformat and overwrite the disk media several times to sanitize the hard drive.
● Reinitialize the storage space of the computer hardware, if possible.
● Break, incinerate, crush, or destroy the storage device.
● Shred audiotapes, microfilm, or microfiche.

YOUR COMPANY NAME
ADDRESS
PHONE/FAX

CONFIDENTIALITY STATEMENT

I, _____ , understand and acknowledge that as a
(Type in individual's name)
principle/employee of _____(company name)_____ my position
as ___(job title)_____ requires that I access and use computer equipment and
software applications owned or leased by___(company name)___ .
I understand that my position as a principle/employee of this company obligates me to abide by
the purchase, lease or rental agreements applicable to this equipment and software.

I understand and acknowledge that my position may require that I handle information regarding
the physicians and medical suppliers who are clients of ___(company name)___ .
I understand and acknowledge that such client information, including financial data, fees,
corporate structure, etc., is privileged and confidential and that I am not at liberty to divulge or
discuss such information with unauthorized individuals within this company or to anyone outside
this company.

I understand and acknowledge that my duties may require me to access and/or process specific
patient data for individuals under the care of___(company name)___ client
physicians and/or medical suppliers. I understand and acknowledge that all patient's data is
protected under federal privacy legislation and that discussion or release of this information in any
form without the patient's express permission is prohibited by federal law and subject to
prosecution and civil monetary penalties for any violation.

I further understand that violations of this confidentiality agreement will result in termination of
employment with___(company name)___ .

My signature below is to verify my understanding and acceptance of the above data
confidentiality requirements and to signify my explicit agreement to abide by these requirements.

_____   _____
Signature   Date

_____   _____
Type Name   Title

FIGURE 8-14 Example of a confidentiality statement for an employee using computer equipment and software. *(From National Association of Claims Assistance Professionals, Inc., Downers Grove, Ill.)*

Electronic Power Protection

Plug equipment into power surge suppressors or, better yet, receptacles with an uninterruptible power supply (UPS) to prevent computer and data file damage. In addition, the entire office should be protected by a surge suppressor installed near the electric circuit breaker panel. This device is called an *all-office* or *whole-office surge suppressor.*

Selection of an Office Computer System

A medical practice wishing to use an in-office computer or an individual wishing to set up his or her own business should consider the following:

1. What is the cost of the basic equipment and will it be purchased or leased?

2. What are the hardware maintenance costs and who will do the repair work?
3. What is the estimated cost of software upgrades and will upgrades require an expanded operating system?
4. How many people on the staff will operate the computer? Will recruitment be necessary? Who will train employees? How much training time is necessary?
5. Will there be insurance and a warranty on the system?
6. How much will the consulting costs be?
7. What is the backup support and response time when there is a system crash (software or hardware)? Who will respond to software problems and who will respond to hardware problems?
8. How much time will it take to convert the current accounting system to the computerized system and who will be doing the conversion?

Major mistakes made by practice administrators and physicians when selecting an office computer system are as follows:

- Practice software process is not structured.
- Specific needs and requirements are not fully addressed.
- Consultant selected for advice is biased.
- Primary users are omitted from purchasing decision process.
- The practice buys more than is required.

- Vendors are allowed to dictate the purchasing process.
- Senior management team finalizes the choice of systems in the process rather than giving end users more input.
- The vendor representative is equated with the product.
- The request for proposal concept is not used (asking the vendor of the software system to submit a proposal for the medical practice that includes features, initial cost, and maintenance of the system in the future).

KEY POINTS

This is a brief chapter review, or summary, of the key issues presented. To further enhance your knowledge of the technical subject matter, review the key terms and key abbreviations for this chapter by locating the meaning for each in the Glossary at the end of this book, which appears in a section before the Index.

1. The American National Standards Institute (ANSI) formed the Accredited Standards Committee X12 (ASC X12), which developed the US standards body for the cross-industry development, maintenance, and publication of electronic data exchange standards.

2. Through HIPAA regulations, standardized transaction and code sets have been implemented to use electronic data interchange effectively.

3. A clearinghouse receives the electronic transmission of claims from the health care provider's office and translates it to a standard format prescribed in HIPAA regulations.

4. Under HIPAA rules, a provider who sends Medicare claims is considered a covered entity that has 10 or more employees and must transmit claims electronically. Medical practices with fewer than 10 employees are not considered covered entities and are not required to submit Medicare claims electronically.

5. Practice management software (PMS) is used to input data, which helps to generate a variety of documents including the 837P (professional) in electronic National Standard Format (NSF), formerly the CMS-1500 (02-12) paper form.

6. When constructing an insurance claim, the supporting code sets are made up of "required" and "situational" data elements identified by the HIPAA standard electronic formats.

7. Ten-character, alphanumeric provider-specialty taxonomy codes are assigned and classify each health care provider. These codes are used when transmitting electronic insurance claims.

8. Employers use their employer identification numbers (EINs) to identify themselves in transactions involving premium payments to health plans on behalf of their employees or to identify themselves to other employers as the source or receiver of information about eligibility. Employers use EINs to identify themselves in transactions when enrolling or disenrolling employees in health plans.

9. HIPAA requires that a National Provider Identifier (NPI), a 10-character numeric identifier, be assigned to each provider to be used in transactions with all health plans.

10. An encoder is helpful because it can reduce the time it takes to build or review a claim and help to improve coding accuracy before batching and transmitting to a third-party payer.

11. An electronic remittance advice (ERA) is the equivalent of a paper summarized statement called an *explanation of benefits (EOB)*, which gives the status of insurance claims with payment details for one or more beneficiaries. It is referred to as *ANSI 835* or *Health Care Claim Payment/Advice (835)*.

12. Several methods are available for submitting claims to either the payer or a clearinghouse, such as cable modem, digital subscriber line (DSL), T-1, direct data entry (DDE), and application service provider (ASP).

13. The HIPAA Security Rule addresses only electronic protected health information (ePHI) and is divided into three sections: administrative safeguards, technical safeguards, and physical safeguards.

14. Computer confidentiality and security measures must be followed at all times to prevent unauthorized disclosure of ePHI.

15. Back up data frequently to prevent loss of files and information.

▣ STUDENT ASSIGNMENT

✔ Study Chapter 8.

✔ Answer the fill-in-the-blank, multiple-choice, and true/false review questions in the *Workbook* to reinforce the theories learned in this chapter and to help prepare for a future test.

✔ Complete the assignments in the *Workbook* to edit and correct insurance claims that have been transmitted and rejected with errors.

✔ Turn to the Glossary at the end of this text for a further understanding of the key terms and key abbreviations used in this chapter.

Receiving Payments and Insurance Problem Solving

Payel Bhattacharya Madero

OBJECTIVES

After reading this chapter, you should be able to:

1. Identify and discuss three health insurance payment policy guidelines.
2. Assess reimbursement payment time frames for all submitted claims.
3. Identify the components of an explanation of benefits document and interpret and post an explanation of benefits document to a patient's account.
4. Discuss secondary insurance and guidelines to billing secondary insurance.
5. List and describe three health insurance claim management techniques.
6. Explain reasons for claim inquiries and identify strategies to discover why payments are delayed.
7. Define terminology pertinent to problem claims filing and discuss types of problems as well as find solutions.
8. Identify specific reasons for rebilling a claim.
9. Describe situations for filing appeals and discuss the review and appeals process.
10. Review Medicare's five levels in the redetermination (appeal) process and determine which forms to use for each level.
11. Review and discuss the TRICARE review and appeal process, including expedited and nonexpedited appeals, as well as reconsideration.
12. List four objectives of state insurance commissioners.
13. Mention seven problems to submit to insurance commissioners.
14. Discuss the type of information necessary to include in an insurance commission request.

KEY TERMS

Advance Beneficiary Notice of Noncoverage
aging report
appeal
delinquent claim
denied claim
explanation of benefits
inquiry

insurance payment poster
insurance payment posting
lost claim
medical necessity
overpayment
peer review
rebill (resubmit)
reimbursement

rejected claim
remittance advice
review
suspended claim
suspense
tracer

KEY ABBREVIATIONS

ABN	DAB	FTC	HO
ALJ	EOB	HIPAA	NPI
CMS	ERISA	HMO	RA

Service to Patients

To reduce insurance problems and obtain correct maximum payments, it is vital to extend service to patients by doing the following:

- Assist patients with in-office registration procedures so that complete and accurate personal and financial data are obtained initially and during follow-up visits to help diminish denied claims.
- Ensure that the patient has provided information about his or her employer, the subscriber, relationship to the subscriber, and the subscriber's date of birth.
- Verify the patient's insurance coverage. If a patient does not have active coverage and services are going to be provided, it is important to communicate that the patient is responsible for all charges and collect payment prior to providing services.
- Post a sign visible to all patients that copayments are collected at the time of the visit. Respectfully inform the patient that the copayment amounts are set by the health insurance carrier and if the patient has concerns about it, he or she should contact the carrier directly.
- Prepare a letter or form for the patient's signature if the patient has a complaint about a third-party payer and send it to the local insurance commissioner explaining the problem and asking for help in resolving it.

RESPONSE FROM A SUBMITTED CLAIM

In the life cycle of a health insurance claim, receiving a response for a submitted claim is vital to the financial success of any medical practice. An insurance company can accept responsibility to pay the claim and reimburse the medical practice, can suspend the claim to investigate the details of the claim further, or can deny the claim for a variety of different reasons. Delay in **reimbursements,** or payments to the medical practice, can also occur when health insurance companies state that they did not receive the claim at all. At times, the insurance company may reimburse claims lower than expected, after which an appeal can be filed. The management of the reimbursement process and insurance company denials is known as follow-up.

This chapter begins with the provisions for payment in the insurance contract and explains how this affects the timeliness for payment. Then the text demonstrates how to interpret the document that accompanies payment and how to manage and organize financial records. To improve cash flow, numerous problems that can occur are presented and some solutions are offered. Finally, the **review** and **appeal** processes for various programs are discussed.

By developing proficient skills and experience in following up on claims, an insurance billing specialist can become a valuable asset to his or her employer and bring in revenue that might otherwise be lost to the medical practice.

CLAIM POLICY GUIDELINES

A patient who seeks medical care with a health insurance card is presenting the contract that he or she has with the insurance company. In other words, the insurance company issued the card to the patient as evidence that it takes responsibility to pay the medical practice for the services the patient receives. As discussed in Chapter 7, in order for the medical practice to get paid for these services, insurance companies require the medical practice to submit a claim form. The insurance company dictates the guidelines for claims submission, such as which services are covered, the reimbursement rates, and time limits for claim submission and payment.

Insured

A patient's insurance card does not specify the detailed benefits and coverages. However, prior to rendering services to the patient, it is in the physician's best interest to be aware of their patients' insurance benefits and coverages. For example, maternity care is an optional benefit; therefore a physician should be aware that by providing maternity care to a patient with no coverage, he or she risks not being reimbursed. Another example is that there may be a provision that the claimant has an obligation to notify the insurance company of a loss (injury, illness, or accident) within a certain period of time or the insurer has the right to deny benefits for that loss.

In some policies, if the insured is in disagreement with the insurer for settlement of a claim, a suit must begin within 3 years after the claim is submitted. Another provision states that an insured person cannot bring legal action against an insurance company until 60 days after a claim is submitted.

Electronic Claims Submission

With the onset and ease of electronic claims submission, many health insurance companies prefer or even require that all claims be sent electronically. The Administration Simplification Compliance Act (ASCA) prohibits payment of initial health care claims not sent electronically as of October 16, 2003, except in limited situations for Medicare and other government-sponsored insurance programs. Most other private health insurance plans have also eliminated the use of paper claims. Workers' compensation insurance plans are the only group that uses paper claims on a regular basis. For more information on electronic claims submission, see Chapter 8.

Capitation Contracts and Fee Schedules

A fee schedule is included when a physician signs a contract with an insurance company or group to become an in-network provider. The physician agrees to the fee schedule, which is typically less than his or her standard fee for service, and agrees not to charge the patient for the difference while the insurance company or group agrees to refer patients to the medical practice. In certain circumstances, medical practices will agree to a contract capitation in which physicians agree to provide services by accepting the patient's copayment and the monthly stipend paid per patient. For more information on contract capitation, see Chapter 11.

Reimbursement Time Frames

All health insurance companies are obligated to reimburse medical practices for services rendered promptly. However, time limits vary in this provision from one third-party payer to another. Specific time limits will be stated in either the insurance contract or the payer's manual outlining claims filing rules. It is reasonable to expect payment within 4 to 12 weeks if claims are submitted on paper or in as little as 7 days when they are transmitted electronically.

If a payment delay occurs and the insurance company is slow or ignores, denies, or exceeds time limits to pay a claim, then it is prudent to contact the insurance company. In the letter, the contracted time limit should be stated, the reason the claim has not been paid should be sought, and a copy should be retained for the physician's files. If the problem persists and there is no favorable response, the state insurance commissioner should be contacted to see whether he or she can take action to improve the situation. A copy of the correspondence should be sent to the state insurance commissioner. Many state insurance commissioners have broad powers to regulate the insurance companies within their state; others have no powers at all. If the carrier is a self-insured plan, a Medicaid or Medicare health maintenance organization (HMO), or an Employee Retirement Income Security Act (ERISA)–based plan, the insurance commissioner will not be able to assist with carrier issues. Claims may be submitted to the insurance company repeatedly with none of them ever being recorded. Often the one claim that makes it to the insurance company is the one that arrives after the self-determined timely filing deadline. If the provider has no contract with the carrier, the provider is not obligated to meet the carrier's deadline. The denial should be appealed and payment demanded.

Managed care plans usually process claims on a daily basis but some plans release payments quarterly. Some plans withhold a percentage that is reserved in a pool and distributed at the end of the fiscal year. In some states, managed care plans do not come under the jurisdiction of the state insurance commissioner. Read through the contract; if you are still unable to determine the responsible entity, check with your state medical society. Because managed care plans vary considerably in payment policies and administrative procedures, Chapter 10 details follow-up procedures and problem-solving techniques.

EXPLANATION OF BENEFITS

An **explanation of benefits (EOB)** is a document issued to both the provider filing the claim and the patient that explains the allowable amount payable, the amount that must be written off, and what the patient is financially responsible for (if any). The EOB also provides details about claims that are denied or delayed and provides the reasons why. Sometimes EOBs will provide details on specific claims that need to be refunded and the reasons why. Finally, if a payment is explained in the EOB, a check will be attached or evidence of an electronic transfer of funds will be evident. An example of an EOB is shown in Figure 9-1. Medicare's version of this document is a **remittance advice (RA)** but the elements of the document are the same; for an example, see Figure 12-14. In this chapter we will refer to the EOB unless the discussion is about Medicare claims, in which case reference to an RA will be made.

A **suspended claim** is one that is processed by a third-party payer but is held in an indeterminate (pending) state regarding payment because of either an error or the need for additional information from the provider of service or the patient. The EOB also states the allowed amount for the service provided based on the contracted fee schedule by the third-party payer, as shown in Figure 9-1. The allowed amount is the maximum dollar value that the insurance company assigns to each medical service. If the health care provider is contracted with the health insurance company, he or she receives a copy of the EOB along with payment. If the provider is not in-network with the insurance company, payment can be sent to the patient, in which case the patient should be billed.

Components of an Explanation of Benefits

At first glance, the EOB may seem difficult to understand. Unfortunately there is no standard format for EOB forms from one carrier to the next but the information contained in each one is usually the same. If one line at a time is read, the description and calculations for each patient may be understood easily. The EOB breaks down how payment was determined and contains the following information in categories or columns:

1. Insurance company's name and address
2. Provider of services
3. Dates of services
4. Service or procedure (CPT) code
5. Amounts billed by the provider

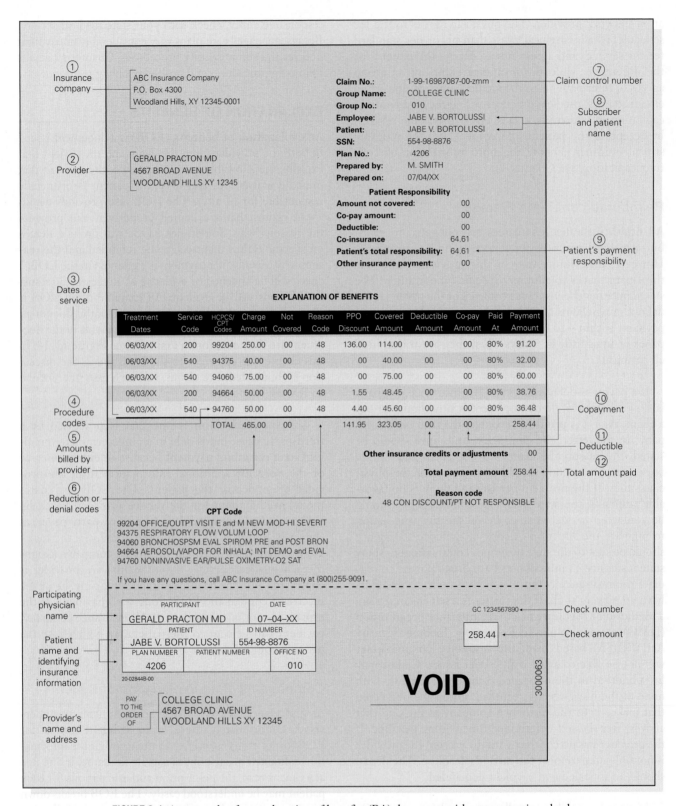

FIGURE 9-1 An example of an explanation of benefits (RA) document with accompanying check that the provider received from a private third-party payer. These payment voucher documents vary among insurance companies.

6. Reduction or denial codes. Comment codes (reasons, remarks, or notes) indicating reasons that payments were denied or reduced, asking for more information to determine coverage and benefits, or stating amounts of adjustment because of payments by other insurance companies (coordination of benefits)
7. Claim control number
8. Subscriber's and patient's name and policy numbers
9. Analysis of patient's total payment responsibility (allowed amount, copayment amount, deductible, coinsurance, other insurance payment, and patient's total responsibility)
10. Copayment amount(s) due from the patient
11. Deductible amounts subtracted from billed amounts
12. Total amount paid by the insurance carrier

Interpreting an Explanation of Benefits

Reading and interpreting an EOB may be overwhelming initially, so take time to read the document carefully. If several patients' claims are submitted to a third-party payer, the EOB may reflect the status of all of those claims and one check voucher may be issued. If the provider has signed a contract agreeing to discount fees with a number of third-party payers and managed care plans, payment amounts may vary along with the percentage of the fee that is adjusted off of the account. In addition, if more than one provider is in the medical practice and the practice is submitting claims using one group tax identification number, more than one patient's claims may appear on a single EOB. The EOB shown in Figure 9-1 should be read line by line to interpret the meanings under each category or column and the numbered explanations should be referred to when necessary. A helpful way to separate patients and their corresponding payments is to use a highlighter or ruler to underline the entire row across the EOB. This helps to reduce errors when posting payments.

Posting an Explanation of Benefits

Insurance payment posting is the process of applying payments to the patient account while writing off all adjustments. Posting of insurance payments is done by line item. In Figure 9-1 each line item, or coded service, is explained separately. The **insurance payment poster,** the individual responsible for posting payments in patient accounts, must be careful to review lines that are posted and lines that are denied. Denials should be presented to the insurance billing specialist's attention as soon as possible; many denials or pending claims have a window of time in which additional information can be forwarded to process the claim.

Patients are then billed for the balance or a secondary insurance is billed. It is during the posting process that payments are evaluated for correctness according to the insurance company contracted requirements. Refer to Chapter 3 and see Figure 3-14, which illustrates a patient's financial accounting record that shows posting of professional service descriptions, fees, payments, adjustments, and running balance due.

If services are reimbursed but you cannot totally understand what appears on an EOB, a phone call to the payer usually clarifies and resolves the problem so that posting can be completed. Most private insurance companies offer secure internet portal access that provides quick reference to the patient's EOB, contracted fee schedule, pending claims, and denied claims.

Claims paid with no errors are designated closed. EOB management can be challenging for a medical office because of the variety of EOB forms. Some EOBs have only one patient while others contain information for multiple patients. The best method to manage EOBs is to create a scanned e-file cabinet in which the patient account in the software system contains a link to the EOB.

Secondary Insurance

In some cases, patients carry secondary insurance to cover the coinsurance for which the patient is responsible. There are some guidelines to billing secondary insurance:
1. The secondary insurance cannot be billed until the primary insurance has paid.
2. Blocks 9a–d of the CMS-1500 (08-05) form should include information about the primary insurance that paid the first part of the claim.
3. Block 30 of the CMS-1500 (08-05) form should reflect the balance after the claim was paid and the amount exceeding the allowable is written off.
4. Depending on the state contractor, Medicare will automatically forward the claim it paid on to the secondary insurance. If the claim was forwarded to the secondary insurance, the EOB will state to which insurance company the EOB was forwarded. An example can be found in Figure 12-16 on the Medicare Remittance Advice. When this happens, there is no need to bill secondary insurance.
5. Reimbursements from secondary insurances should be designated separately from primary insurance payments on patient account statements.

Paid claims that have an outstanding balance should be kept aside to monitor secondary insurance payments, especially when Medicare forwards the claim to these carriers. In some cases, more commonly when Medicaid is assigned as the secondary insurance, secondary insurances may claim that the amount paid by the primary insurance exceeds their allowable for the service, so the balance should be written off.

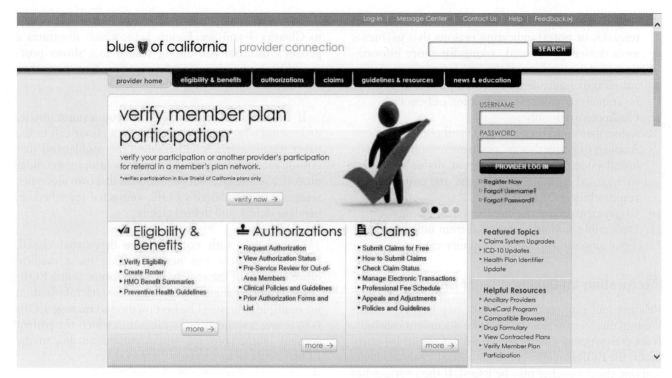

FIGURE 9-2 Online health insurance provider portals provide quick and easy access to patient eligibility, authorization for services, insurance claim status, and RAs.

EOB Management

After posting payments and adjustments to applicable patient accounts, the paper EOB should be filed in a designated area clearly marked in a folder. Some offices may group these remittances by payer, by month received, or by some other method. If your office receives electronic EOB forms and you print them out, manage them accordingly. Some practice management systems allow for paper EOB forms to be scanned into the software and some do automatic posting of payment by downloading electronic files that work in sync with the format of the remittances.

CLAIM MANAGEMENT TECHNIQUES

Insurance Claims Register

Since most claims are submitted electronically, it is vital to check Batch Claim Reports and Scrubber Reports (see Figures 8-10 and 8-11) on a scheduled basis. An acknowledgement report from the clearinghouse will list each insurance claim submitted per patient; this report should be followed up on each week to ensure that every claim is processed to prevent **delinquent claims,** or claims that are not paid within 30 days of the service date. Once the insurance company confirms receipt of the claim,

insurance billing specialists can view and confirm patient claim status using secure internet portals (Figure 9-2).

Purging Paid Files

When claims are paid off and have a zero balance, they are purged, or removed in bulk, from the insurance claim file. Some medical offices remove files when EOBs are posted but this process can be time consuming. Scheduling regular purging of the paid claims reduces the resources needed for the payment posting process. Most medical software programs offer practice management reports that can be used to track insurance payments. The most efficient way to purge patient accounts it to run an **aging report** and remove all accounts that have a zero balance (Figure 9-3). Once insurance payment posters have this report, they can forward the aging report with current balances to the follow-up specialist to obtain the status of the outstanding claims.

Aging Reports

Each month an aging report should be run. This report will indicate which claims are outstanding. The aging report categorizes outstanding claims as current, 30 days, 60 days, 90 days, and 120 days. After running the report,

AETNA									
Patient Name	Acct #	Primary Insurance	Secondary Insurance	Aging Analysis					Total Balance
				0-30	31-60	61-90	91-120	over 120	
Bassett, Eleanor	75846	AETNA		$145.00	$0.00	$0.00	$0.00	$0.00	$145.00
Herron, John	83029	AETNA		$0.00	$42.41	$0.00	$0.00	$0.00	$42.41
Holt, Maxine	64739	AETNA	BLUE SHIELD	$145.00	$0.00	$0.00	$0.00	$0.00	$145.00
Kellog, Keenan	24537	AETNA		$0.00	$0.00	$145.00	$0.00	$0.00	$145.00
Lincoln, Frank	85940	AETNA		$0.00	$15.00	$0.00	$0.00	$0.00	$15.00
Markham, Melanie	14263	AETNA	MEDICARE	$0.00	$0.00	$0.00	$260.00	$0.00	$260.00
McDonald, Lydia	56374	AETNA		$260.00	$0.00	$0.00	$0.00	$0.00	$260.00
McLean, Mary	24395	AETNA		$0.00	$0.00	$0.00	$0.00	$260.00	$260.00
Aetna Aging Total :				**$550.00**	**$57.41**	**$145.00**	**$260.00**	**$260.00**	**$1,272.41**

FIGURE 9-3 The aging report shows patient account balances according to the number of days after the date of service.

proper follow-up should be made by inquiring why a claim has not yet been paid. The insurance billing specialist can write notes on the aging report documenting phone calls to the payer or adjustments made or include notes in the patient's medical billing software profile. For example, a note indicating that the claim is to be corrected and rebilled would be helpful; many software systems allow the user to create alerts for when the status of the claim should be reviewed again. The key to getting the most reimbursements is clear and regular documentation.

Because time is of the essence, it is wise to be aggressive on claims that are outstanding for more than 60 days, especially when there are issues concerning timely filing.

Using the practice management software's monthly reporting capabilities is useful when tracking the payment history of insurance companies. This is an easy method to discover which companies pay slowly or pay less on certain services and it provides excellent reports for tax purposes or to understand trends in the financial operations of the health care office. An analysis of which insurance companies pay for various procedures can assist the medical office staff to prepare negotiations of future managed care insurance contracts.

An insurance company payment history system can help to avoid potential problems and pinpoint requirements that must be met to secure additional payment on a reduced or denied claim.

CLAIM INQUIRIES

When reviewing an aging report, unpaid claims that are more than 30 days old require that an **inquiry** on claim status be made to the health insurance company. These claims could be delayed because they may not have been received by the insurance company or for other reasons relating to the member's health plan. Different types of claim inquiries can focus on denial codes on the EOB

or can be related to patient coinsurance or deductible responsibilities. To reduce the number of phone calls to the insurance companies, many private insurance organizations have set up online physician web portals that allow insurance billing specialists to review patient claim status and benefit information. If more information about the claim is needed beyond the scope of the online portal, insurance benefit specialists can be reached by calling the member services number on the back of the patient's ID card. The following are reasons for making inquiries:

● There was no response to a submitted claim within 30 to 45 days.
● Payment was not received within the time limit for the plan or program.
● Payment is received but the amount is incorrect.
● Payment is received but the amount allowed and the patient's responsibility is not defined.
● A duplicate payment or overpayment was made.
● Payment received was for a patient not seen by the provider. It is possible to receive a payment check made out to a payee's name that is different from the patient's name. Making a call may quickly clarify for whom the payment is being made.

In addition to nonpayment or reduced payment, there are other reasons for inquiries to an insurance company, including the following:
● EOB shows that a professional or diagnostic code was changed from what was submitted.
● EOB shows that the service was disallowed when it was a benefit.
● EOB shows that additional information was needed and it was sent in a timely manner but payment has not been sent.
● The claim should be revised and resubmitted. Check to see whether the procedure codes were correct and that the services listed were described fully enough to justify the maximum allowable benefits. If services were coded correctly and a particular service was

COLLEGE CLINIC
4567 Broad Avenue
Woodland Hills, XY
12345-0001
Telephone 555/486-9002
Fax (555) 487-8976

Committee on Physician's Services

Re: Underpayment
Identification No.: _____ M18876782 _____
Patient: _____ Peaches Melba _____
Type of Service: _____ Plastic & Reconstructive Surgery _____
Date of Service: _____ 1 - 3 - XX _____
Amount Paid: _____ $ 75.00 _____
My Fees: _____ $ 180.00 _____

Dear Sirs:

Herewith a request for a committee review of the above-named case, since I consider the allowance paid very low having in mind the location, the extent, the type, and the necessary surgical procedure performed: The skin graft, one inch in diameter, included the lateral third of eyebrow and was full thickness to preserve hair follicles.

Operative report for the surgery has been sent to you with the claim.

Considering these points I hope that you will authorize additional payment in order to bring the total fee to within reasonable and customary charges.

Sincerely,

Cosmo Graff, M.D.

Cosmo Graff, M.D.

mf
enclosure

FIGURE 9-4 A letter signed by the physician appealing a fee reduction. This letter lists information specific to the patient claim in question and is sent to the third-party payer after payment has been received and the physician feels that the reimbursement should be higher.

disallowed, be sure to meet the requirements of your office in documenting this situation.

• There is an error on the EOB.
• The check received was issued to the wrong physician.

Inquire about the claim if any of these situations occurs. While there are many online provider web portals for private insurance claims inquiry, sometimes government health plans do not offer the same online tools. For this reason, government health plans have their own inquiry or **tracer** forms available online that needs to be submitted in writing along with a copy of the claim. If a claim must be reviewed after payment has been rendered, send the letter as shown in Figure 9-4. Remember that effective follow-up centers around effective documentation, so document the name of the person spoken to, date and time of call, department or extension of the person, and an outline of the conversation and save these notes in the patient account of the practice management software.

PROBLEM CLAIMS

Problems in claims filing will result in late reimbursement payments, so any issues need to be addressed urgently. While physicians may be anxious to receive reimbursements in a timely manner, it is not efficient for the medical office to follow up on claims less than 60 days after the date of service. Many types of problem claims (for example, delinquent, in **suspense** [pending], lost, rejected, denied, downcoded, partial payment, payment lost in the mail, payment made to patient, and **overpayment**) exist. Table 9-1 contains a complete list of the types of problems and their descriptions.

To keep accounting accurate and up to date, these problems require some type of follow-up action. The claim status may be indicated on an EOB; however, sometimes a claim is submitted and no status is reported. As mentioned, visiting the online insurance provider web

Table 9-1	Insurance Claim Processing Problems
TYPE	**DESCRIPTION**
Delinquent claims	• Payment overdue from nonpayer
Denied claims	• Lack of insurance coverage (canceled, service provided before effective insurance, or lapsed beyond renewal date)
	• Selected diagnoses not covered
	• Frequency limitations or restrictions per benefit period
	• Procedure performed by ineligible specialty provider (for example, podiatrist would not be paid for neurosurgery)
	• Bundled with other services
	• Payable only in certain locations (for example, outpatient only)
	• Prior approval needed and not obtained
	• Service or procedure not justified by diagnosis
	• Missing or incorrect POS code
	• Missing physician signature
	• Missing necessary and/or requested medical documentation
	• Insurance policy issue (preexisting condition or preauthorization required under plan)
	• Experimental procedure not reimbursable
	• Incorrect code for service rendered
	• Code selected from incorrect system (CPT code instead of HCPCS Level II national code)
	• Unbundled codes when one code should have been submitted
	• Unspecified diagnostic code reported
Downcoded claims	• Computer software selects procedure code at lower level than medical service requires
Lost claims	• Claim not received by third-party payer
Overpayment	• Third-party payer pays more than the bill or the allowed amount
	• Third-party payer pays more than one's fee or contract rate
	• Third-party payer sends provider payment intended for patient
	• Provider receives duplicate payments from two or more insurance companies or from the patient and one or more third-party payers
	• Provider receives payment for someone who is not the provider's patient
Payment errors	• Third-party payer sends provider payment intended for patient
	• Patient paid by third-party payer when provider should have been paid
Pending (suspense) claims	• Claim has an error
	• Additional information required
	• Claim review needed by third-party payer (complex procedure, high reimbursement, utilization management)
Rejected (soft denial) claims	• Claim contains technical error (missing or incorrect information, numbers transposed, invalid diagnostic or procedural code numbers, duplicate charges, duplicate dates of service, and so on)
	• Third-party payer instructions not followed
Two-party check	• Check written to both the provider and the hospital
Underpayment	• Third-party payment at less than negotiated contract rate

CPT, Current Procedural Terminology; *HCPCS*, Healthcare Common Procedure Coding System; *POS*, place of service.

portal is the most efficient way to view claim status. For government-sponsored insurances, calling to confirm claim status is the most efficient step.

To prevent repeated claims errors, if the office manager understands and has a good overview of the insurance claims process, he or she should identify the source of the errors within the medical office. Often a claim may be denied because of an error that occurred when collecting registration information at the front desk or when posting charges to the account. Other errors occur because of wrong procedure or diagnostic codes, incorrect provider numbers, and a variety of situations mentioned in prior chapters. Many claims are denied for wrong gender and wrong year of birth. The more unusual or foreign-sounding a name is, the more denials occur on the basis of gender. Be aware that some names

(for example, Alex and Cameron) could be either male or female.

The individual working at the front desk must collect insurance information accurately and update patient demographic information (for example, insurance identification number and address) at every office visit or medical encounter. The person posting to accounts must be certain to post to the correct patient account and ensure that secondary insurances are billed after the primary insurance company has paid. Identified errors should be brought to the attention of the responsible individuals to improve accuracy of outgoing claims and avoid future problems.

There is a significant difference in the way problem claims are handled when filed by paper or filed electronically. Since most health insurance claims should be submitted electronically, the problems and solutions listed will focus mainly on electronic submission.

Types of Problems

The following are specific claim problems and possible solutions.

Delinquent, Pending, or Suspense

PROBLEM: Delinquent claims are typically beyond 60 days overdue on the aging report. The nonpayer can be an insurance company; managed care plan; or intermediary for the Medicaid, Medicare, or TRICARE programs. Sometimes nonpayment is caused by a claim in review or in suspense because of an error or the need for additional information. The carrier may be investigating a claim because of preexisting conditions or possibly because the patient may have a work-related injury. If a service is not covered, sometimes there is no response; however, a follow-up should be initiated to further investigate.

SOLUTION: Use claim management techniques to keep on top of delinquent claims so that follow-up can be accomplished in a timely manner. If the office handles a large volume of claims, divide the unpaid claims into four groups, one for each of the three largest insurers and the fourth for all others. Work on one group each week so that the work is spread out over the 4 weeks in each month. Routinely visit the online provider web portals to check for claims status and look for evidence of the claim being submitted while reconciling the electronic data interchange (EDI) clearinghouse acknowledgement report for up-to-date information. If the claim was submitted and confirmed received, it is wise to look at how the claim was billed (for example, accurate coding). If this information is correct and the dates on the claim are correct, contact the payer to find out what information is holding up the claim or why the claim was denied. If the claim was not successful in being received by the clearinghouse and there is no clear reason on reports or on investigating the claim data showing exactly what information was amiss, then perhaps there was a problem with the format. Contacting the clearinghouse gives you more insight as to why the claim was not successfully received or was rejected. The insurance billing specialist can contact the payer immediately after finding out that the claim is delinquent or the payer can be contacted after initial steps of investigation take place, such as in-house editing and contacting the clearinghouse.

Lost Claims

PROBLEM: Lost claims are more common with paper claim submission; sometimes managing large volumes of claims leads to some getting lost from time to time. Paper claims can get lost in the mail, be sent to the incorrect address, or be mismanaged through the health insurance mail management system.

SOLUTION: The insurance company should be contacted if there has been no response to a claim that has aged 60 days. The first step is to check claim status with the private insurance company online through the online provider web portal or to call the local government agency office. If there is no record of the claim, all lost claims should be resubmitted. If a claim is determined to be lost, submit a copy of the original claim referencing it as "copy of the original claim submitted on (date)"; on rare occasions, insurance companies may accept the resubmission of a claim in the form of a fax if the fax references the original submission date. Before sending it, verify the correct mailing address (for example, post office box number and zip code).

Ask if there is a backlog of claims to resolve the situation. This indicates that the claim probably has not been logged into the system. Always verify that the patient is insured by the insurance company and is covered for the basic benefits claimed.

Lost claims are especially crucial to managed care plan insurance claim filings; many of these have deadlines to file claims within 30 days after the date of service. If there is a possibility that claims have been mishandled, gather documentation and send a letter to the state insurance commission as well as a letter to the third-party payer about the action taken.

Always retain the electronic response or confirmation from the carrier saying that it received the specific claim. Keep all clearinghouse reports that confirm received transmissions and relay information regarding claim status. Practice management software programs display the date of every claim submitted. Tamper-proof data recorded by the computer may be used as a legal form of proof that the claim was submitted to the third-party payer. Unfortunately this does not "prove" that the payer received the claim, so some payers do not always accept this. Send a printed copy of the electronic proof of timely filing to the third-party payer. Alternately, you may send a letter with the proof of filing, a copy of the claim, and a copy of the denial if you received one for exceeding the timely filing limit.

Rejected Claims

Chapter 7 discusses some common reasons why paper claims are rejected or delayed. A **rejected claim** is a submitted claim that does not follow specific third-party payer instructions or contains a technical error. Such

Box 9-1	Common Reasons Why Health Insurance Claims Are Rejected

Box 9-1   Common Reasons Why Health Insurance Claims Are Rejected

Code description does not match services rendered
Duplicate charges
Duplicate dates of service
Incorrect dates of service
Incorrect electronic submission code
Incorrect number of days in the month (for example, February)
Incorrect year of service
Incorrect, invalid, nonspecific, or missing diagnostic code numbers
Mismatch of POS to type of service
Missing NPI number for the provider and/or facility
Missing or invalid POS
Missing or invalid provider number when the patient was referred
Missing referring physician when billing tests
Missing required HIPAA transaction code sets
Missing subscriber date of birth
Missing, invalid, or incorrect procedure codes and modifiers
Missing physician signature
Transposed numbers

HIPAA, Health Insurance Portability and Accountability Act; *NPI,* National Provider Identifier; *POS,* place of service.

claims may be disapproved or discarded by the system and returned to the biller. Technical errors consist of missing or incorrect information and are found through computer edits, screening processes for benefit provisions, and proofreading. Medicare-mandated prepayment screens are discussed in Chapter 12. Common reasons why health insurance claims are rejected can be found in Box 9-1.

PROBLEM: Paper or electronic claim rejections may occur due to one or more of the following:

- Transposed numbers
- Missing required Health Insurance Portability and Accountability Act (HIPAA) transaction code sets
- Missing subscriber date of birth
- Missing, invalid, or incorrect procedure codes and modifiers
- Missing or invalid place of service (POS)
- Mismatch of POS to type of service
- Missing referring physician when billing tests
- Missing or invalid provider number when the patient was referred
- Incorrect, invalid, nonspecific, or missing diagnostic code numbers
- Incorrect dates of service
- Incorrect year of service
- Incorrect number of days in the month (for example, February)
- Code description does not match services rendered
- Duplicate dates of service
- Duplicate charges

SOLUTION: Likely, an electronic claim will not make it into a batch to be transmitted to the payer if a series of computer edits have been performed before batching (that is, grouping claims together). The system will flag this particular claim as needing edits and will not batch it with the rest. If the claim does go through to the payer and is reported as being rejected, review the rejection reason code and correct the field. Then resubmit the claim. Never send a corrected claim for review or appeal because this type of claim should always be resubmitted.

PROBLEM: A claim is submitted for several services. One line item is rejected for incomplete information but the other services are paid.

SOLUTION: Generate a new claim for the rejected services online and note in Block 19 that it is a resubmission.

PROBLEM: Third-party payer requests further information or information about another insurance carrier.

SOLUTION: A common mistake during the patient registration process is not obtaining the insurance subscriber's name, employer, and date of birth. It is important to verify insurance information with the patient (including confirmation of the patient's primary, and possibly secondary, insurance information), obtain a signed patient release of information form that follows Health Insurance Portability and Accountability Act (HIPAA) guidelines, and call or mail the information to the insurance company. Identify the subscriber, subscriber ID number, and date of service on all correspondence.

PROBLEM: Resubmitted claim is returned a second time.

PAPER CLAIM SOLUTION: Review the EOB statement to determine whether there is a denial code or narrative explanation. Examine the claim for missing, incomplete, or incorrect information and, if found, correct it. Evaluate the claim to determine whether it is a candidate for the appeal process. Determine whether a specific appeal form must be submitted. Submit chart notes, a detailed summary, or a copy of the operative or pathology report, as applicable, to clearly identify the procedure or service. Enclose a cover letter with the resubmitted data. The letter must specifically state what course of action is being requested (that is, review) and it must have the name and signature of the person requesting the review.

A common denial reason is **medical necessity,** which means that the insurance company is denying that the patient needed the medical service performed. These types of denials are caused by diagnosis and procedure code not matching. An example of this would be a denial for hammertoe surgery with a broken wrist diagnosis. Because these denials are related to faulty coding, they should be returned to the original coder to be corrected and resubmitted.

Denied Claims

A **denied claim** occurs due to denial of health insurance benefits coverage policy issues. It stands to reason that insurance companies save money when a claim is denied and only a small percentage of individuals pursue appeals. State laws require insurance companies to notify the insured of a denial and state why the claim was denied. It is possible that payment can be received even after a claim has been denied in whole or in part.

When a claim is denied and the responsible party is found to be the patient, transfer the entire balance to the patient's account. However, an exception is a Medicare patient, who must have signed an **Advance Beneficiary Notice of Noncoverage (ABN)** acknowledging that Medicare will not pay for the specific medical service and that the patient is responsible for the fee. If the insurance company has not contacted the patient, notify the patient by phone or mail as soon as possible to keep him or her informed. Always retain the correspondence from the insurance company so that it can be retrieved quickly in case a patient inquires and has additional questions. The recourse to a denied claim is to appeal and request a review of coverage in writing.

Service to Patients

At times patients need a medical service that is not covered by Medicare. At this point, patients need to be guided through the process of obtaining care. One-on-one counseling for patients who need to sign an Advance Beneficiary Notice of Noncoverage (ABN) is necessary so that patients understand that the possibility is high that they will be held financially responsible for the services rendered. At this time, it is wise to make payment arrangements with the patient to prepare for Medicare denying payment for services. Refer to Chapter 12 and to Figure 12-9 for an example of a completed ABN.

The appeals process varies among third-party payers. A Medicare claim may be redetermined (appealed) by requesting a review in writing and federal laws require that an explanation be given for each denied service. In Medicare Part B redetermination cases, carriers have been instructed to pay an appealed claim if the cost of the hearing process is more than the amount of the claim.

Some reasons why insurance claims are not paid because of denial are:
- Selected diagnoses not covered
- Frequency limitations or restrictions per benefit period
- Procedure performed by ineligible specialty provider (for example, a podiatrist would not be paid for neurosurgery)
- Bundled with other services

- Payable only in certain locations (for example, outpatient only)
- Prior approval needed and not obtained
- Service or procedure not justified by diagnosis
- Missing or incorrect place-of-service (POS) code

When the claim is denied, simply changing information on the claim and resubmitting will not resolve the problem. Additional examples with suggested solutions are as follows:

PROBLEM: The medical service provided was not covered for the patient (for example, routine physical examination, routine tests, routine foot care, routine dental care, cosmetic surgery, custodial care, eye or hearing examinations for glasses or hearing aids, and some immunizations). Plastic surgery and maternity care can be considered a general exclusion in many insurance policies.

SOLUTION: Send the patient a statement with a notation of the response from the insurance company. Before providing services, always verify coverage for routine physical examinations or tests and services by calling or checking the online provider web portal as to whether the health insurance will accept financial responsibility. Discuss this with the patient before service is provided and advise of the likelihood of the claim being denied; in these instances it may be appropriate to request payment at the time of service. Refer to the Service to Patients box about ABNs for more information.

PROBLEM: Insurance coverage is canceled or temporarily lapsed prior to date of service.

SOLUTION: It is a good practice to verify insurance coverage for each patient prior to his or her appointment for services by visiting the online provider web portal or by calling to verify coverage. If the claim is then denied after services were rendered, send the patient a statement with notation of the insurance determination on the bill.

PROBLEM: Health insurance company indicates that the provided service was not medically necessary. "Medical necessity" has become the encompassing denial reason that indicates that the insurance company does not agree with the services provided to the patient because they were not necessary. This makes clearing the medical necessity denial reason most challenging to overturn. The following are a few reasons why insurance companies deny medical necessity:
- The diagnosis code and the procedure code do not match
- The procedure code and the place or type of service do not match
- The procedure is performed by a physician of a different specialty
- The frequency of the same procedure rendered is more than authorized

● The procedure is experimental and has not yet been approved for reimbursement by the insurance company
● Physician documentation is unclear or limited

SOLUTION: Determine under what circumstances the third-party payer considers the service to be medically necessary. It is vital that the physician's documentation be specific enough to support the necessity of the services provided. If the physician believes that the patient's condition supported the medical necessity for the service, send an appeal for review to the insurance company, explaining in detail the reasons why the service was necessary. Keep a list of codes that have been denied for medical necessity and what further determinations were made in the insurance company payment history. Check the insurance contract to determine whether the patient may be billed. Consider asking patients to sign an ABN or Waiver of Liability form before treatment. Beware that you do not have every patient sign such documents because then these documents would be considered a blanket waiver; if the claim is denied, bill the patient.

PROBLEM: Service was for an injury that is approved and covered under workers' compensation. Create a workers' compensation information sheet asking the employee and employer to fill out separate sections with space for the following: explanation of the injury, insurance information, claim adjuster's name and telephone number, and claim or case number.

SOLUTION: Since most workers' compensation insurance companies typically accept paper claims, all correspondence should be made directly with the claims adjuster via phone or mail. Locate the carrier for the industrial injury, request permission to treat, and send the carrier a report of the case with a bill. Notify the patient's health insurance carrier monthly about the status of the case.

PROBLEM: Service was not preauthorized for a surgery, hospitalization, or diagnostic procedure.

SOLUTION: Contact the insurance company or check the online provider web portal to determine whether preauthorization was necessary for the service or if any sanctions were imposed. The office may want to institute a standard procedure that all surgical procedures and durable medical equipment and supplies be confirmed with insurance companies prior to rendering services. Document the contact name, date, and time of the call or if using the online provider portal, print out the preauthorization information for the patient's chart. If there were problems or difficulties with the case leading to the reason that precertification was not obtained, write a letter of appeal noting the history. Insurance payers can change their policies on certain procedure codes throughout the year.

PROBLEM: Deductible was not met.

SOLUTION: Prior to rendering services to the patient, confirm with the insurance company the patient's current deductible and the amount for which the patient will be financially responsible for medical services. Inform the patient at the prescreening appointment that the deductible must be collected at that appointment or the procedure should be rescheduled.

PROBLEM: Elective surgery or procedures that are not typically covered by health insurance.

SOLUTION: Inform the patient prior to scheduling the appointment that he or she is responsible to pay for services upfront, prior to the procedure.

PROBLEM: Claim is incomplete and denied because essential elements are missing and/or inaccurate.

SOLUTION: Measures to Prevent Denied Claims

Prevention measures to avoid denied claims are as follows:
1. Be proactive and verify insurance coverage prior to the first visit; this saves time and prevents surprises for everyone. Ensure that the demographic information is current at each visit.
2. Include progress notes and orders for tests for extended hospital services.
3. Submit a letter from the prescribing physician documenting necessity when ambulance transportation is used.
4. Clarify the type of service (for example, primary surgical services versus assist-at-surgery services).
5. Use modifiers to further describe and identify the exact service rendered.
6. Keep abreast of the latest policies for all contracted payers as well as for the federal programs by going to the Centers for Medicare and Medicaid Services (CMS) website to read currently posted Medicare Transmittals (formerly called Program Memorandums). For example, know the Medicare local coverage determinations (LCDs) and national coverage determinations (NCDs) that state which conditions and services are covered and limitations on coverage. Read news releases from the Blue Plans, Medicaid, TRICARE, workers' compensation insurance companies, and managed care plans.
7. Obtain current provider manuals for all contracted managed care payers as well as the Blue Plans, Medicaid, Medicare, and TRICARE for quick reference. When bulletins or pages are received from these programs during the year, keep the manuals up to date by inserting the current material.
8. Become familiar with the modifier descriptions and their appropriate use and verify that the payer recognizes them.

Downcoding

Reduced reimbursement is the result of downcoding.

PROBLEM: The procedure or diagnosis code used is general or unspecified.

SOLUTION: Be sure to read through all procedure notes and provider orders to determine the most specific diagnosis code related to the patient's condition. If the patient experiences complications, these should be added to the code. If the physician's notes are not specific enough to determine a more specific diagnosis, emphasize to them the importance of specificity, especially regarding diagnosis. Include modifiers when necessary to provide more specification for procedures.

Payment Made to Patient

PROBLEM: An insurance payment sent to the patient instead of the provider can occur for two reasons, either the provider is considered out of network from the patient's health plan or the assignment of benefits was not signed by the patient.

SOLUTION: Call the insurance company or visit the online provider web portal to verify whether the payment was made, to whom, for which dates of service, the amount, the check number, and the date of issue. If the provider has a participating agreement, the insurance company is obligated to pay the provider and must proceed by correcting the error. The following are two different courses of action to take after this has been verified:

1. Call the patient, explain that the insurance company sent payment to the patient in error, and ask when full payment can be expected. Document the commitment in the patient's financial record. If the patient cannot be reached by telephone, send a letter by certified mail to the patient. Document each effort that was made toward collection of the payment from the patient and the patient's responses. Then discuss with the physician whether he or she wishes to discharge the patient from the practice.

2. Send a letter to the insurance company, including a copy of the claim with EOB indicating that payment was made to the patient and a copy of the assignment of benefits. Demand payment from the insurance company, stating the need to honor the assignment and the signed participation agreement. The insurance company must recover the payment from the patient. If a dead end is reached after pursuing reimbursement from the insurance company, file a complaint with the state insurance commissioner. After receiving the physician's complaint, the commissioner will write to the insurance company and request a review of the claim. If the insurance company admits that there is an assignment of benefits and that it inadvertently paid the patient, the insurance company must pay the physician within 2 to 3 weeks and honor the assignment even before it recovers its money from the patient. The insurance company then files for payment from the patient.

Two-Party Check

PROBLEM: This is a situation in which a received check is made out to both the physician and the hospital and only part of the sum is the physician's payment. This might occur when the provider is contracted with the hospital.

SOLUTION: If you do not receive an EOB containing the breakdown of both parties' payments, call the insurance company and ask how much should be retained by the physician. Request that the allocation be sent in writing. Ask whose tax identification number will be used on the 1099 form for reporting income to the Internal Revenue Service (IRS). The hospital's income should not be reflected on the physician's 1099 form. To avoid another problem like this, inquire why the insurance company paid in this manner and ensure that all future claims are sent with an employer identification number (EIN) or Tax ID number different from the hospital's.

Underpayment

It is important that the insurance billing specialist perform random checks and monitor large claim payments made during the first 3 months of a new contract to ensure that the third-party payer's system has the contracted payment fee schedule correctly loaded into the software. Track the charge, allowable, deductible, and paid amount to determine whether the amounts are correct (Figure 9-5).

PROBLEM: Underpaid claims.

SOLUTION: Print the incorrectly paid claims and send them by mail to the third-party payer's contract negotiator to be resolved. Ask them to re-adjudicate the claims on the basis of the agreed-upon contracted amount; include a letter with the claims clearly stating that they are not duplicate claims but do need to be reviewed for appropriate payment. Use codes or notations on the claims to indicate that they are updated.

Overpayment

Overpayments can happen for a variety of reasons but handling them can be challenging. Overpayments can happen for any one of the following reasons:

• A payment was made twice for the same date of service. This usually happens when a claim is rebilled prior to receiving confirmation of health insurance receipt.

Method for Calculating Over- and Underpayments						
Third-party payer: _____						
Patient name	Procedure/ service	Claims paid date	Provider charge	Allowed amount	Amount paid	Overpayment (+) Underpayment (−)
May Ito	Colonoscopy	5/2/20XX	$1500	$900	$2000	$1100+

FIGURE 9-5 Audit method used for calculating overpayments and underpayments. Subtract the allowed amount, which is the insurance contract's fee schedule amount minus any patient co-payment or deductible from the amount paid. Any positive (+) number is an overpayment and any negative (−) number is an underpayment.

- A payment was made that was above the contracted allowable amount.
- A payment was made for a patient and date of service that does not exist.
- A payment was made for a service that was not performed for the specific patient.

An overpayment is a sum of money paid by the insurance company or patient to the provider of service that is more than the account balance or more than the allowed amount. The insurance payment poster usually discovers overpayments when payments are posted in patient accounts. The Office of the Inspector General (OIG) strongly advises providers to return overpayments promptly. Not doing so can lead to severe fines and implicate fraudulent activity.

Some states have laws or court decisions restricting managed care plans and other insurers from recovering payments made in error from providers. Other states will not allow insurers to recover if the provider "changed its position" by relying on the payment (that is, the provider spent the money to pay its bills). It is essential to research the law pertaining to the handling of overpayments in the state in which the medical provider practices. First, determine whether an overpayment exists by reviewing the available financial documents on the case in question. Then decide how to handle the overpayment. Be sure to get the physician's attorney's advice on the extent to which you can challenge a plan's demand for repayment on the basis of state law or court decisions.

It is wise to develop an overpayment policy and procedure for each type of insurer, program, or managed care plan and for every type of overpayment situation that may occur.

PROBLEM: Overpayment scenarios that may occur are as follows:
- Receiving more than one's fee from a third-party payer
- Receiving more than the contract rate from a managed care plan

- Receiving payments that should have been paid to the patient
- Receiving duplicate payments from two or more insurance companies or from the patient and one or more third-party payers
- Receiving payment made for someone who is not the provider's patient

SOLUTION: When an overpayment occurs, post the activity to the appropriate patient account with additional notation that it was received in error and a refund was made. Creating an account specifically for overpayments is advisable to track all funds in this category. In any type of overpayment situation, cash the third-party payer's check and make out a refund check payable to the originator of the overpayment. Keep a copy of the third-party payer's check before it is deposited. The refund check should always be sent to the attention of a specific person at the insurance company. In case of an audit, this establishes documentation showing that the problem has been resolved. Usually insurance companies process a credit of the overpayment amount to the next check voucher.

Refund checks should be given top priority and written as soon as reasonably possible. Ensure that the office policy is clearly stated and adhered to in all cases. If the patient pays and a third-party pays and the overpayment must be refunded to the patient, always write a check—never refund in cash. Send the patient a letter with a check to explain the overpayment. If the patient pays by credit card, wait until the charges have cleared to draft a check or preferably process a credit card refund to the credit card company.

If the patient cannot be located to return the money, send a check by registered mail to the patient's last known address. When it comes back marked "undeliverable," retain the document as legal proof that an honest effort was made to return the overpayment. The money should be listed as taxable income and put in the bank.

Commercial Carriers

Problem: An overpayment made by a commercial health plan such as Blue Plan.
Solution: First, call and notify the patient; then proceed cautiously before refunding money by doing the following:
- Investigate the refund request by sending a letter to the insurance payer disputing the recoupment. Include documentation as proof (for example, operative report, health record, or bundling guidelines).
- Obtain documentation from the insurance payer to prove why the refund is legitimate.
- The general rule is to not pay old recoupments dating back more than 4 or 5 years.
- If two or more third-party payers send duplicate payments, write a letter to each explaining the situation and let them straighten it out. Then send a refund to the correct third-party payer to the attention of a specific person after receiving a letter explaining to whom the money should be sent.

Managed Care Plan

Problem: An overpayment from a managed care plan is discovered.
Solution: Review the payer's policy about overpayments and be sure it is clearly documented in the provider's contract. Address this issue if the payer does not define it. Follow your office protocol for documenting overpayments.

Medicare

Problem: A Medicare patient makes an overpayment.
Solution: For assigned claims, if Medicare sends a letter to the physician, respond with a letter and overpayment check to the patient within 15 days. For nonassigned claims, if Medicare sends a letter to the physician, a refund check must be made within 15 days or the physician may be subject to civil monetary penalties and sanctions. If Medicare feels that there is an overpayment, they will exercise their right to recoup the payment from a future reimbursement.

REBILLING

If a claim has not been paid within a reasonable amount of time, do not automatically **rebill (resubmit)** the third-party payer without researching the reason why it is still outstanding. Simply rebilling claims can be considered duplicate claims and the insurance company may audit the physician's practice for trying to collect duplicate payment unless it is marked "Possible duplicate." Instead, follow up on the claim as indicated in the previous section. If it is discovered that an error has been made in completing the insurance claim form, make the changes and resubmit the form, indicating that the new claim is corrected.

Patient accounts with a balance should be billed on a monthly basis, even when insurance payment is expected, so that they understand what has been submitted and what is pending. The statement should clearly identify the claim that has been submitted and what action is expected from the patient. If collection becomes a problem, action can be referenced to the date of service if the patient has been billed consistently.

In December 2004, the CMS implemented a process that allows providers to resubmit corrected claims that have been rejected for minor errors or omissions rather than appealing those claims. For example, claims with missing or incorrect provider numbers, claims with incorrect modifiers, or claims with keying errors (incorrect date or POS) can be rebilled. These claims can be corrected through the clearinghouse and resubmitted electronically.

REVIEW AND APPEAL PROCESS

An appeal is a request for payment by asking for a review of a claim that has been underpaid, incorrectly paid, or denied by an insurance company. In the Medicare program, appeals are referred to as redeterminations. Usually there is a time limit for appealing a claim. Before starting the appeals process for a claim, check every private third-party payer, Medicare, TRICARE, managed care, and workers' compensation reimbursement against the appropriate fee schedule to determine whether the benefits were allowed correctly. To determine this information, read the payment voucher document or refer to provider manuals for the various insurance programs.

Appeals can be time consuming and costly, so it may be a good idea to see if the insurance company will settle the claim prior to an appeal filing. An appeal on a claim should be based not only on billing guidelines but also on state and federal insurance laws and regulations. There may be a discrepancy in the way the physician's office and insurance company interpret a coding guideline. The decision to appeal a claim should be based on several factors. The provider should determine that there is sufficient information to back up the claim and the amount of money in question should be sufficient in the physician's opinion. Ultimately, the decision to appeal rests in the physician's hands, not the insurance billing specialist's. To proceed, make a telephone call to the insurance company. It may save time and money and an expert who is able to solve the problem may be reached. The following are basic guidelines:

● Assemble all documents needed (for example, patient's medical record, copy of the insurance claim form, and EOB).
● Remain courteous at all times.
● Obtain the name and extension number of the insurance claims representative or adjuster and keep this with the telephone records. After developing rapport, you may wish to call on him or her in the future for help. Ask for any toll-free numbers that the company may have and keep these for future reference.
● Listen carefully. Jot down the date and take notes of how to solve the problem. This may be of help if another problem of the same type occurs.

An appeal is filed in the following circumstances:
● Payment is denied and the reason for denial is not known.
● Payment is received but the amount is incorrect. Verify that initially the correct amount was billed. Perhaps there was an excessive reduction in the allowed payment.
● The physician disagrees with the decision by the third-party payer about a preexisting condition.
● Unusual circumstances warranted medical treatments that are not reflected in the payment.
● Precertification was not obtained within contract provisions because of extenuating circumstances and the claim was denied.
● Inadequate payment was received for a complicated procedure.
● "Not medically necessary" is stated as the reason for denial and the physician disagrees.

FILING AN APPEAL

Refer to Procedure 9-1 at the end of this chapter for the procedure to follow when filing an appeal that is not a Medicare case.

If the appeal is won but copies of the same documents must be submitted each time this issue arises, ask the third-party payer how future claims with the same issue may be handled. Keep track of this information in a file.

Appeals must be in writing but some programs require completion of special forms. Always send a copy of the original claim, EOB, and any other documents to justify the appeal.

It is important to keep track of the status after inquiry or appeal until payment for the case is resolved. Use the insurance claims register mentioned in Chapter 3 or a separate active file labeled "Appeals Pending."

If an appeal is denied, the physician may want to proceed to the next step, which is to request a **peer review.** A peer review is an evaluation done by a group of unbiased practicing physicians to judge the effectiveness and efficiency of professional care rendered. This group determines the medical necessity and subsequent payment for the case in question.

Additional information on tracing delinquent claims, appealing or reviewing a claim, or submitting a claim for a deceased patient can be found in the chapters on Medicaid (Chapter 13), Medicare (Chapter 12), TRICARE (Chapter 14), and workers' compensation (Chapter 15).

Medicare Review and Redetermination Process

A physician or beneficiary has the right to appeal a claim after payment or denial. The Medicare program has five levels of redetermination and special guidelines to follow:
● Level 1: Redetermination (telephone, letter, or CMS-20027 Form)
● Level 2: Reconsideration (hearing officer [HO] hearing)
● Level 3: Administrative law judge (ALJ) hearing
● Level 4: Medicare Appeals Council
● Level 5: Federal District Court

Table 9-2 illustrates the Medicare Part B appeals process. Because Medicare guidelines change frequently, refer to their website www.cms.gov.

Redetermination (Level 1)

On October 1, 2004, the redetermination step became effective; redetermination is the first step to resolve a

Table 9-2	Medicare Part B Redetermination Process			
LEVEL	TIME LIMIT FOR REQUEST	AMOUNT IN CONTROVERSY	JURISDICTION	FORM
1	Redetermination (telephone, letter, or CMS-20027 form)	120 days from initial claim determination	None	Medicare carrier/ MAC	CMS-20027 form CMS-1500 (02-12) corrected claim resubmitted
2	Reconsideration (QIC)	180 days from receipt of MRN	None	Carrier/QIC	CMS-20033
3	ALJ hearing	60 days from receipt of the Hearing Officer's (HO's) determination	$150 or more (2015)	Carrier/Social Security Bureau of Hearings and Appeals	CMS-5011A/B
4	Medicare Appeals Council	60 days from receipt of hearing decision	None	Federal District Court	
5	US District Court	60 days from receipt of the Departmental Appeals Board's (DAB's) decision	At least $1460 (2015) increased annually		

ALJ, Administrative law judge; *CMS*, Centers for Medicare and Medicaid Services; *DAB*, departmental appeal board; *HO*, hearing officer; *MAC*, Medicare administrative contractor; *MRN*, Medicare Redetermination Notice; *QIC*, Qualified Independent Contractor.

denied claim. Information about the denied claim is found on the Medicare RA. A written request for redetermination must include the following information if the CMS-20027 form is not used:

● Beneficiary name
● Medicare Health Insurance Claim (HIC) number
● Specific service and/or item(s) for which a redetermination is being requested
● Specific date(s) of service
● Name and signature of the party or the representative of the party

If the claim was denied because of a simple error made by the insurance billing specialist, such as omission of the National Provider Identifier (NPI) of the referring physician or failure to code a diagnosis, then complete a CMS-20027 form and resubmit a corrected claim (Figure 9-6). Include only the denied services and indicate in Block 19 "resubmission, corrected claim." In the event that the third-party payer made an error (for example, a procedure code was different from what was submitted or the date of service was entered incorrectly from the paper claim to the payer's computer), then resubmit the claim with an attachment explaining the error. If response to the resubmission indicates that the claim has been "processed" previously, go to the next appeal level. A notice must be mailed by the Medicare intermediary within 60 days of receipt of a request from a beneficiary or provider. It must include reasons for the decision, a summary of clinical or scientific evidence used in making the redetermination, a description of how to obtain additional information, a notification of the right to appeal, and instructions on how to appeal the decision to the next level. If requested, the Medicare intermediary must provide information about the policy, manual, or regulation used in making the redetermination decision.

The decision must be written in language that the beneficiary can understand.

Reconsideration (Level 2)

The physician may ask for a review when a claim is assigned. The request must be within 6 months from the date of the original determination shown on the RA. Figure 9-7 shows Form CMS-20033, which may be used in requesting a reconsideration of Medicare Part B claims. However, some state Medicare contractors have developed their own request forms. Contact the carrier to find out the necessary form to use. Review the RA for the denial code or narrative stating why the claim has been denied. Check the claim for accuracy of diagnostic, procedural, or Healthcare Common Procedure Coding System (HCPCS) codes or missing modifiers as well as for any other item that might be incorrect or missing.

Attach the following with the reconsideration request:
1. Copy of the original insurance claim
2. Copy of the RA showing the denial
3. Photocopy of other documents, such as operative or pathology report or detailed summary about the procedure, with appropriate words highlighted to help the reviewer
4. The reconsideration form with explanation of the procedure indicating justification for the services and the reason that the provider should receive more reimbursement

Mail the documents by certified mail with return receipt requested and retain copies of all documents sent to the carrier in the provider's pending file.

If a claim is unassigned, the beneficiary (patient) can pursue the review or appoint the physician as an authorized representative. The patient completes form

DEPARTMENT OF HEALTH AND HUMAN SERVICES
CENTERS FOR MEDICARE & MEDICAID SERVICES

MEDICARE REDETERMINATION REQUEST FORM – 1ST LEVEL OF APPEAL

1. Beneficiary's name: Carolyn N. Harvey

2. Medicare number: 072-XX-1461

3. Item or service you wish to appeal: Office Visit (99215)

4. Date the service or item was received: 07-24-20XX

5. Date of the initial determination notice (please include a copy of the notice with this request):
   (If you received your initial determination notice more than 120 days ago, include your reason for the late filing.)

   09-02-20XX

   5a. Name of the Medicare contractor that made the determination (not required):

   Palmetto GBA

   5b. Does this appeal involve an overpayment? ☐ Yes ☒ No
   (for providers and suppliers only)

6. I do not agree with the determination decision on my claim because:

   Established patient is 60 years old and has diabetic nephropathy with increasing edema and dyspnea.

7. Additional information Medicare should consider:

   Comprehensive history and comprehensive examination was performed because patient had not been seen for a
   year. Her case had to be discussed with a cardiologist because of possibility of congestive heart failure condition.

8. ☒ I have evidence to submit. Please attach the evidence to this form or attach a statement explaining what
   you intend to submit and when you intend to submit it. You may also submit additional evidence at a
   later time, but all evidence must be received prior to the issuance of the redetermination.

   ☐ I do not have evidence to submit.

9. Person appealing: ☐ Beneficiary ☒ Provider/Supplier ☐ Representative

10. Name, address, and telephone number of person appealing: Gerald Practon, MD

    4567 Broad Avenue, Woodland Hills, XY 12345 555-486-9002

11. Signature of person appealing: *Gerald Practon, MD*

12. Date signed: 10-04-20XX

PRIVACY ACT STATEMENT: The legal authority for the collection of information on this form is authorized by section 1869 (a)(3) of the Social Security
Act. The information provided will be used to further document your appeal. Submission of the information requested on this form is voluntary, but failure
to provide all or any part of the requested information may affect the adjudication of your appeal. Information you furnish on this form may be disclosed
by the Centers for Medicare and Medicaid Services to another person or government agency only with respect to the Medicare Program and to comply
with Federal laws requiring or permitting the disclosure of information or the exchange of information between the Department of Health and Human
Services and other agencies. Additional information about these disclosures can be found in the system of records notice for system no. 09-70-0566, as
amended, available at 71 Fed. Reg. 54489 (2006) or at http://www.cms.gov/PrivacyActSystemofRecords/downloads/0566.pdf

Form CMS-20027 (12/10)

FIGURE 9-6 Medicare Redetermination Request Form—1st Level of Appeal, CMS-20027,
which can be used by the Medicare beneficiary or physician when requesting a redetermination
of a submitted claim.

DEPARTMENT OF HEALTH AND HUMAN SERVICES
CENTERS FOR MEDICARE & MEDICAID SERVICES

MEDICARE RECONSIDERATION REQUEST – 2ND LEVEL OF APPEAL

1. Beneficiary's name: _____Jose F. Perez_____

2. Medicare number: _____032-XX-6619_____

3. Item or service you wish to appeal: _____Electrocadiographic Monitoring, 24 hrs (93224)_____

4. Date the service or item was received: ___01-21-20XX_____

5. Date of the redetermination notice (please include a copy of the notice with this request):
   (If you received your redetermination notice more than 180 days ago, include your reason for the late filing.)
   _____03-24-20XX_____

   5a. Name of the Medicare contractor that made the redetermination (not required if copy of notice attached):
   Palmetto GBA

   5b. Does this appeal involve an overpayment?   ☐ Yes ☒ No
   (for providers and suppliers only)

6. I do not agree with the redetermination decision on my claim because:
   Patient had heart palpitations, tachycardia, and lightheadedness (near syncopal episode). Although patient had a
   previous Holter monitor within the 60 months time limitation, it did not provide any clinical evidence of disease.
   Patient underwent recent monitoring after experiencing additional symptoms that were more severe then the inital.

7. Additional information Medicare should consider:
   _____
   _____
   _____

8. ☒ I have evidence to submit. Please attach the evidence to this form or attach a statement explaining what
        you intend to submit and when you intend to submit it. You may also submit additional evidence at a
        later time, but all evidence must be received prior to the issuance of the reconsideration.

   ☐ I do not have evidence to submit.

9. Person appealing: ☐ Beneficiary   ☒ Provider/Supplier   ☐ Representative

10. Name, address, and telephone number of person appealing: ___Gerald Practon, MD_____

    _____4567 Broad Avenue, Woodland Hills, XY 12345_____555-486-9002_____

11. Signature of person appealing: _____*Gerald Practon, MD*_____

12. Date signed: ___06-05-20XX_____

Form CMS-20033 (12/10)

FIGURE 9-7 Medicare Reconsideration Request Form—2nd Level of Appeal, CMS-20033, which can be used when requesting a reconsideration of Medicare Part B claims.

SSA-1696 (Rec 06/12) (Figure 9-8) and obtains the physician's acceptance signature. Decisions on unassigned claims are sent to the patient.

Send all requests to the review department. Most insurance companies have an address or post office box for review of requests that is different from initial claim submissions, so be sure to send it to a correct current address.

The third-party payer usually completes a review within 30 to 45 days. Make a follow-up inquiry if no response is received in that time frame.

If certain procedures are consistently denied, ask the carrier what information is necessary to process the claim. If the provider is not satisfied with the results of the review, move to the next level.

Department of Health and Human Services
Centers for Medicare & Medicaid Services

Form Approved OMB
No. 0938-0950

Appointment of Representative

Name of Party Carol T. Usner	Medicare or National Provider Identifier Number 432XX9821A

Section 1: Appointment of Representative
To be completed by the party seeking representation (i.e., the Medicare beneficiary, the provider or the supplier):
I appoint this individual, ___Gene Ulibarri, MD___ to act as my representative in connection with my claim or asserted right under title XVIII of the Social Security Act (the "Act") and related provisions of title XI of the Act. I authorize this individual to make any request; to present or to elicit evidence; to obtain appeals information; and to receive any notice in connection with my appeal, wholly in my stead. I understand that personal medical information related to my appeal may be disclosed to the representative indicated below.

Signature of Party Seeking Representation *Carol T. Usner*	Date 08-03-20XX
Street Address 530 Hutch Street	Phone Number (with Area Code) (555)-386-0122

City Woodland Hills	State XY	Zip Code 12345

Section 2: Acceptance of Appointment
To be completed by the representative:
I, ___Gene Ulibarri, MD___, hereby accept the above appointment. I certify that I have not been disqualified, suspended, or prohibited from practice before the Department of Health and Human Services; that I am not, as a current or former employee of the United States, disqualified from acting as the party's representative; and that I recognize that any fee may be subject to review and approval by the Secretary.

I am a / an ___Non-Attorney eligible for direct payment.___

(Professional status or relationship to the party, e.g. attorney, relative, etc.)

Signature of Representative *Gene Ulibarri, MD*	Date 08-03-20XX
Street Address 4567 Broad Avenue	Phone Number (with Area Code) (555) 486-9002

City Woodland Hills	State XY	Zip Code 12345

Section 3: Waiver of Fee for Representation
Instructions: This section must be completed if the representative is required to, or chooses to waive their fee for representation. (Note that providers or suppliers that are representing a beneficiary and furnished the items or services may not charge a fee for representation and must complete this section.)
I waive my right to charge and collect a fee for representing ___Carol T. Usner___ before the Secretary of the Department of Health and Human Services.

Signature *Gene Ulibarri, MD*	Date 08-03-20XX

Section 4: Waiver of Payment for Items or Services at Issue
Instructions: Providers or suppliers serving as a representative for a beneficiary to whom they provided items or services must complete this section if the appeal involves a question of liability under section 1879(a)(2) of the Act. (Section 1879(a)(2) generally addresses whether a provider/supplier or beneficiary did not know, or could not reasonably be expected to know, that the items or services at issue would not be covered by Medicare.)
I waive my right to collect payment from the beneficiary for the items or services at issue in this appeal if a determination of liability under §1879(a)(2) of the Act is at issue.

Signature *Gene Ulibarri, MD*	Date 08-03-20xx

Form CMS-1696 (Rev 06/12)

FIGURE 9-8 Form CMS-1696 (Rev 06/12) completed by a Medicare patient appointing the physician as his or her authorized representative.

Administrative Law Judge Hearing (Level 3)

A request for a hearing before an ALJ may be made if the amount still in question is $150 or more (usually in combined claims). The request must be made within 60 days of receiving the reconsideration officer's decision (Figure 9-9). It may take 18 months to receive an ALJ assignment. Proof that the claim represents an unusual case and warrants special consideration may lead to a successful conclusion. However, the decision might be reversed, allow partial

adjustment of the carrier's payment, or deny payment. If the final judgment is not satisfactory, proceed to the next level.

Medicare Appeals Council (Level 4)

The Medicare Appeals Council is part of the Office of Hearings and Appeals of the Social Security Administration. A request must be made within 60 days of the ALJ decision; if there is a question that the final judgment was

DEPARTMENT OF HEALTH AND HUMAN SERVICES
OFFICE OF MEDICARE HEARINGS AND APPEALS

REQUEST FOR MEDICARE HEARING BY AN ADMINISTRATIVE LAW JUDGE
Effective July 1, 2005. For use by party to a reconsideration/fair hearing determination issued by a Fiscal Intermediary (FI), Carrier, or Quality Improvement Organization (QIO) (Amount in controversy must be $100 or more.)

☐ Part A
☒ Part B

Send copies of this completed form to:
Original – The FI, Carrier, or QIO that issued the Reconsideration/Fair Hearing Notice
Copy – Appellant

Appellant *(The party appealing the reconsideration determination)* Gaston Input, MD	
Beneficiary *(Leave blank if same as the appellant.)* Deborah P. Sawyer	**Provider or Supplier** *(Leave blank if same as the appellant.)*
Address 1605 Evans Road	Address

City Woodland Hills	State XY	Zip Code 12345	City	State	Zip Code
Area Code/Telephone Number (555) 742-1821	E-mail Address dpsawyer@gmail.net		Area Code/Telephone Number	E-mail Address	

Health Insurance (Medicare) Claim Number 481-XX-6491	Document control number assigned by the FI, Carrier, or QIO 320-486-9002

FI, Carrier, or QIO that made the reconsideration/fair hearing determination Medicare Blue Cross/Blue Shield of North Dakota	Dates of Service From 02/03/20XX To 06/03/20XX

I DISAGREE WITH THE DETERMINATION MADE ON MY APPEAL BECAUSE:
Complications arose during surgical procedure requiring additional procedures to be performed. See attached chart notes and medical reports.

You have a right to be represented at the hearing. If you are not represented but would like to be, your Office of Medicare Hearings and Appeals Field Office will give you a list of legal referral and service organizations. *(If you are represented and have not already done so, complete form CMD-1696.)*

Check Only One Statement:	☐ I <u>wish</u> to have a hearing. ☒ I <u>do not wish</u> to have a hearing and I request that a decision be made on the basis of the evidence in my case. *(Complete form HHS-723, "Waiver of Right to an ALJ Hearing.")*	Check Only One Statement:	☒ I <u>have</u> additional evidence to submit. ☐ I <u>have no</u> additional evidence to submit.

The appellant should complete No. 1 and the representative, if any, should complete No. 2. If a representative is not present to sign, print his or her name in No. 2. Where applicable, check to indicate if appellant will accompany the representative at the hearing.   ☐ Yes   ☐ No

1. (Appellant's Signature) *Gaston Input, MD*	Date 10/11/20XX	2. (Representative's Signature/Name)	Date
Address 4567 Broad Avenue		Address	☐ Attorney ☐ Non-Attorney
City Woodland Hills	State XY	Zip Code 12345	City	State	Zip Code
Area Code/Telephone Number (555)486-9002	E-mail Address inputclinic@cmail.net.		Area Code/Telephone Number	E-mail Address

Answer the following questions that apply:
A) Does request involve multiple claims?   ☐ Yes ☒ No
   (if yes, a list of all the claims must be attached.)
B) Does request involve multiple beneficiaries?   ☐ Yes ☒ No
   (If yes, a list of beneficiaries, their HICNs and the dates of the applicable reconsideration determinations must be attached.)
C) Did the beneficiary assign his or her appeal rights to you as the provider/supplier?   ☒ Yes ☐ No
   (If yes, you must complete and attach form CMS-20031. Failure to do so will prevent approval of the assignment.)
D) If there was no assignment, are you a physician being held liable pursuant to 1842(I)(1)(A) of the Social Security Act?   ☐ Yes ☒ No

CMS-5011A/B U2 (08/05) EF 08/2005 ATTACH A COPY OF THE RECONSIDERATION/FAIR HEARING DETERMINATION (IF AVAILABLE) TO THIS COPY.

FIGURE 9-9 Request for Medicare Hearing by an Administrative Law Judge, CMS-5011A/B.

not made in accordance with the law, the council by its own election may review the ALJ decision. If the council denies a review, the provider may file a civil action for a federal district court hearing.

Federal District Court (Level 5)

The amount in controversy must be at least $1400 (in 2014 and increased annually) and an attorney must be hired to represent the provider and manage the case. The case may

be filed where the physician's business is located. Contact the local medical society for suggestions of names of attorneys experienced at this level of the appeals process.

Centers for Medicare and Medicaid Services Regional Offices

One final suggestion (and this can be done with steps for a hearing or a review) is to write or telephone the medical director at one of the CMS regional offices. Sometimes a regional officer intercedes or takes steps to correct problems or inequities. CMS regional offices may be located by accessing the Medicare website.

Medigap

Insurance companies that sell Medigap (MG) policies must be certified before being allowed to sell in each state. The certification can be lifted from any insurer that does not honor its contract agreements. Only the state insurance commissioner can exert pressure on MG insurance companies. If payment is slow in coming or is not received from an MG insurer, first try the paper or electronic claim solutions for delinquent claims mentioned previously in this chapter. As a last resort, tell the insurer, "If I do not receive payment, I will have no alternative but to contact the state insurance commissioner."

When the MG insurance is Medicaid, in most cases the secondary payment is written off. This occurs because the Medicare prospective payment fee schedule is higher than the Medicaid fee schedule. Therefore Medicaid states that since the amount paid by Medicare is above its regular fee schedule, the balance of the claim should be written off.

TRICARE Review and Appeal Process

A provider who treats a TRICARE patient but is out of network is not able to obtain information from TRICARE. Contact the patient for his or her assistance. Also, out-of-network providers who wish to treat an obstetric case may need a nonavailability request form completed and processed before a patient can receive care. There must be a reason the patient cannot go to a providing facility and TRICARE determines whether it will approve the request. Otherwise, claims will be denied.

All TRICARE inquiries are done through the online provider portal or the automated phone system. TRICARE managed care contracts have been adopted throughout the United States and the appeals procedures that TRICARE contractors use in these areas may vary. For information on how to file reviews and appeals for those contracts, ask the contracting insurance company for instructions and forms.

There are two types of TRICARE appeals, expedited and nonexpedited. Expedited appeals must be filed within 3 days of the receipt of the initial denial. These appeals should include an expedited review of a prior authorization denial. This process varies slightly depending on the regional contractor, so research the appeals process with your local TRICARE contractor.

Nonexpedited appeals must be filed no more than 90 days after the receipt of the initial denial. The steps to file a nonexpedited appeal follow:

1. Send a letter to the regional TRICARE contractor at the address specified in the notice to appeal. The appeal letter must be submitted no more than 90 days after the date of the RA. Include in the appeal the RA stating the denial, along with a claim form and all medical documentation relating to the claim. If for some reason essential paperwork for the insurance claim is not available to be sent, include this reason in the appeal letter. Keep copies of all paperwork for future reference and follow-up.
2. The TRICARE contractor will review the case and make a decision. If the decision is not favorable, the next level of appeal is TRICARE Quality Monitoring Contractor (TQMC).
3. Send a letter to TQMC including all of the documentation from the original appeal and the decision received from the regional TRICARE contractor. The letter must be received by TRICARE no more than 90 days after the date of the appeal decision. Again, if all documentation is not available to be sent along with the appeal, include the reasons why in the appeal letter. Keep your paperwork for future reference and follow-up.
4. The TQMC issues a second reconsideration decision. If the claim is for less than $300, the TQMC decision is final. If there is still a dispute about a claim that is more than $300, you may request that the TRICARE Management Activity (TMA) schedule an independent hearing.

Reconsideration

Participating providers may appeal certain decisions made by TRICARE and request reconsideration. Providers who do not participate may not appeal but TRICARE Standard patients and parents or guardians of patients younger than 18 years of age who seek care from nonparticipating providers may file appeals. Providers who do not participate may not receive any information about a particular claim without the signed authorization of the patient or the patient's parent or guardian.

Matters that can be appealed include the following:
1. Medical necessity disagreements (inappropriate care, level of care, investigational procedures)
2. Factual determinations (hospice care, foreign claims, provider sanction cases)
   a. Denials or partial denials of requests for preauthorization for certain services or supplies
   b. Coverage issues—notification that TRICARE will not pay for services before or after a certain date

Matters that cannot be appealed include the following:

1. Denial of services received from a provider not authorized to provide care under TRICARE
2. A specific exclusion of law or regulation
3. Allowable charges for particular services
4. Issues relating to the establishment and application of diagnosis-related groups
5. Decisions by the claims processor to ask for additional information on a particular case
6. A determination of a person's eligibility as a TRICARE beneficiary

The TRICARE department that handles appeals also collects and organizes all information necessary to review the case effectively. Usually a determination decision is made within 60 days from receipt of the appeal. Disagreements about the amount allowed for a particular claim may be reviewed by the claims processor to determine whether it was calculated correctly. However, an individual cannot appeal the amount that the TRICARE contractor determines to be the allowable charge for a certain medical service.

Requests must be sent to the claims processor of the state in which services were provided and must be postmarked within 90 days of the date the provider receives the Summary Payment Voucher (formerly referred to as an RA). Include photocopies of the claim, the Summary Payment Voucher, and other supporting documents with the request form or letter. The claim identification number assigned by the claims processor should be included in any inquiry concerning payment of the claim. If TRICARE denies the initial request, the other two levels of review—formal review and hearing—may be pursued.

STATE INSURANCE COMMISSIONER

Commission Objectives

The insurance industry is protected by a special exemption from the Federal Trade Commission (FTC) under the McCarran-Ferguson Act of 1945. Under the exemption, the FTC cannot attack unfair or deceptive practices if there is any state law about such practices. The regulations vary widely from state to state and by no means are all 50 states equally strict. If a complaint arises about an insurance policy, medical claim, or insurance agent or broker, the insurance department of the state of residence or the state in which the insurance company's corporate office is headquartered should be contacted. Sometimes this department is referred to as the *insurance commission of the state*. State insurance departments usually have various objectives, including the following:

- To make certain that the financial strength of insurance companies is not unduly diminished

- To monitor the activities of insurance companies to ensure that the interests of the policyholders are protected
- To verify that all contracts are carried out in good faith
- To ensure that all organizations authorized to transact insurance, including agents and brokers, are in compliance with the insurance laws of that state
- To release information on how many complaints have been filed against a specific insurance company in a year
- To help explain correspondence related to insurance company bankruptcies and other financial difficulties
- To assist if a company funds its own insurance plan
- To help resolve insurance conflicts

The insurance commissioner can hold a hearing to determine whether licensed insurers, agents, or brokers are in compliance with the insurance laws of the state but the commissioner does not have the authority vested in a court of law to order an insurance company to make payment on a specific claim.

The insurance commissioner reviews the policy to determine whether the denial of a claim by the insurance company was based on legal provisions of the insurance contract and advises the patient if there is an infraction of the law. If there is an infraction, the patient should consult an attorney to determine whether the claim should be submitted to a court of law.

Types of Problems

Problems that should be submitted to the insurance commissioner are as follows:

1. Improper denial of a claim or settlement for an amount less than that indicated by the policy, after proper appeal has been made
2. Delay in settlement of a claim, after proper appeal has been made
3. Illegal cancellation or termination of an insurance policy
4. Misrepresentation by an insurance agent or broker
5. Misappropriation of premiums paid to an insurance agent or broker
6. Problems about insurance premium rates
7. Two companies that cannot determine which is primary

COMMISSION INQUIRIES

An insurance billing specialist may not be in a position to know the particulars about a case and should never assume or accuse unless he or she is certain or has concrete evidence. Remember, "Jump to conclusions, suffer contusions."

Requests to the insurance commissioner must be submitted online. In some states, the insurance commissioner requires that the complaint come from the patient even if an assignment of benefits form has been signed. In such a case, a letter or form should be prepared for the patient to sign and then submit. Depending on the circumstances of the case, one may wish to send copies to the state medical association or an attorney. Mail may be sent certified, return receipt requested. The request should contain the following information:

1. The inquiring person's (patient) or policyholder's name because the commissioner's responsibility is to the patient (the consumer), not the physician
2. The policyholder's address
3. The policyholder's telephone number
4. The insured's name
5. Name, address, and title of the insurance agent or official of the insurance company
6. A statement of the complaint including, if possible, a copy of the policy, medical bills, unpaid medical insurance claim, canceled checks, and any correspondence from the company pertaining to the claim
7. The patient's signature
8. The name and address of the insurance company, agent, or broker or name and address of the finance company if the premium was financed
9. The policy or claim number
10. The date of loss
11. The date on which the patient signed the complaint form

If an insurance company is continually a slow payer, one method to speed up payments is to include a note to the carrier that reads, "Unless this claim is paid or denied within 30 days, a formal written complaint will be filed with the state insurance commissioner."

Another method is to send a letter to the insurance commissioner with a copy notation inserted at the end to the insurance company. It might read, "The attached claim has been submitted to the XYZ Insurance Company. It has not been paid or denied. Please accept this letter as a formal written complaint against the XYZ Insurance Company."

Insurance companies are rated according to the number of complaints received about them, so they do not want the insurance commissioner to be alerted to any problems. Some states have information available to the public on how many claims have been submitted against a company if this information is necessary.

PROCEDURE 9-1

File an Appeal

OBJECTIVE: To compose, format, key, proofread, and print a letter of appeal and attach photocopies of information to substantiate reimbursement requested

EQUIPMENT/SUPPLIES: Typewriter or computer, printer, letterhead paper, envelope, attachments (if necessary), thesaurus, English dictionary, medical dictionary, and pen or pencil

DIRECTIONS: Follow these basic step-by-step procedures, which include rationales, to learn this skill and practice it by completing the *Workbook* assignment.

1. Refer to Figure 9-10 and Procedure 4-2 at the end of Chapter 4 and follow the procedure to compose, format, key, proofread, and print a letter.
2. Include the beneficiary's name, health insurance claim number, date of initial determination, dates of service in question, items or services in question, name and address of the provider, and signature of appellant.
3. Compose a letter with an introduction that stresses the medical practice's qualifications, the physician's commitment to complying with regulations and providing appropriate services, and the importance of the practice to the payer's panel of physicians or specialists.
4. Provide a detailed account of the necessity of the treatment given and its relationship to the patient's problems and chief complaint. You might cross-reference the medical record and emphasize parts of it that the reviewer may have missed.
5. Explain the reason why the provider does not agree with the claim denial listed on the EOB or RA.
6. Abstract excerpts from the coding resource book and attach a photocopy of the article or pertinent information showing the name of the article, coding resource, and date of publication.
7. Send copies of similar cases with increased reimbursement from the same insurance company if available from the insurance company payment history file.
8. Call the insurance company and speak to the individual responsible for appeals; explain what the resubmission is trying to accomplish. Direct the correspondence to this person.
9. Retain copies of all data sent for the physician's files.
10. Use a method that confirms the payer received the letter, such as a certified return receipt or signature using Federal Express or Airborne Express services.

Continued

PROCEDURE 9-1—cont'd

PHYSICIAN'S LETTERHEAD

January 2, 20XX

Committee on Physician's Services
Medicare
Street address of fiscal intermediary
City, State, ZIP Code

Dear Madam or Sir:

Re: Underpayment

Identification No.:	1910-2192283-101
Patient:	Mrs. Sarah C. Nile
Type of Service:	Exploratory laparotomy
Date of Service:	December 1, 20XX
Amount Paid:	$000.00
My Fees:	$0000.00

Herewith a request for a committee review of the above-named case,
since I consider the allowance paid very low having in mind the patient's
condition prior to surgery, the location, the extent, the type, and the
necessary surgical procedure performed.

Enclosed are photocopies of the history and physical showing the grave
status of the patient prior to surgery, operative report, pathology report,
and discharge summary. The Medicare Remittance Advice and the
Medicare CMS-1500 claim originally submitted are also enclosed.

Considering these points, I hope that you will authorize additional
payment in order to bring the total fee to a more reasonable amount.

Sincerely,

Hugh R. Aged, MD
Hugh R. Aged, MD
NPI# 73542109XX

mf

FIGURE 9-10 A cover letter signed by the physician appealing a claim.

KEY POINTS

This is a brief chapter review, or summary, of the key issues presented. To further enhance your knowledge of the technical subject matter, review the key terms and key abbreviations for this chapter by locating the meaning for each in the Glossary at the end of this book, which appears in a section before the Index.

1. Payment from a third-party payer after submission of a paper claim should occur within 4 to 12 weeks and of an electronic claim should occur within 7 days. When a payment problem develops and the insurance company is slow, ignores, denies, or exceeds time limits, contact the third-party payer.

2. An explanation of benefits (EOB) or electronic Medicare remittance advice (RA) should be read and interpreted line by line and checked to establish whether the amount paid is correct. Amounts should then be posted to each patient's financial account.

3. Routine periodic checks of the insurance claims electronic tracking report or insurance paper claims register (log) should be done to follow up on delinquent claims.

4. The individual handling the front desk must collect insurance information accurately and update patient demographic information routinely to avoid future collection problems.

5. To avoid denied claims and assist in solving claim problems, keep abreast of the latest policies for all contracted payers as well as for the federal programs.

6. A decision to appeal a claim should be based on whether there is ample information to back up the claim and if a substantial amount of money is in question.

7. The levels of a Medicare appeal are (1) redetermination by telephone, letter, or form; (2) reconsideration by a hearing officer; (3) hearing by an administrative law judge; (4) review by the Medicare Appeals Council; and (5) judicial review in the Federal District Court.

8. The types of a TRICARE appeal are expedited and nonexpedited.

9. To complain about a problem with an insurance contract or claim involving a private third-party payer or a Medigap (MG) supplemental plan, the state insurance commission must be contacted.

10. Always file the appropriate form or write a letter to begin the appeal process for resolving an insurance problem or complaint.

🖥 STUDENT ASSIGNMENT

✔ Study Chapter 9.

✔ Answer the fill-in-the-blank, multiple-choice, and true/false review questions in the *Workbook* to reinforce the theory learned in this chapter and to help prepare you for a future test.

✔ Complete the assignments in the *Workbook* to fill in a form for tracing a delinquent claim, locate errors on a returned claim, and complete a form to appeal a Medicare case.

✔ Turn to the Glossary at the end of this text for a further understanding of the key terms and key abbreviations used in this chapter.

Office and Insurance Collection Strategies

Payel Bhattacharya Madero

OBJECTIVES

After reading this chapter, you should be able to:

1. Explain the cash flow cycle in a medical office.
2. Define *accounts receivable* and explain how it is handled.
3. Describe procedures collecting complete and accurate patient information.
4. State medical office policies for managing patient accounts and collection.
5. Describe guidelines for missed appointments.
6. Recite and discuss types of fee adjustments available to patients.
7. Discuss fees with patients.
8. Name and describe payment options available to patients.
9. Define how to use the *aging account receivable report* effectively in collections.
10. Discuss dun messages, electronic media, and manual and computer billing, as well as state the role of a billing service in the collection process.
11. List the names of the federal credit laws applicable to a physician office setting.
12. Explain statutes of limitations of three kinds of financial accounts.
13. Perform oral and written communication collection techniques.
14. Describe insurance collection from the patient and from third-party payers.
15. State and discuss the role of a collection agency in the collection process.
16. Explain the purpose of small claims court in the collection process.
17. Name and discuss basic actions in tracing a debtor who has moved and left no forwarding address.
18. Identify and describe special collection issues.

KEY TERMS

accounts receivable	creditor	itemized statement
age analysis	cycle billing	lien
American Medical Association Code of Ethics	debit card	netback
	debt	no charge
automatic stay	debtor	nonexempt assets
balance	discount	professional courtesy
bankruptcy	dun messages	reimbursement
bonding	embezzlement	secured debt
cash flow	estate administrator	skip
Code of Medical Ethics	estate executor	statute of limitations
collateral	fee schedule	unsecured debt
collection ratio	financial accounting record	write-off
credit	garnishment	
credit card	insurance balance billing	

KEY ABBREVIATIONS

A/R	FACT	FTC	TILA
ATM	FCBA	HMO	W2
CMS	FCRA	N/A	
e-check	FDCPA	NC	
ERISA	FEHBA	NSF	

Service to Patients

Explain fees and answer questions at initial encounter or during registration, or both, to establish the patient's responsibility for the service to be rendered. Offer payment options to the patient who is experiencing financial problems. If you can make the financial aspect of the medical service go smoothly, you can ease a patient's troubles. Patients rely on the insurance billing specialist for timely, accurate reporting of services. This helps to avoid making patients pay for your mistakes and adding expense and causing delays in payment.

CASH FLOW CYCLE

The practice of medicine in the United States is both a profession and a business. Although the physician decides what type of medicine he or she will practice, it is often the practice administrator who takes over the responsibilities for the business portion of the practice. It is extremely important for the physician and insurance billing specialist to work together to provide all patients with the best possible medical care and ensure that the physician is paid fairly for services rendered.

Today this process has become increasingly complex. Physician office and billing practices have evolved from the barter system of days past. Since the Great Depression, the availability of **credit** and **credit cards** has become a common feature of the financial marketplace. The word *credit* comes from the Latin word *credere*, which means "to believe" or "to trust." This trust is in an individual's business integrity and his or her financial ability to meet obligations when they become due. For many, the idea of credit has changed and may simply mean to put off paying today what one can pay tomorrow.

A large percentage of **reimbursement** to physicians' offices is generated from third-party payers (private insurance, government plans, managed care contracts, and workers' compensation). The physician, the practice administrator responsible for financial affairs, and the patient must understand these insurance contracts, which list the following:

● Reimbursement provisions
● Preauthorization for services
● Medical services not covered
● Portion of the bill for which the patient is responsible
● Process for reimbursing the office

Figure 10-1 shows a flow chart and overview of a medical practice's billing procedures that illustrates the sequence from beginning to end.

ACCOUNTS RECEIVABLE

Accounts receivable (A/R) include the unpaid **balances** due from patients and third-party payers for services that have been rendered. Each medical practice has a policy about handling A/R. The effectiveness of this policy and its enforcement are reflected in the practice's cash flow. The **cash flow** is the ongoing availability of actual cash in the medical practice. When charges are collected at the time of service, the A/R is zero. In an ideal situation, all outstanding balances are paid within 60 days; however, this is not possible for the following reasons:

1. Health care expenses have increased and exceed the expenses the patient pays for everyday living.
2. The public seems to have the attitude that it is a right, rather than a privilege, to receive the best possible health care. Therefore care of the indigent becomes an unreimbursable expense in the medical office.
3. Legal proceedings often delay the payment of medical expenses.
4. Third-party payers do not always pay claims in a timely manner, resulting in further delays in the collection of patient copayments.
5. Managed care plans seek discounted rates for their members obtaining medical services.

By monitoring A/R, the insurance billing specialist is able to evaluate the effectiveness of the collection process. Later in this chapter, A/R ratio formulas are presented in the section titled "Accounts Receivable and Age Analysis by Aging Report."

The best way to keep A/R down is to verify insurance benefits before providing care to the patient (if possible), collect copayments and deductibles at the time of service, obtain authorizations for noncontracted health maintenance organization (HMO) patients, and monitor A/R weekly. Set up automatic alerts when patients with a balance in their account want to schedule an appointment. This reminds the receptionist to ask for a copayment, deductible, or noncovered fee. Electronic claims that have not been paid within 30 days

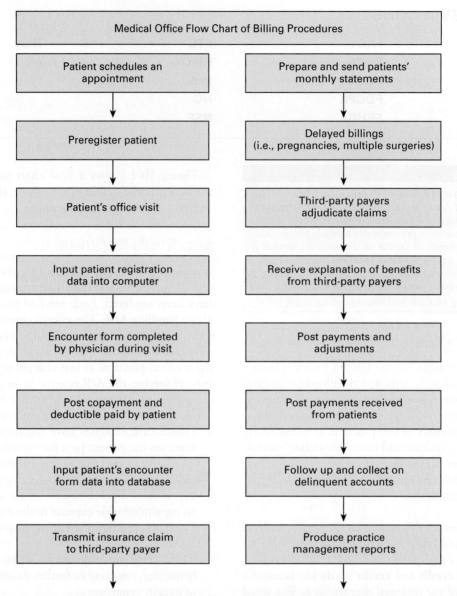

FIGURE 10-1 Medical office flow chart showing a medical practice's billing procedures from scheduling the patient's appointment to producing practice management reports.

of submission may have problems that can range from the carrier asking for additional information from the patient to the patient not being one of the carrier's insured (Chapter 9 reviews problems with electronic claims submission).

The **collection ratio** is the relationship of the amount of money owed to a physician and the amount of money collected on the physician's A/R. A collection rate of 100% is obviously desirable, although unrealistic, and should always be sought as a goal for the person managing collections in the physician's office. To calculate the collection ratio for a 1-month period, divide the amount of monies collected during the current month by the total amount of A/R.

PATIENT EDUCATION

While most Americans feel that health insurance is a right, most do not understand how it works, so the burden of educating them falls on the medical office. The medical assistant works with the front office medical staff to educate the patient in the following aspects of health care:

● Benefits, including how many appointments are allowed per year, copays, and deductibles
● The approximate out-of-pocket expense for patients after insurance has paid
● The cost of medications, medical equipment, and ambulatory services
● The difference between emergency and urgent care and the costs involved

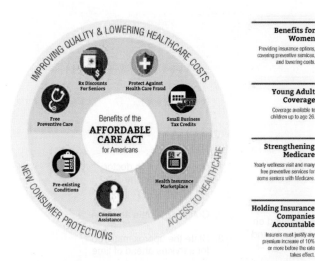

FIGURE 10-2 The Affordable Care Act is focused on improving quality of patient care, reducing costs of health care, protecting patients' right to access care, and other consumer protections.

The Affordable Care Act of 2013 was enacted to allow more Americans access to quality health care. Some of the provisions include free preventive care, elimination of preexisting conditions, expanded Medicaid coverage, and discount medications for seniors (Figure 10-2).

The Affordable Care Act also provides subsidized health insurance for lower-income individuals and allows young adults up to age 26 to remain on their parent's health care plan. Currently this Act does not affect how physicians are reimbursed; probably the biggest change that the medical office will experience is that the number of self-pay patients will decrease.

A new patient information packet should be provided to the patient on the initial visit that contains information about the medical office payment policies. This decreases the number of billing statements sent and increases collections. Never allow a patient to believe that he or she is not responsible for the bill; some medical offices prefer to post a sign stating the office policy (Figure 10-3). Discuss copayment requirements (see Chapter 3) with patients who are enrolled in managed care plans and convey the office policy of collecting this amount when registering the patient for the office visit. A new patient information pamphlet or brochure and confirmation letter (Figure 10-4) may be e-mailed as an attachment or sent to welcome the new patient to the practice. This message or letter informs the patient about the practice, clearly outlines payment expectations, provides collection policies and procedures in printed form, includes a missed appointment clause, establishes a contact person, invites questions, and confirms all specific details discussed.

YOUR CO-PAY IS EXPECTED AT THE TIME OF SERVICE, UNLESS PRIOR FINANCIAL ARRANGEMENTS HAVE BEEN MADE.

FIGURE 10-3 Signs for payment like this are commonly found in the medical office.

Patient Registration Form

There is no substitution for good information-gathering techniques at the time of initial patient registration because this assists later in billing and collection. Always obtain complete and accurate demographic and identifying information from the patient on the first visit and confirm the accuracy of that information on each subsequent visit. Chapter 3 describes the data that should be obtained from the patient; Figure 3-6 is an example of a patient registration information form, also called a *patient information sheet*. For commercial insurance plans, have the guarantor agree in writing to pay for all medical treatment. By obtaining the guarantor's signature, he or she is then bound by contract to pay the bill.

Learn as much as possible about the patient before any services are provided. This is when the patient is likely to be the most cooperative. Information provided on the patient information sheet will prove critical to any billing and collection efforts. The patient should be instructed to answer all questions and indicate any spaces on the form that do not apply by marking N/A (not applicable). A helpful tip is to assist the patient to focus on vital information needed by using a yellow highlighter and blocking all necessary information. One field often overlooked is the subscriber information and his or her date of birth, even though dependents may have insurance cards issued in their name. Reviewing the completed patient information sheet ensures that all blanks have been addressed and accurate information has been collected. It also alerts office staff of an account that may be a future problem. Items often overlooked are the street address, when a post office box is given; an apartment or mobile home park number; a cellphone number; and a business telephone number with department and extension. These help you to trace a patient who has moved. If a patient refuses to divulge any information, invoking privacy laws, it should be policy to require payment for services at the time that care is rendered. A potential nonpaying patient may be recognized at this time. Some indications to look for include:

- Incomplete information on the registration form
- Multiple changes of residence
- Questionable employment record
- No telephone numbers (business, cell, or home)

COLLEGE CLINIC
4567 Broad Avenue
Woodland Hills, XY 12345-0001
Tel. (555) 486-9002
FAX (555) 487-8976

February 3, 20XX

Mrs. Mary M. McLean
4919 Dolphin Way
Woodland Hills, XY 12345-0001

Dear Mrs. McLean:

Thank you for making an appointment with Dr. Ulibarri and entrusting us with your personal health care. Your appointment has been scheduled on _____ (date) at ___ o'clock (time). Please arrive 15 minutes early and bring the completed patient registration and history form.

The fee for your physical examination is approximately $_____ (charge). If laboratory tests, an electrocardiogram, or any procedures are necessary, there will be additional charges. For patients covered by insurance, our office policy requires all copayments at the time of service, so please expect to pay this on the day of your visit. For more information about your copayment responsibility, contact your insurance carrier prior to the office visit. All deductibles and/or coinsurance payments are expected soon after your insurance company has paid their portion of service charges. For your convenience, we accept cash, checks, and credit cards (Visa, American Express, and MasterCard).

Please contact us 24 hours prior to cancel your appointment or there will be a $25 missed appointment fee charged.

Enclosed is a brochure with information regarding our medical practice and a map on the back for your convenience. We look forward to your visit. Please call me at (555) 486-9002 if you have any questions.

Sincerely,

Fran Staple, CMA
Office Manager

Enc: brochure, patient registration, history form

1. State with which doctor the patient has the appointment.

2. Confirm the date and time.

3. State the approximate fee for services ahead of time.

4. Alert the patient that additional charges may be added for additional services.

5. Offer payment options.

6. Enclose patient brochure, patient registration, and history form.

7. Establish a contact person and invite questions.

FIGURE 10-4 New patient confirmation letter emphasizing information to incorporate when writing to a new patient.

- Post office box listed with no street address
- A motel address
- Incomplete insurance information or no insurance coverage
- No referral information or authorization from a primary care physician (PCP) for patients enrolled in a managed care plan

Employers are changing health plans with increasing frequency and patients are more transient than ever, so update this form each time the patient is seen. This can be done by printing out a data sheet or having the patient review a copy of his or her registration form. The patient should sign or initial any changes or corrections.

FEES

Fee Schedule

Most medical practices operate with a set of fees that must be applied uniformly to all patients in the practice; these fees are set by the physician and are loosely based on the Medicare physician payment fee schedule. As discussed in Chapter 6, a **fee schedule** is a listing of accepted charges or established allowances for specific medical procedures. Always quote fees and state policies about the collection of fees to the patient at the initial visit. Under federal regulations, a list of the most common services the physician offers, including procedure code numbers with a description of each service and its price, must be available to all patients.

Missed Appointments

Missed appointments are expensive for providers, so patients should be informed of the importance of keeping appointments. The medical staff should inform patients from the very first visit about the missed appointment fee, which is typically $35 to $50. Regardless of the type of insurance the patient carries, he or she should be held responsible for the fee if the appointment is missed without calling in. Missed appointment charges should not be billed to the insurance company; the patient is responsible for these fees regardless of the insurance he or she carries. To avoid possible discrimination or civil rights violations, ensure that the missed appointment fee is applied to all patients of the medical office.

Some medical offices hold a specific 24- to 48-hour appointment cancellation policy. As a professional courtesy to patients, the medical office should call or contact patients to remind them of the date and time of the appointment just prior to this cancellation period. The medical office staff should also inform the patient of the cancellation fee if the patient was to miss the appointment.

Fee Adjustments
Discounted Fees

A physician may choose to discount his or her fees for various reasons but this practice is ill-advised and may be illegal in some circumstances. A **discount** is a reduction of the normal fee based on a specific amount of money or a percentage of the charge. When a physician offers a discount, it must apply to the total bill, not just the portion that is paid by the patient (copayment or coinsurance amount). By following this rule, the physician is giving a discount to both the patient and the insurance company but the same discount must be given to each member of the insurance plan. This practice could reduce the physician's payment fee schedule with the insurance company and trigger a reduction in the physician's allowable reimbursement schedule; therefore the physician should weigh the long term outcome of discounting fees. All discounts must be electronically posted to the patient's **financial accounting record** and any financial reasons or special circumstances should be documented in the patient's medical record. This ensures complete record keeping and safeguards any questions that may be asked during a financial audit.

Cash Discounts

Cash discounts may be offered to patients who pay the entire fee, in cash, at the time of service (Figure 10-5). If a cash discount system is offered, this policy should be posted in the office and every active patient sent notification. Research your state laws because some states do not allow cash discounts and check the medical practice's insurance contracts to determine whether they are affected. Also, refer to your office's compliance protocol to ensure that any such discounts do not implicate fraud.

Financial Hardship

Financial hardship cases are the most difficult for the physician to determine. The insurance billing specialist should never assume anything about a patient's financial status, nor judge a patient's ability to pay based on his or her appearance. The Department of Health and Human Services (DHHS) annually publishes a guideline on poverty income (Figure 10-6), which is used to determine eligibility for uncompensated services under the Hill-Burton, Community Services Block Grant, and Head Start programs. Physicians may choose to follow these guidelines to direct patients to government-sponsored programs, obtain public assistance, and determine who is eligible for a hardship waiver. A hardship waiver can vary from 25% to 100% of the bill. Various financial forms are available to obtain this information; a copy of the patient's wage and tax statement (W2) or income tax return should be examined to make a reliable decision. The patient also should sign a written explanation to verify true financial hardship. This helps in the collection process and allows the physician to accept the insurance as payment in full, in certain circumstances, without being suspected of insurance fraud. The reason for a fee reduction must be documented in the patient's medical record. Very large medical organizations or medical practices whose services may not be covered by insurance create and use a sliding scale fee schedule based on federal poverty levels and patients pay according to their financial situation.

Be careful about giving a discount because it can be construed as discriminatory if not given to other patients consistently. To avoid problems, develop a written policy about what qualifies a patient for a financial hardship discount.

Write-Off or Courtesy Adjustment

A **write-off** or *courtesy adjustment* (the preferred term) is a **debt** that has been determined to be uncollectable and is taken off (subtracted/credited) the accounting books. It is considered lost income but may not be claimed as a loss for tax purposes. The insurance billing specialist should obtain financial information on all patients who request a write-off. Office policies about adjustments and all discounts should be in writing and all staff members should be informed. The physician must approve all discounts, adjustments, and special payment arrangements prior to patient contract signature.

STATEMENT

College Clinic
4567 Broad Avenue
Woodland Hills, XY 12345-0001
Telephone: (555) 486-9002
Fax: (555) 487-8976

Jake Herron
439 Zinfendale Lane
Woodland Hills, XY 12345

Phone No. (H) _____555/862-4193_____ (W) 555/862-5900_____   Birthdate: __02/12/79__

Insurance Co. _____None_____   Policy No. _____

DATE	REFERENCE	PROFESSIONAL SERVICE DESCRIPTION	CHARGE		CREDITS		CURRENT BALANCE	
					PAYMENTS	ADJUSTMENTS		
3-3-XX	99203	OV Level 3, NP	70	92			70	92
3-6-XX	81000	UA	8	00			78	92
3-6-XX	93000	ECG Hosp admit, C Hx PX	34	26			113	18
4-6-XX		Billed pt. **We can clear this account on MasterCard, Visa, or Discover.** Please authorize this by giving us your account number, expiration date, type of card, and the amount you would like to charge.						← 1. First dun message
4-26-XX	Ck #602	ROA Pt			50	00	63	18
5-6-XX		Billed pt. **PLEASE NOTE**—This account is Past Due. Your prompt attention is courteously requested.					63	18 ← 2. Second dun message
6-6-XX		Billed pt. **FINAL NOTICE**—If we do not hear from you within 10 days, this account will be turned over to our collection agency.					63	18 ← 3. Third dun message
6-29-XX	Ck #639	ROA Pt			50	00	13	18
7-29-XX	Ck #701	ROA Pt			13	18		0
8-14-XX	99213	OV Level 3	40	20			40	20
8-14-XX	Cash	ROA Pt (20% Cash discount)			32	16	8 04	0 ← 4. Cash discount

Due and payable within 10 days.   **Pay last amount in balance column.**

Key: PF: Problem-focused   SF: Straightforward   CON: Consultation   ED: Emergency Dept.
      EPF: Expanded problem-focused L : Low complexity   HX: History   HCD: House call
      D: Detailed   M: Moderate complexity   PX: Phys Exam   HV: Hospital visit
      C: Comprehensive   H: High complexity   OV: Office visit

FIGURE 10-5 Electronic hard copy of a patient's financial accounting record showing dun messages, posted payments, and cash discount.

HIPAA Compliance Alert COMPLIANCE GUIDELINES FOR DEVIATIONS FROM STANDARD COLLECTION PROCEDURES

The Office of the Inspector General issued guidance to providers that they are free to use whatever policy they want on charity care, discounts, write-offs, and collections, as long as it is done consistently and the reasons for granting these are documented (for example, in the medical practice's compliance manual). Ensure that these deviations from standard collection procedures are not tied to or conditional on referrals or use of the provider's services. Ensure that office policy states the minimum effort in collection of debts, such as one or more letters or telephone calls. The provider who uses minimum collection efforts can waive the obligations of patients in financial need in accordance with office policy and try to collect more aggressively from other patients who are not financially needy.

2015 Guidelines on Poverty Income			
Size of Family Unit	48 Contiguous States and D.C.	Alaska	Hawaii
1	$11,770	$14,720	$13,550
2	15,930	19,920	18,330
3	20,090	25,120	23,110
4	24,250	30,320	27,890
5	28,410	35,520	32,670
6	32,570	40,720	37,450
7	36,730	45,920	42,230
8	40,890	51,120	47,010
For each additional person add	$4,160	$5,200	$4,780

FIGURE 10-6 Department of Health and Human Services (DHHS) 2015 guidelines on poverty income, http://aspe.hhs.gov.

The physician must approve the portion of the charge to be credited to the financial record before the debt is forgiven. A write-off is possible in three circumstances. The first is as stated in the preceding discussion, when the patient has proved a financial hardship. The second is when it will cost more to bill the balance than what is owed. For example, the balance may be $1.05. It will cost the practice more than this amount to collect the balance. This type of write-off is known as a *small balance write-off.* The third situation is when the provider has made a good faith effort to collect the balance with no success. In this case, the balance is written off and the account may or may not be sent to a professional collection agency depending on whether the agency accepts balances less than, for example, $35 for collection.

Professional Courtesy

Professional courtesy is a concept attributed to Hippocrates but the foundations actually are derived from Thomas Percival's *Code of Medical Ethics,* written in 1803. The *American Medical Association (AMA) Code of Ethics,* formulated and adopted in 1847, closely mirrored Percival's code. The practice of professional courtesy served to build bonds between physicians and reduce the incentive for physicians to treat their own families. Most physicians agree that one of the greatest honors and privileges in the practice of medicine is to be asked to care for a physician and his or her family members. The practice of professional courtesy often was extended to others in the health care profession and members of the clergy. Most hospitals and many surgeons have given up the practice of free care today because most physicians now have insurance coverage for medical expenses.

Professional courtesy means either a discount or an exemption from charges that may be given to certain people at the discretion of the physician rendering the service.

An interim rule from the Centers for Medicare and Medicaid Services (CMS), effective September 5, 2007, identifies proper ways to offer professional courtesy.
1. The professional courtesy is offered to all physicians on the entity's bona fide medical staff or in the entity's local community or service area without regard to volume or value of referrals or other business generated between the parties.
2. The health care items and services provided are of a type routinely provided by the entity.
3. The entity's professional courtesy policy is written and approved in advance by the entity's governing body.
4. The professional courtesy is not offered to a physician (or immediate family member) who is a federal health care program beneficiary unless there has been a good faith showing of financial need.
5. If the professional courtesy involves any whole or partial reduction of any coinsurance obligation, the insurer is informed in writing of the reduction.
6. The arrangement does not violate the Anti-Kickback statute (section 1128B(b) of the Act) or any federal or state law or regulation governing billing or claims submission.

Physicians must examine their policies on professional courtesy to ensure that they do not violate the contractual terms in private, managed care or government sponsored insurance policies. If the treating physician does not bill the physician-patient for services rendered, the third-party payer is relieved of its contractual obligation. If the treating physician waives the deductible and copayment, the physician may be accused of not treating others with the same insurance coverage in an equal manner. Although there may be some situations in which it is defensible to not charge for services to health care professionals, the physician should ensure that this professional courtesy is not linked to patients who have been referred to the practice. Laws prohibit any inducement or kickbacks from physicians (or others) that could influence the decision of a physician (or other) to refer patients or that may affect a patient's decision to seek care.

> **HIPAA Compliance Alert**
> **PROFESSIONAL COURTESY GUIDELINES**
>
> Professional courtesy may violate fraud and abuse laws depending on how the recipients of the professional courtesy are selected and how the courtesy is extended. If selection depends on referral of individuals, it may implicate the Anti-Kickback statute. An insurance claim submitted as a result of such a professional courtesy may also be affected by the False Claims Act.

Copayment Waiver

Waiving copayments is another way that physicians have reduced the cost of medical care for patients in the past. In doing so, the physician accepts the insurance payment only. In most situations, both private insurers and the federal government ban waiving the copayment, so it is not recommended. Waiving copayments could violate the contract between the patient and third-party payer. If the physician has contracted with a third-party payer, waiving the copayment may be a violation of the physician and managed care contract. Some insurance companies look at this as a means of recouping its losses by undergoing litigation against the provider or demanding the return of all payments made to the provider.

No Charge

No charge (NC) means waiving the entire fee for professional care. This is permitted as long as it is not part of a fraudulent scheme and is offered to all patients. All NC visits must be fully documented in the clinical portion of the patient's medical and account record. As a way of trying to satisfy a patient's deductible, a physician or insurance billing specialist cannot assess a fee for services that the insurance company or third-party payer does not cover.

Another instance when "NC" occurs on a patient's account is when follow-up visits are posted after a patient undergoes surgery considered under a surgical package or Medicare global fee structure. When posting such charges in a medical billing system, Current Procedural Terminology (CPT) code 99024 (postoperative follow-up visit included in global fee) may be used.

Reduced Fee

Precautions should be taken before reducing the fee of a patient who dies. The doctor's sympathy in this case could be misinterpreted and result in a malpractice suit. A fee reduction should never be based on a poor result in the treatment of a patient.

If a patient disputes a fee and the physician agrees to settle for a reduced fee, the agreement should be in writing in the patient account file.

> **HIPAA Compliance Alert**
> **DISCUSSION OF FINANCIAL MATTERS WITH PATIENTS**
>
> Because the patient's financial history is personal, in-the-office conversations about fees must be private so that other individuals cannot overhear. The patient should be made to feel comfortable so that he or she feels free to discuss any financial problems. Be firm. Use tact. Always use a courteous but businesslike approach when discussing financial matters.

Discussing Fees

People have a difficult time asking each other for money and talking about financial obligations. Financial arrangements should be discussed up front and in great detail before any services are provided. Many medical practices create their own collection problems by not being clear about how and when they expect to be paid. If patients are not told that payment is due at the time of service, most assume they can pay at a later time. Patients are unaware of additional absorbed services given to patients during an office visit. Figure 10-7 presents a detailed description of some of those tasks that may be pointed out to patients so that they have a better understanding of the time expended by the provider and staff. The following are some guidelines to help you communicate effectively about money.

1. Be courteous at all times but express a firm, businesslike approach that will not offend the patient.
2. Never badger or intimidate a patient into paying; merely state the payment policy and educate the patient.
3. Inform the patient of his or her full financial responsibility and balance due in a clear manner.
4. Verify the patient's copayment listed on his or her insurance card and collect this amount before the patient's office visit.
5. Make it easier for the patient to pay rather than leave without making payment.

ABSORBED MEDICAL SERVICES

✔ Create and maintain patient's permanent medical records.

✔ Order, review/interpret, document/file, and telephone laboratory test results to the patient.

✔ Order x-rays, review/interpret, compare with previous studies if abnormal, consult with radiologist, document/file, and telephone results to the patient.

✔ Write and send consultation reports/letters to referring or consulting physicians and other providers.

✔ Telephone consultations with physicians.

✔ Complete family medical leave forms, disability forms, waivers for handicapped plates, waivers of insurance premiums, automotive forms, life insurance premium forms, travel insurance forms, and school, camp, or athletic participation forms.

✔ E-mail responses to patients.

✔ Write letters of referral to specialists.

✔ Create patient education materials.

✔ Conduct medical research pertinent to the patient's case.

✔ Write prescriptions and communicate with pharmacies about patients' prescriptions.

✔ Transmit (or complete) patients' insurance claim forms and complete insurance application forms.

✔ Conduct utilization review negotiations with hospitals and insurance companies.

✔ Review and maintain documentation for patients' hospital medical records.

✔ Write medical orders for hospitalized patients and orders for those in nursing facilities.

✔ Write letters to obtain medical services, instruments, or equipment for patients.

✔ Arrange for hospital admissions and follow-up consultations with nurses and other physicians.

FIGURE 10-7 Details of additional absorbed medical services the provider and staff give to patients during an office visit, depending on the complexity of a medical problem.

6. Do not give the patient an option by asking if he or she would like to pay now or have a bill sent.
7. Motivate the patient to pay by appealing to his or her honesty, integrity, and pride.

The following are examples of communicating in a positive manner and letting the patient know exactly what is expected:

• "The office visit is $62, Mrs. Smith. Would you like to pay by cash, check, credit card, or debit card?"
• "Your copayment for today's visit is $20, Mr. Jones, and you can pay by cash, check, credit card, or debit card."
• "Your insurance policy shows a $100 deductible that is your responsibility and currently has not been met, Miss Rodriguez. You must pay the full fee today, which is $100."

• "Mrs. Merryweather, I must collect $4.77 today for your vitamin B_{12} injection. The injection is not covered by your insurance policy."
• "We look forward to seeing you on Tuesday, March 3, at 10 AM, Mr. Gillespie. The consultation fee will be approximately $150 and payment is expected at the time of service. We accept cash, check, credit cards, or debit cards for your convenience."

Collecting Fees

Payment at the Time of Service

Collecting applicable copayments and other amounts due from the patient on each office visit is strongly recommended. To avoid difficulties in collecting at a future date, ask for fixed copayments before the patient is seen by the provider. This will alleviate billing for small amounts or possible problems with collection if statements are sent by mail after the visit. The importance of collecting outstanding bills, coinsurance amounts, and money from cash-paying patients up front should be communicated to office staff. One-on-one communication is the best way to motivate a **debtor.** Each patient's account balance (amount due) should be reviewed before his or her appointment. If the appointment schedule is on a computer system, print the account balance by each patient's name. If an appointment book is used, make a copy of the page showing the day's schedule. Write overdue balances by the patient's name after obtaining overdue amounts from each patient's financial accounting record. This information also should be recorded on the transaction slip for that day's visit and may be "flagged" when the transaction slips are printed or written. Treat this information confidentially, and keep it out of view of other patients. When a patient arrives whose name is "flagged," alert the patient accounts manager.

To do effective preappointment collection counseling, the patient should be taken to a quiet area away from the general activity of the office. Sit down with the patient and discuss the situation. Use an understanding attitude and helpful nature while verbalizing phrases such as "I understand" and "I can help." Ask direct questions to learn exactly what problems the patient is facing. Answers to questions such as "When do you expect your next paycheck?" and "How much are you able to pay today?" help to determine the strategy. The goal should be to collect the full amount. If that is not possible, try to collect a portion of the balance. Get a promise to pay for the remaining balance by a specific date. If the patient is unable to comply, set up a payment plan. The chances of reaching a mutually satisfactory resolution are greatly improved when the two parties are face to face. Refer to Procedure 10-1 to create an a financial agreement with the patient.

A face-to-face interview is better than a telephone interview because a financial agreement can be signed when the debtor is present (Figure 10-8), resulting in a better follow-up response. Let the patient know that the practice is willing to help and that the debtor should inform the insurance billing specialist if he or she runs into further problems making the payment. This personal contact helps if a renegotiation of the agreement is necessary. A medical practice cannot refuse to let an established patient see the doctor because of a debt but the office staff has every right to ask for payment while the patient is in the office.

Encounter Forms. Multipurpose billing forms (see Chapter 3) are known by many names, including *encounter form.* These forms are helpful when collecting fees at the time of service. Encounter forms can be given to patients to bill their insurance companies, used to inform patients of current charges and outstanding balances, and used as receipts for payment (Figure 10-9).

Patient Excuses for Nonpayments. Nonpayers tend to dismiss financial arrangements with curt remarks. Look directly at the patient, confidently expecting payment. Demonstrate to the patient the right to request payment. Be ready if excuses are offered. Table 10-1 shows examples of patients' excuses and possible responses.

When a patient chatters nervously, it may be a way of setting up reasons to rationalize not paying. Do not let this be distracting. Pause after asking for payment and do not say another word until the patient responds. Many people feel uncomfortable with silence but pauses may work to your advantage and help to complete a transaction. The cash flow and collection ratio are increased by taking this approach, while decreasing billing chores and collection costs. The quick identification of nonpayers may be obtained and the person responsible for collections notified.

Credit and Debit Cards

The current economic trend is heading toward the use of credit and debit cards. Patients find these easier to use and tend to always have them on hand. Accepting credit cards can improve a medical practice's financial management in many ways:

● Lower risk of embezzlement by current employees
● Fewer trips to the banks for deposit; funds are electronically transferred to the physician's account
● Fewer concerns about check fraud
● Convenient for patients

Credit card payment is an option that provides patients with an alternative to clear their account balances. Credit cards are issued by organizations that entitle the cardholder to credit at their establishments. This method of payment may be most useful as a down payment on uninsured or elective procedures. According to a survey by American Express, 33% of patients said they would use a credit card to pay for health care–related expenses if the option were given. Credit cards can help to manage A/R by improving cash flow, reducing billing costs, lowering overhead, and reducing the risk of bad debts. If a practice accepts credit cards, advise all patients in the following ways:

● Display a credit card acceptance sign.
● Include an insignia or message on the patient account statement.
● Include the credit card policy in the new patient brochure or new patient welcome letter.
● Have staff members verbalize to patients that this option is available.

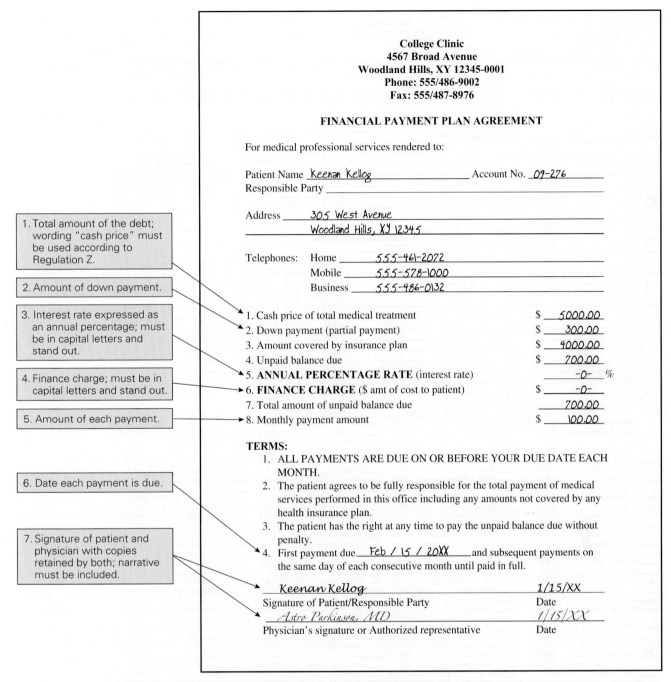

College Clinic
4567 Broad Avenue
Woodland Hills, XY 12345-0001
Phone: 555/486-9002
Fax: 555/487-8976

FINANCIAL PAYMENT PLAN AGREEMENT

For medical professional services rendered to:

Patient Name _Keenan Kellog_   Account No. _09-276_
Responsible Party _____

Address _305 West Avenue_
Woodland Hills, XY 12345

Telephones: Home _555-461-2072_
          Mobile _555-578-1000_
          Business _555-486-0132_

1. Total amount of the debt; wording "cash price" must be used according to Regulation Z.

2. Amount of down payment.

3. Interest rate expressed as an annual percentage; must be in capital letters and stand out.

4. Finance charge; must be in capital letters and stand out.

5. Amount of each payment.

6. Date each payment is due.

7. Signature of patient and physician with copies retained by both; narrative must be included.

1. Cash price of total medical treatment $ _5000.00_
2. Down payment (partial payment) $ _300.00_
3. Amount covered by insurance plan $ _4000.00_
4. Unpaid balance due $ _700.00_
5. **ANNUAL PERCENTAGE RATE** (interest rate)   _-0-_ %
6. **FINANCE CHARGE** ($ amt of cost to patient) $ _-0-_
7. Total amount of unpaid balance due   _700.00_
8. Monthly payment amount $ _100.00_

TERMS:
1. ALL PAYMENTS ARE DUE ON OR BEFORE YOUR DUE DATE EACH MONTH.
2. The patient agrees to be fully responsible for the total payment of medical services performed in this office including any amounts not covered by any health insurance plan.
3. The patient has the right at any time to pay the unpaid balance due without penalty.
4. First payment due _Feb / 15 / 20XX_ and subsequent payments on the same day of each consecutive month until paid in full.

Keenan Kellog   _1/15/XX_
Signature of Patient/Responsible Party   Date
Astro Parkinson, MD   _1/15/XX_
Physician's signature or Authorized representative   Date

FIGURE 10-8 Financial payment plan agreement that provides full disclosure of all information by the Truth in Lending Act, Regulation Z.

Patients may prefer to clear a debt immediately and make monthly payments to the credit card company instead of owing money to their doctor.

Verifying Credit Cards. The insurance billing specialist should check credit card warning bulletins to ensure that the card has not been canceled or stolen. Large practices may have an electronic credit card machine that allows the insurance billing specialist to swipe the card through the machine, which is linked to the credit card company. Transactions are then approved, processed, and deposited in a bank account, usually in 2 working days. A receipt is generated for the patient.

Verifying Credit Card Holders. Always verify the cardholder by asking for photo identification, such as a

STATE LIC.# C1503X
SOC. SEC. # 000-11-0000
PIN # _____

College Clinic
4567 Broad Avenue
Woodland Hills, XY 12345-4700

Phone: 555-486-9002

☐ Private   ☐ Bluecross   ☐ Ind.   ☐ Medicare   ☐ Medi-cal   ☐ HMO   ☒ PPO   → 1. Insurance identifying data

| Patient's last name *McDonald* | First *Lydia* | | Account #: *3794* | Birthdate *01/06/80* | Sex ☐ Male ☒ Female | Today's date *05/06/XX* |
| Insurance company *XYZ Insurance Company* | Subscriber *Lydia McDonald* | | | Plan # *ABC* | Sub. # | Group *340* |

ASSIGNMENT: I hereby assign my insurance benefits to be paid directly to the undersigned physician, I am financially responsible for non-covered services.
SIGNED: Patient, or parent, if minor) *Lydia McDonald*   Today's date *05/06/XX*

RELEASE: I hereby authorize the physician to release to my insurance carriers any information require to process this claim.
SIGNED: Patient, or parent, if minor) *Lydia McDonald*   Today's date *05/16/XX*

→ 2. Assignment of medical benefits

X	DESCRIPTION	CODE	FEE	X	DESCRIPTION	CODE	FEE	X	DESCRIPTION	CODE	FEE
	OFFICE VISITS	NEW	EST.		Venipuncture	36415			OFFICE PROCEDURES		
	Blood pressure check		99211		TB skin test	86580			Anoscopy	46600	
	Level II	99202	99212		Hematocrit	85013			Ear lavage	69210	
	Level III	99203	99213		Glucose finger stick	82948			Spirometry	94010	
	Level IV	99204	99214		IMMUNIZATIONS				Nebulizer Rx	94664	
X	Level V	99205	99215	$132.28	Allergy inj. X1	95115		X	EKG	93000	$34.26
	PREVENTIVE EXAMS	NEW	EST.		Allergy inj. X2	95117			SURGERY		
	Age 65 and older	99387	99397		Trigger pt. inj.	20552			Mole removal (1st)	17100	
	Age 40 - 64	99386	99396		Therapeutic inj.	96372			(2nd to 14th)	17003	
	Age 18 - 39	99385	99395		VACCINATION PRODUCTS				Flat warts (1st - 14th)	07110	
	Age 12 - 17	99384	99394		DPT	90701			15 or more	17111	
	Age 5 - 11	99383	99393		DT	90702			Biopsy, 1 lesion	11100	
	Age 1 - 4	99382	99392		Tetanus	90703			Addt'l. lesions	11101	
	Infant	99381	99391		MMR	90707			Endometrial Bx	58100	
	Newborn ofc		99432		OPV	90712			Skin tags to 15	11200	
	OB/NEWBORN CARE				Polio inj.	90713			Each addt'l. 10	11201	
	OB package		59400		Flu	90662			I & D abscess	10060	
	Post-partum visit N/C				Hemophilus B	90645			SUPPLIES/MISCELLANEOUS		
	LAB PROCEDURES				Hepatitis B vac.	90746			Surgical tray	99070	
	Urine dip	81000			Pheumovax	90670			Handling charge	99000	
	UA qualitative	81005			VACCINE ADMINISTRATION				Special report	99080	
	Pregnancey urine	81025			Age: Through 18 yrs. (1st inj.)	90460			DOCTOR'S NOTES:		
	Wet mount	87210			Age: Through 18 yrs. (ea. addt'l. inj.)	90461					
	kOH prip	8722			Adult (1st inj.)	90471					
	Occult blood	82270			Adult (ea. addt'l. inj.)	90472					

→ 3. Procedure codes

	DIAGNOSES	ICD-10-CM						
	Abdominal pain/unspec.	R10.9		Colitis/unspec.	K51.90		FUO	R50.9	Osteoarthritis (site)	M19._

DIAGNOSES   ICD-10-CM

Abdominal pain/unspec... R10.9	Colitis/unspec. K51.90	FUO R50.9	Osteoarthritis (site)...... M19._
Absess .... L02._	Confusion R41.0	Gastritis K29.70	Otitis media .... H66.9_
Allergic reaction .... T78.40_	CHF I50.9	Gastroenteritis (colitis)... K52.9	Parkinson's disease ... G20
Alzheimer's disease G30	Constipation K59.00	G.I. bleed K92.2	Pharyngitis, acule J02.9
Anemia/unspec. D64.9	COPD J44.9	Gout/unspec. M10.9	Pleurisy R09.1
Angina/unspec. I20.9	Cough R05	Headache R51	Pneumonia J18.9
Anorexia R63.0	Crohn's disease/unspec. .. K50.90	Health exam .... 200._	Pneumonia, viral J12.9
Anxiety/unspec. F41.9	CVA I63.9	Hematuria/unspec. R31.9	Prostatitis/unspec. N41.9
Apnea, sleep G47.30	Decubitus ulcer .... L89._	Herpes simplex B00.9	PVD I73.9
Arrhythmia, cardiac I49.9	Dehydration E86.0	Herpes zoster B02.9	Radiculopathyp .... M54.1_
Arthritis, rheumatoid.... M06.9	Dementia/unspec. F03	Hiatal hernia K44.9	Rectal bleeding K62.5
Asthma/unspec. J45.909	Depression, major/unsp.. F32.9	HTN (HBP) I10	Renal failure N19
Atrial fibrillation I48.0	Diab I, no complications .. E10.0	Hyperlipidemia/unspec... E78.5	Sciatica .... M54.3_
B-12 deficiency E53.8	Diab II, no complications .. E11.9	Hypothyroidism/unspec.. E03.9	Shortness of breath R03.02
Back pain, low M54.5	w/kidney complic. .... E11.2_	Impotence .... N52._	Sinusitis, chr./unspec.... J32.9
BPH N40	w/ophthalmic compl... E11.3_	Influenca, respiratory J10.1	Syncope R55
Bradycardia/unspec. R00.1	w/neurolog complic. ... E11.4_	Insomnia G47.0	Tachycardia/unspec. R00.0
Broncitis, acute........ J20._	w/circulatory cmpl.... E11.5_	IBS, diarrhea .... K58.	Tachy., supraventric I47.1
Bronchitis, chronic J42	Insulin use Z79.4	Lupus, systemic erythim. M32.9	Tendinitix/unspec....... M77.9
Bursitis/unspec. M71.9	Diarrhea/unspec. R19.7	MI, acute .... I21._	TIA G45.9
CA, breast .... C50._	Diverticulitix K57.92	MI, old I25.2	Ulcer, duodenal/unspec... K26.9
CA, lung .... C34._	Diverticulosis K57.90	Migraine G43.9	Ulcer, gastric/unspec.... K25.9
CA, prostate C61	Dizziness R42	Myalgia M79.1	Ulcer, peptic/unspec. ... K27.9
Cellulitis .... L03._	Dysuria R30.0	Neck pain M54.2	URI/unspec. J06.9
☒ Chest pain/unspec..... R07.9	Edema/unspec. R60.9	Neuropathy G62.9	UTI N39.0
Cirrhosis, liver/unspec... K74.60	Endocarditis I38	Nausea R11.1	Vertigo R42
Cold, common J00	Esophageal reflux K21.0	Nausea/vomitting R11.0	Weight gain R63.5
	Fatigue (lethargy) R53.83	Obesity/unspec. E66.9	Weight loss R63.4

→ 4. Diagnostic codes

Diagnosis/additional description:

Doctor's signature/date
P. Cardi, MD

→ 5. Patient's previous balance

Return appointment information: -with whom   Self/other

Days _____   Wks. 2   Mos. _____

PLEASE RMEMBER THAT PAYMENT IS YOU OBLIGATION, REGARDLESS OF INSURANCE OR OTHER THIRD PARTY INVOLVEMENT.

Rec'd. by:		
☒ Cash	Total today's fee	$166.54
☐ Check # _____	Amount rec'd. today	$10.00

→ 6. Total charges and payments received

FIGURE 10-9 Encounter form; diagnostic codes from *International Classification of Diseases,* Tenth Revision, Clinical Modification (ICD-10-CM) and procedural codes for professional services from Current Procedural Terminology (CPT). *(Courtesy Bibbero Systems, Inc., Petaluma, Calif.; telephone: 800-242-2376; fax: 800-242-9330; www.bibbero.com.)*

Table 10-1	**Possible Responses to Patients' Excuses for Avoiding Payment**
EXCUSE	**RESPONSE**
"Just bill me."	"As we explained when we made your appointment, Mr. Barkley, our practice bills for charges more than $50. Amounts less than $50 are to be paid at the time of the visit. That will be $25 for today's visit, please."
"I have insurance to cover this."	"We will be billing your insurance for you, Miss Butler, but your policy shows a deductible in the amount of $300 that still must be met. We must collect the full fee for today's visit, which is $150 to meet that deductible responsibility."
"I get paid on Friday; you know how it is."	"I understand. Why don't you write the check today and postdate it for Saturday. We will hold the check and deposit it on the next business day." (Depending on office policy.)
"If I pay for this, I won't be able to pay for the prescription."	"Our payment policy is very much like the pharmacy's: we expect payment at the time of service. Let me check and see if the doctor can dispense some medication samples to last until you can get your prescription filled."
"I don't have that much with me."	"How much can you pay, Mrs. Fish? I can accept $10 now and give you an envelope to send us the balance within the week or I can put it on your credit or debit card." (Get a commitment and write the balance due under the sealing flap of the envelope. Also write the date on a tickler calendar or the patient's financial accounting record while the patient is watching.)
"I'll take care of it."	"I know you will, Mr. Stone; I just need to know when that will be so that I can document your intentions for our bookkeeper." (Get a commitment and input the date in the patient's financial accounting record while the patient is watching. Hand him an envelope with the amount due written under the sealing flap.)
"I forgot my checkbook."	"We take Visa, MasterCard, and American Express, Mr. Storz." (If the patient still does not pay, provide him with a self-addressed envelope and write the patient's name, account number, date of service, amount due, and expected payment date under the sealing flap. Restate the expected payment date as you hand the patient the envelope. Input the date in the patient's financial accounting record while the patient is watching.)

driver's license. Examine the card carefully and observe the following guidelines:

- Accept a credit card only from the person whose name is on the card.
- Match the name on the card with the patient's other identification and ensure that the expiration date has not passed.
- Look on the back of the card for the word "void." This is an alert that the card has been heated, which is a method used to forge a signature.
- Check the "hot list" for problem cards.
- Verify all charges regardless of the amount and get approval from the credit card company.
- Compare the signature on the credit card receipt against the signature on the card (Figure 10-10, *A* and *B*).

Credit Card Fees. Most banks directly deposit the amount on the credit card receipt and subtract the monthly fees from the practice's bank account. A statement from the bank indicates how much has been credited to the account. The fees can be negotiated on the basis of volume but usually range from 2% to 10% on each transaction. Some medical practices charge patients a service fee for using credit cards. Do not issue cash or check refunds for any payments made by credit card. Patients who want to make payments may have their credit cards charged for each scheduled payment. Some medical practices choose to impose a nominal fee (50 cents) for all credit and debit card transactions to recoup the fee charged by the credit card company.

Currently, simple credit card reader terminal devices attached to a smartphone or tablet are available on the market (Figure 10-11).

Credit Card Options. Online bill payment or e-payment, such as PayPal, is another way patients can pay their medical office bills. It is done through the medical practice's secure website. Payment can be verified immediately and deposited directly into the medical office bank account.

Other cards are used for credit in a physician's office. Automated teller machine (ATM) cards are sometimes accepted for medical care if the practice has a credit card scanner. An ATM card is a magnetically encoded bankcard used to make deposits and withdraw cash from checking or savings accounts. Private-label cards are credit vehicles that can be used only to pay for health care. Some large practices offer their own private-label health cards. Smart cards also are used in some locations. They are small credit or debit cards that contain a computer chip that can store money in the form of electronic data. Special-use smart cards for telephone calls, gas stations, and fast food are now in use, as are common cards having multiple uses. These cards may also contain patient health care data.

Visa offers a credit card service unique to the health care market. It has a preauthorized health care form that allows patients to authorize the medical office to bill their

```
        COLLEGE CLINIC                          COLLEGE CLINIC
        4567 Broad Avenue                       4567 Broad Avenue
      Woodland Hills, XY 12345-0001           Woodland Hills, XY 12345-0001

05/26/20XX              09:39:14        05/26/20XX              09:39:14
Merchant ID:    00000000262026XX        Merchant ID:    00000000262026XX
Terminal ID:         038802XX           Terminal ID:         038802XX
0150302859XX                            0150302859XX

        CREDIT CARD                             CREDIT CARD

          MC SALE                                 MC SALE

CARD#           XXXXXXXXXX4021          CARD#           XXXXXXXXXX4021
INVOICE              009                INVOICE              009
Batch #:           00716                Batch #:           00716
Approval Code:      4123P               Approval Code:      4123P
Entry Method:      Swiped               Entry Method:      Swiped
Mode:              Online               Mode:              Online

SALE AMOUNT        $70.00               SALE AMOUNT        $70.00

                                               CUSTOMER COPY
    _____
      Customer Signature

A       MERCHANT COPY                 B
```

FIGURE 10-10 A, Merchant copy of a credit card receipt showing the patient's signature. **B,** Customer copy of a credit card receipt.

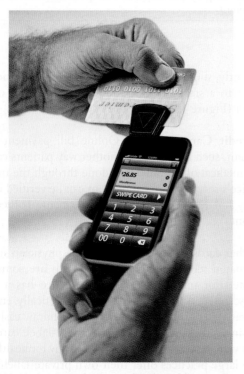

FIGURE 10-11 Square it device used with a tablet to collect credit card payments. (*Photo copyright* iStock.com.)

account directly for copayments and the balance not covered by insurance. Patients who need a series of treatments, such as allergy injections or chemotherapy, can fill out one form designating these services, which authorizes the staff to charge the patient's account directly.

Debit Cards. A **debit card** is a card that permits bank customers to withdraw cash at any hour from any affiliated

ATM in the country. The holder may make cashless purchases from funds on deposit without incurring revolving finance charges for credit. Medical practices that offer credit card payment may use the same electronic credit card machine to swipe the debit card for verification and approval. Separate debit card machines are also available for businesses that do not accept credit cards. Debit cards take the place of check writing; however, once the debit card is approved for a certain amount, the bank that issued the debit card is responsible for paying the funds that were approved. There are no returned checks for nonsufficient funds (NSF) with this method of payment.

Payment by Check

E-Checks. Another payment option that is becoming popular is payment by e-check. With an e-check, the patient gives his or her checking account information, such as account number and bank routing number. A signature to confirm the electronic transaction is required and the check is deposited immediately.

Paper Check Verification. Check verification requires the insurance billing specialist to become familiar with the appearance of a good check. A personal check is the most common method of payment in most medical offices but it is not a personal guarantee of payment. A driver's license and one other form of identification always should be required. Check these against existing records. Call the bank to verify all out-of-state and suspicious checks. A verification service (which is a private company with resources to identify patient information quickly over the telephone) or a check authorization system may be worthy of consideration for clinics and larger group practices.

Check Forgery. *Forgery* is false writing or alteration of a document to injure another person or with intent to deceive (for example, signing another person's name on a check to obtain money or pay off a debt without permission). To guard against forgery, always check that the endorsement on the back of the check matches the name on the front. Be suspicious if the beneficiary or provider states that he or she did not receive the check but the third-party payer shows it as being cashed, or if the payee of the check claims that the signature is not his or hers.

Payment Disputes. Problem checks appear in many forms. One is the check for partial payment when the debtor (the patient) writes "payment in full" on the check. If the **creditor** (the medical office) cashes the check, it may be argued that the debt is paid in full. A legal theory called *accord and satisfaction* may apply to this situation if the debt is truly disputed by the debtor. If the check is retained (and cashed) by the physician, it can be considered "accord and satisfaction" and the physician cannot procure the balance from the patient. The operative words are "truly disputed." If there is a legitimate, genuine dispute over the amount of the bill and an amount less than the full amount of the bill is accepted, the physician could be precluded from seeking the balance. However, acceptance of payment does not necessarily mean acceptance of the "paid in full" remark. Even if a check marked "paid in full" is accidentally cashed, 90 days may be available to rectify the situation by returning the funds to the patient and informing him or her that the accord and satisfaction is not acceptable. A patient who is paying less may be dissatisfied with the practice in some way. This may help to defuse any lurking issues and address the patient's underlying problem.

Postdated Checks. Checks dated to be payable 3 to 6 months in the future are not honored by the bank. Always read the date on every check. Federal collection law states that if a check dated more than 5 days in advance is accepted, the patient must be notified no more than 10 days and no less than 3 days before the check is deposited. State laws vary but some states have regulations in addition to federal laws.

Unsigned Checks. Another problem is unsigned checks. Ask the patient to come to the office and sign the check or send a new one. If you are unable to reach the patient or if there is a transportation or time limitation problem, write the word "over" or "see reverse" on the signature line on the front of the check. On the back of the check, where the endorsement should appear, write "lack of signature, guaranteed," the practice's name, and one's own name and title. This endorsement in effect is a guarantee that the practice will absorb the loss if the patient's bank or the patient does not honor the check.

Returned Checks. When the physician's office receives notice that a check was not honored, the reason should be stated on the back of the check. The most common reason is NSF. Call the bank to find out if there are adequate funds in the account to cover the check and take the NSF check to the bank immediately. You might telephone the patient to see if they suggest redepositing it. Check the state laws about NSF checks. There is a time limit for making the check good and there are additional charges (up to 10% of the value of the check) that the patient must make to restore the check. If the patient does not respond, the matter may be turned over to a regional district attorney or satisfaction may be obtained through small claims court. An NSF demand letter (Figure 10-12) should be sent by certified mail with return receipt requested and include the following:

1. Check date
2. Check number
3. Name of the bank where the check is drawn
4. Name of person the check was payable to
5. Check amount
6. Any allowable service charge
7. Total amount due
8. Number of days the check writer has to take action

Future payments should be in the form of cash, money order, or a cashier's check. If the patient wants the check to be returned, be sure to photocopy it and keep it in the financial record because it serves as an acknowledgment of the debt. The bad check may be returned to the patient after it has been replaced with a valid payment. Place a notation on the patient's record to this effect.

If notified that the checking account is closed, send a demand letter immediately. In most states, legal action can be taken if the patient does not respond in 30 days. Consider filing a claim in small claims court. Most states have written codes or statutes pertaining to bad checks. Often legislation allows the creditor to add punitive damages to the amount of the debt being collected, sometimes up to three times the amount of the check.

When a patient stops payment on a check, it is usually done to resolve a good faith dispute. In this case, the patient believes that he or she has legal entitlement to withhold payment. The physician may want to contact a lawyer to discuss his or her legal rights and responsibilities before sending a demand letter and trying to collect.

Itemized Patient Statements

Every patient receives an **itemized statement** (Figure 10-13) of his or her account showing the dates of service, a list of detailed charges, copayments and deductibles paid, the date the insurance claim was filed (if appropriate),

COLLEGE CLINIC
4567 Broad Avenue
Woodland Hills, XY 12345-0001
Tel. (555) 486-9002
FAX (555) 487-8976

August 15, 20XX

Mrs. Maxine Holt
444 Labina Lane
Woodland Hills, XY 12345-0001

Dear Mrs. Holt:

The following check has been dishonored by the bank and returned without payment:

Date:	08/04/20XX
Check No.:	755
Amount:	$106.11
Payable to:	Perry Cardi, MD
Bank:	Woodland Hills National Bank
Reason:	Nonsufficient funds

This is a formal notice demanding payment in the amount of $106.11 within 15 days from today's date or your account will be considered for legal action.

Please make payment immediately by cash, cashier's check, or money order at the above address. Your immediate attention will be appreciated.

Sincerely,

Delores Yee, CMA-A

Patient Accounts Manager
for Perry Cardi, MD

FIGURE 10-12 Demand letter for returned check. This letter serves as a formal notice to collect payment and notifies a patient of impending legal action.

applicable adjustments, and the account balance. These items also are listed on the patient's account or financial accounting record card (see Figures 3-14 and 10-5). Timeliness, accuracy, and consistency have a significant effect on the cash flow and collection process when sending itemized statements. A credit card option should be printed on the statement to encourage easier and faster payment.

Professional bills are a reflection of the medical practice. The billing statement should be patient-oriented and easy to read and understand. Avoid technical terms and abbreviations that might lead to misunderstandings and confusion. Enclose a return envelope with the address payments should be mailed to or that have a window that displays the medical office's mailing address. Addressed envelopes should contain the statement "Forwarding Service Requested" so that the postal service can forward the mail and provide the physician's office with a notice of the patient's new address. When this notice is received in the physician's office, it should be circulated to all necessary departments to record the new information.

Patients can be oriented to the billing process by having the insurance billing specialist electronically generate a printed statement as the patient leaves the office that explains pertinent information, such as account number, dates of service, payments, procedures, interest fees, copayments, and deductibles. Patients may choose to receive their statements electronically, so ask software providers for this component. If using standard mail, patient information pamphlets about common health concerns (such as blood pressure, cholesterol, or back pain) can be sent with the bill to convey a caring attitude.

The office is likely to experience an increase in telephone calls from inquiring patients when statements go out in the mail. A patient account representative or department should handle all billing questions, ensuring a consistent response.

Accounts Receivable and Age Analysis by Aging Report. Age analysis is a term used for the procedure of systematically arranging the A/R by age from the date of service. Accounts are usually aged in periods

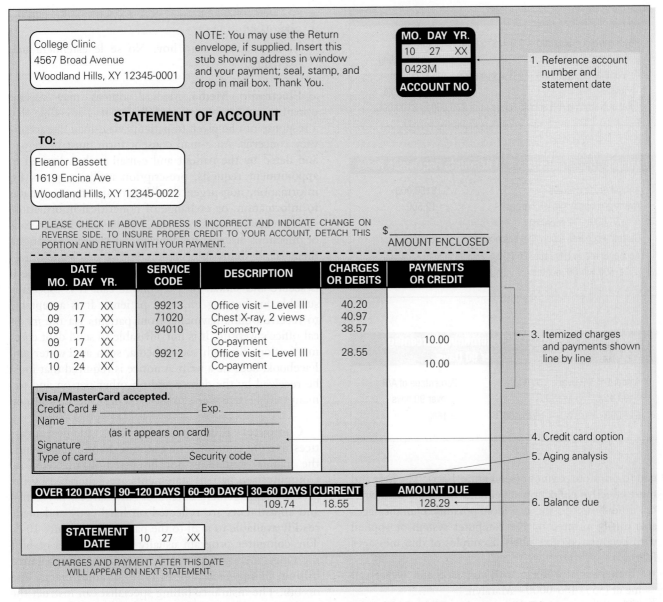

FIGURE 10-13 Patient account statement. A credit card option should be printed near the bottom of the statement to encourage payment. *(Form adapted courtesy Bibbero Systems, Inc., Petaluma, Calif.; telephone: 800-242-2376; fax: 800-242-9330; www.bibbero.com.)*

of 30, 60, 90, and 120 days and older, as shown at the bottom of Figure 9-3. An aging report can be generated by the practice management system or by other software in a computer system. This helps collection follow up by providing easy recognition of overdue accounts and allows the insurance billing specialist to determine which accounts need action in addition to a regular statement.

The formula for determining the A/R ratio is to divide the month-end A/R balance by the monthly average charges for the prior 12-month period. An average total A/R (all monies not collected at the time of service) should be one and a half to two times the charges for 1 month of services (Examples 10-1 and 10-2).

Accounts that are 90 days or older should not exceed 15% to 18% of the total A/R. To calculate this figure, divide the total amount of A/R by the amount of accounts that are 90 days old and older (Example 10-3). The practice management system should calculate this automatically when an aging report is required.

A decision tree showing time frames for sending statements and making telephone calls is presented in Figure 10-14.

Dun Messages

Dun messages are phrases printed on statements to inform or remind a patient about a delinquent account

Example 10-1	Formula	
Physician's	$50,000 × 1.5 = $75,000	Total
Charges	Or	Outstanding
Monthly	$50,000 × 2.0 = $100,000	Accounts
Total		Receivable
Total outstanding A/R should range from $75,000 to $100,000.		

Example 10-2	Calculation of Accounts Receivable Ratio
Annual gross charges	$150,000
Average monthly gross charges	12,500
(150,000 ÷ 12 months)	
Current accounts receivable balance	20,000
Accounts receivable ratio: 20,000 ÷ 12,500 = 1.60 months	

Example 10-3	Formula for Determining Percentage of Accounts over 90 Days		
Amount of A/R over 90 days	A/R total		Percentage of A/R over 90 days
$12,000	÷	$75,000	= 16%

and to promote payment (see Figure 10-5). The best and most effective collection statements include a handwritten note; however, this is seldom possible. Dun messages also can be printed by the computer system or applied with brightly colored labels. Examples of dun messages follow:

- "If there is a problem with your account, please call me at (555) 486-0000—Maralyn."
- "This bill is now 30 days past due. Please remit payment."
- "This bill is now 60 days past due. Please send payment immediately."
- "Your account is 90 days past due. Please remit payment now to avoid collection action."
- "FINAL NOTICE: If we do not hear from you within 10 days, this account will be turned over to our collection agency."

Do not send intimidating, impatient, or threatening statements. These serve only to antagonize patients. Dun messages should be printed in different languages and sent to patients who speak English as a second language. Examples are as follows:

- "No payment yet; your payment by return mail will be appreciated."
  - "No hemos recibido pago. Agracieramos remita por correo."

- "Payment needed now. No further credit will be extended."
  - "Se requiere pago hoy. No se le estendera mas credito."

Electronic Media. Medical offices may receive e-mail messages about their bills but it is advisable that a response not be given to patients via e-mail due to privacy concerns. An e-mail consent form must be signed and dated by the patient and e-mail is then limited to appointment requests, prescription refills, requests for information, non-urgent health care questions, updates to information, or exchange of noncritical information, such as changes in office hours, holiday schedules, recalls or infectious diseases, immunizations, insurance changes, financial eligibility information, and so on. Some offices use their websites for live chat with patients because it is secure and similar to a telephone call. It is especially suitable for hearing impaired patients. It is acceptable to receive online payments from patients via the medical office's website. It is not advisable to send debt communications through social media, such as Twitter and Facebook, because a written notice is required that must be received by the debtor and no other person and too many people have access to social media over the internet.

Computer Billing. Because most medical practices use the computer to generate billing statements, the manual system is not discussed in this edition. Computerized patient statements are generated by the practice management software. All charges, payments, and adjustments are reflected on hard copy and made readily available to mail to the patient (see Figure 10-5) The computer program usually offers choices of billing types, including patient billing, **insurance balance billing,** billing according to types of adjustments, and no bill. The insurance billing specialist can instruct the computer to print all bills of a specific type. The computer also can be instructed to print bills according to specific accounts, dates, and insurance types. Accounts are automatically aged and standard messages can be printed on the statements for each of the aged dates (that is, 30, 60, 90, or 120 days). Some systems allow personalized messages to be inserted that override the standard messages.

Billing Services. Billing services can be contracted by medical practices to reduce administrative paperwork by taking over the task of preparing, submitting, and following up for third-party health insurance companies and patient. They may provide data entry of patients' demographic and billing information, charges, receipts, and adjustments; tracking of payments from patients and third-party payers; production of management reports; purging of inactive accounts; and collection of accounts.

Collection Decision Tree

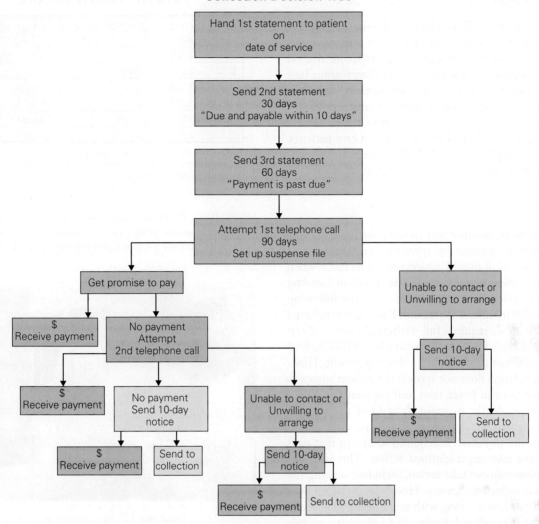

FIGURE 10-14 Collection decision tree. This is a quick reference used to help determine when to send statements, make telephone calls, and send accounts to a collection agency.

Some advantages of billing services are advanced technology, professional and understandable bills, experts answering all billing-related telephone inquiries, and no downtime caused by vacations or medical or personal leave. This service allows the medical office to have fewer disruptions and freedom from worry about financial matters when trying to provide medical care.

The physician's office sends billing and receipt information to the system daily. This may be done in writing or through a computer system. The billing service then prepares the bills, mails them, and also may receive payments. Regular reports, whether weekly or monthly, are sent to the physician summarizing the transactions. Billing services may offer full account management services and in many cases customize a service that meets the needs of the provider. Most medical billing services charge a percentage of every claim collected, typically 5%

to 10%. Using a billing service company is most commonly referred to as *outsourcing*. When choosing a billing service, make a list of important questions and visit the facility. Also ask for references so that you may obtain valuable feedback from other provider offices that have used the same billing service.

HIPAA Compliance Alert

GUIDELINES WHEN CONTRACTING WITH A BILLING SERVICE

Have a written directive in place that gives the billing company permission to communicate directly with the insurance company and a Medicare administrative contractor (MAC) about denied or problem claims. When changing billing services, be sure to revoke such authorizations with each carrier and MAC.

Billing Guidelines

Billing procedures are determined by the size of the practice, number of accounts, and number of staff members assigned to the collection process. Adopt a specific method of handling accounts and decide which billing routine best fits the practice. Check insurance and managed care contracts carefully to determine which circumstances allow for patients to be billed. Be sure to conform to federal guidelines if there is a need to bill managed care patients. See Procedure 10-2 at the end of this chapter for the procedure for seven-step billing and collection guidelines.

Payment Plans

Payment plans are another way to offer the patient a way of paying off an account by spreading out the amount due over a period of time. Caution should be taken when offering patients a payment plan. The Truth in Lending Consumer Credit Cost Disclosure law (see the following section titled "Credit and Collection Laws"), also referred to as *Regulation Z*, requires full written disclosure about the finance charges for large payment plans involving four or more installments, excluding a down payment. However, this regulation does not apply if the patient agrees to pay in one sum or in fewer than four payments and then decides independently to make drawn-out partial payments. Patients often think that if they make any amount of payment, the physician is required to accept that payment and not take any additional action. This is incorrect. The physician can take action, including sending the account to a collection agency. Have a written payment plan schedule when working with accounts in which payment plans may be offered. Figure 10-15 illustrates sample guidelines that may be used or revised according to individual practice and management policies (Figure 10-16).

When patients seek care from the medical practice but are honest about their financial status, it is necessary to develop a financial payment plan agreement. This agreement (see Figure 10-8) provides the patient a clear understanding of all fees, the agreed-upon monthly payment amount, and the monthly due date. It may be wise to set up an automatic monthly withdrawal from the patient's bank account or credit card to ensure receipt of the patient's payment. A statement that provides the account balance should be sent to the patient every month after a payment is made.

CREDIT AND COLLECTION LAWS

The following laws are important because they provide the legal framework within which the insurance billing specialist must execute the physician's collection policy. In addition, each state may have specific collection laws that must be researched and obeyed. Most states have

PAYMENT PLAN SCHEDULE

Balance due amount	Minimum monthly payment	Time frame for full payment
$0 – $200	$35	6 months
$201 – $500	$50	1 year
$501 – $1000	$100	1 year
$1001 – $3000	$125	2 years
$3001 – $5000	$150	2 years
>$5001*	$200	5 years

*Accounts over $5000 must complete credit card application to certify minimum required payment and are subject to approval by office manager.

FIGURE 10-15 Payment plan schedule used in the physician's office to negotiate monthly payments shows balance due amounts, minimum monthly payment, and payment time frames.

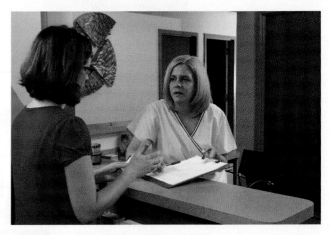

FIGURE 10-16 Insurance billing specialist setting up a payment plan with a patient.

prompt payment laws designed to govern actions of insurers and third-party payers to pay insurance claims in a timely manner. See Example 10-4 for wording an appeal letter citing your state's prompt payment law. Box 10-1 includes names and descriptions of the federal credit and collection laws that affect medical practices.

> **HIPAA Compliance Alert** **RED FLAGS RULE**
>
> The Red Flags Rule is a set of Federal Trade Commission (FTC) requirements for businesses that have more than 20 employees and issue credit to their clients. This rule aims to prevent fraud and identity theft of a person's personal data for illegal use. A health care provider must create a plan to help recognize warning signs (or "red flags") associated with fraud and identity theft or face civil penalties for violation. A medical practice must notify patients if their data were stolen.

| Example 10-4 | Sample Appeal Letter Citing State Prompt Payment Law |

Date

To Whom It May Concern:

Thank you for the opportunity to submit this denied claim for reconsideration of payment. We are contacting you about the professional services rendered to [patient's name, date of service, and medical services].

We request immediate payment of the above-referenced claim. According to our records, this claim was filed on [date of filing] but payment has not been received.

Failure to release payment may be a violation of [name of state and code number]. [Insert wording of the state's code.] Please adjudicate this claim immediately based on this state's mandate.

Thank you for your reconsideration.

Sincerely, [your name], Account Representative

Statute of Limitations

A formal regulation or law setting time limits on legal action is known as a **statute of limitations.** Regarding collections, the statute of limitations is the maximum time during which a legal collection suit may be rendered against a debtor. However, for a lawsuit to be successful, a concerted effort should be made to collect on an account from the time services are rendered. The patient should receive regular statements indicating that if the insurer does not pay, the patient will be held responsible.

Statutes vary according to the following three kinds of accounts:

1. *Open book accounts* (also called *open accounts*) are open to charges made from time to time. Payment is expected within a specific period but credit has been extended without a formal written contract. Physicians' patient accounts are usually open book accounts.
2. *Written contract accounts* have a formal written agreement in which a patient signs to pay his or her bill in more than four installments (see the "Truth in Lending Act" section in Box 10-1).
3. *Single-entry accounts* have only one entry or charge, usually for a small amount.

THE COLLECTION PROCESS

For collections to be handled effectively, staff members should be trained in collection techniques. Most insurance billing specialists can be trained to be efficient collectors when given the correct tools. New collectors need time to gain confidence, which is an important aspect of being a good collector.

Telephone Collection Procedures

Telephone collections are made easier if the insurance billing specialist is convinced that he or she can collect before trying to convince the patient to pay. Two important factors to consider are the insurance billing specialist's ability to contact the patient and the patient's ability to pay the bill. The following are helpful suggestions for using the telephone to address a collection problem:

- Contact the patient in a timely manner at the first sign of payment delay. Prepare before making a telephone collection call by reviewing the account and noting anything unusual. Locate information as to where the patient is employed (or if unemployed) by reviewing the patient registration form.
- Decide what amount will be settled for if payment cannot be made in full. Make the first call count. Act in a calm, businesslike manner and combine empathy with diligence. Be positive and persuasive. Listen to what the patient has to say, even if he or she gets angry and raises his or her voice. Lower the volume of your own voice and respond in a composed manner. Try to pick up clues from what the patient is saying; he or she may be giving the real reason for nonpayment.
- Ask questions, show interest, and let the patient know that he or she is being listened to.
- Respond in a respectful manner and carefully word the reply; when patients are distressed, they do not always make sense. The goal is to encourage the patient to pay, not agitate the patient.
- Use all resources and learn to negotiate.

Office Policy

The most organized approach to making collection calls is to print out the aging report and target accounts in the 60- to 90-day categories. The most effective results come from this group. Prior to making each call, review the patient's financial account in the practice management software for notes on previous patient encounters. Start with the largest amount owed and work the accounts in decreasing amounts owed. After this category has been completed, move on to the 90- to 120-day accounts. Finally, go after accounts that are more than 120 days old.

Most state collection laws allow telephone calls to the debtor between 8 AM and 9 PM. Never call between 9 PM and 8 AM because to do so may be considered harassment. However, according to collection experts, the best time to telephone is between 5:30 PM and 8:30 PM on Tuesdays and Thursdays and between 9 AM and 1 PM on Saturdays. However, regardless of when the call is made, track the times when the most patients are contacted and adjust the calling schedule accordingly. Perhaps the physician's office

Box 10-1   Federal Credit and Collection Laws

Equal Credit Opportunity Act (ECOA)

Prohibits discrimination in all areas of granting credit. Detailed credit information should be obtained before performing services to prevent accusations of impartiality. New patients should be informed that payment is due at the time of service and that they should arrive 20 minutes early to fill out a credit application if they wish to establish credit for treatment. Data, such as the patient's address, previous addresses, length of residence, employment history, and approximate wage, can be verified with a credit bureau. The report will also contain the patient's name changes, the patient's bill-paying history, and any history of bankruptcy. If the patient has a poor credit rating, credit may be denied and the patient then has 60 days to request the reason in writing. The law prohibits discrimination against any applicant for credit for the following reasons:

- Age, color, marital status, national origin, race, religion, or sex
- Receiving income from alimony or any public assistance program

Fair Credit Reporting Act (FCRA)

Regulates agencies that either issue or use reports on consumers (patients) in connection with the approval of credit. Credit reporting agencies can provide reports only when the following occurs:

- A court order is issued.
- The report is requested by the consumer (patient) or instructions are given by the patient to provide the report.
- There is a legitimate business need for the information.

If credit is refused, the physician must provide the patient with a reason credit was denied and the name and address of the agency from which the report came. Specific information about what the report contains is not necessary and should not be given. The patient must have an opportunity to correct any inaccuracies if they occur.

Fair and Accurate Credit Transactions (FACT) Act (Public Law 108-159)

Establishes (as of December 4, 2003) medical privacy provisions as part of consumer credit law. The bill amends the FCRA to include improved medical privacy protections and protections against identity theft. Credit bureaus and creditors must comply with a number of medical privacy restrictions that ban the sharing of medical information. Title IV of the FACT Act limits the use and sharing of medical information in the financial system and provides an expanded definition of medical information. For military personnel, it provides an active-duty alert that can be placed on the credit file for a year at the three major credit bureaus. This means that a creditor cannot issue new credit or a card without first contacting the active-duty individual whose name is on the card.

Fair Credit Billing Act (FCBA)

Applies to "open end" credit accounts, such as credit cards and revolving charge accounts for department store accounts. It does not cover installment contracts, such as loans or extensions of credit you repay on a fixed schedule. Consumers often buy cars, furniture, and major appliances on an installment basis and they repay personal loans in installments as well. The FCBA settlement procedures apply only to disputes about "billing errors," such as unauthorized charges. Federal law limits the consumer's responsibility for unauthorized charges

to $50; charges that list the wrong date or amount; charges for goods and services that the consumer did not accept or were not delivered as agreed; math errors; failure to post payments and other credits, such as returns; failure to send bills to the current address, provided the creditor receives the change of address, in writing, at least 20 days before the billing period ends; and charges for which an explanation or written proof of purchase along with a claimed error or request for clarification are requested. The consumer must write to the creditor at the address given for "billing inquiries," not the address for sending payments, and include one's name, address, account number, and a description of the billing error. Send the letter so that it reaches the creditor within 60 days after the first bill was mailed that contained the error. Send the letter by certified mail, return receipt requested, for proof of what the creditor received. Include copies (not originals) of sales slips or other documents that support the position. Keep a copy of the dispute letter. The creditor must acknowledge the complaint in writing within 30 days after receiving it, unless the problem has been resolved. The creditor must resolve the dispute within two billing cycles (but not more than 90 days) after receiving the letter. Payment may be withheld on the disputed amount (and related charges) during the investigation. Any part of the bill not in question must be paid, including finance charges on the undisputed amount.

The creditor may not take any legal or other action to collect the disputed amount and related charges (including finance charges) during the investigation. Although the account cannot be closed or restricted, the disputed amount may be applied against the credit limit. If the creditor's investigation determines that the bill is correct, one must be told promptly and in writing how much is owed and why. Copies of relevant documents may be requested. At this point the disputed amount is owed plus any finance charges that accumulated while the amount was in dispute. The minimum amount that was missed because of the dispute may have to be paid. If the results of the investigation are disputed, the creditor may be written to within 10 days after receiving the explanation and the disputed amount may be refused. At this point the creditor may begin collection procedures. Any creditor who fails to follow the settlement procedure may not collect the amount in dispute, or any related finance charges, up to $50, even if the bill turns out to be correct. For example, if a creditor acknowledges the complaint in 45 days—15 days too late—or takes more than two billing cycles to resolve a dispute, the penalty applies. The penalty also applies if a creditor threatens to report, or improperly reports, one's failure to pay to anyone during the dispute period.

Electronic Fund Transfer Act (EFTA)

Limits consumers' liability if there has been an unauthorized use of an ATM card, debit card, or other electronic banking device.

Truth in Lending Act (TILA)

Applies to anyone who charges interest or agrees to payment of a bill in more than four installments, excluding a down payment. When a specific agreement is reached between patient and physician, Regulation Z of this consumer protection act requires that a written disclosure of all pertinent information be made, regardless of the existence of a finance charge (see Figure 10-8). This full disclosure must be discussed at the time

Box 10-1   Federal Credit and Collection Laws—cont'd

the agreement is first reached between patient and physician and credit is extended. According to the Federal Trade Commission (FTC), the Truth in Lending provision is not applicable and no disclosures are necessary if a patient decides on his or her own to pay in installments or whenever convenient.

It is essential to include the following items:

1. Total amount of the debt
2. Amount of down payment
3. Finance charge
4. Interest rate expressed as an annual percentage
5. Amount of each payment
6. Date each payment is due
7. Date final payment is due
8. Signature of patient and physician with copies retained by both
9. Account balance with total interest and total amount paid by the patient at the end of the contract

Medical practices that implement late payment charges that meet the criteria defined in the TILA as a finance charge must comply with a host of requirements that revolve around proper disclosure to patients.

Charges must meet the following criteria to qualify as late payment charges:

1. The account balance must be paid in full at the time of initial billing.
2. The account is treated as delinquent when unpaid.
3. The charge is assessed to a patient's account only because of his or her failure to make timely payments.
4. Installments are limited to no more than three.
5. The creditor (physician or insurance billing specialist) makes a "commercially reasonable" effort to collect these accounts.

When a physician continues to treat a patient with an overdue account, the courts have viewed this as continuation of care and an extension of credit. Patients who fall into this delinquent status should be referred elsewhere. See Figure 4-20 for instructions on sending a discharge letter. After the patient has paid the overdue amount, the patient can be taken back and treated on a cash-only basis.

Truth in Lending Consumer Credit Cost Disclosure

Requires businesses to disclose all direct and indirect costs and conditions related to the granting of credit. All interest charges, late charges, collection fees, finance charges, and so forth must be explained up front, before the time of service. Include the following on all statements to charge interest and bill the patient monthly:

- Amount of each payment
- Due date
- Unpaid balance at the beginning of the billing period
- Finance charges
- Date balance is due

Fair Debt Collection Practices Act (FDCPA)

Addresses the collection practices of third-party debt collectors and attorneys who regularly collect debts for others. Although this Act does not apply directly to physician practices collecting for themselves, a professional health care collector must avoid the actions that are prohibited for collection agencies. The main intent of the Act is to protect consumers from unfair, harassing, or deceptive collection practices. Refer to the guidelines in Box 10-2, which are taken from the FDCPA, to help avoid illegalities, enhance collections, and maintain positive patient relations. For more information about collection laws in your state, contact your state attorney general's office. The stricter law prevails if there is a conflict between state and federal laws.

---

hours should be increased to include one evening a week or Saturday mornings to make collection calls. Another option is the use of flex time, in which the employee can choose his or her own working hours from within a broad range of hours approved by management. Use a private telephone away from the busy operations of the office to eliminate interruptions. Patients may be embarrassed about not being able to pay their bills and patient confidentiality must be maintained. Follow the guidelines stated in the Fair Debt Collection Practices Act (Box 10-2).

Some medical practices have found success in reaching patients by text messaging. The medical office must receive permission to text the patient during the initial patient encounter prior to using this tool. There are many online companies that will text patients with appointment reminders. Be careful not to include any information that will violate the privacy of the patient, so keep the messages general, such as "Dr. Leonard Baskin's office has a message for you about your account; please call (888) 873-9472."

Be alert for new ideas or approaches to collection by watching how banks and other retailers implement sophisticated collection skills. Decide whether any of these could be used to the medical practice's advantage and present the techniques to the office manager. Keep abreast of improvements made to collection software that improve collection results and allow more collectors to work from their homes. Other advances (for example, call block, which is an expanded telephone service) have made it more difficult to make collection calls. This service was originally intended to screen out unwanted telemarketing calls by intercepting blocked, unlisted, or unknown numbers. Standard numbers are usually allowed to go through. The key to averting a block is to ensure that the number the call is being placed from is listed and within the patient's area.

For a step-by-step procedure on making telephone collection calls, see Procedure 10-3 at the end of this chapter.

Telephone "Don'ts". Communication is important, especially when trying to work with a patient on difficulties in making payments. Remain professional at all times and treat the patient with respect. The following is a list of *don'ts* for telephone collections:

- Do not raise your voice and antagonize the patient.
- Do not accuse the patient of dishonesty or lying.

Box 10-2   Fair Debt Collection Practices Act Guidelines

1. Contact debtors only once a day; in some states, repeated calls in 1 day or the same week could be considered harassment.
2. Place calls after 8 AM and before 9 PM.
3. Do not contact debtors on Sunday or any other day that the debtor recognizes as a Sabbath.
4. Identify yourself and the medical practice represented; do not mislead the patient.
5. Contact the debtor at work only if unable to contact the debtor elsewhere; no contact should be made if the employer or debtor disapproves.
6. Contact the attorney if an attorney represents the debtor; contact the debtor only if the attorney does not respond.
7. Do not threaten or use obscene language.
8. Do not send postcards for collection purposes; keep all correspondence strictly private.
9. Do not call collect or cause additional expense to the patient.
10. Do not leave a message on an answering machine indicating that you are calling about a bill.
11. Do not contact a third party more than once unless requested to do so by the party or the response was erroneous or incomplete.
12. Do not convey to a third party that the call is about a debt.
13. Do not contact the debtor when notified in writing that a debtor refuses to pay and would like contact to stop, except to notify the debtor in writing that there will be no further contact or that there will be legal action.
14. Stick to the facts; do not use false statements.
15. Do not prepare a list of "bad debtors" or "credit risks" to share with other health care providers.
16. Take action immediately when stating that a certain action will be taken (for example, filing a claim in small claims court or sending the patient's case to a collection agency).
17. Send the patient written verification of the name of the creditor and the amount of debt within 5 days of the initial contact.

- Do not act like a "tough guy" or threaten a patient.
- Do not consent to partial payments until payment in full has been asked for and do not agree to a long string of small partial payments.
- Do not engage in a debate.
- Do not report a disputed account to a collection agency or bureau until the patient's dispute is disclosed as part of the record.

Telephone collection calls are effective on the day before patients are due for their appointments. State the date and time of the appointment and then remind the patient of the balance owed and ask whether he or she could please bring payment to the appointment.

Telephone Collection Scenarios

The most difficult part of one-on-one collections is preparing for the many situations that may be encountered and the various responses the patient may make. Table 10-2 lists some statements that patients make about not paying

an account and examples of responses that the insurance billing specialist can make.

Collection Letters

Collection letters are another method of reaching patients and reminding them of their debt. Knowledge of the patient base and of individual patients may help to determine the effectiveness of collection letters. Every medical practice is unique and the number of accounts, the geographic spread of patients, the staff size, and the amount of time collectors have to spend on individual accounts helps to determine which collection method best suits the practice.

The positive aspect of collection letters is that they can reach a large number of patients rapidly and the cost is relatively low, especially if form letters are used (Figure 10-17).

Collection letters have some negative aspects, such as the following:
- Letters usually take 2 or 3 days to reach the patient and may lie unopened for a week or more.
- Letters are one-way communication and thus lack the ability to provide the reason for nonpayment.
- Response and recovery through letters are relatively poor.
- Manual preparation takes time (especially if a decision must be made before sending each letter).
- The costs of postage and supplies are increasing.

The insurance billing specialist is often the one who composes collection letters and devises a plan for collection follow-up. A series of collection letters may be written using varying degrees of forcefulness, starting with a gentle reminder. When a collection letter is written, use a friendly tone and ask why payment has not been made. Imply that the patient has good intentions to pay. This may be done by suggesting that the patient has overlooked a previous statement. Communicate the doctor's sincere interest in the patient. Always invite the patient to explain the reason for nonpayment in a letter, telephone call, or office visit. It should sound as though the patient is eager to clear the debt.

When collection letters are sent toward the end of the year, include a statement letting the patient know that if the account is paid in full by the end of the year, the medical expense may be used as an income tax deduction. Another tactic is to send a notice advising the patient that he or she may skip December's payment because of increased expenses during the holidays. This tactic may be used as an opportunity to build patient relationships but the collector must be firm and clear when offering such leeway. Collection letters sent after the first of the year can suggest that the patient clear the debt by using an income tax refund check.

Table 10-2 Telephone Collection Scenarios

STATEMENT	RESPONSE
"I can't pay anything now."	"Are you employed? Are you receiving unemployment compensation, welfare, or Social Security benefits?" You are determining the patient's ability to pay.
"I can't pay the whole bill now."	"How long will it take you to pay this bill?" Ask this question instead of "How much can you pay?"
"I can pay but not until next month."	"When do you get paid?" Ask for payment the day after payday. "Do you have a checking account?" Ask for a postdated check.
"I have other bills."	"This is also one of your bills that should be paid now. Let's talk about exactly how you plan payment."
"How about $10 a month (on a $300 bill)?"	"I'd like to accept that but our accountant does not allow us to stretch out payments beyond 90 days, which would be $100 a month." This adheres to (Truth in Lending Law) regulations for collecting payment in installments without a written agreement. If the patient tries to cooperate, then compromise. If not, turn the account over to a collection agency.
"I sent in the payment."	"When was the payment sent? To what address was it sent? Was it a check? On what bank was it drawn and for what amount? What is the canceled check number?" Investigate to determine whether the check was posted to a wrong account. If not, call the patient back and ask if he or she would call his or her bank to see if it cleared; if it has not cleared, the patient should stop payment. Ask the patient to call back and verify the status of the check. If the patient is not being truthful, he or she will not follow through. Ask for a new check and tell the patient that a refund will be made if the other one shows up.
"I cannot make a payment this month."	"The collection agency picks up all of our delinquent accounts next Monday. I don't want to include yours but I need a check today."
"The check is in the mail."	"May I have the check number and date it was mailed?" Call back in 3 days if not received.
"I'm not going to pay the bill because the doctor didn't spend any time with me."	"May I confirm the doctor you saw, the date, and time? For what reason did you see the doctor? Do you still have the problem for which you saw the doctor?" Get as much information as possible and research the office schedule on the day the patient was seen. Let the doctor know about the patient's complaint and inquire how he or she would like to handle the complaint.
"I thought the insurance company was paying this."	"Your insurance paid most of the bill; now the balance is your responsibility. Please send your check before Friday to keep your account current." Explain why (deductible, copayment benefit) the service is not covered under the insurance plan.

Types of Collection Letters

A form letter saves time and can go out automatically at specific times during the billing cycle (Figure 10-18).

Collection letters should contain the following information:

● Full amount owed
● Services performed
● What action the patient should take
● Time frame in which the patient should respond
● How the patient should take care of the bill
● Why the patient should take care of the bill
● Address to which the patient should send payment
● Telephone number to contact the office
● Contact person's name
● Signature, which can be listed as "Financial Secretary," "Insurance Billing Specialist," "Assistant to Doctor _____," or one's name and title with the physician's name below it

When pursuing collection, the insurance billing specialist should stay within the authorization of the physician. All letters should be noted on the back of the financial accounting record, in the collection log, or in the computer comment area. Abbreviations can be used to indicate which letter was sent (Table 10-3) as well as the date on which the letter was mailed. Letters can be sent in brightly colored envelopes to attract attention. The envelope should include "Address Service Requested" or "Forwarding Service Requested" on the outside to ensure that the letter is forwarded if the patient has moved so that the office will be notified of the patient's new address. Always include a self-addressed stamped envelope.

Collection Abbreviations

Collection abbreviations can be used to save time and space while documenting efforts to collect and patients' responses. A few of the most common abbreviations are listed in Table 10-3. Always use standard abbreviations so that anyone

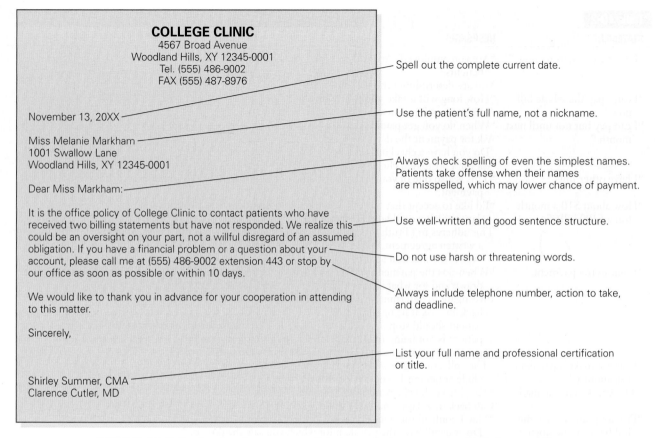

COLLEGE CLINIC
4567 Broad Avenue
Woodland Hills, XY 12345-0001
Tel. (555) 486-9002
FAX (555) 487-8976

November 13, 20XX ———— Spell out the complete current date.

Miss Melanie Markham ———— Use the patient's full name, not a nickname.
1001 Swallow Lane
Woodland Hills, XY 12345-0001

Dear Miss Markham: ———— Always check spelling of even the simplest names. Patients take offense when their names are misspelled, which may lower chance of payment.

It is the office policy of College Clinic to contact patients who have received two billing statements but have not responded. We realize this ———— Use well-written and good sentence structure.
could be an oversight on your part, not a willful disregard of an assumed obligation. If you have a financial problem or a question about your ———— Do not use harsh or threatening words.
account, please call me at (555) 486-9002 extension 443 or stop by our office as soon as possible or within 10 days.

We would like to thank you in advance for your cooperation in attending ———— Always include telephone number, action to take, and deadline.
to this matter.

Sincerely,

———— List your full name and professional certification or title.

Shirley Summer, CMA
Clarence Cutler, MD

FIGURE 10-17 Collection form letter sent to all patients who have not responded after two billing cycles.

working on the account will know exactly what attempts have been made to collect and what action has been taken.

Insurance Collection

Most patients carry some form of insurance; however, filing an insurance claim is only the first step in collecting fees owed. Good follow-up techniques (see Chapter 9) are necessary to ensure payment from the third-party payer and copayment or coinsurance payment from the patient.

First, affirm that a clean insurance claim was submitted electronically with all necessary preauthorization and documentation for services. Next, follow up in a timely manner with electronic submission reports from the clearinghouse. Track all denials to learn what services are being denied and which insurance companies are denying payment. It is worth investing money and staff resources to identify the cause of claim denials.

History of Accounts

If the third-party payer seems to be ignoring all efforts to trace the claim, an exact history of the account may be the best weapon with which to proceed. A history of the account is a chronologic record of all events that have

occurred. Keep all communications received from the third-party payer, note all telephone calls, and keep copies of all documents sent. Send a copy of the history of the account directly to the third-party payer and demand a reply. This may also be done in the case of an insurance company dispute or a refusal to pay.

Coinsurance Payments

Use a letter or statement to collect from patients who have insurance coverage. Clearly indicate to the patient that the insurance billing specialist has submitted an insurance claim and advise the patient what action is expected. The status of the insurance claim should be noted on all statements. Notify patients promptly when insurance payment has been received. Ask patients to get involved in the insurance process or to pay the bill within 10 days if a problem exists. The following are examples of notations on statements for patients with insurance coverage:

● "We have received payment from your insurance company. The balance of $_____ is now your responsibility."
● "Your insurance company has paid its share of your bill. This statement is for the amount payable directly by you."
● "Your insurance company has paid $_____ for the above services. The remaining portion of $_____ is now your responsibility."

COLLEGE CLINIC
4567 Broad Avenue
Woodland Hills, XY 12345-0001
Tel. (555) 486-9002
FAX (555) 487-8976

March 16, 20XX

Mr. Frank Lincoln
3397 Westminster Avenue
Woodland Hills, XY 12345-0001

Account No.   593287
Amount Due: $ _____

Dear Mr. Lincoln:

The care of our patients is more important than writing letters about overdue accounts. Yet, as you must realize, the expense of furnishing care can only be met by payments from appreciative patients.

Your account is seriously past due and has been removed from our current files because of its delinquent status. Our office policy indicates that your account should be placed with a collection agency. However, we would prefer to hear from you regarding your preference in this matter.

Enclosed is a current statement of your account. Please indicate your payment choice.

☐ I would prefer to settle this account immediately. Please find payment in full enclosed.

☐ I would prefer to make monthly payments (up to six months). To exercise this option, please call and make arrangements to come into our office to sign a financial agreement.

☐ Please charge the full amount to my credit card. (We accept American Express, MasterCard, and Visa). To exercise this option, please telephone our office or fill in the enclosed form and return it with the envelope provided.

_____   _____
          Signature   Date

Please select one of the three options above, sign the form, and return this notice within 10 days from the date indicated in the letter. A postmarked return envelope is provided. Failure to respond will result in an automatic referral to our collection agency. Please do not hesitate to call if you have any questions regarding this matter.

Sincerely,

Gil Steinberg
Office Manager

Enc. Envelope, Credit Card Agreement Form

FIGURE 10-18 Multipurpose collection letter with checklist. This advises the patient of a seriously past due account, offers the patient three payment options, and warns the patient that failure to respond will result in a referral to a collection agency.

- "The balance of this account is your share of the cost. Please remit today. For questions, call 486-9002."
- "Your insurance company has not responded. The account is due and payable. Please contact your insurance company about payment. Thank you for your assistance."

Insurance Checks Sent to Patients

Send a letter immediately to notify patients who receive insurance checks (see Chapter 9). Advise such patients that they have received payment from their insurance company and that their account is due and payable within 10 days. Do not send continuous monthly bills; instead, speed up the collection process. If the patient refuses to pay and the physician does not want the patient to return, send a 10-day notification advising the patient that the account will go to a collection agency. If there is no response, ask the physician whether he or she wishes to discharge the patient from the practice.

Table 10-3	Collection Abbreviations		
ABBREVIATION	**DESCRIPTION**	**ABBREVIATION**	**DESCRIPTION**
Atty	Attorney	NSN	No such number
B	Bankrupt	OFC	Office
Bal	Balance	OOT	Out of town
Bk*	Bank	OOW	Out of work
BLG	Belligerent	PA	Payment arrangement
BTTR	Best time to reach	PH or PH'D	Phoned
CB	Call back	Ph/Dsc*	Phone disconnected
CLM	Claim	PIF	Payment in full
DA*	Directory assistance	PIM	Payment in mail
DFB	Demand for balance	PMT	Payment
DNK	Did not know	POE	Place of employment
DSC	Disconnected	POW	Payment on way
EMP	Employed	PP	Promise to pay or partial payment
EOM	End of month	PT	Patient
EOW	End of week	RCD	Received
FA	Further action	R/D*	Reverse directory
FN	Final notice	RE	About
H	He (or husband)	RES	Residence
HHCO	Have husband call office	S	She (or wife)
HSB	Husband	SEP	Separated
HTO	He phoned office	SK*	Skip or skipped
HU	Hung up	SOS	Same old story
INS	Insurance	SP/DEL*	Special delivery
L1, L2	Letter one, letter two (sent)	STO	She phoned office
LB	Line busy	TB	Phoned business
LD	Long distance	TR	Phoned residence
LM	Left message	TXT	Texted
LMCO	Left message, call office	TT	Talked to
LMVM	Left message, voice mail	TTA	Turned to agency
LTR	Letter	UE or U/Emp	Unemployed
MR	Mail return	UTC	Unable to contact
N1, N2	Note one, note two (sent)	VFD	Verified
NA	No answer	Vfd/E	Verified employment
NFA*	No forwarding address	Vfd/I	Verified insurance
NHD*	Never heard of debtor	W/	Will
NI	Not in	WCO	Will call office
NLE	No longer employed	WCIO	Will come in office
NPL	No phone listed	W/I	Walk-in
NPN	Non-published number	WVO	Will visit office
NR	No record	X	By
NSF	Nonsufficient funds		

*Used in skip tracing.

Managed Care Organizations

When a medical practice deals with several managed care organizations, trying to remember all of the contract information can be confusing. A managed care desk reference (see Chapter 11) can help staff members to find information quickly. "Promised payment date" along with all the other information on the desk reference grid or matrix can be easily referred to by the insurance billing specialist when trying to collect from managed care organizations.

Ensure that all referral authorizations are in place before the patient is to be seen. If a patient shows up without a referral, offer to reschedule or inform the patient that the visit must be paid for in cash before leaving the office. If the patient has no money, a promissory note may be executed but this action is not preferred and would be carried out as a last option.

When dealing with managed care contracts, do not sign any contract that holds a third party "harmless." The "hold harmless" clause is a way for one party to shift financial responsibilities to another party. Such "hold harmless" clauses often include phrases that state that the third party is "held harmless" to pay claims, liabilities, costs, expenses, judgments, or damages awarded by any court to all patients who bring any legal action against the medical practice. If the third party goes out of business or goes bankrupt before the contract is honored, the physician cannot collect any money from the patient that the third party was to have paid. To avoid such possibilities, ensure that payments from all managed care organizations are current.

Check to see that all third-party payers are insured by a federal agency. Such insurance would pay the physician in the event that the managed care organization could not. Managed care bankruptcy is discussed in Chapter 11.

Medicare

A provider must make genuine efforts to collect the unpaid deductible and coinsurance amounts from all Medicare patients. Reasonable efforts must include subsequent billings, telephone calls, and in-person collection efforts done in the same manner as with all patients. Accounts may not be written off until sequential statements (spaced 15 to 30 days apart) have been sent, with an increasing intensity in the collection message. A telephone call should be placed to the debtor asking for payment; a request for payment should be made when the patient is seen in person as well.

Medigap Insurance

When a patient has Medigap (MG) insurance, ensure that the patient's signature appears in Block 13 of the CMS-1500 (02/12) insurance claim form. Do not routinely enter "signature on file" unless the insured has signed an insurance-specific statement authorizing assignment of benefits to the physician named on the claim form. A signed statement allowing the physician to bill and receive payment for MG-covered services until the beneficiary revokes authorization is preferred. A Medicare "signature on file" is not sufficient.

Workers' Compensation

Verify the validity of work-related injury and illness through the patient's employer and obtain accurate billing information, including the date of injury. Send timely bills and reports using the correct coding system and fee schedule. Always keep the adjuster assigned to the case informed of ongoing treatment. The patient and employer should both be notified if a problem exists. Document all correspondence, including telephone authorizations for treatment and any tracing efforts. Any disputed or unresolved workers' compensation cases may be revised to self-pay or referred to a financial service representative or the proper state-level authority. The physician may file for mediation on behalf of the patient if proper authorization was obtained and a claim form sent at the time of the patient's treatment. A claim may also be filed with the state labor board, naming the patient's employer and workers' compensation carrier, whenever there is difficulty getting full payment. The industrial board has the employer pressure the carrier to resolve the matter. If an insurance company has not paid or has sent a written notice of nonpayment, the provider may file a request for default judgment from the state authority. If the judgment is in the provider's favor, the payer is ordered to pay in full. See Chapter 15 for more information on delinquent workers' compensation claims.

Suing a Third-Party Payer

As stated in the section titled "Statute of Limitations," there are time periods during which an insured person may sue the insurance company to collect the amount that the claimant believes is owed. An insured person may not initiate a legal action against the insurer until 60 days after the initial claim has been submitted. A lawsuit against the insurer must be filed within 3 years of the date on which the initial claim was submitted for payment.

When the insurance company does not respond to reason or negotiation after the physician's office has tried to collect from an insurance plan, the only alternatives are surrender or litigation. A lawsuit may be worthwhile if a high-dollar claim is in question. Third-party payers may be sued for payment under two circumstances: claim for plan benefits or breach of contract and claim for damages.

Claims for plan benefits are used when the claim is governed by the Employee Retirement Income Security Act (ERISA), and Federal Employee Health Benefit Act (FEHBA). ERISA governs health insurance that is provided as a benefit of employment. FEHBA governs all health insurance provided as a benefit to federal employees.

An insured person is entitled to appeal a denied claim under these two federal laws. A timely request must be filed to sue for payment. The time limit for ERISA is within 60 days of denial; the time limit for FEHBA is within 6 months. Federal laws apply across the country and overrule all state laws. Suits based on claims for plan benefits may be made when denial is based on the following:

● Medical necessity
● Preexisting condition
● Usual and customary rate issues
● Providers or facilities that are not covered
● Services that fall within an exclusion to coverage
● Failure to offer Consolidated Omnibus Budget Reconciliation Act (COBRA) coverage by a plan administrator

When the claim falls outside the scope of these federal laws, it is possible to sue if the conduct of the payer constitutes a violation of state laws relating to unfair insurance practices.

Suing based on claim for damages falls entirely under state law in the state where the physician practices. This is most likely to occur if the patient has no plan benefit but the patient or physician's office is led to believe so by the insurer or plan administrator. Examples include the following:

● Insurer misquoting benefits during a verification of those benefits
● Denial of payment because of lack of medical necessity when preauthorization of treatment was obtained

Collection Agencies

Delinquent accounts should be turned over to a collection agency only after all reasonable attempts have been made to collect by the physician's office. Knowing when to turn accounts over helps to determine the success of the collection agency. The longer the unpaid balance remains in the physician's office, the less chance the agency has to collect the account, so the determination that an account is uncollectable should be made quickly. Some guidelines follow:

● When a patient states that he or she will not pay or there is a denial of responsibility
● When a patient breaks a promise to pay
● When a patient makes partial payments and 60 days have lapsed without payment
● When a patient fails to respond to the physician's letters or telephone calls
● When payment terms fail for no valid reason
● When a check is returned by the bank because of NSF and the patient does not make an effort to rectify the situation within 1 week of notification
● When delinquency coexists with marital problems, divorce proceedings, or child support agreements

● When a patient is paid by the insurance company and does not forward the payment to the physician (This constitutes fraud and may be pursued with legal action.)
● When a patient gives false information
● When a patient moves and the office has used all resources to locate the patient

Not all accounts should go to a collection agency. Such accounts include those of personal friends and elderly widows or widowers living on pensions and accounts with balances under $25. Many physicians prefer to adjust small bad debts off of the books rather than increase administrative costs. All disputed accounts should be reviewed and approved by the physician before they are sent to collection; to expedite the collection process, it is important for the physician and the office manager to establish a standard policy for deciding which accounts are sent to collections. There should be a systematized approach for turning accounts over to a collection agency that still allows room for exceptions.

Choosing an Agency

The collection agency is a reflection of the medical practice, so it is important to choose one wisely. Choose a reputable agency that is considerate and efficient, with a high standard of ethics. The agency should specialize in physician accounts and have an attitude toward debtors with which the physician agrees. Find out how long the agency has been in business and request a list of at least 10 references and statistics on their collection effectiveness. The average collection rate varies greatly but falls between 20% and 60% on assigned accounts. Ensure that the reported rate includes all accounts more than 1 year old and does not exclude accounts with small balances.

An agency's performance can be evaluated by the amount collected, less the agency's fees, which is called the **netback.** For instance, if a collector recovered 25% of $5000 ($1250) and takes a 50% commission, the physician's netback is $625. If a different collector recovered 25% of the $5000 ($1250) and charged a 30% commission, the netback is $375. Although the second agency collected the same amount, its lower commission afforded the physician more money.

When choosing a collection agency, make sure (1) to set up a separate post office box or lock box for the collection project; (2) to set up a separate bank account for the collection project; (3) that the contract stipulates that all correspondence be sent to the post office box (no correspondence is sent to the collection agency's physical or payment address); (4) that all e-checks and credit card receipts are deposited into the physician's bank account;

and (5) that under no circumstance is the collection agency to receive any payments.

If collected funds go directly to the collection agency (whether insured, bonded, registered, or licensed), there is nothing to stop the agency from stealing the physician's money. The collection agency also could have a hidden lawsuit against it or an income tax lien and the physician may lose all of his or her money if the money goes to the agency's bank account. Do not put "hold harmless" clauses in contracts. Hold the collection agency responsible for its actions. Many states do not regulate collection agencies and simply require that these agencies be registered. In addition to checking references, check with the state's Department of Corporations to determine whose name is on the collection agency's registration, if the tax identification number is correct and current, and if the address listed is different from the one the agency gave. Contact the circuit court to determine whether there are any lawsuits or judgments against the collection agency. Find out how many of the collection agency's employees will be assigned to the account, then monitor them once the contract is signed. They may have the best credentials and references and belong to all of the correct organizations but if they acquire an increasing number of accounts and the amount of recoupment remains constant each month or is less than the national average, they may be picking and choosing the accounts. This is especially true when they are overanxious to receive a new file. If this happens, consider looking for another collection agency. Ensure that an account can be recalled without a penalty. The patient may have coverage with an insurance carrier that the provider has a contract with, so find out if the collection agency has the ability to resend a claim or if the billing company or office staff handles this. If so, does the contract have provisions for this and does the collection agency receive recoupment for obtaining insurance information?

The biggest key to the agency's effectiveness is the doctor's own credit and collection policy. A comprehensive patient registration form, along with verifying employment, turning accounts over quickly when they qualify, and giving the agency all available information, helps the agency to pick up the paper trail and secure payment. A good collection agency has membership in a national collection society and the approval of the local medical society. Review the agency's financial statement and ensure that the agency is licensed, bonded, and carries "hold harmless clause" insurance. If a patient should sue because of harassment, this insurance will protect the physician from being sued as well. The local bar association and state licensing bureaus can be contacted to determine whether any complaints have been lodged against the agency or law firm. Find out if the agency reports uncollectable debtors ("deadbeats") to a credit bureau and investigate which one is used.

Types of Agencies

There are local, regional, and national agencies. National agencies and those that use the internet may have better results when tracing **skips** (patients who owe balances on their accounts and move without leaving a forwarding address). Local agencies are more aware of the socioeconomic status of patients. Some agencies pay their staff commissions and bonuses for high productivity and others are low key and more customer-oriented. Find out the experience level of the staff and ensure that the agency values the physician's business.

Another option is to use a collection service, such as CollectNet, which gives small and midsized facilities with limited budgets the collection capabilities of large collection systems by connecting to databases. The medical practice is able to make calling lists, print collection letters, search for telephone numbers and addresses, access patient credit reports, write and format reports, monitor collection progress, and set automatic callback reminders. Optional features include BankruptcyNet, SkipNet, LetterNet, and BureauNet. Collection agencies use this service but it is also available to large groups and clinics.

Agency Operating Techniques

Collection agencies must follow all of the laws stated in the Fair Debt Collection Practices Act. They may not "harass" the debtor or make false threats and they may not use letters that appear to be legal documents. A provision should be included for the agency to seek permission from the physician's office before suing a debtor in municipal court and charging a percentage of the judgment. A progress report should be provided to the physician's office on a regular basis at least monthly. The agency also should return any uncollectable accounts to the physician's office within a reasonable time and not charge for these accounts. If a debtor moves, ask if the account is then forwarded to another collection office. All procedures used to make collections should be shown to the physician's office, including collection letters and telephone scripts. The physician's office should be aware if the agency uses a personalized or standard approach. A personal visit to the premises of the collection agency can provide a first-hand view of its operating techniques.

Agency Charges

Agencies may be paid a flat rate on all accounts according to volume. Some agencies may leave the accounts in the control of the physician's office, where the staff speaks with the patient and posts all delinquent incoming monies. Other agencies charge a commission on the basis of a percentage of an account and the physician's office refers all calls to the agency once the account is turned over to it.

A standard rate needed for most agencies to break even is one third of all monies collected and an average rate charged is 50%. Make sure the commission is based on how much is collected on the overdue accounts and not the total amount of overdue accounts turned over to the agency.

Agency Assigned Accounts

Patients' accounts turned over to a collection agency should have a letter of withdrawal sent by certified mail (see Figures 4-20 and 4-21). Place a note on all financial accounting records indicating the date on which the account was assigned. Once an account has been given to a collection agency, it is illegal to send the patient a monthly statement. Financial management consultants usually recommend that the patient's balances be written off the A/R at the time the account is assigned. A portion of the account balance can be written back on if and when the agency collects on the debt. Accounts also should be listed in a separate journal to help track the effectiveness of the agency. Allow enough columns to show the future date, amount, and percentage of an account collected by the agency as well as the total account balance.

Each patient account that has been sent to collection should have an alert pop up every time the file is opened in the practice management software. This will alert all medical staff of the situation if the patient calls on short notice or walks in to be seen. If the patient sends payment to the physician's office after the account has been turned over to an agency, notify the collection agency immediately. Any calls about accounts that have gone to collection should be referred to the agency.

Small Claims Court

Small claims court is a part of our legal system that allows laypeople access to a court system without the use of an attorney. Some advantages are a modest filing fee, minimal paperwork, exclusion of costly lawyers, and a short time frame from filing the action to trial date. Incorporated physicians are usually represented by an attorney and the agency must file in a municipal or justice court if an account has already been sent to a collection agency.

Most states have small claims courts (also called *conciliation courts*, *common pleas*, *general sessions*, *justice courts*, or *people's courts*). Each state has monetary limits on the amount that can be handled in small claims court and accounts should be reviewed for eligibility. The dollar amount varies from state to state and sometimes from one county to another. The national median small claims jurisdiction is $5300. Several legislative bills being considered by the US Senate and House committees address raising the dollar limit. Several states have already had such bills signed into law. The new limits in these states vary from $3000 to $25,000. There also may be limits on the number of claims filed per year that are for more than a specific dollar amount.

When filing a claim, the person filing the petition (the physician's office) is referred to as the *plaintiff* and the party being brought to suit (the patient) is called the *defendant*. It is generally recommended that the plaintiff send a written demand to the defendant before filing a lawsuit to give the defendant a final opportunity to resolve the claim.

For a step-by-step procedure on filing a claim in small claims court, see Procedure 10-4 at the end of this chapter.

After filing a claim, a trial date will be set and both plaintiff and defendant will be ordered to appear before the judge. Often a postcard is sent notifying the plaintiff when the defendant has been served. If the amount of delinquent debt is more than the monetary limit for small claims court, consider "cutting the claim to fit" the limit. For example, if the amount of debt is $2757 and the state limit is $2500, consider waiving (giving up) the $257 (difference) to bring the amount down to the limit. The claim cannot be divided into two different suits of $1378.50 and suing twice on the same claim is not allowed.

Claim Resolutions

The defendant has the following four options after he or she is served:
1. **Pay the claim.** The court clerk will receive the money and forward it to the physician's office but the filing fee or service charges will not be refunded.
2. **Ignore the claim.** The judge may ask the physician's representative to state the physician's side but the physician will win by default. The judgment will be awarded in the physician's favor, usually including court costs.
3. **Answer the petition.** A contested court hearing will be held. The plaintiff (physician) has the burden of proving his or her claim to the court. A counterclaim may be filed by the patient at this time.
4. **Demand a jury trial.** The case will be taken out of small claims court and the physician will be notified by the county clerk to file a formal complaint in a higher court. An attorney must represent the physician if this occurs.

Trial Preparation

The plaintiff and defendant must both appear on the trial date or the claim will be dismissed and cannot be refiled.

Instead of attending the trial in person, the physician may send a representative, such as his or her assistant or bookkeeper. If the claim is settled before trial, a dismissal form should be dated, signed, and filed with the clerk.

Preparation for the trial is essential and can mean the difference between success and failure. Decide what the judge should hear to conclude in the physician's favor. Although being represented in court by a lawyer is not allowed, a lawyer can be asked for advice before going to court. Recommendations to help prepare for trial are as follows:

1. Be on time; otherwise, the court may give a judgment in the defendant's favor.
2. Be ready to submit the basic data required by the court: the physician's name, address, and telephone number; the patient's name and address; the delinquent amount being claimed; and a brief summary of the claim.
3. Show all dates of service and amounts owed, the date on which the physician's bill was due (if a series of treatments is involved), the date of the last visit, the date of the last payment (if any payment was made), and the amount still unpaid.
4. Include all attempts to collect the debt and organize all exhibits in chronologic order. Include documentation, such as copies of statements, letters, notes, receipts, contracts, dishonored checks, telephone calls, other discussions with the patient, and other evidence to present to the court. A timeline showing the sequence of events may be useful.
5. Speak slowly and clearly, present the case in a concise manner, and use a businesslike approach. Answer all questions accurately but briefly.
6. Present a witness if live testimony is relevant. A notarized statement from a witness is admissible but not as effective.
7. Try to anticipate the opposing party's evidence and arguments so that a rebuttal may be prepared. Keep in mind that a third party will be making the decision.

The judge will question the physician or representative and the patient, review the evidence, and then make a ruling. Winning the case gives the physician the right to attach a debtor's bank assets, salary, car, personal assets, or real property. The small claims office can show the assistant how to execute a judgment. Judgments are usually effective for many years. There is a small charge if the physician decides to execute against the patient's assets but this charge is recoverable from the defendant.

A losing defendant may appeal and request a new trial in superior court. The defendant may ask the judge to make small installment payments but not all judges order this alternative. If the defendant fails to pay, a writ of execution may be obtained from the clerk's office to enforce judgment. This writ of execution permits the marshal to obtain funds from a losing party's bank account or take items of the losing party's property to satisfy the judgment.

Federal Wage Garnishment Laws

Federal wage **garnishment** laws provide a limit on the amount of employee earnings withheld in a work week or pay period when a debtor's future wage is seized to pay off a debt. They also protect the employee from being dismissed if his or her pay is garnished for only one debt, regardless of the number of levies that must be made to collect. This law is enforced by the compliance officers of the Wage and Hour Office of the US Department of Labor. The laws do not apply to federal government employees, court-ordered support of any person, court orders in personal bankruptcy cases, or state or federal tax levies. The patient's employer becomes involved as the "trustee" because the employer owes money to the debtor for wages earned.

Once a garnishment has been ordered by the court, an employer has to honor it by satisfying the terms of garnishment before wages can be paid to the debtor. Only a percentage of the wage (usually 25%) is garnished and paid to the creditor. This amount is determined from the employee's disposable earnings. Disposable earnings are the amount left after Social Security and federal, state, and local taxes are deducted. The statute resulting in the smaller garnishment applies when state garnishment laws conflict with federal laws. This method of collection should be considered a last resort for the medical office and used only with large bills.

Tracing a Skip

A patient who owes a balance on his or her account and moves but leaves no forwarding address is called a *skip*. In these cases, an unopened envelope is returned to the office marked "Returned to Sender, Addressee Unknown." Place the words "Forwarding Service Requested" below the doctor's return address on the envelope and the post office will make a search and forward the mail to the new address. The physician's office will be informed of this new address for a nominal fee. Complete a Freedom of Information Act form at the post office if the address is a rural delivery box number and the US Postal Service will provide the physical location of a person's residence. When patients send payments by mail, precautions must be taken to avoid discarding envelopes with a change of address. Always match the address on the envelope, along with the check, against the patient's account. One staff person should be responsible for updating all patients' addresses in all locations to prevent this problem.

Box 10-3   Search Techniques Used to Trace a Debtor

1. Cross-check the address on the returned envelope with the patient registration form and account to ensure that it was mailed correctly.
2. Check the zip code directory to determine whether the zip code corresponds with the patient's street address or post office box.
3. File a request with the local post office to obtain a new or corrected address.
4. Call the primary care physician (PCP) for updated information when investigating for a physician specialist or any referring practice.
5. Determine whether the patient has been seen at the hospital; if so, speak to someone in the accounts department.
6. Inquire at the patient's place of employment. If the patient is no longer employed, ask to speak to the personnel department in an effort to locate the patient. Do not divulge the reason for the call.
7. Contact persons listed on the patient registration form, including personal referrals.
8. Request information from the Department of Motor Vehicles if a driver's license number is available.
9. Request information from utility companies.
10. Inquire at the patient's bank to determine whether he or she is still a customer.
11. Obtain the services of a local credit bureau to check reports and receive notification if the patient's Social Security number shows up under a different name or at a new address.
12. Check public records, such as tax records, voter registration, court records, death and probate records, hunting and fishing licenses, and marriage licenses.

Skip Tracing Techniques

Once it is determined that a patient is a skip, tracing should begin immediately. Office policies should be established stating how the skip will be traced, whether he or she is to be traced in the office or at what point the account will be sent to a collection agency. Some offices choose to make only one attempt whereas others prefer to do most of the detective work themselves. Box 10-3 lists techniques that can be used to initiate the search for the debtor.

Never state one's business with the patient when trying to make any of these contacts. Keep all information confidential. A good skip tracer should have patience and the ability to pursue all necessary steps with tenacity and tact. A good imagination, a detective's instincts, and the ability to get along with people help in this tedious job.

Skip Tracing Services

There are several outside services from which to choose. Some agencies offer customized service with several levels of skip tracing available. Each level is more extensive and costly. The physician's office decides at which

level it would like the search conducted. The first level usually involves verifying the patient's information and checking for typographical errors. The highest level uses every resource available to find the patient. The age of the account, the account balance, and the cost of the level of skip tracing service are all considerations when deciding which level to choose. A collection agency or credit bureau (as mentioned) may offer the services of skip tracing as well.

Search via Computer

Another method of skip tracing is to use electronic databases or online services. "Information wholesalers" also exist. They cater to bill collectors and similar interested parties. Currently there are a number of bills pending in Congress aimed at restricting the flow of personal data in cyberspace. Perhaps in the future this information will not be so easy to obtain; however, conducting a successful electronic search is relatively easy at present. The following are several methods used to search electronic databases to locate a debtor's address and home telephone number:

● *Surname scan* can be done locally, regionally, or nationally using data banks that have been compiled from public source documents.
● *Address search* provides property search and any change of address from all suppliers of data to the database, including the US Postal Service. Names of other adults in the household who may have the debtor's telephone number listed under their name may be included.
● *Credit holder search* is used to establish occupation.
● *Phone number search* permits access to the names of other adults within the same household who have a telephone number.
● *Neighbor search* displays the names, addresses, and telephone numbers of the debtor's former neighbors.
● *Zip code search* provides the names, addresses, and telephone numbers of everyone within that zip code who has the same last name as the debtor.
● *City search* locates everyone with the same last and first name within a given city as well as all people who live in that city.
● *State search* finds all people with the same last name or same last and first name within the state and lists their addresses and telephone numbers.
● *National search* operates the same way as the state search. It is recommended for people with unusual last names.
● *Business search* lists all the names of the businesses in the neighborhood of the patient's last known residence. This search may help find where the patient has relocated or verify the patient's place of employment.

Explore several directories to cross-check results because data change frequently. Information is not secure when using the internet. The patient's right to privacy must never be violated.

Special Collection Issues

Bankruptcy

Bankruptcy laws are federal laws applicable in all states that ensure equal distribution of the assets of an individual among the individual's creditors. There are two kinds of bankruptcy petitions: voluntary and involuntary. A voluntary petition is one filed by a person asking for relief under the Bankruptcy Reform Act (the Code). An involuntary petition is one filed against a person by his or her creditors requesting that a person obtain relief under the Code.

When a patient files for bankruptcy, he or she becomes a ward of the court and has its protection. The patient is granted an **automatic stay** against creditors, which means that the physician may contact the patient only for the name, address, and telephone number of his or her attorney. The insurance billing specialist should no longer send statements, make telephone calls, or attempt to collect the account. A creditor can be fined for contempt of court if he or she continues to proceed against the debtor. If a collection agency has the account and has been notified of the bankruptcy, the situation is the same as if the physician has been notified. If the physician is notified first, the collection agency should be called and informed of the bankruptcy. Notification of bankruptcy does not have to be in writing; verbal communication is valid (for example, if a patient contacts the doctor's office to inform him or her of the bankruptcy). Bankruptcy remains part of the debtor's permanent credit record for 10 years.

After a patient informs the physician's office of the bankruptcy, determine what type of bankruptcy the debtor has filed. Refer to Box 10-4 for a listing of the five types of bankruptcy cases.

Bankruptcy Rules. Under the bankruptcy rules effective October 17, 2005, debtors have to meet an income test and must have insufficient assets to be eligible for filing a Chapter 7 bankruptcy. Otherwise they are forced into Chapter 13 bankruptcy, in which a debt repayment plan is ordered.

When filing a claim, the proper form may be obtained from a stationery store or by writing to the presiding judge of the bankruptcy court. If a creditor fails to file a claim, the creditor will lose his or her right to any proceeds from the bankruptcy. A plan for payment will be approved by the court. The trustee may be contacted from time to time to check the status of the claim and the payments that should be expected. Once a patient has obtained credit counseling and petitioned for bankruptcy, there must be a time lapse of 6 years before he or

---

Box 10-4   Types of Bankruptcy Cases

Chapter 7 Case

This is sometimes called a *straight petition in bankruptcy* or *absolute bankruptcy*. In this case, all of the **nonexempt assets** of the bankrupt person are liquidated and distributed according to the law to the creditors. Secured creditors are first in line for payment of all **secured debt.** Unsecured creditors are last. A person declares those to whom he or she owes money and is not required to make payment, thus eliminating all of the debtor's outstanding legal obligations for **unsecured debt.** Most medical bills are considered unsecured debt because they are not backed by any form of **collateral.** The only debt that is discharged in Chapter 7 bankruptcy is the debt that had been incurred up to the point of filing for protection under Chapter 7. So, if a patient files before services are rendered, the bankruptcy laws do not apply for the treatment provided. A Chapter 7 bankruptcy does not necessarily result in the discharge of all debts. If the patient lies about his or her financial status, the debt may not be dischargeable. If the debt incurred was for a luxury service (for example, facelift), immediately preceding the filing, it is possible that it may not be discharged. Consult the practice's attorney before adjusting the debt off the books in such a situation. All creditors are notified by the Administrator in Bankruptcy as to the proceedings and may choose either to attend the proceedings or to make a claim against whatever assets remain.

Chapter 9 Case

This case is used for reorganization proceedings when a city or town is insolvent or unable to meet its debts. A plan is put into effect to adjust such debts.

Chapter 11 Case

This case is used for reorganization of a business enterprise when the company is unable to meet its debts but would like to continue business and would be unable to do so if creditors took away its assets. A plan of arrangement is confirmed by the court and each class of creditor must accept the plan or receive at least that which it would receive on liquidation of the company.

Chapter 12 Case

This case is used for reorganization when a farmer is unable to meet his or her debts.

Chapter 13 Case

This is sometimes called a *wage earner's bankruptcy*. It is designed to protect the wage earner from creditors while allowing the wage earner to make arrangements to repay a portion of his or her bills (about 70%) over a 3- or 5-year period. The debtor pays a fixed amount agreed on by the court to the trustee in bankruptcy. A claim needs to be filed as directed by the debtor's attorney.

---

she can file again. The only exception to this is Chapter 13 bankruptcy.

Terminally Ill Patients

Although it may be difficult to collect from patients who are terminally ill, it is usually harder to collect from the estates after they have died. When a patient is too sick or scared to communicate necessary information, consult the physician about whether to obtain the patient's permission to speak to family members and stress the need for help. Usually, terminally ill patients want to do the right thing. Call the patient before he or she comes in to receive service. Ensure that the patient is aware of the existing balance and try to work with the patient to eliminate at least a portion of the balance before the next appointment. Estimate costs and prepare a plan that is agreeable to both the physician and the patient.

Estate Claims

Great care and sensitivity should be taken when trying to collect on a deceased patient's account. When you discover that a patient has died, first pursue insurance or managed care plan coverage. The entire probate system was set up to help protect families from painful involvement in estate settlements. Do not offend the deceased's family by making contact during the time of bereavement. However, file a claim after the first or second week so that the physician's name can be added to the list of creditors.

Refer to Procedure 10-5 at the end of this chapter for filing an estate claim.

After filing, the claim is denied or accepted. If accepted, an acknowledgment of the debt is sent to the physician's office. Many delays arise because of the legal complications of settling an estate but the debts are paid according to a priority system when the estate is settled. Usually funeral expenses are paid first; following in order are estate administration expenses, claims due for the deceased person's last illness, and taxes and other debts. Any amounts left are divided among family members. A lien or lawsuit may be filed against the estate in the rare case of a rejection of the claim.

Various state time limits and statutes govern the filing of a claim against an estate. Check with the county court in your state to obtain filing deadlines. Deadlines may range from 2 months to 3 years but must be adhered to for successful collection from an estate.

Litigation

A difficult question arises when the physician is advised that a patient is involved in a pending litigation related to the services provided to the patient. It may not be necessary to wait until the litigation is resolved to pursue payment. Assess whether the patient has the ability to pay before possibly receiving a settlement in a lawsuit. Before withholding collection activity, the medical practice should get a guarantee that the physician will be paid in full before the patient (debtor) receives money from a settlement. The agreement must be guaranteed by the lawyer representing the patient. If the patient is working, regular payments should be required pending the settlement of the patient's litigation. It is always advisable to contact a malpractice attorney in such cases.

Liens. A **lien** is a claim on the property of another as security for a debt. This may include a claim on a future settlement of a lawsuit. The physician may be asked to accept a lien by a patient or the patient's attorney when the patient has been involved in an automobile accident and is awaiting a settlement (Figure 10-19). In litigation cases, a lien is a legal promise to satisfy a debt owed by the patient to the physician out of any proceeds received on the case. See Chapter 15 for further details about industrial cases.

Patient Complaints

It is generally in the physician's best interest to resolve patient complaints and billing disputes quickly, accurately, and amicably. Always address collection complaints seriously. Listen to the patient with an open mind. Note specifically what the patient is saying and what the patient wants to do. Look beyond the complaint to determine what caused the problem. The source of the problem, not just the symptom of the problem, should be resolved. A patient complaint form may be adapted to prompt staff to pay close attention to positive customer relations. This form may help to screen poor collection techniques by staff members, pinpoint billing department problems, and identify policies and procedures that need improvement.

The patient may refuse to pay the physician if the patient's complaint is not addressed. Some guidelines to follow when a patient calls or writes a letter complaining about the physician or the medical practice are:
1. Listen carefully (or read the letter carefully) and establish exactly what the patient complaint is and what the patient wants done about it.
2. Thank the person for calling (or writing); demonstrate appreciation of his or her input on the situation.
3. Apologize, regardless of whether the patient is right or wrong.
4. Answer the complaint. Explain what happened, if applicable, and state what is being done about it.
5. Use a professional and sincere approach. If the patient is wrong, state that the complaint is unjustified but first explain your estimation of the situation and its resolution. Otherwise, the patient is likely to become quite upset. Do not be sarcastic, condescending, or insulting.
6. Take all complaints seriously. Do not respond in a lighthearted manner or use humor; it will only serve to upset the patient.

REQUEST FOR ALLOWANCE OF LIEN
ASSIGNMENT AND AUTHORIZATION

WHEREAS, I have a right or cause of action out of personal injury, to wit:

I, _____ hereby authorize _____ ,
     patient's name   physician's name

to furnish upon request, to my attorney, _____ , any and all medical records, or reports of examination, diagnosis, treatment, or prognosis but not necessarily limited to those items as set forth herein, in addition to an itemized statement of accounts for services rendered therefore or in connection therewith, which my attorney may from time to time request in connection with the injuries described above and sustained by me on the _____ day of _____ , 20XX.

I hereby irrevocably authorize and direct my said attorney set forth herein to pay to _____ all charges for attendance in court,
          patient's name

if required as an expert witness whether he testifies or not; reports or other data supplied by him; depositions given by said doctor; medical services rendered or drugs supplied; and any other responsible and customary charges incurred by my attorney as submitted by _____ and in
                      physician's name

connection with said injury. Said payment or payments are to be made from any money or monies received by my attorney whether by judgment, decree, or settlement of this case, prior to disbursement to me and payment of the amount as herein directed shall be the same as if paid by me. This authorization to pay the aforementioned doctor shall constitute and be deemed as assignment of so much of my recovery I receive. It is agreed that nothing herein relieves me of the primary responsibility and obligation of paying my doctor for services rendered, and I shall at all times remain personally liable for such indebtedness unless released by the aforementioned doctor or by payment disbursed by my attorney. I accept the above assignment:

Dated: _____ Patient: _____

As the attorney of record for the above-named, I hereby agree to observe the terms of this agreement, and to withhold from any award in this case such sums as are required for the adequate protection of Dr. _____ ,

Date: _____ Attorney: _____

FIGURE 10-19 A patient's authorization to release information to an attorney and grant lien to the physician against proceeds of settlement in connection with accident, industrial, or third-party litigation cases.

7. **Respond in letter form.** Whether the complaint has been received by telephone or by letter, take the time to write to answer the complaint. This indicates that the matter is not being taken lightly.
8. **Be cordial and sincere.** Express to the patient the hope of continuing a friendly relationship but that payment is necessary. Treat the patient with respect, good will, and sincere appreciation. Often, kindness can turn a negative into a positive. The complaint can be turned into a payment.
9. **Follow up** after the complaint has been resolved by looking at the root of the problem and taking the necessary time to communicate this to the office manager.

This follow-up allows creation of a plan of action that can help to prevent the same type of problem from recurring.

Bonding

Insurance billing specialists, claims assistance professionals, or anyone who handles checks or cash should be bonded or insured. A practice that carries a fidelity or honesty bond means that an insurance company will prosecute any guilty employees. **Bonding** is an insurance contract by which a bonding agency guarantees payment of a certain sum to a physician in case

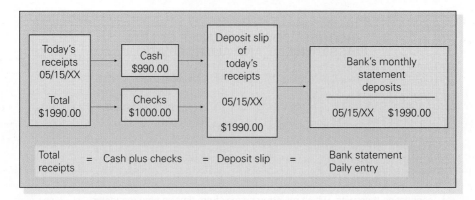

FIGURE 10-20 Auditing the daily collection in the medical office to reconcile with the bank deposit.

of a financial loss caused by an employee or some contingency over which the payee has no control. Bonding methods for a practice with three or more office employees are as follows:

- *Position-schedule bond* covers a designated job, such as a bookkeeper or nurse, rather than a named individual. If one employee in a category leaves, the replacement is automatically covered.
- *Blanket-position bond* provides coverage for all employees regardless of job title.
- *Personal bond* provides coverage for those who handle large sums of money. A thorough background investigation is required.

Such bonding contracts may be obtained from a casualty insurance agent or broker. Bond coverage should be reviewed periodically with the insurance agent to ensure that coverage is keeping pace with the expansion of the business.

Collection Controls

Embezzlement. Embezzlement is stealing money that has been entrusted in one's care. In many cases of insurance claims embezzlement, the physician is held as the guilty party and has to pay huge sums of money to the third-party payer when false claims are submitted by an employee. If an undiscovered embezzler leaves the employer and you are hired to replace that person, you could be accused some months later of doing something that you did not do. Take precautions as an employee and to protect the medical practice.

Precautions for Financial Protection. To prevent the temptation to steal from a medical practice, the following office policies should be routinely practiced. The physician or supervisor must approve all entries posted about adjustments, discounts, and write-offs. If a patient owes money to the physician that is uncollectable and adjusted off, be sure that the physician has approved and the balance due has been brought to zero. Ask the physician, an auditor, or an outside consultant to occasionally check an entire day's records (the patient sign-in log and appointment schedule) with the daysheet, patients' financial accounting records, encounter forms, and cash receipt slips. A daily trail of the balance of A/R, including daily deposit of checks and cash, can assist in reviewing monthly income and aid in discovering embezzlement. Audit the daily collection in the medical office to reconcile the bank deposit (Figure 10-20). If poor bookkeeping and record keeping are noticed, bring this to your employer's attention.

All insurance payment checks should be immediately stamped within the endorsement area on the back "For Deposit Only," called a *restrictive endorsement*. The bank should be given instructions never to cash a check made payable to the physician.

Encounter forms, transaction slips, and cash receipts should be pre-numbered. If a mistake is made when completing one, void it and keep the slip as part of the financial records. It is especially imperative to have pre-numbered insurance forms if the physician's practice allows the use of a signature stamp when submitting claims. Thus filing of fictitious insurance claims can be totally eliminated.

As a precautionary measure, always type your initials at the bottom left or top right corner of the insurance claim forms that you submit. This will indicate to office personnel who did the work. Always retain the explanation of benefits (EOB) or remittance advice (RA) documents that accompany checks from insurance companies.

Only a few of the many precautions for protection are mentioned here; embezzlement can occur in A/R, accounts payable, with petty cash, with use of computers, and in various other aspects of a medical practice.

PROCEDURE 10-1

Create a Financial Agreement with a Patient

OBJECTIVE: To assist the patient in making credit arrangements by completing and signing a Truth in Lending form

EQUIPMENT/SUPPLIES: Patient's financial accounting record (ledger), calendar, Truth in Lending form, typewriter or computer, calculator, and quiet private room

DIRECTIONS: Follow the step-by-step procedures, which include rationales, to learn this job skill. An assignment is presented in the *Workbook* to practice this skill.

1. Explain the patient's balance due and answer questions about credit.
2. Inform the patient of the medical practice's office policy about extending credit payments.
3. Discuss an installment plan concerning the amount of the total debt, the down payment, the amount and date of each installment, and the date of final payment.
4. Subtract the down payment from the total debt. Divide the remaining amount by the number of months the debt is being carried to determine the monthly installment amounts and date of final payment.
5. Complete a Truth in Lending form after mutually agreeing on the terms if the payments require more than four installments. This procedure complies with Regulation Z.
6. Review the completed Truth in Lending form with the patient.
7. Ask the patient to sign the Truth in Lending form.
8. Make a photocopy of the Truth in Lending form for the patient to retain.
9. File the original Truth in Lending form in the patient's financial file in the office.

PROCEDURE 10-2

Seven-Step Billing and Collection Guidelines

OBJECTIVE: To properly bill and collect payments for professional services rendered to patients

EQUIPMENT/SUPPLIES: Patients' financial accounting statements, envelopes, calendar, and telephone

DIRECTIONS: Follow these step-by-step procedures and guidelines, which include rationales, to learn this job skill.

1. Present the first statement at the time of service. This can be a formal statement or an encounter form (multipurpose billing form).
2. Mail the second itemized statement within 30 days of treatment. The phrase "due and payable within 10 days" should be printed on each statement. Local paycheck issuing patterns should be considered before selecting a date for statements to be mailed. Choose which billing routine the office will use.
   a. *Monthly billing. Using the monthly billing system, all statements are mailed at the same time during the month. Choose a mail-out day at the beginning of the month so that the patient will receive the bill near the 15th or send statements near the end of the month so that the patient receives the bill on the 1st.*
   b. *Cycle billing.* **Cycle billing** *is a system of billing accounts at spaced intervals during the month based on a breakdown of accounts by alphabet, account number, insurance type, or date of first service. This relieves the pressure of having to get all statements out at one time and allows collection at a faster, more organized rate than accounts collected at random. It also allows continuous cash flow throughout the month and distributes the influx of incoming calls from patients about problem accounts. The number of cycles may be determined by how the collector wishes to divide the workload. Using two cycles per month, statements would be sent on the 25th to arrive by the 1st and on the 10th to arrive by the 15th of the month. Using four cycles per month, statements should be sent every Tuesday or Wednesday to arrive at the end of the week. If a cycle that was established by the first date of service is used and the patient was first seen on the 11th of the month, then he or she should receive a bill every month on the 11th.*
3. Send the third statement 30 days after the second statement was sent. Indicate that the payment is past due.
4. If there is no response to the third statement, place the first telephone call to the patient depending on office policy (7 to 14 days). Ask if there is a problem. Ask for a payment commitment and set up a suspense file. Accounts are put in a suspense file for active follow-up. Action must be taken within the time frame mentioned, after the patient has been so advised.
5. Check for payment as promised. Allow 1 day for mail delay. Place the second telephone call to the patient and ask for payment. Set up a new payment date. Allow 5 days.

Continued

PROCEDURE 10-2—cont'd

6. Check for payment as promised. Send a 10-day notice advising the patient that unless payment is received in 10 days, the account will be turned over for legal action.
7. Check for payment. Promptly surrender the account for collection or legal action. Figure 10-15

shows a collection decision tree to be used when determining when to send statements, 10-day notices, and accounts to a collection agency and when to make telephone calls.

PROCEDURE 10-3

Telephone Collection Plan

OBJECTIVE: To obtain payment of a delinquent account balance due by making the first collection telephone call

EQUIPMENT/SUPPLIES: Telephone, pen or pencil, patient's financial accounting record, computerized account, or collection telephone log

DIRECTIONS: Follow these step-by-step procedures and guidelines, which include rationales, to learn this job skill.

1. Set the mood of the call by the manner of speech and tone of voice. The first 30 seconds of the call sets the scene for the relationship with the patient. Follow the Fair Debt Collection Practices Act when making a telephone call.
2. State the name of the caller and the practice represented and identify the patient. Be certain the debtor is being spoken to before revealing the nature of the call.
3. Identify oneself and the facility.
4. Verify the debtor's address and any telephone numbers.
5. State the reason for the call by asking for full payment and stating the total amount owed. Ask for payment courteously but firmly.
6. Take control of the conversation and establish urgency by asking for full payment now. Speak slowly in a low voice; staying calm and polite prevents quarreling.
7. Ask when payment will be made, how it will be made, and if it will be sent by mail or in person.
8. Pause for effect. This turns the conversation back to the patient to respond to the demand or explain why payment has not been made. Never assume that if a patient does not respond, it means "no."
9. Find out if the patient needs clarification of the bill.
10. Inquire if the patient has a problem. Ask if the practice can be of assistance, especially when the patient is unable to give a reason for nonpayment.

11. If the patient is reluctant to agree to an amount, question him or her by asking one of the following: "How much are you willing to pay?" "Do you have a regular paycheck?" "Will payment be made through a checking account?"
12. Obtain a promise to pay with an agreeable amount and a due date; be clear how and when payment is expected but give the patient a choice of action. Set immediate deadlines for payment.
13. Ask for half of the amount if full payment is not possible.
14. Discuss a payment plan if the patient is not able to pay half of the balance owed. Be realistic and reasonable. It is self-defeating to set up payment arrangements the patient cannot afford. Advise the patient that the entire balance will become due and payable if the payment is even 1 day late. Ask the patient to please call before the due date with an explanation if any problems arise to prevent payment.
15. Restate the importance of the agreement.
16. Tell the patient to write down the amount and due date.
17. Document the agreement on the patient's financial accounting record by inserting the date of the call and abbreviated notations, in the computer system, or in a collection telephone log. Note the time the patient was spoken to.
18. Send confirmation of the agreement (Figure 10-21) as a follow-up to the telephone call.
19. Check the account the day after the payment was due; allow 1 day for mail delay. If the patient fails to make payment as promised, make another telephone call and ask the patient if there is still a problem. Get a new commitment to pay and confirm again. If the patient continues to avoid payment, advise the patient that the account will be turned over to a collection agency and follow through as stated.

COLLEGE CLINIC
4567 Broad Avenue
Woodland Hills, XY 12345-0001
Tel. (555) 486-9002
FAX (555) 487-8976

October 2, 20XX

Mr. Leonard Blabalot
981 McCort Circle
Woodland Hills, XY 12345-0001

Dear Mr. Blabalot:

I am glad we had an opportunity to discuss your outstanding balance with our practice during our phone conversation on October 1, 20XX. This will confirm and remind you that you agreed to pay $100 on your account on or before October 15, 20XX.

A return envelope is enclosed for your convenience.

Sincerely,

Charlotte Rose Routingham
Business Office

Enc. envelope

FIGURE 10-21 Letter confirming telephone payment discussion sent to remind patient of the payment terms agreed upon.

PROCEDURE 10-4

File a Claim in Small Claims Court

OBJECTIVE: To file a claim to obtain payment for a delinquent or uncollectable financial account in small claims court

EQUIPMENT/SUPPLIES: Small claims court filing form, photocopy of the patient's financial accounting record, computer or typewriter, pen or pencil, envelope, and check for filing fee

DIRECTIONS: Follow these step-by-step procedures and guidelines, which include rationales, to learn this job skill.

1. Obtain a Claim of Plaintiff or Plaintiff's Original Petition form to notify the patient that action is being filed. This can be obtained from the clerk's office located at the municipal or justice court. Obtain booklets and material to help guide the claimant through the process.
2. Complete and file the papers with the small claims court; make sure to have the patient's correct name and street address.
3. Make a photocopy of the small claims court form for the office files.

4. Pay the clerk the small filing fee. Filing fees vary by state, by county within some states, and by the amount of the claim.
5. Make arrangements to serve the defendant. The summons or citation can be served on the patient by a sheriff or court-appointed officer by paying a small fee plus mileage for the constable who serves it. The person serving the defendant must fill out a proof of service form.
6. After being served, a patient has one of four options.
   a. *Pay the claim to the court clerk. This will be forwarded to the physician but the filing fee or service charge will not be refunded.*
   b. *Ignore the claim. The physician will win by default. In some states, a judgment may be requested in writing, but in other states, the physician or the physician's representative (medical employee) must appear on a specified date. If the patient does not appear, the judgment is granted in the physician's favor and usually court costs are included in the judgment.*

Continued

PROCEDURE 10-4—cont'd

c. *Request a small claims hearing. The court clerk will let both parties know when to appear. The patient may file a counterclaim against the physician at this time.*

d. *Demand a jury trial. The case will be taken out of small claims court. The physician will be notified by the court clerk to file a formal complaint in a higher court and an attorney must represent the physician.*

7. Appear in court (physician or the physician's medical employee or representative) on the specified date; otherwise, the claim will be dismissed and cannot be refiled.

8. Basic information required by the court follows:
   a. *Physician's name, address, and telephone number*
   b. *Patient's name and address*
   c. *Delinquent amount*
   d. *Summary of the claim, including the date the physician's bill was due, date of the last visit, date of the last payment, unpaid amount, and all records of telephone contacts and letters sent*

9. Determine what the judge needs to hear to decide a favorable case. Good preparation for the trial can make the difference between success and failure.

10. Organize all exhibits in a notebook, in chronologic order. A timeline showing the sequence of events can be useful.

11. Take a businesslike professional approach at the hearing by giving concise and accurate answers to the judge's questions, speaking slowly and clearly. The physician or assistant must bring any witnesses, statements, receipts, contracts, notes, dishonored checks, or other evidence to court. The judge will question the physician's medical employee or representative or physician and the patient, review the evidence, and then make a ruling.

12. Put a lien on the debtor's wages, automobile, bank or personal assets, or real property if the judgment, which is usually effective for many years, is in the physician's favor. This is the physician's legal right. The small claims office will show the physician's medical employee or representative or physician how to execute a judgment.

13. Pay a small fee if the physician decides to execute against the patient's assets. It is recoverable from the patient.

PROCEDURE 10-5

File an Estate Claim

OBJECTIVE: To file a claim on an estate for a deceased patient who has an outstanding balance on his or her financial accounting record

EQUIPMENT/SUPPLIES: Statement of Claim form, computer or typewriter, pen or pencil, photocopy machine, patient's financial accounting record, US Postal Service certified mail forms, and envelope

DIRECTIONS: Follow these step-by-step procedures and guidelines, which include rationales, to learn this job skill.

1. Confirm the date and place of death with the hospital, nursing home, or funeral home.

2. Pursue payment from all third-party payers first.

3. Contact the Register of Wills office in the county where the patient lived or the probate department of the superior court, County Recorder's Office. Request a Statement of Claim form or the county's proper document to formally register a claim against an estate.

4. File the claim according to the instructions received with the claim form. When probate is filed, a notification will be sent advising the court of probate, the attorney representing the estate, and the **estate executor** or **estate administrator.** Perhaps a small fee should be included for court costs.

5. Send a photocopy of the patient's financial accounting record (itemized statement) by certified mail, return receipt, to the attorney and copies to the executor and the court. If the physician treated the deceased patient's last illness, that fact should be clearly indicated on the statement.

6. Allow the legal system to take its course. A call to the executor can be made periodically to check on the status of the estate.

KEY POINTS

This is a brief chapter review, or summary, of the key issues presented. To further enhance your knowledge of the technical subject matter, review the key terms and key abbreviations for this chapter by locating the meaning for each in the Glossary at the end of this book, which appears in a section before the Index.

1. The physician, the practice administrator responsible for financial affairs, and the patient must understand insurance contracts, which list payment provisions, medical services not covered, the portion of the bill for which the patient is responsible, and the process for reimbursing the office.

2. The insurance billing specialist must monitor the A/R weekly to determine the effectiveness of collection. An average A/R should be one and a half to two times the charges for 1 month of services.

3. Collect copayments and deductibles from patients at the time service is rendered. The medical practice can charge a missed appointment fee regardless of the health insurance the patient carries; the patient is responsible for paying the missed appointment fee.

4. Under HIPAA, physicians are free to use whatever policies they want on charity care, discounts, write-offs, and collections but this must be done consistently and the reasons must be documented. Professional courtesy should be kept to a minimum.

5. When payments are made by check, require two forms of verification. Always take immediate action when the bank returns a check for NSF. When payments are made by credit card, require picture ID verification.

6. Online services such as Square can be used to accept credit cards at any time. Fees vary depending on the amount of transactions for the medical practice. It is customary for the medical practice to impose a nominal fee on the patient for credit transactions.

7. Recognize overdue accounts to determine when to send dun messages on statements, make telephone calls, or send to a collection agency.

8. Use alternative payment methods to help cash flow and reduce collection costs such as credit card payments, debit cards, e-checks, and payment plans.

9. Follow all federal and state laws that affect collection of delinquent accounts.

10. Contact the patient in a timely manner by telephone at the first sign of payment delay and then send a collection letter as a reminder.

11. Delinquent accounts should be turned over to a collection agency only after all reasonable attempts have been made to collect.

12. Learn and use all techniques in skip tracing a debtor.

13. It is in the physician's best interest to resolve patient complaints and billing disputes quickly, accurately, and amicably.

💻 STUDENT ASSIGNMENT

✔ Study Chapter 10.

✔ Answer the fill-in-the blank, multiple-choice, and true/false review questions in the *Workbook* to reinforce the theory learned in this chapter and to help prepare you for a future test.

✔ Complete the assignment in the *Workbook* to give you hands-on experience in selecting a dun message, posting a courtesy adjustment and insurance or patient payment, composing a collection letter and accepting three methods of credit card payments.

✔ Turn to the Glossary at the end of this text for a further understanding of the key terms and key abbreviations used in the chapter.

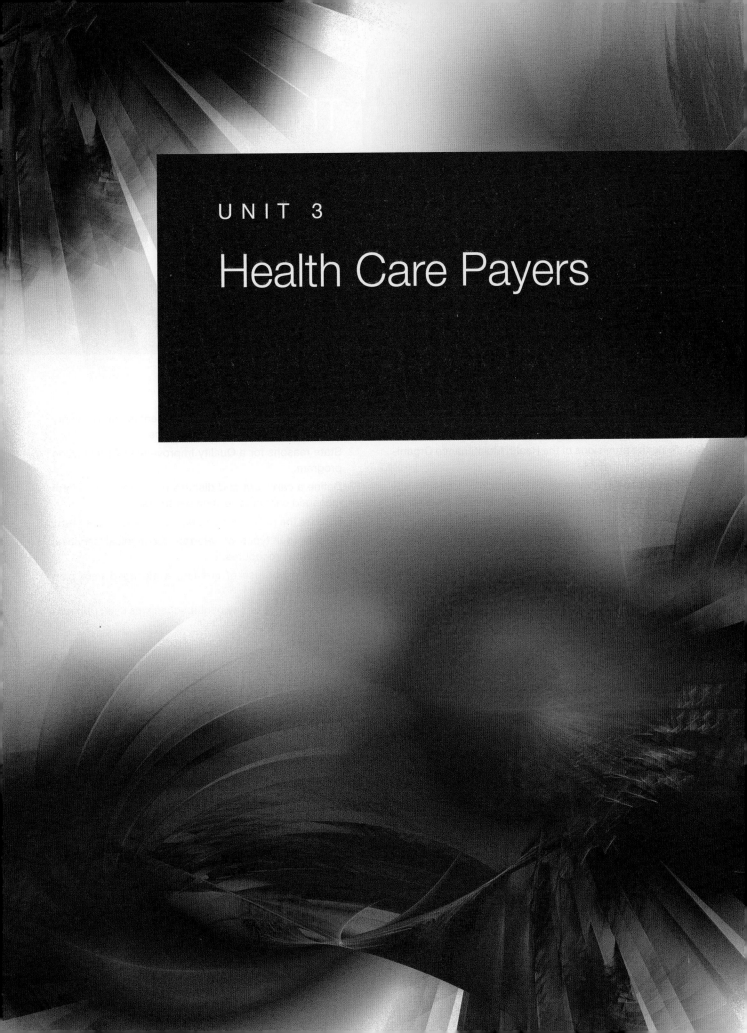

UNIT 3

Health Care Payers

The Blue Plans, Private Insurance, and Managed Care Plans

Marilyn Takahashi Fordney

OBJECTIVES

After reading this chapter, you should be able to:

1. Discuss the difference between a traditional indemnity insurance plan and a managed care plan.
2. State the provisions of the Health Maintenance Organization Act of 1973.
3. Explain health maintenance organization benefits, eligibility requirements, and the various HMO models.
4. List features of an exclusive provider organization.
5. List two types and two different functions of foundations for medical care.
6. Define and discuss independent practice associations.
7. Name the features of preferred provider organizations.
8. Describe the features of a physician provider group.
9. Explain the features of a point-of-service plan.
10. Discuss triple-option health plans, provider-sponsored organizations, and religious fraternal benefit societies.
11. Explain how the Employee Retirement Income Security Act affects managed care insurance.
12. State reasons for a Quality Improvement Organization program.
13. Define a *carve out* and discuss how carve outs affect managed care organization contracts.
14. Discuss the patient information letter and its contents.
15. Identify four types of referrals for medical services, tests, and procedures.
16. State the purpose of creating a managed care plan reference guide.
17. Describe types of payment mechanisms used for managed care plans.

KEY TERMS

ancillary services
buffing
capitation
carve outs
churning
claims-review type of foundation
closed panel program
comprehensive type of
    foundation
copayment
deductible
direct referral
disenrollment

exclusive provider organization
fee-for-service
formal referral
foundation for medical care
gatekeeper
health maintenance organization
in-area
independent (or individual) practice association
managed care organization
participating physician
per capita
physician provider group

point-of-service plan
preferred provider organization
prepaid group practice model
primary care physician
self-referral
service area
staff model
stop-loss
tertiary care
turfing
utilization review
verbal referral
withhold

KEY ABBREVIATIONS

copay	HEDIS	PCP	QISMC
EBP	HMO	POS	UR
EPO	IPA	PPG	
ERISA	MCO	PPO	
FMC	NCQA	QIO	

Service to Patients

Carefully follow guidelines for each managed care contract regarding preauthorization for certain tests and services, hospital admissions, inpatient or outpatient surgeries, elective procedures, or when the patient must be seen by someone other than the primary care physician (PCP). If authorization is obtained in a timely manner, the patient's health care will not be delayed and payment will be forthcoming. These policies and procedures provide good service to the patient.

PRIVATE INSURANCE

Numerous private insurance companies across the United States (US) offer health insurance to individuals and groups. Most offer a variety of managed care plans. However, with the passing of the Affordable Care Act, significant changes from fee-for-service medicine to a value-based health care system are taking place. This chapter describes the difference between private insurance and managed care. **Fee-for-service** reimbursement was discussed in previous chapters. A number of value-based reimbursement methods are being introduced across the United States. However, this chapter explains managed care capitation as a form of reimbursement and will introduce some of the value-based systems that are being contemplated in some regions.

Blue Cross and Blue Shield Plans

Blue Cross/Blue Shield is a pioneer in private insurance and had a nonprofit status that made them unique among all private insurance carriers for many years. Blue Cross/Blue Shield is the largest insurance company in the US. Each plan is independently owned and operated in each state. The plans work together in a network similar to a spider web. Originally, Blue Cross plans were developed to cover hospital expenses and Blue Shield plans were established primarily to cover physician services. Different plans have been developed to allow members to seek treatment from Blue Cross/Blue Shield providers anywhere in the US. With so many different plans, it is difficult for the insurance billing specialist to know which type the member is enrolled in. However, the patient's identification card is important and helpful in obtaining the correct information needed for billing purposes. The identification number consists of 9 to 12 numbers and 1 to 3 alpha characters. The patient may have a traditional plan or a managed care plan (for example, preferred provider organization [PPO], point-of-service [POS] plan, independent [or individual] practice association [IPA], **health maintenance organization [HMO],** or Medicare HMO). Plans are different and may have diverse names in each state (for example, Premera in Alaska and Washington state; Care First in Maryland, northern Virginia, Washington, DC, and Delaware; and Horizon in New Jersey). This chapter describes these managed care systems.

Nationally, the Blue Cross/Blue Shield Association is a single corporation administering the rules and regulations for the regional plans to follow. The regional plans process claims for members who have plan coverage for hospital expenses, outpatient care, other institutional services, home care, dental benefits, and vision care. Most of the affiliated organizations have converted to for-profit status and operate in much the same way as other private insurance carriers. In some areas, Blue Cross and Blue Shield are separate organizations and in some situations they may compete against each other. They have plans that are similar to other private insurance companies and they do not have standardized claim form guidelines. In addition, Blue Cross/Blue Shield may act as a Medicare administrative contractor (fiscal intermediary) in certain regions. An experienced insurance billing specialist should be aware of the many problems these circumstances cause. For example, the policy number may require the claim to be sent to the home plan or to be sent through the provider's state carrier. Blue Cross/Blue Shield realizes that this is a problem, so the organization is developing a product called Blue Plan that incorporates all products. The intent is to help the patient avoid making payments. Always verify the mailing address for claims and the address for sending appeals, because these may not always be the same. Some plans may have a form that should be used as a cover sheet when submitting an appeal.

There are other unique situations with Blue Cross/Blue Shield regarding contracts. Blue Cross/Blue Shield would like to have contracts with both medical groups and the providers that work for the group. This poses unique problems when the group and provider are contracted, when the group is contracted and the provider is not, and when there is no contract with either the provider or the group. Each situation has a different effect on claims processing and payment. A provider must be individually contracted with Blue Cross/Blue Shield to receive reimbursement as a member physician. In some places, areas have been divided into regions and all physicians within a given region are called in-network and those outside of the designated area are called out of network. **Deductibles** and **copayments** vary according to the patient's plan and whether a patient sees an in-network physician versus one that is out of network.

Because Blue Cross/Blue Shield contracts are like other types of private and managed care plans, in this text the organization is not listed separately in the description of types of fee structures, network physicians, managed care plans, and guidelines for completing the CMS-1500 (02-12) insurance claim form or electronic claims processing. A medical practice should have available for reference the current provider manual for its state's Blue Cross/Blue Shield plans. When filing a claim, two of the most important elements to obtain from the member's/subscriber's card are their ID number and group number (Figure 11-1).

MANAGED CARE

Until the early 1970s, most health insurance was delivered through traditional fee-for-service plans. This scenario

has changed from indemnity plans to managed health care plans, such as HMOs. In an indemnity plan, also referred to as *traditional insurance*, the insured pays a fixed monthly premium and 100% of all medical bills until he or she reaches the annual deductible; then the insurance company pays a percentage of covered benefits up to a maximum amount. The insured may obtain care from any health care provider and the provider is paid each time a service is rendered on a fee-for-service basis. In a managed care plan, a specified set of health benefits is provided in exchange for a yearly fee or fixed periodic payments to the provider by the plan. The patient pays a smaller monthly premium and may be restricted as to which health care provider to seek care from. In addition to HMOs, other types of **prepaid group practice models** that use a managed care approach and are operated by **managed care organizations (MCOs)** are discussed in this chapter.

In prepaid group plans, patients join the plan and pay monthly medical insurance premiums individually or through their employer. The physician renders service to the patient and the patient usually pays a small copayment and occasionally a deductible as required by the plan. Providers that join the plan are paid using the capitation method. **Capitation** is a system of payment used by managed care plans in which physicians and hospitals are paid a fixed **per capita** amount for each patient enrolled over a stated period of time, regardless of the type and number of services provided.

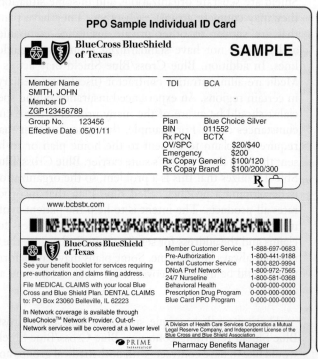
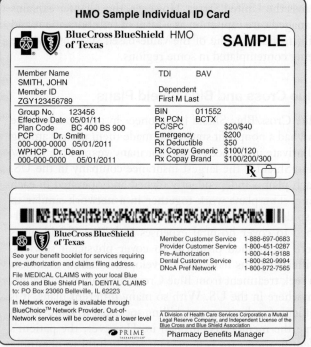

FIGURE 11-1 Examples of BlueCross BlueShield of Texas member's/subscriber's cards showing ID numbers and group numbers, two of the most important elements. BCA = Blue Choice PPO Network, and BAV = Blue Advantage HMO Network.

Prepaid Group Practice Health Plans

The *Ross-Loos Medical Group* in Los Angeles was America's oldest privately owned prepaid medical group. It was founded in 1929 by Drs. Donald E. Ross and H. Clifford Loos and existed only in southern California, where it expanded to 17 medical group locations. In 1975, the Ross-Loos Medical Group formed a corporation and received a federal grant to develop a health care system under the federal Health Maintenance Organization Act of 1973. In 1980, INA Healthplan, Inc. of Philadelphia merged with Ross-Loos. Ross-Loos is now known as *CIGNA Healthplans of California*.

Most CIGNA patients are served under a prepayment (capitation) group plan; they pay a monthly premium and receive hospital, surgical, and professional benefits from a CIGNA staff physician or CIGNA Health Care Center. Several thousand other CIGNA patients are private and are treated on a fee-for-service basis. In the case of an emergency when the patient is outside the area of a CIGNA Health Care Center, he or she may seek professional or hospital care in other facilities but CIGNA must be notified as soon as possible. A dental plan and Medicare supplemental plan are available through CIGNA as well.

Another pioneer of the prepaid group practice concept is the *Kaiser Permanente Medical Care Program*. It began in 1933 when Dr. Sidney R. Garfield and a few physicians working for him gave combined industrial accident and personal medical care to approximately 5000 workers building a fresh-water aqueduct across the California desert to Los Angeles. Dr. Garfield charged the insurance carriers $1.50 per worker per month and the workers 5 cents per day. In return, he provided comprehensive health care. Then, in 1938, Henry J. Kaiser and his son, Edgar, started a joint venture to complete the Grand Coulee Dam in Washington and invited Dr. Garfield to form a medical group to furnish care to the workers for 7 cents per day prepaid by the employer. The group expanded to include the workers' wives and children.

Kaiser Permanente now has centers in 12 regions covering 16 states. Patients are served under a prepayment group plan and receive hospital, surgical, and professional benefits from physicians located at the Kaiser Permanente Medical Care Centers. In most regions, the Kaiser Permanente Medical Plan is a **closed panel program** composed of multispecialty physicians and limits the patient's choice of personal physicians to those practicing in one of the 12 geographic regions.

In January 1994, Kaiser Permanente announced a venture with Pacific Mutual Life Insurance Company to give Kaiser's 4.6 million California patients the option of using physicians and medical facilities outside the vast Kaiser network. This was the first time that Kaiser allowed certain member groups of its two California HMOs to seek medical help from non-Kaiser physicians and it was termed a *POS option* (see the section titled "Point-of-Service Plans" later in this chapter). In this option, Kaiser pays up to a specified amount and the patient pays the rest depending on the contract. Kaiser does not provide care on a fee-for-service or cost reimbursement basis.

In emergency situations when patients cannot reach a Kaiser Center, they may seek the services of outside facilities or physicians. They are transferred to a Kaiser facility when their condition stabilizes.

Health Maintenance Organization Act of 1973

An HMO is a prepaid group practice that can be sponsored and operated by the government, medical schools, clinics, foundations, hospitals, employers, labor unions, community or consumer groups, insurance companies, hospital medical plans, or the US Department of Veterans Affairs (VA).

In 1973, Congress passed the Health Maintenance Organization Act of 1973 (Public Law 93-222), creating authority for the federal government to assist HMO development in a number of ways, including (1) providing grants, loans, and loan guarantees to offset the initial operating deficits of new HMOs that meet federal standards (for example, are federally qualified) and (2) requiring most employers to offer an HMO to their employees as an alternative to traditional health insurance.

Accreditation

The National Committee for Quality Assurance (NCQA) is a not-for-profit organization that accredits HMOs, including traditional staff and group model HMOs, network and IPA model HMOs, mixed models, and open-ended HMOs. This means that the HMO has met certain quality standards. Receiving a seal of approval means that the HMO has met state and federal requirements allowing them to participate in Medicaid and other managed care programs. NCQA developed the Health Plan Employer Data and Information Set (HEDIS), which is a set of data reporting standards that compares performance between plans.

Eligibility

Those who have voluntarily enrolled in an HMO plan from a specific geographic area (**in-area** or **service area**) or who are covered by an employer that has paid an established sum per person to be covered by the plan are eligible. The law states that an employer employing 25 or more persons may offer the services of an HMO as an alternative health treatment plan for employees. Medicare and Medicaid beneficiaries also may become members of managed care plans, whether retired or employed. The federal government reimburses the HMOs on a per capita basis, depending on the size of the enrollment. This means that the HMO is paid a fixed per capita amount (also known as *capitation*) for each patient served without considering the actual number or nature of services provided to each person.

To qualify as an HMO, an organization must present proof of its ability to provide comprehensive health care. To retain eligibility, an HMO must render periodic performance reports to the offices of the Department of Health and Human Services (DHHS). Thus accurate and complete medical records are imperative to the survival and cost control of an HMO.

Primary Care Physician. Most managed care plans use a **primary care physician (PCP)** as a gatekeeper. A **gatekeeper** is a physician who controls patient access to specialists and diagnostic testing services. Usually PCPs are physicians who practice in the fields of internal medicine, family practice, general practice, or pediatrics. Although obstetrics/gynecology is considered specialty care, the obstetrician/gynecologist may be contracted as a PCP and, when not, it is common for MCOs to allow self-referral by members to obstetricians/gynecologists for certain services (for example, Pap tests).

Identification Card. Each enrollee of a managed care plan is given an identification card. To see an example of a card from this type of plan, refer back to Figure 3-8. The card usually lists the patient's name, member number, group number, and primary care physician's name. The name of the MCO and type of plan with the amount of copayment for various outpatient services (for example, office visit, emergency department, urgent care center, and pharmacy) may be included by some plans.

Both sides of the patient's card should be photocopied because the insurance address, telephone numbers used for inquiries and authorizations, and other important information may be listed on the front and back of the card.

Benefits

Benefits under the HMO Act fall under two categories, basic and supplemental health service, and are listed in Box 11-1.

MANAGED CARE SYSTEMS

Health Maintenance Organizations

The oldest of all prepaid health plans is the HMO. An HMO is a plan or program by which specified health

---

Box 11-1   **Health Maintenance Organization Act Benefits of 1973**
Basic Health Services
Alcohol, drug abuse, and addiction medical treatment
Dental services (preventive) for children younger than age 12 years
Diagnostic laboratory, x-ray, and therapeutic radiology services
Emergency health services in or out of the HMO service area
Family planning and infertility services
Health education and medical social services
Home health services
Hospital services (inpatient and outpatient)
Mental health services on an outpatient basis, short-term (not to exceed 20 visits) ambulatory, evaluative, and crisis intervention
Physicians' services and consultant or referral services without time or cost limits
Preventive health services (for example, physical examinations for adults, vision and hearing tests for children through age 17 years, well-baby care, immunizations, health education)
Supplemental Health Services
Dental care not included in basic benefits
Extended mental health services not included in basic benefits
Eye examinations for adults
Intermediate and long-term care (nursing facilities and nursing homes)
Prescription drugs
Rehabilitative services and long-term physical medicine (for example, physical therapy)

---

services are rendered by physicians or providers to an enrolled group of persons. Fixed periodic payments are made in advance to providers of services (**participating physicians**) by or on behalf of each person or family. If a health insurance carrier administers and manages the HMO, it contracts to pay in advance for the full range of health services to which the insured is entitled under the terms of the health insurance contract.

HMO Models

There are important differences in the structure of various HMOs that influence the way physicians practice and perhaps the quality of medical care delivered. Following are several types of HMO models.

Prepaid Group Practice Model. The *prepaid group practice model* delivers services at one or more locations through a group of physicians who contract with the HMO to provide care or through its own physicians who are employees of the HMO. For example, Kaiser Permanente is a prepaid group practice model wherein physicians form an independent group (Permanente) and contract with a health plan (Kaiser) to provide medical treatment to members enrolled by the plan. Although the physicians work for a salary, it is paid by their own independent group and not by the administrators of the health plan. This design permits the physicians to concentrate on medicine.

Staff Model. The **staff model** is a type of HMO in which the health plan hires physicians directly and pays them a salary instead of contracting with a medical group.

Network HMO. A *network HMO* contracts with two or more group practices to provide health services. It is common for those physicians to see both HMO and non-HMO patients in their own offices. Network physicians are typically paid a capitation amount for the care of each HMO patient in their panel of patients, regardless of whether the patient is actually seen by the physician in any given month.

Direct Contract Model. A common type of model in open-panel HMOs is the *direct contract model.* This type of managed care health plan contracts directly with private practice physicians in the community rather than through an intermediary such as an IPA or a medical group. Contracted health care services are delivered to subscribers by individual physicians in the community.

The Office of Health Maintenance Organizations can provide further information on HMOs.*

Exclusive Provider Organizations

An **exclusive provider organization (EPO)** is a type of managed care plan that combines features of HMOs (for example, enrolled population, limited provider panel, gatekeepers, utilization management, capitated provider reimbursement, and authorization system) and PPOs (for example, flexible benefit design, negotiated fees, and fee-for-service payments). It is referred to as exclusive because employers agree not to contract with any other plan. The member must choose medical care from network providers with certain exceptions for emergency or out-of-area services. If a patient decides to seek care outside the network, generally he or she is not reimbursed for the cost of the treatment. Technically, many HMOs can be considered EPOs. However, EPOs are regulated under insurance statutes rather than federal and state HMO regulations.

Foundations for Medical Care

A **foundation for medical care (FMC)** is an organization of physicians sponsored by a state or local medical association concerned with the development and delivery of medical services and the cost of health care. The first foundation for medical care was established in 1954 in Stockton, California. Foundations have sprung up across the US and some comprehensive foundations have assumed a portion of the underwriting risk for a defined population. Foundations deal primarily with various groups—employer groups, government groups, and county and city employees. Some plans are open to individual subscribers but these instances usually represent a small percentage of the foundation activity.

Two basic types of foundations for medical care operations exist and each functions differently: (1) a **comprehensive type of foundation,** which designs and sponsors prepaid health programs or sets minimum benefits of coverage; and (2) a **claims-review type of foundation,** which provides evaluation of the quality and efficiency of services by a panel of physicians to the numerous fiscal agents or carriers involved in its area, including those processing Medicare and Medicaid. Reviews are done for services or fees that exceed local community guidelines.

A key feature of the foundation is its dedication to an incentive reimbursement system. For a participating physician, income is received in direct proportion to the number of medical services delivered (for example, fee-for-service) rather than payment through capitation. The FMC offers a managed care plan fee schedule to be used by member physicians. In some areas, foundation physicians agree to accept the foundation allowance as payment in full for covered services. The patient is not billed for the balance. However, the patient is billed for non-benefit items, a deductible, and coinsurance.

The patient may select any member or nonmember physician he or she wishes. Member physicians agree to bill the foundation directly and a nonmember physician may wish to collect directly from the patient. Many foundations submit claims on the CMS-1500 (02-12) form and others transmit data electronically. The foundation movement has a national society, the American Managed Care and Review Association (AMCRA), which can provide further information on AMCRA or on foundations in an individual state.†

Independent Practice Associations

Another type of MCO is the **independent (or individual) practice association (IPA),** in which the physicians are not employees and are not paid salaries. Instead, they are paid for their services on a capitation or fee-for-service basis out of a fund drawn from the premiums

---

*Centers for Medicare and Medicaid Services, Room 4350, Cohen Building, 330 Independence Ave., SW, Washington, DC 20201.

†1227 25th St., NW, #610, Washington, DC 20037 (formerly known as the American Association of Foundation for Medical Care)

collected from the subscriber, union, or corporation by an organization that markets the health plan. A withheld amount of up to 30% is used to cover costs of operating the IPA. IPA physicians make contractual arrangements to treat HMO members out of their own offices. A participating physician may also treat non-HMO patients.

Preferred Provider Organizations

A **preferred provider organization (PPO)** is another type of managed care plan. A PPO contracts with a group of providers (designated as "preferred") to deliver care to members. PPO members have the freedom to choose any physician or hospital for services but they receive a high level of benefits if the preferred providers are used. There are usually coinsurance requirements and deductibles and claims have to be filed. Occasionally the PPOs pay 100% of the cost of care but most do not. As with major medical policies, coinsurance requires the patient to pay 20% to 25% of the allowed amount up to a certain point and then the PPO pays 80% to 100% of the balance. Predetermination of benefits may be required, as well as fee limits, quality control, and utilization review (UR). Some hospital indemnity plans pay fixed fees for various services. The patient pays the difference if the charges are higher.

Silent Preferred Provider Organizations

Sometimes preferred provider payers and plan administrators purchase existing preferred provider networks without talking to those providers who have signed contracts. These may be referred to as *silent, blind,* or *phantom PPOs, discounted indemnity plans, nondirected PPOs,* or *wraparound PPOs.* They gain the ability to limit reimbursement (lower or discount payments) without the provider's knowledge or consent. Providers that are taken in by silent PPOs are unable to get paid out of network, which reduces their income. Silent PPOs complicate the appeal process because it may be difficult to contact another payer directly and claims may be lost because of timely filing laws. Silent PPOs are considered legitimate in most states. Whenever you see "network discount applied" on an explanation of benefits document, investigate the claim further to determine whether a silent PPO is operating. To discover silent PPOs, always precertify procedures and look at patients' insurance cards even if the patients are established.

Physician Provider Groups

A **physician provider group (PPG)** is a physician-owned business entity that has the flexibility to deal with all forms of contract medicine and still offer its own packages to business groups, unions, and the general public. One division may function as an IPA under contract to an HMO. Another section may act as the broker or

provider in a PPO that contracts with hospitals, as well as other physicians, to market services or medical supplies to employers and other third parties. Still another portion might participate in joint ventures with hospitals, freestanding imaging centers and laboratories, purchase of diagnostic equipment, retail medical equipment as a corporate subsidiary, and so on. The sideline businesses do not pay dividends but provide income to make future assessments to participating physicians unnecessary. The difference between an IPA and a PPG is that member physicians may not own an IPA whereas a PPG is physician owned.

The ability of PPGs to combine services (joint purchasing, marketing, billing, collections, attorneys, and accountant fees) is an advantage because it cuts down on the cost of running a business and allows each physician to retain his or her own practice in addition to these joint ventures. The physicians turn over a small percentage of their income to the PPG for expenses. Patients call one telephone number to make appointments and the billing is done in one location.

Point-of-Service Plans

The typical **point-of-service (POS) plan** combines elements of an HMO and a PPO while offering some unique features. It is basically an HMO consisting of a network of physicians and hospitals that provides an insurance company or an employer with discounts on its services. In a POS program, members choose a PCP who manages specialty care and referrals. A POS plan allows the covered individual to choose services from a participating or nonparticipating provider with different benefit levels. The POS program pays members a higher level of benefits when they use program (network) providers. The member may use providers outside the network but higher deductibles and coinsurance percentages for out-of-network services act as incentives for members to stay within the network.

The POS plan may also provide nonparticipating benefits through a supplemental major medical policy. The key advantage of POS programs is the combination of HMO-style cost management and PPO-style freedom of choice.

Triple-Option Health Plans

Triple-option health plans allow members to select from three choices: HMOs, PPOs, or "traditional" indemnity insurance. Some of these plans allow the employee to change plans more often than traditional arrangements. They incorporate cost containment measures, such as precertification for hospital admission, hospital stays, and second surgical opinions.

Table 11-1	Types of Managed Care Organizations and Their Characteristics	
PLAN TYPE	**MEMBER ADVANTAGES**	**MEMBER DISADVANTAGES**
HMO	• Low cost for benefits • Preventive health care • No claim forms • Fixed, low copayments • Low monthly premium • Less out-of-pocket regardless of usage	• Restricted access to providers, tests, hospitals, and treatments except in emergencies or pay a penalty
Group model (open or closed panel)	• Providers care only for plan members	• Must use gatekeeper, approved providers
Staff model	• Providers on staff of HMO	• Must use gatekeeper, approved providers
Network model	• Providers see plan and nonplan patients • Small copayment per office visit • Providers receive capitation fee	• Must use gatekeeper, approved providers
Direct contract model	• Contracted health care services to members by private practice physicians in the community	
EPO	• Flexible benefit design • Providers give negotiated discounts	• Must use gatekeeper, approved providers except in emergencies • Employer contracts only with one plan • Patient who seeks care outside the network is not reimbursed
IPA	• Can use services from several affiliated providers, hospitals, or facilities • Out-of-pocket expenses minor	• Must use gatekeeper, approved providers
POS	• Patients choose network or non-network providers • Providers give negotiated discounts • More flexible than basic HMO • Can bypass gatekeeper to see specialist	• Pay more if member sees non-network provider
PPO	• More flexible than HMO • Does not require gatekeeper • Patients may choose network or non-network providers • Providers give negotiated discounts for each service and patients pay a small percentage • Pay less for network provider • Reduced costs for drugs	• Pay more if member sees non-network provider • Preventive services may not be covered • Patients pay a deductible • Claims must be filed • Possible predetermination of benefits • Pay fixed fees and patient pays the difference if bill is higher

EPO, Exclusive provider organization; *HMO*, health maintenance organization; *IPA*, independent (or individual) practice association; *POS*, point-of-service plan; *PPO*, preferred provider organization.

Provider-Sponsored Organization

A *provider-sponsored organization (PSO)* is a managed care plan that is owned and operated by a hospital and provider group instead of an insurance company.

Religious Fraternal Benefit Society

A *religious fraternal benefit society (RFBS)* is a managed care option that is associated with a church, group of churches, or convention. Membership is restricted to church members and is allowed regardless of the person's health status.

Tables 11-1 and 11-2 give an overview or summary of five of the most common types of managed care plans.

Employee Retirement Income Security Act

The insurance billing specialist should be aware that no matter what the type of plan, coverage is either purchased by an individual or paid by an employer. This is extremely important to know because when an employer

pays for the plan, it is regulated by the Employee Retirement Income Security Act (ERISA). However, after the passing of the federal legislation known as the *Patient Protection and Affordable Care Act (Affordable Care Act)* and H.R. 4872, the Health Care and Education Reconciliation Act of 2010 (the Reconciliation Act), beginning in 2014 almost everyone was required to be insured or they must pay a fine. Small businesses, the self-employed, and the uninsured may pick plans offered through state-based purchasing pools. Large employers with more than 50 employees must pay a $2000-per-employee fee, excluding the first 30 employees from the assessment, if the government subsidizes their workers' coverage. ERISA regulates all managed care insurance paid by the employer or supplemented by the employee for the employee's spouse or children, which today is about 85% of the claims that are non-Medicare/Medicaid/workers' compensation. ERISA is regulated by the Department of Labor; if the plan is an ERISA plan, the State Insurance Commissioners have no power to help with insurance carrier issues. Consequently, if the MCO is "related to" an employee benefit plan (EBP),

Table 11-2	Financial Systems of Managed Care Plans					
	Network					AUTHORIZATION
PLAN	IN	OUT	COPAY DEDUCTIBLE	PAYMENT METHOD		REQUIRED
HMO	X		Fixed copay	Capitated Fee-for-service (carve outs)		X
PPO	75%/25% 80%/20% 90%/10%	60%/40% 70%/30%	Fixed copay Deductible	Fee-for-service		X
IPA	Limit Large group		Fixed copay	Capitated Fee-for-service (carve outs)		X
EPO	X		Fixed copay	Fee-for-service Capitated		X
POS	X	X	Fixed copay Deductible	Fee-for-service Capitated		X

EPO, Exclusive provider organization; *HMO,* health maintenance organization; *IPA,* independent (or individual) practice association; *POS,* point-of-service plan; *PPO,* preferred provider organization.

the requirements of ERISA and its regulations are of overriding importance and severely restrict patient rights.

No employer is obligated to establish an EBP. To encourage them to do so, Congress has given them, their plans, their HMOs and insurers, and their administrators substantial immunities from liability. State regulation of HMOs administered by self-insured EBPs is preempted by ERISA; therefore employees cannot be protected by those state laws that limit the excesses of other HMOs not subject to ERISA.

Any case "relating to" an EBP falls under federal jurisdiction and is always moved from state court to federal court when a lawsuit is initiated. There the patient and provider will find that the usual state law tort claims are also preempted by ERISA; therefore any claims against the HMO or EBP for medical malpractice, wrongful death, fraud, nonpayment or incorrect payment of claims, and so on will be summarily dismissed if filed in state courts. Effective January 1, 2003, changes to ERISA took effect regarding time limitations on claims processing and the appeals process. Therefore you should know whether the policy is paid for by the patient or employer. Refer to the resources at the end of this chapter for more information on ERISA.

At the printing of this edition, the health care reform legislation has not been completely finalized and its impact on ERISA has not been stated. To keep you up to date as legislation is passed, additional provisions will be placed on the Evolve website.

MEDICAL REVIEW

Quality Improvement Organization

A *Quality Improvement Organization (QIO)* program (formerly known as *professional* or *peer review organization*) contracts with the Centers for Medicare and Medicaid

Services (CMS) to review medical necessity, reasonableness, appropriateness, and completeness and adequacy of inpatient hospital care for which additional payment is sought under the outlier provisions of the prospective payment system (PPS). Generally, it operates at the state level. A review addresses whether the services met professionally recognized standards of health care and may include whether the appropriate services were provided in appropriate settings. The QIO's professional medical staff performs these reviews. The results of the reviews are submitted to CMS. A review is an evaluation of the quality and efficiency of services rendered by a practicing physician or physicians within the specialty group. Practitioners in a managed care program may come under peer review by a QIO. A review may be used to examine evidence for admission and discharge of a hospital patient and to settle disputes over fees (see Chapter 17). QIOs are not restricted to MCO programs and also play a role in Medicare inpatient cases.

Quality Improvement System for Managed Care

Quality Improvement System for Managed Care (QISMC) is a CMS initiative to strengthen MCO efforts to protect and improve the health and satisfaction of Medicare and Medicaid beneficiaries. QISMC adopts a broad definition of "quality" to include the "measurement of health outcomes, consumer satisfaction, accountability of MCOs for achieving ongoing quality improvement, the need for intervention to achieve this improvement, and the importance of data collection, analysis, and reporting."

Utilization Review of Management

A management system called **utilization review (UR)** is necessary to control costs in a managed care setting. UR is a formal assessment of the cost and use of components of the health care system. The UR committee reviews individual cases to determine medical necessity for medical tests and procedures. It also watches over how providers use medical care resources. If medical care, tests, or procedures are denied, the patient must be informed of the need for the denied service and the risks of not having it. The written reasons for denial let the patient know his or her rights to receive the service and obligation to pay before obtaining such services.

Emphasis is placed on seeing a high volume of patients in a performance-based reimbursement system. **Churning** occurs when a physician sees a patient more than medically necessary, thus increasing revenue through an increased number of services. Churning may be seen in fee-for-service practices as well as in some managed care environments. **Turfing** is the term used when the sickest high-cost patients are transferred to other physicians so that the provider appears to be a low utilizer. **Buffing** is the term for making this practice look justifiable to the plan. All of these situations may affect UR.

MANAGEMENT OF PLANS

Contracts

Nationwide data from Medirisk, Inc.* can be used to make a knowledgeable financial decision on how a managed care plan will affect an existing medical practice. Data supplied by this company can help a practice to evaluate existing fees, negotiate with managed care firms, and weigh practice expansions (for example, add partners or a satellite office). A physician should have the contract reviewed by an attorney before signing a contract with a managed care plan.

Carve Outs

When an MCO contracts with a physician group, the following important considerations should be known:
1. How many patients will the MCO provide?
2. What is the per capita rate (capitation amount per patient)?
3. What services are included in the capitated amount?

Medical services not included in the contract benefits are called **carve outs** (not included within the capitation rate) and may be contracted for separately. For example, if an internist contracts with an MCO, all evaluation and management services, as well as electrocardiograms, spirometries, hematocrits, fasting blood sugar tests, and urinalyses, might be included in the capitation amount that is received per person, per month, regardless of whether any of these services were rendered. However, sigmoidoscopies and hospital visits might be "carved out" of the

contract and paid on a fee-for-service basis. Generally, physicians prefer carve outs for expensive procedures when contracting with MCOs.

PLAN ADMINISTRATION

Patient Information Letter

Inform managed care subscribers in writing what is expected from them and what they can expect in turn. The patient information letter should outline possible restrictions, noncovered items, expectations for copayment, and names of the managed care plans in which the physician is currently participating. Note that if the patient neglects to notify the office of any change in eligibility status in the plan, such as **disenrollment,** the patient is then held personally responsible for the bill. Also mention that the managed care patient must inform the office if hospitalization, surgery, or referral to a specialist is necessary. State that because of restrictions, failure to do so will make the patient liable for denied services. This letter may be referred to as a *waiver of liability* and in the Medicare program is called an *Advance Beneficiary Notice of Noncoverage (ABN)*. Post a sign in the waiting room advising managed care patients to check with the receptionist about participating plans.

Figure 11-2 shows a sample letter of appropriate wording and content. File a copy of the letter given to the patient in the patient's medical record. If the patient refuses to agree with managed care policy, document this in the medical record. Reimbursement may depend on the documentation.

> **HIPAA Compliance Alert**
> ### RIGHT TO AUDIT RECORDS
>
> When patients are members of a managed care organization (MCO) and the physician has signed a contract with the MCO that has a clause stating "for quality care purposes, the MCO has a right to access the medical records of their patients and for utilization management purposes," the MCO has a right to audit those patients' financial records that relate only to the medical services provided to the member by the physician.

Medical Records
When using an electronic medical record (EMR) system, the patient's account may be identified with a patient type that corresponds with the insurance plan the patient has joined.

Scheduling Appointments
Screen patients when they call for appointments to determine whether they belong to the same prepaid health plan as the physician. Ask the patient to read from the

*5901 Peachtree Dunwoody Road, NE, Suite 455, Building B, Atlanta, GA 30328.

XYZ MEDICAL GROUP, INC.
1400 Avon Road, Suite 200
Woodland Hills, XY 12345

January 1, 20XX

TO: OUR PATIENTS

RE: PREFERRED PROVIDER ORGANIZATIONS

The following is a list of the PPOs and health insurance plans that we are members of and, therefore, will bill for you:

1. Georgia County Foundation
2. VIP Health Plan
3. Blue Cross Prudent Buyer Plan
4. Georgia County PPO
5. Northwest PPO
6. Blue Shield PPO

We are participating providers in several different PPOs. In order that we may maintain proper records for referrals and/or hospitalization, we request that each patient who is enrolled in a specific PPO keep our office currently informed regarding his or her eligibility status in that plan. Each time you are in the office for a visit, please verify with the receptionist that we have the correct coverage information.

If you have not informed us of changes in the status of your eligibility within the plan, you will be held responsible for any outstanding balance on your account due to that change.

Additionally, when your physician feels it is necessary to either hospitalize you or refer you to another physician outside this group, it is your responsibility to inform your physician that you belong to a specific PPO, as there may be restrictions imposed by that PPO regarding admission and referrals. If you fail to inform your physician at the time of referral or admission, our group may not be held responsible for noncoverage charges due to these restrictions.

If you have any questions regarding the above, please ask to speak to our insurance specialist.

I have read and understand the above text.

Signed: _____   Date: _____
                    Patient (subscriber)

FIGURE 11-2 Letter to preferred provider organization (PPO) subscribers outlining restrictions and noncovered services.

---

insurance card to determine whether the physician's name is listed as the patient's PCP. Keep on hand an alphabetic list and profile of all plans with which the practice has a signed contract. It might also be useful to have a list of plans to which the practice does not belong. If the patient is not in a participating plan and still wishes to schedule a visit, inform him or her that payment at the time of the appointment is necessary and the amount is determined by the private fee schedule. This is an excellent idea if the patient is not a member of an HMO. In some states (Florida, for example), an HMO patient cannot be billed for services that are covered. The provider must obtain authorization to treat the patient if the person is an HMO patient and the provider is not a participating provider because collecting from the HMO patient could "backfire" on the provider. The patient will pay for the visit and

then send a copy of the receipt to his or her HMO. The HMO could file a complaint with the appropriate HMO regulatory agency because the provider treated its client without authorization and billed the client for the balance. The HMO could request a claim form from the provider and the provider would enter his or her private fee, which is more than the provider billed the HMO for another patient. This would open the door to possible fraud and abuse charges. The HMO could contact the patient, stating that he or she should not have had to pay for the visit because the patient was in an HMO. Finally, the patient could demand a refund and the provider would have no choice but to refund the money because the patient could turn the provider over to the HMO regulatory agency. The assignment of benefits must be checked on the claim form, either to the provider or to the patient.

Encounter Form

Many managed care plans use an internal document on which the services rendered to the patient are checked off (charge ticket, encounter form, routing slip). It also may be used as a billing statement. The original is forwarded to the health plan's administrative office and a copy is retained in the physician's files. Some plans require data from such documentation on a CMS-1500 (02-12) Health Insurance Claim form. Examples of encounter forms are shown in Figures 3-11, 8-3, and 10-9.

Preauthorization or Prior Approval

Some managed care plans require preauthorization for certain services or referral of a patient to see a specialist. The following are several types of referrals that a plan may use.

1. **Formal referral.** An authorization request is required by the MCO contract to determine medical necessity. This may be obtained via telephone or a completed authorization form (Figure 11-3) mailed or transmitted by fax or e-mail.
2. **Direct referral.** An authorization request form is completed and signed by the physician and handed to the patient. Certain services may not require completion of a form and may be directly referred (for example, obstetric care, dermatology).
3. **Verbal referral.** The PCP informs the patient and telephones the referring physician to inform that the patient is being referred for an appointment.
4. **Self-referral.** The patient refers himself or herself to a specialist. The patient may be required to inform the PCP.

Patients may be unaware of preapproval requirements. A good precaution is to ask the patient about insurance coverage at the time the appointment is made. If the patient is a member of a managed care plan, carefully review the patient's preauthorization requirements. If approval is necessary for certain situations, inform the patient of this before he or she sees the physician. If a patient has obtained the written authorization approval, ask the patient to fax or mail you a copy because it may have an expiration date noted on it. Even if preapproved, the treatment must be medically necessary or payment may be denied after submission of a claim. If an authorization is delayed and the patient comes in for the appointment, the plan should be called to obtain a verbal authorization. The date, time, and name of the authorizing person should be documented; otherwise, the patient's appointment should be rescheduled. A referral recommendation must be documented in the patient's record and, if applicable, sent to the referring physician.

A tracking system, such as a referral tracking log, should be in place for pending referrals so that care may be rendered in a timely manner and patients do not get "lost" in the system (Figure 11-4). This log should include the date on which the authorization is requested, the patient's name, procedure or consultant requested, insurance plan, effective and expiration dates, dates of follow-up, name of person who approved or denied the request, and appointment date for consult or procedure. Sometimes authorization approvals are sent to the PCP and not to the referring or ordering physician. In these cases, follow-up must be made with the PCP. A maximum 2-week turnaround time should be allowed and all authorization requests should be tracked.

If a managed care plan refuses to authorize payment for recommended treatment, tests, or procedures, have the PCP send a letter to the plan that is worded similarly to that shown in Figure 11-5. Include medical documentation, such as office visit notes, laboratory reports, and x-ray reports, to support the insurance claim. Then, after all efforts have been exhausted, send a letter such as the one shown in Figure 11-6 to the patient informing him or her of this fact and asking the patient to appeal the denial of benefits.

In some managed care plans, when a PCP sends a patient for consultation to a specialist who is not in the managed care plan, the specialist bills the PCP. This is done because the PCP receives a monthly capitation check from the plan and any care for the patient must come from the capitation pool. This type of plan encourages PCPs not to refer patients so that they can retain profits.

If a specialist recommends referral to another specialist (**tertiary care**), ensure that the recommendation is provided in writing. Call the specialist at a later date to determine whether the recommendation was acted on. If the patient refuses to be referred, ensure that this is documented. If a referral form is necessary, do not telephone or write a letter. The managed care plan may refuse payment if the proper form is not completed.

When a referral authorization form is received, make a copy of the form for each approved office visit, laboratory test, or series of treatments. Then use the form as a reference to bill for the service. All copies being used indicates that all services that the patient's plan has approved are completed. Ask the PCP or the managed care plan for a new authorization to continue treatment on the patient. The request should be generated in a timely manner so that treatment is not delayed.

Diagnostic Tests

Many managed care plans require that patients have laboratory and radiology tests performed at plan-specified

College Clinic
4567 Broad Avenue
Woodland Hills, XY 12345-0001
Telephone: (555) 486-9002
Fax: (555) 487-8976

MANAGED CARE PLAN AUTHORIZATION REQUEST

**TO BE COMPLETED BY PRIMARY CARE PHYSICIAN
OR OUTSIDE PROVIDER**

☐ Health Net   ☐ Met Life
☒ Pacificare   ☐ Travelers
☐ Secure Horizons   ☐ Pru Care
☐ Other

Member/Group No.: __54098XX__

Patient Name: __Louann Campbell__   Date: __7-14-20XX__

☐ Male   ☐ Female   Birthdate: __4-7-1952__   Home Telephone Number: __(555) 450-1666__

Address: __2516 Encina Avenue, Woodland Hills, XY 12345-0439__

Primary Care Physician: __Gerald Practon, MD__   Provider ID #: __TC 14021__

Referring Physician: __Gerald Practon, MD__   Provider ID #: __TC 14021__

Referred to: __Raymond Skeleton, MD__   Office Telephone number: __(555) 486-9002__

Address: __4567 Broad Avenue, Woodland Hills, XY 12345__

Diagnosis Code: __724.2__   Diagnosis __Low back pain__

Diagnosis Code: __722.10__   Diagnosis __Sciatica__

Treatment Plan: __Orthopedic consultation and evaluation of lumbar spine; R/O herniated disc L4-5__

Authorization requested for: ☐ Consult only   ☐ Treatment only   ☐ Consult/Treatment
                               ☐ Consult/Procedure/Surgery   ☐ Diagnostic Tests

Procedure Code: __99244__   Description: __New patient consultation__

Procedure Code: _____   Description: _____

Place of service: ☒ Office ☐ Outpatient ☐ Inpatient ☐ Other   Number of Visits: __1__

Facility: _____   Length of Stay: _____

List of potential future consultants (i.e., anesthetists, surgical assistants, or medical/surgical):

Physician's Signature: __Gerald Practon, MD__

TO BE COMPLETED BY PRIMARY CARE PHYSICIAN

PCP Recommendations: __See above__   PCP Initials: __GP__

Date eligibility checked: __7-14-20XX__   Effective Date: __1-15-20XX__

TO BE COMPLETED BY UTILIZATION MANAGEMENT

Authorized: _____ Auth. No. _____ Not Authorized _____

Deferred: _____   Modified: _____

Effective date: _____ Expiration date: _____ Number of visits: _____

FIGURE 11-3 A managed care plan treatment authorization request form completed by a primary care physician (PCP) for preauthorization of a professional service.

facilities. These are referred to as *network facilities*. Obtain the necessary authorizations for such services and allow sufficient time to receive the test or x-ray results before the patient's return appointment. When verifying benefits, ask if the deductible applies; that is, if a provider orders a radiology service that is on site, the deductible may not apply, but if the patient is sent to an outside facility, the deductible applies.

Inform the patient ahead of time when there is doubt about coverage for a test or the managed care plan indicates that a test is not covered. Disclose the cost and have

AUTHORIZATION REQUEST LOG

Date requested	Patient name	Procedure/ consult	Insurance plan	1st F/U	2nd F/U	3rd F/U	Approved	Scheduled date
2/8/XX	Juan Percy	Bone scan- full body	Health Net	2/20			J. Smith	2/23/XX
2/8/XX	Nathan Takai	MRI-L-knee	Pru-Care	2/20	3/3			
2/9/XX	Lori Smythe	Consult Neuro G. Frankel MD	FHP	2/22			T. Hope	2/26/XX
2/10/XX	Bob Mason	Cervical collar	Secure Horizons	2/22	3/5	3/19		

FIGURE 11-4 An authorization request log to be used as a system for tracing referral of patients for diagnostic testing, procedures, and consultations.

Ms. Jane Smith
Chairperson
Utilization Review Committee
ABC Managed Care Plan
111 Main Street
Anytown, XY 12345-0122

Dear Ms. Smith:

On _____ I prescribed_____ for_____.
      Date   List treatment, test, procedure   Patient's name

On _____ you refused to authorize for that treatment. I find that I
      Date
must take issue with your determination for the following reasons:

In my medical judgment, the treatment is a very important part of my overall care of_____
_____. This patient suffers from_____. The treatment is
Patient's name   Describe condition
necessary to _____. Failure to perform the treatment could
                    Describe why necessary
result in the following problem(s):

Enclosed are copies of the laboratory and radiological reports. For these reasons, I urge you to reconsider your refusal to authorize payment for the procedure I have prescribed.

By copy of this letter to_____ I am reiterating my suggestion that
                            Patient's name
he/she obtain the treatment despite your refusal to authorize payment, for the reasons I
have set forth in this letter and in prior discussions with _____.
                                                      Patient's name
Yours truly,

John Doe, MD
Enclosures
cc: (Name of patient)

FIGURE 11-5 A letter to a managed care plan when there is a refusal to authorize payment for a recommended treatment, test, or procedure.

Mr. Avery Johnson
130 Sylvia Street
Anytown, XY 12345-0022

Dear Mr. Johnson:

On ———————— I prescribed ———————————— for you. On ——————— ,
        Date   Treatment, test, procedure   Date

——————————————————— refused to authorize for same. On that basis,
     Name of Managed Care Plan
you have informed me of your decision to forego the treatment I have prescribed. I
expressed my concerns regarding your decision during our discussion on ——————— about
                                                                          Date
the potential ramifications of your refusal to undergo the treatment.

The purpose of this letter is to recommend that you appeal ———————————————
                                                            Name of Managed Care Plan's
denial of benefits and reconsider your decision to forego the treatment in light of the
potential consequences of your refusal.

Should you wish to discuss this further, please do not hesitate to contact me.

Sincerely yours,

John Doe, MD

FIGURE 11-6 A letter sent by the provider to inform the patient about refusal of payment for treatment, test, or procedure by the managed care plan.

the patient sign a waiver agreement to pay for the service, thus enabling the billing of the patient for the service. If an authorization is denied because a test is deemed "medically unnecessary" and the physician wishes to appeal, the physician can present clinical reasons to the MCO's medical director to receive approval and bring attention to possible expansion of benefits for future patients.

Managed Care Guide

Creating a grid or matrix of all MCOs with which the practice has contracts can help you to keep up with the growth of local managed care plans and remember which physician belongs to which plan in the practice. Use a sheet of paper and list each plan with the billing address vertically in a column to the left. Then list significant data horizontally across the top. Suggested titles for column categories are as follows: eligibility telephone numbers, copayment amounts, preauthorization requirements, restrictions on tests frequently ordered, participating laboratories, participating hospitals, and the contract's time limit for promised payment. Referring to this grid can provide specifics about each plan's coverage and copayment amounts at a glance (Figure 11-7). Some practices keep this information in a three-ring binder with dividers for each insurance plan. A good procedure is to include this information on each patient's data sheet when benefits are verified.

FINANCIAL MANAGEMENT

Payment

Deductibles

Usually there is no deductible for a managed care plan. However, if there is one, be sure to verify with the insurance company, ask patients if they have met their deductibles, and collect them in the early months of the year (January through April). Deductibles are applied to claims as they are received and processed by the plan.

Copayments

In a managed care plan, a copayment is a predetermined fee paid by the patient to the provider at the time service is rendered. It is commonly referred to as a *copay* and is a form of cost sharing because the managed care plan or insurance company pays the remaining cost. Remember to verify the copayment amount when inquiring about insurance plan benefits. Always collect the copay at the time of the patient's office visit. Billing for small amounts is not cost effective. Copays are commonly made for office visits, prescription drugs, inpatient mental health services, urgent care visits, and emergency department visits. However, the amount may vary according to the type

MANAGED CARE PLAN REFERENCE GUIDE

Plan name/address	Telephone eligibility	Copay	Preauthorization requirements	Test restrictions	Contracted lab(s) radiology	Contracted hospital(s)	Promised payment
Aetna PPO POB 43 WH XY 12345	555-239-0067	$5	hosp/surg/all dx tests	PE 1/yr	ABC Labs	College Hosp	30 days
Blue PPO POB 24335 WH XY 12345	555-245-0899	$8	referral specialist	PE 1/yr	Main St. Lab	St. John MC	30 days
Health Net POB 54000 WH XY 12345	555-408-5466	$5	hosp/surg see check list referrals	Mammo-gram 1/yr	Valley Lab	St. Joseph MC	45 days
Travelers MCO POB 1200 WH XY 12345	555-435-9877	$10	surg/hosp admit referrals	Pap >50 q3yr <50 q1yr	College Hosp Metro Lab	College Hosp	30 days

FIGURE 11-7 Managed care plan quick reference guide to help keep track of specifics for each managed care plan in which the physician participates.

of service. In some plans there may be a separate copayment for x-ray studies and durable medical equipment.

Payment Models and Mechanisms

Concierge Medicine. Because insurance companies are paying less for services and there is an increase in documentation and paperwork, some physicians have opted to collect a monthly and/or annual retainer fee from patients. This system may be referred to as "concierge medicine" or "direct pay." A monthly fee can range from $50 to $150 or an annual fee can range from $1200 to $10,000. Services might include same-day appointments, more time for an office visit, and contact with physicians via telephone, e-mail, and text messaging. If the patient also has an insurance plan, the patient may have to do the paperwork and file the insurance claim.

Cash-Only Practices. Some physicians have decided not to join a network and prefer to have patients pay cash. If the patient has insurance, some physicians generate a completed CMS-1500 claim form so that the patient can submit the claim to the insurance company.

Value-Based Reimbursement. With the advent of the Affordable Care Act, medical providers are beginning to move away from long-standing volume-based health care models toward value-based care models. For example, the fee-for-service model rewards volume and intensity of service so that more procedures and hospital admissions give more money to the provider versus value-based health care, which aligns payment and measures objectively the

clinical quality of health care. Some of these value-based models are listed here.

Pay for Performance. Providers receive fee-for-service payments and also receive compensation or bonuses for complying with certain clinical goals. For example, a goal might be to immunize 80% of the practice's patients by age 2 using nationally approved guidelines. If the provider exceeds that goal, reaching a higher percentage, then the medical practice receives a bonus.

Bundled Payment/Episode of Care. Providers agree to accept a single negotiated fee to deliver all medical services for one patient for a specified procedure or condition (for example, hip replacement surgery, pregnancy and birth, certain cardiac procedures). This can reduce costs for payers and increase payment to providers. The provider tries to improve efficiency and quality within episodes. However, one must watch that the costs of services for the procedures or conditions do not exceed the agreed-upon reimbursement amount.

Patient-Centered Medical Home (PCMH). The medical home consists of a single team managing with better coordination of medical care that agrees to provide more services. It is paid a negotiated fee-for-service plus a monthly payment based on per-member-per-month (PMPM) and/or a pay-for-performance incentive. The team or group must show certain organizational and structural capabilities (for example, extended office hours, use of electronic health records, e-prescribing, patient disease registries).

Shared Savings (One-Sided Risk). A combination of payment systems (fee-for-service, pay for performance, bundled payments, global payments, or capitation) that rewards providers that reduce total health care spending on their patients below an expected level set by the payer. Providers receive a share of the savings.

Shared Risk. Providers receive performance-based incentives to share cost savings combined with disincentives to share the excess costs of health care delivery. There is an agreed-upon budget with the payer and the provider must cover a portion of costs if savings targets are not achieved (for example, a percentage of premium or a set amount [50/50 sharing of excess costs]). If the payer wants the provider to accept more risk, the provider can either obtain stop-loss insurance or carve out certain patients or conditions. Another way of limiting risk would be to include a risk corridor arrangement. A corridor protects from high loss but at the same time obstructs opportunities for gains.

Provider-Sponsored Health Plans (PSHPs). A large provider network or hospital system assumes 100% of the financial risk for insuring the patient population. It collects premiums from employers or individuals and directs how care is delivered to patients and how much is spent on giving that care. To set this up, the organization must have an insurance license and obtain approval as a health plan for the state in which it operates commercial, Medicare Advantage, or Medicaid plans. Such systems have responsibilities, such as claims payment, customer service, insurance reporting, and so on.

Full Risk: Capitation Models. These value-based systems involve managed care plans that can range from fee-for-service and capitation to salaried physicians. Details about other payment mechanisms follow.

Contact Capitation. Contact capitation is based on the concept of paying physicians for actual patient visits or "contacts." A scenario under this payment method occurs when a patient is referred to a specialist for care. A "contact" occurs when the patient visits the specialist for treatment. The patient is assigned to the specialist for a defined period of time called the *contact period.* The length of the contact period is set in advance for each type of specialty by the participating specialty physician panel and MCO and it may be tailored to the demographic and practice needs of the group. Each new patient visit during a contact period initiates a "contact point." Contact points determine how much to pay each physician. The average contact point value is determined by dividing the net specialty capitation pool or total amount of money set aside to be used for a particular specialty by the number of contacts in a certain time period. The average contact

value is used to determine the amount paid to each specialist during each month in the contact period.

Case Rate Pricing. For specialists, another payment method is case rate pricing. This means that the specialist contracts with the managed care plan for an entire episode of care. This may be done for certain high-volume, expensive surgical procedures (for example, knee surgery, cataracts, bypass surgery).

Stop-Loss Limit. Some contracts have a **stop-loss** section, which means that if the patient's services are more than a certain amount, the physician can begin asking the patient to pay (fee-for-service). Monitor each patient's financial accounting record in those instances.

Contract Payment Time Limits

Usually state laws dictate the time limit within which a managed care plan must pay. The contract may or may not state the terms of payment, time limits, and late payment penalties, all of which can vary from one plan to another. Prompt payment laws require payment within 30, 45, 55, or 60 days. To diminish late payment of claims, a contract can specify that late claims accrue interest (for example, 5% interest for claims paid after the payment time limit has elapsed). Some states have enacted laws enforcing interest penalties for late payment for either or both private payers, as well as managed care plans. Therefore know the laws for the pertinent state. A time limit payment provision is an important factor to consider when reviewing a contract before a medical practice participates.

Monitoring Payment

Monitor payments made from all managed care plans and note whether the payment received is less than the agreed amount as stated in the contract. If payment has been reduced, send a letter to the plan citing, "As per contract, see page xx about the fee for the consultation."

Sometimes a procedure (for example, angioplasty with an assistant) may be done and the plan will not pay for an assistant, stating that it is not usual practice. However, perhaps the standard practice in a specific region is to always use an assistant for an angioplasty. When this is emphasized, the plan may remit additional payment.

Some states may have screening fees for emergency services and may or may not require prior approval for such services as defined by the Consolidated Omnibus Budget Reconciliation Act of 1985 (COBRA). Some states have adjudication laws with penalties if the managed care plan does not pay promptly. The following steps should be taken if claims are not paid in a timely manner (30 days):

1. Write to the plan representative and list unpaid claims, claims paid after the payment time limit, and claims paid in error.
2. Send a statement to the director of the managed care plan notifying him or her that if the bill is not paid, the employer's benefits manager or patient will be contacted and alerted to outstanding, slow-paying accounts. Explain that this will prevent the physician from renewing the plan's contract and ask the recipient to contact the plan's representative. The consumer has a choice of managed care plans; if the present plan does not fulfill his or her expectations, the managed care plan loses members because of dissatisfaction.
3. Take examples and statistics to the next renegotiating session when the physician's contract is expiring.

Chapters 9 and 10 present information on how to handle slow or delinquent managed care plan payers.

Statement of Remittance

Managed care plans pay either by a capitation system (monthly check for the number of patients in the plan) or on the basis of the services given to the patient (monthly check with a statement of remittance or explanation of benefits [EOB]).

In the capitation system, a monthly check arrives written out for the total amount of monthly capitation. The accompanying paperwork lists all eligible patients being paid for on a per capita basis divided into two groups: commercial and senior. Patients categorized as commercial are usually younger than age 65 and are paid at a lesser rate because their risk is lower (for example, they do not need to see the doctor frequently). The senior patient category includes those older than 65 years of age; these are paid at a higher rate because of the increased risk. Always verify the individual capitated amounts listed by each name on the accompanying paperwork against the monthly eligibility list to balance the amount of the check. Contact the MCO if an error appears. If a specialist is capitated, there may be thousands of patients on the capitation plan and a list of patients will not be provided. The capitation amount for a specialist may be only a few cents per month calculated according to the risk of the patient needing specialty services.

In the system where payment is based on services rendered and a statement of remittance or EOB is generated, such statements itemize services that have been rendered to patients and usually indicate the amount billed, amount allowed, amount paid, and any copayment to be made by the patient (Figure 11-8). Generally patients under

STATEMENT OF REMITTANCE

PATIENT NAME (ID NUMBER)	SERVICE DATE MO. DAY YR	POS	NO SVC	PROCEDURE NUMBER AND DESCRIPTION	AMOUNT BILLED	AMOUNT ALLOWED	RISK WITHHELD	CO PAY	AMOUNT PAID	ADJ. CODE
380224171-01 ALAN E.				CLAIM NO. 62730406 ACCOUNT NO.						
	092620XX	03	1	81000 URINALYSIS-ROUTINE	1000	1000	100	0	900	
	092620XX	03	1	82270 OCCULT BLOOD ANY S	1200	1200	120	0	1080	
	092620XX	03	1	99243 COMPRE RE-EXAM OR	6500	6500	650	0	5850	
	092620XX	03	1	36415 VENIPUNCTURE W/CEN	1700	1700	170	0	1530	
				CLAIM TOTALS =10400	10400	10400	1040	0	9360	
558700321-01 RONALD B.				CLAIM NO. 62730407 ACCOUNT NO.						
	092520XX	03	1	90050 LIM EXAM EVAL A/O	3000	3000	300	300	2400	
				CLAIM TOTALS = 3000	3000	3000	300	300	2400	
473760096-01 DORMA L.				CLAIM NO. 62730408 ACCOUNT NO.						
	092520XX	03	1	90050 LIM EXAM EVAL A/O	3000	3000	300	300	2400	
				CLAIM TOTALS = 3800	3000	300	380		3120	

VENDOR SUMMARY: TOTAL AMOUNT PAID $1,638.96   TOTAL WITHHELD $194.39
AMOUNT PAID YEAR-TO-DATE: $42,411.95   AMOUNT WITHHELD YEAR-TO-DATE $5,109.94

Adjustment Code Legend
A = Adjusted: Billed amount exceeds VIP allowed.
O = Claim for service denied. Charges for this service included in other benefit payment. No patient liability.

FIGURE 11-8 Statement of remittance or explanation of benefits for noncapitated patients or contracted fee-for-service indicating the amount billed, amount allowed, amount paid, and any copayment to be made by the patient.

managed care plans do not receive an EOB. Payments are checked against the managed care contract for verification and then posted to the patients' accounts. An error should be brought to the attention of the plan's administrator and, depending on the circumstances, appealed.

Accounting

Managed care plans vary in their financial reimbursement structure and careful accounting procedures are required. Accounting can become a confusing issue because of a mixture of private and managed care patients with copayment requirements, coinsurance amounts, deductibles, and withholds. Good practice management software is designed to handle each plan in the computer separately to eliminate mistakes.

Fee-for-Service

Some medical practices handle managed care patient accounts the same as fee-for-service patient accounts. If coinsurance payment is necessary at the time of service,

post first the charge and then the coinsurance prepayment, calculated based on either the percentage of the charge the plan allows or the flat copayment amount (for example, $15 for each office visit). After receiving the EOB document from the insurance plan, post an adjustment entry of the disallowed amount, which is calculated on a percentage of the MCO's allowable charge to balance the account (Figure 11-9). An overpayment should be shown as a refund or credit to the account.

Year-End Evaluation
Withhold

Depending on the contract, a managed care plan may retain a percentage of the monthly capitation payment or a percentage of the allowable charges to physicians until the end of the year to cover operating expenses. This is known as **withhold**. A statement of remittance from the MCO shows the risk amounts withheld for each patient's visit in the eighth column of Figure 11-8. The withhold plus interest is returned to the physician at the

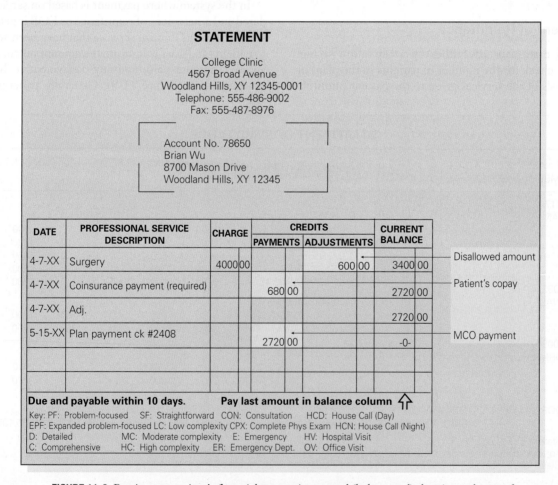

STATEMENT

College Clinic
4567 Broad Avenue
Woodland Hills, XY 12345-0001
Telephone: 555-486-9002
Fax: 555-487-8976

Account No. 78650
Brian Wu
8700 Mason Drive
Woodland Hills, XY 12345

DATE	PROFESSIONAL SERVICE DESCRIPTION	CHARGE	CREDITS		CURRENT BALANCE	
			PAYMENTS	ADJUSTMENTS		
4-7-XX	Surgery	4000 00		600 00	3400 00	← Disallowed amount
4-7-XX	Coinsurance payment (required)		680 00		2720 00	← Patient's copay
4-7-XX	Adj.				2720 00	
5-15-XX	Plan payment ck #2408		2720 00		-0-	← MCO payment

Due and payable within 10 days.   Pay last amount in balance column ⇑

Key: PF: Problem-focused   SF: Straightforward CON: Consultation   HCD: House Call (Day)
EPF: Expanded problem-focused LC: Low complexity CPX: Complete Phys Exam HCN: House Call (Night)
D: Detailed   MC: Moderate complexity   E: Emergency   HV: Hospital Visit
C: Comprehensive   HC: High complexity   ER: Emergency Dept.   OV: Office Visit

FIGURE 11-9 Posting to a patient's financial accounting record (ledger card) showing a charge of $4000. The plan allows $3400; therefore the patient's prepaid coinsurance amount is $680 (20% of $3400). The managed care plan sent a check for $2720 (80% of $3400) and the disallowed amount ($600) is adjusted off the account, which brings the account balance to zero.

DEBIT						
Date	Patient	Service	Charge	Withhold	Disallow	
5/15/20XX	Mason	99204	106.11	5.94	21.22	Disallowed amounts
5/15/20XX	Mason	93000	34.26	1.92	3.43	
5/15/20XX	Mason	81000	8.00	.38	2.40	
5/15/20XX	Self	93501	1500.00	240.00	300.00	
Total			1648.38	248.24	327.05	Total withheld amount owed by MCO

FIGURE 11-10 A managed care plan when payment is on a fee-for-service basis. Note the disallowed portion of the charge, which is based on the plan's allowable charge. A portion of the allowable charge is withheld.

end of the plan year if the budgeted services for the plan are not overused. However, the withhold or a portion of it is retained by the plan if services are overused. Thus physicians share in any surplus or pay part of any deficit at year's end. This risk sharing creates an incentive for limiting care by the gatekeeper and limiting referrals to specialists, thereby keeping medical costs down. The withhold can cover all services or be specific to hospital care, **ancillary services** (laboratory, x-ray use), or specialty referrals.

A managed care plan that withholds a percentage of the allowable charge must be tracked in the physician's accounts receivable so that it is not prematurely written off as a bad debt. To do this, develop a capitation accounting worksheet listing the dates of service, patients' names, Current Procedural Terminology (CPT) code for the service rendered, fee-for-service charges, withheld amounts, and disallowed amounts (Figure 11-10). Then total all columns. The total of the withheld column is a debit entry that indicates what the managed care plan owes to the medical practice pending its year-end reconciliation. If and when the withheld amount arrives, the accounting worksheet can be compared with the amount withheld during the year. The amount of withholds that are not returned to the physician is adjusted once withholds are settled. The total of the column for disallowed amounts shows the amount written off by the medical practice. Combine the withheld returned amount with the managed care payment for the year to determine whether it is worthwhile for the practice to participate in the plan. Some practices can use the information to renegotiate increased fees when the managed care contract is to be renewed.

Capitation versus Fee-for-Service

Financial management reports are generated via computer and are the responsibility of the manager or accountant in most medical practices. However, it can be an asset for an insurance billing specialist to have some knowledge of the content of these reports. Most medical practices monitor plan payments for profit or loss by comparing actual income from managed care patients with what would have been received from fee-for-service plans. To do this, one designs a capitation accounting sheet for each capitated plan. This sheet shows a listing of dates of service and professional service descriptions (procedures, injections, and laboratory work) as well as charges and payments (Figure 11-11). As managed care plan patients receive services, actual service fees are posted in a charge column from the office fee schedule as if the patient were a private payer. In a payment column, office visit, copayments, and the monthly capitation payment are posted. Then all columns are totaled. It is necessary to apply a discount to the total charged amount for a realistic comparison because the physician is usually paid on an allowed amount rather than an actual charge. Calculate the difference between the actual charge and the average allowed amount to do this.

Compare the capitated payment amounts plus copayment amounts with the total discounted charges at the end of the year. This gives an accurate idea of whether the capitated payment received is adequate for the services the physician performed. Compiling monthly records and reviewing them at the end of the year helps a medical practice to assess the gain or loss of each capitation plan.

Bankruptcy

If an MCO declares bankruptcy, such as through a Chapter 11 filing, it is obligated to pay all bills incurred before the filing. However, in some situations, another entity may take over the plan and all services incurred after filing are paid by the new payer. If the patient had treatment before the filing, a delay in getting reimbursed may occur because the MCO cannot repay debts incurred before its filing until it has worked out a reorganization plan. Physicians under contract with the MCO are obligated to honor their

CAPITATION ACCOUNTING WORKSHEET

NAME OF PLAN ABC Managed Care Plan

DATE OF SERVICE	PROFESSIONAL SERVICE DESCRIPTION	CHARGES Services Fees	PAYMENTS Capitation	Copay	
20XX 1/15	Capitation (105 members) @ $8 ea		840.00		Capitation payment
2/15	Capitation (115 members)		920.00		
2/20	Sanchez OV/Copay	35.00		5.00	Copayment amount
2/22	Jones OV/Copay	35.00		5.00	
2/23	Davis OV/Copay	35.00		5.00	Actual fee-for-service charge
3/6	Evans OV/Copay	35.00		5.00	
3/15	Capitation (130 members)		1040.00		
4/10	Wu OV/Copay	35.00		5.00	
4/15	Capitation (135 members)		1080.00		
	May through December are not shown				
END OF YEAR TOTALS		3500.00	6880.00	500.00	

FIGURE 11-11 An accounting sheet for a capitation plan from January through April showing dates of service, professional service descriptions, members' charges, and capitation payments and copayments received by the medical practice. Charges and payments columns may be totaled at the end of the year to compare capitation with fee-for-service earnings.

contractual commitments. If their contracts expire or if they have escape clauses, they may be required to continue accepting patients, depending on the contract provisions.

Some clauses allow a physician to withdraw from seeing managed care patients or leave if the MCO is in bankruptcy proceedings for more than 4 months. However,

bankruptcy courts have broad powers to prevent physicians from leaving MCOs in bankruptcy proceedings if the court deems such actions to be detrimental to the rehabilitation of the debtor.

For additional information on bankruptcy, see Chapter 10.

KEY POINTS

This is a brief chapter review, or summary, of the key issues presented. To further enhance your knowledge of the technical subject matter, review the key terms and key abbreviations for this chapter by locating the meaning for each in the Glossary at the end of this book, which appears in a section before the Index.

1. Providers must be contracted with Blue Cross/Blue Shield to receive payment as a member physician. Patients may have a traditional fee-for-service or one of many types of managed care plans. Plan benefits and coverage, as well as deductibles and copayments, vary.

2. Managed care plans are prepayment health care programs in which a specified set of health benefits is provided in exchange for a yearly fee or fixed periodic payments to the provider of service. Patients join the plan and pay monthly medical insurance premiums individually or through their employer. Patients pay a small copayment and sometimes a deductible for medical services.

3. Primary care physicians (PCPs) act as gatekeepers who control patient access to specialists and diagnostic testing services.

4. Health maintenance organizations (HMOs) have models, such as prepaid group practice model, staff model, network HMO, and direct contract model.

5. The Patient Protection and Affordable Care Act (the Affordable Care Act) and H.R. 4872, the Health Care and Education Reconciliation Act of 2010 (the Reconciliation Act), have provisions effective within a year that include the following: forbids insurers from canceling insurance coverage (rescission), eliminates preexisting condition exclusions, ends lifetime limits on benefits, gives tax credits to small businesses that offer coverage, provides temporary insurance until 2014 for people who have been denied because of their health status, allows young people to remain on their parents' insurance until age 26, requires

insurers to use a high percentage of premiums for benefits instead of profits or overhead, makes some preventive measures free, and almost everyone is required to be insured or they will pay a fine.

6. Types of managed care plans are the exclusive provider organization (EPO), foundation for medical care (FMC), independent (or individual) practice association (IPA), preferred provider organization (PPO), silent PPO, physician provider group (PPG), point-of-service (POS) plan, triple-option health plan, provider-sponsored organization (PSO), and religious fraternal benefit society (RFBS).

7. Managed care plans, such as employee benefit plans (EBPs) purchased by employers, must comply with the federal regulations of the Employee Retirement Income Security Act (ERISA) and do not fall under state laws.

8. The Quality Improvement Organization (QIO) program (formerly the peer review organization) evaluates cases to determine appropriateness, medical necessity, and quality of care.

9. Utilization review (UR) is a process based on established criteria for evaluating and controlling the medical necessity of services and providers' use of medical care resources to curb expenditures.

10. Some managed care plans may require prior approval for certain medical services or referral of a patient to a specialist. Four types of referrals are formal referral, direct referral, verbal referral, and self-referral.

11. If a contract has a stop-loss limit, it means that the provider can begin asking the patient to pay the fee for the service when the patient's services are more than a specific amount.

12. A managed care plan that has a withhold provision may retain a percentage of the monthly capitation payment or a percentage of the allowable charges to physicians until the end of the year to cover operating expenses.

🖥 STUDENT ASSIGNMENT

✔ Study Chapter 11.
✔ Answer the fill-in-the-blank, multiple-choice, and true/false review questions in the *Workbook* to reinforce the theory learned in this chapter and to help prepare you for a future test.
✔ Complete the assignments in the *Workbook* to give you hands-on experience in abstracting information

from a medical record to complete treatment authorization forms for prepaid health insurance cases.
✔ Turn to the Glossary at the end of this text for a further understanding of the key terms and key abbreviations used in this chapter.

Marilyn Takahashi Fordney

OBJECTIVES

After reading this chapter, you should be able to:

1. Explain eligibility criteria for Medicare.
2. Name important information to abstract from a patient's Medicare card.
3. Identify the benefits and nonbenefits of Medicare.
4. List five federal laws adopted to increase health benefits for employed elderly individuals.
5. Explain various Medicare and other insurance coverage combinations.
6. Differentiate between an HMO risk plan and an HMO cost plan.
7. Name the conditions under which an HMO-Medicare patient can be seen by a nonmember HMO physician.
8. Name the federal program that relates to utilization and quality control of health services.
9. State the name of the federal act applicable to reducing fraud and abuse.
10. State the benefits for a participating versus nonparticipating physician.
11. Explain when to obtain a patient's signature on an Advance Beneficiary Notice of Noncoverage or waiver of liability agreement.
12. Define and discuss a Medicare-mandated prepayment screen.
13. Discuss three initiatives and how they affect Medicare.
14. Explain the resource-based relative value scale system that Medicare uses to establish fees.
15. List situations for obtaining an annual patient's signature authorization.
16. Determine the time limit requirements for transmitting a Medicare claim.
17. Explain claims submission for individuals who have Medicare with other insurance.
18. List CMS-1500 (02-12) block numbers that require Medigap information when transmitting a Medicare/Medigap claim.
19. Discuss the two ways in which to submit billing for a deceased patient.
20. State the components of a Medicare remittance advice.
21. Post information on the patient's financial accounting record after a Medicare payment has been received.

KEY TERMS

Advance Beneficiary Notice of Noncoverage
approved charges
assignment
benefit period
Centers for Medicare and Medicaid Services
Correct Coding Initiative

crossover claim
diagnostic cost groups
disabled
end-stage renal disease
formulary
hospice
hospital insurance
intermediate care facilities

limiting charge
medical necessity
Medicare
Medicare administrative contractors
Medicare/Medicaid
Medicare Part A
Medicare Part B

Medicare Part C
Medicare Part D
Medicare secondary payer
Medicare Summary Notice
Medigap
national alphanumeric codes
nonparticipating physician
nursing facility
participating physician

Physician Quality Reporting
   Initiative
premium
prospective payment system
Quality Improvement
   Organization
qui tam action
reasonable fee
Recovery Audit Contractor
   Initiative

relative value unit
remittance advice
resource-based relative value
   scale
respite care
Supplemental Security Income
volume performance standard
whistleblowers

KEY ABBREVIATIONS

ABN	ICFs	NF	PQRI
CAP	ICU	nonpar physician or	PSO
CCI	LCDs	provider	QIO
CLIA	LGHP	OASDI	RA
CMS	MAAC	OBRA	RAC Initiative
COBRA	MAC	OCNA	RBRVS
DC	Medi-Medi	OIG	RFBS
DCGs	MG	OR	RVU
DEFRA	MMA	par physician or	SOF
DME	MSA	provider	SSI
EGHP	MSN	PAYRID	TEFRA
ERA	MSP	PFFS plan	VPS
ESRD	NCDs	PIN	
GPCIs	NEMB	PPS	

Service to Patients

Remind the patient to bring in his or her insurance identification card or cards. Give assistance to patients who may be visually impaired or have hearing impairment and need to complete registration forms for filing insurance claims. Work closely with caregivers and be aware of each patient's limitations, caring for each one with dignity.

Answer the patient's questions about Medicare Summary Notice (MSN) documents because these can be confusing to patients and can lead to misunderstandings about payments for services rendered.

BACKGROUND

Although Social Security is one of the United States' important domestic programs, this system is by no means the first. A number of social insurance programs existed throughout Europe and Latin America before the Social Security Act was signed into law in 1935. Before the United States had Social Security, 20 other nations already had similar systems in operation. Another 30 countries had different social insurance programs in place, such as workers' compensation.

POLICIES AND REGULATIONS

Medicare is administered by the **Centers for Medicare and Medicaid Services (CMS).** It is subdivided into three divisions with the following responsibilities:

1. The Center for Medicare Management oversees traditional fee-for-service Medicare, including development of payment policy and management of fee-for-service contractors.
2. The Center for Beneficiary Choices provides beneficiaries with information on Medicare, Medicare Select, and Medicare Plus (+) Choice programs and **Medigap (MG)** options. It also manages the Medicare+Choice plans, consumer research, and grievance and appeals functions.
3. The Center for Medicaid and State Operations focuses on federal-state programs such as Medicaid, the State Children's Health Insurance Program, insurance regulations, and the Clinical Laboratory Improvement Amendments (CLIA).
4. CMS also enforces the insurance portability and transaction and code set requirements of the Health Insurance Portability and Accountability Act (HIPAA).

Eligibility Requirements

The Social Security Administration (SSA) offices take applications for Social Security, control the eligibility process, and provide information about the Medicare program. If an individual already receives Social Security or Railroad Retirement benefits, he or she is automatically enrolled in Medicare Parts A and B starting on the first day of the month that the individual turns 65 years of age with enough applicable work credits that are equal to 10 years of full-time employment. In 2000, the retirement age gradually increased for people born in 1938 or later. By 2027, full-time retirement age will be 67 for people born after 1959. Benefits may increase if retirement is delayed beyond full retirement age. As of this edition, Medicare still may begin at age 65. Those who apply for Social Security early (at age 62 years) do not receive Medicare but receive monthly reduced Social Security benefits. If an individual is younger than 65 years of age and **disabled,** he or she will automatically get Medicare Parts A and B after getting Social Security disability or Railroad Retirement benefits for 24 months. An individual does not have to be retired to receive Medicare benefits.

Medicare is a federal health insurance program for the following categories of people:
1. People 65 years of age or older who are on Social Security
2. People 65 years of age or older who are retired from the railroad or Civil Service
3. Disabled individuals who are eligible for Social Security disability benefits* and who are in the following categories:
   a. Disabled workers of any age
   b. Disabled widows of workers who are fully or currently insured through the federal government, Civil Service, SSA, **Supplemental Security Income (SSI),** or Railroad Retirement Act and whose husbands qualified for benefits under one of these programs
   c. Adults disabled before age 18 years whose parents are eligible for or retired on Social Security benefits
4. Children and adults who have chronic kidney disease requiring dialysis or who have **end-stage renal disease (ESRD)** requiring a kidney transplant
5. Kidney donors (All expenses related to the kidney transplantation are covered.)

All persons who meet one of the previously stated eligibility requirements determined by SSA are eligible

*In the disabled categories, a person must be disabled for not less than 12 months to apply for disability benefits. A disabled beneficiary must receive disability benefits for 24 months before Medicare benefits begin. See Chapter 16 for further information on this topic.

for **Medicare Part A** (hospital coverage) at no charge. Those who qualify for full Medicare benefits may also elect to take **Medicare Part B** (outpatient coverage). Medicare Part B recipients pay annually increasing basic **premiums** to the SSA and some pay a Medicare surtax on federal income tax payments. This premium may be deducted automatically from the patient's monthly Social Security check if he or she wishes. Those individuals not eligible for Medicare Part A **(hospital insurance)** at 65 years of age may purchase Part B from the SSA.

Illegal Immigrants

An illegal immigrant is an individual who is not a citizen or national of the United States but belongs to another country or people. In the Medicare program, an illegal immigrant may be eligible for Part A or B coverage. To be eligible, the applicant must have lived in the United States as a permanent resident for 5 consecutive years. It is usually not necessary to state on the CMS-1500 (02-12) form or ASC X12 version 5010 electronic claims transmission that the patient is an alien when billing Medicare.

Health Insurance Card

The patient should present his or her Medicare health insurance card. It indicates the patient's name. Beginning in 2015, a federal law was adopted to prevent medical identify theft; thus, Medicare cards that are issued will not display, code, or embed Social Security numbers of beneficiaries. Over a period of 4 to 8 years, the Department of Health and Human Services will update and distribute replacement cards to Medicare beneficiaries. During this transition period, some patients may present cards showing an insurance claim number (Figures 12-1 and 12-2) that usually is abstracted from the card and used when transmitting a claim. Generally, the claim number is the Social Security number of the wage earner with an alpha suffix. The card indicates hospital and medical coverage, effective date, and patient status. Verify effective date because Part A and Part B may have different effective dates. If a beneficiary applies after his or her eligibility date, Part B could have a future date shown on the card. When a husband and wife both have Medicare, they receive separate cards and claim numbers. However, a spouse's card might have the husband's claim number if she has never worked and has no SSA work credits. Medicare cards are red, white, and blue and cards issued after 1990 are plastic. In addition, ask to see the patient's Part D card for prescription coverage. Medicare Prescription Drug Plans (sometimes called PDPs) add drug coverage to original Medicare, Medicare Cost Plans, some Medicare Fee-for-Service (PFFS) plans, and Medicare Medical Savings Account (MSA) plans.

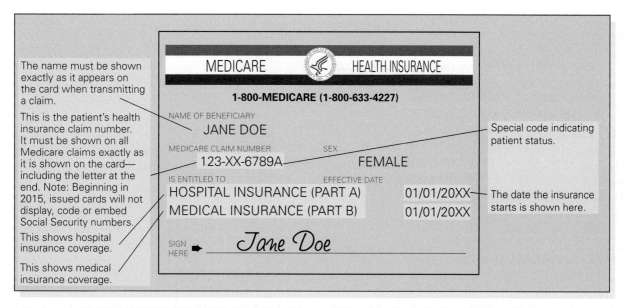

The name must be shown exactly as it appears on the card when transmitting a claim.

This is the patient's health insurance claim number. It must be shown on all Medicare claims exactly as it is shown on the card—including the letter at the end. Note: Beginning in 2015, issued cards will not display, code or embed Social Security numbers.

This shows hospital insurance coverage.

This shows medical insurance coverage.

Special code indicating patient status.

The date the insurance starts is shown here.

MEDICARE **HEALTH INSURANCE**

1-800-MEDICARE (1-800-633-4227)

NAME OF BENEFICIARY
JANE DOE

MEDICARE CLAIM NUMBER   SEX
123-XX-6789A   FEMALE

IS ENTITLED TO   EFFECTIVE DATE
HOSPITAL INSURANCE (PART A)   01/01/20XX
MEDICAL INSURANCE (PART B)   01/01/20XX

SIGN
HERE ➡ *Jane Doe*

FIGURE 12-1 Important information on a patient's Medicare health insurance identification card.

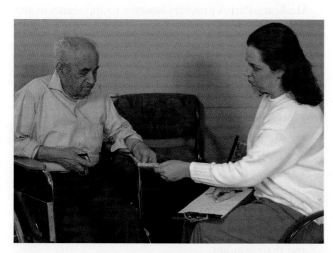

FIGURE 12-2 Insurance billing specialist obtaining the identification card from a disabled Medicare patient.

If the card shows a health maintenance organization (HMO) (for example, Kaiser or Secure Horizons), then you know that the patient signed up and is covered by a managed care plan and not the Medicare standard program. The physician may or may not have a contract with that plan, so coverage for services would be in question. Then ask to see the insurance card for the managed care plan.

The letters after the Medicare number on the patient's identification card indicate the patient's status as follows (this is only a partial listing):

A = wage earner (shown in Figure 12-1)
B = husband's number (wife 62 years or older)
D = widow

HAD = disabled adult
C = disabled child
J, Kl, or Jl = special monthly benefits, never worked under Social Security
M = Part B benefits only
T = entitled to hospital and/or medical insurance benefits but is not entitled to monthly Social Security benefits

A patient whose Medicare card claim number ends in "A" has the same Social Security and claim numbers. A patient whose Medicare card claim number ends in "B" or "D" has *different* Social Security and claim numbers. A quick check between Social Security and card claim numbers may identify a submission error and forestall a claims rejection.

The letters preceding the Medicare number on the patient's identification card indicate railroad retirees:
A = retired railroad employee
Examples: A 000000 (6 digits); A 000-00-0000 (9 digits)

MA = spouse of a retired railroad employee

WA/WD = widow or widower of deceased employee (age or disability)

Examples: WA000000 (6 digits); WA000-00-0000 (9 digits)

CA = child or student

WCA/WCD = widow of retiree with child in her care or disabled child of deceased employee

PA/PD = parent of deceased employee (male or female)

H = Railroad Retirement Board pensioner before 1937

MH = wife of Railroad Retirement Board pensioner before 1937

WH = widowed wife of Railroad Retirement Board pensioner before 1937

WCH = widow of Railroad Retirement Board pensioner with child in her care

PH = parent of Railroad Retirement Board pensioner before 1937

JA = widow receiving a joint and survivor annuity

X = divorced spouse's annuity, for use on forms AA-3 and AA-7 only

Example: CA 123-45-6789C

Enrollment Status

Under Medicare Part B, if an individual receiving Social Security or Railroad Retirement benefits did not sign up for Medicare at the time of eligibility, then the individual is eligible to enroll in Medicare 3 months before his or her 65th birthday. The enrollment period ends 3 months after the month in which the person turns 65. If the enrollment period is missed, the individual must wait until the next general enrollment period, January 1 through March 31, of the following year.

A telephone hotline, or in some states a modem connection, is available to verify the enrollment status. This is useful because patients can switch coverage to a senior managed care plan on a month-to-month basis. Most carriers also allow information on deductible status. The patient's numeric information (Medicare number and date of birth) is entered into the telephone system and the digital response indicates how much of the deductible has been satisfied. Contact the local Medicare administrative contractor (MAC) for information about this service.

Benefits and Nonbenefits
Medicare Part A: Hospital Benefits

Part A of Medicare is hospital insurance benefits for people 65 years of age or older, for people younger than age 65 with certain disabilities, or for people with ESRD. Funds for this health service come from special contributions from employees and self-employed persons, with employers matching contributions. These contributions are collected along with regular Social Security contributions from wages and self-employment income earned during a person's working years.

A **benefit period** begins on the day a patient enters a hospital and ends when the patient has not been a bed patient in any hospital or **nursing facility (NF)** (formerly called *skilled nursing facility*) for 60 consecutive days. It also ends if a patient has been in an NF but has not received skilled nursing care for 60 consecutive days. An NF offers nursing or rehabilitation services that are medically necessary to a patient's recovery. Services provided are not custodial. Custodial services are those that assist the patient with personal needs (for example, dressing, eating, bathing, and getting in and out of bed). Hospital insurance protection is renewed every time the patient begins a new benefit period. There is no limit to the number of benefit periods a patient can have for hospital or NF care. However, special limited benefit periods apply to hospice care.

Medicare Part A provides benefits to applicants in any of the following situations:

1. A bed patient in a hospital (up to 90 hospital days for each benefit period).
2. A bed patient in an NF receiving skilled nursing care (up to 100 extended care days for each benefit period).
3. A patient receiving home health care services.
4. A patient who needs care in a psychiatric hospital (up to 190 days in a lifetime).
5. A terminally ill patient diagnosed as having 6 months or less to live who needs hospice care. A **hospice** is a public agency or private organization that is primarily engaged in providing pain relief, symptom management, and supportive services to terminally ill people and their families.
6. A terminally ill patient who needs **respite care.** Respite care is a short-term inpatient stay that may be necessary for the terminally ill patient to give temporary relief to the person who regularly assists with home care. Inpatient respite care is limited to stays of no more than 5 consecutive days for each respite period.

Figure 12-3 contains information on five major classifications of inpatient hospital cost-sharing benefits for Medicare Part A. Miscellaneous hospital services and supplies might consist of intensive care unit (ICU) costs, blood transfusions, drugs, x-ray and laboratory tests, medical supplies (casts, surgical dressings, and splints), use of wheelchair, operating room (OR) and recovery room costs, and therapy (physical, occupational, and speech language). There are no benefits for personal convenience items (television, radio, and telephone), private

MEDICARE (PART A): HOSPITAL INSURANCE–COVERED SERVICES FOR 2015

Services	Benefit	Medicare Pays	Patient Pays
HOSPITALIZATION Semiprivate room and board, general nursing and miscellaneous hospital services and supplies. (Medicare payments based on benefit periods.)	First 60 days	All but $1260	$1260 deductible
	61st to 90th day 91st to 150th day[1]	All but $315 a day	$315 a day
	60-reserve-days benefit	All but $630 a day	$630 a day
	Beyond 150 days	Nothing	All costs
NURSING FACILITY CARE Patient must have been in a hospital for at least 3 days and enter a Medicare-approved facility generally within 30 days after hospital discharge.[2] (Medicare payments based on benefit periods.)	First 20 days	100% of approved amount	Nothing
	21st to 100th day	All but $157.50 a day	Up to $157.50 a day
	Beyond 100 days	Nothing	All costs
HOME HEALTH CARE Part-time or intermittent skilled care, home health aide services, durable medical equipment and supplies, and other services.	Unlimited as long as Medicare conditions are met and services are declared "medically necessary."	100% of approved amount; 80% of approved amount for durable medical equipment.	Nothing for services; 20% of approved amount for durable medical equipment.
HOSPICE CARE Pain relief, symptom management, and support services for the terminally ill.	If patient elects the hospice option and as long as doctor certifies need.	All but limited costs for outpatient drugs and inpatient respite care.	Limited cost sharing for outpatient drugs and inpatient respite care.
BLOOD	Unlimited if medically necessary.	All but first 3 pints per calendar year.	For first 3 pints.[3]

[1] This 60-reserve-days benefit may be used only once in a lifetime.
[2] Neither Medicare nor private Medigap insurance will pay for most long-term nursing home care.
[3] To the extent the blood deductible is met under Part B of Medicare during the calendar year, it does not have to be met under Part A.

FIGURE 12-3 Five major classifications of Medicare Part A benefits. *(Updated from Medicare & You 2015, US Government Printing Office.)*

duty nurses, or a private room unless the private room is determined medically necessary. Similar benefits also relate to nursing facilities.

Benefits for hospice and respite care consist of nursing and physicians' services, drugs, therapy (physical, occupational, and speech-language pathology), home health aide, homemaker services, medical social services, medical supplies and appliances, short-term inpatient care, and counseling.

Medicare Part B: Medical and Preventive Care Benefits

Part B of Medicare is medical insurance (MI) benefits for the aged and disabled. Funds for this program come equally from those who sign up for it and the federal government. A medical insurance premium is automatically deducted from monthly checks for those who receive Social Security benefits, Railroad Retirement benefits, or a Civil Service annuity. Others pay the premium directly to the SSA. In some states, when a person is eligible for Medicare Part B and Medicaid, Medicaid pays for the monthly Part B premiums.

Table 12-1 contains information on medical and preventive care benefits for Medicare Part B. In addition to medical and surgical services by a doctor of medicine (MD), doctor of osteopathy (DO or MD), or a doctor of dental medicine or dental surgery (DDS), certain services by a doctor of podiatric medicine (DPM) and limited services by a doctor of chiropractic (DC) are paid for. Dental care is covered only for fractures or surgery of the jaw. Optometric examinations are provided if a person has aphakia (absence of the natural lens of the eye). In 2010 the Patient Protection and Affordable Care Act (the Affordable Care Act) made preventive measures such as screenings for colon, prostate, and breast cancers free to Medicare beneficiaries.

Nonbenefits. Nonbenefits, also referred to as *noncovered services*, consist of routine foot care, eye or hearing

Table 12-1   Medicare Part B: Medical Insurance—Covered Services and Preventive Care Benefits

SERVICES	COVERAGE REQUIREMENTS AND LIMITATIONS	MEDICARE PAYS	PATIENT PAYS
Abdominal aortic aneurysm screening	One-time screening on referral	100% of approved amount	Nothing for screening test
Alcoholic misuse screening and counseling	One screening per adult per year	100% of approved amount if doctor accepts assignment	Nothing for screening or counseling in primary care setting
Ambulance services	For transportation to a hospital or skilled nursing facility (NF)	80% of approved amount after deductible	Current annual deductible* plus 20% of approved amount or limited charges†
Ambulatory surgery center	Facility fees are covered for approved services	80% of approved amount after deductible	Current annual deductible plus 20% of approved amount
Blood	Pints of blood as an outpatient or as part of a Part B–covered service	80% of approved amount	First 3 pints plus 20% of approved amounts for additional pints (after current annual deductible)‡
Bone mass measurement	Once every 24 months for qualified individuals and more frequently if medically necessary	100% of approved amount	Nothing for test
Cardiac rehabilitation	Includes exercise, education, and counseling	80% of approved amount after deductible	Current annual deductible plus 20% of approved amount
Cardiovascular disease (behavioral therapy)	One visit per year	100% of approved amount if doctor accepts assignment	Nothing for visit
Cardiovascular screening	Every 5 years to test cholesterol, lipid, and triglyceride levels for heart attack or stroke prevention	100% of approved amount	Nothing for test
Chemotherapy	In doctor's office	80% of approved amount after deductible	Current annual deductible plus 20% of approved amount
Chiropractic services	Limited services to correct subluxation using manipulation	80% of approved amount after deductible	Current annual deductible plus 20% of approved amount
Clinical laboratory services	Includes blood tests, urinalysis, and some screening tests	100% of approved amount	Nothing for tests
Clinical trials	Tests new types of medical care to prevent, diagnose, or treat diseases	80% of approved amount after deductible	Current annual deductible plus 20% of approved amount
Colorectal Cancer Screening (one or more of the following tests may be covered)§			
Fecal occult blood test	Once every 12 months	100% of approved amount	Nothing for test
Flexible sigmoidoscopy	Once every 48 months if age 50 or older, or every 120 months when used instead of a colonoscopy for those not at high risk	100% of approved amount	Nothing for test
Screening colonoscopy	Once every 120 months (high risk every 24 months)	100% of approved amount	Nothing for test
Barium enema	Once every 48 months if age 50 or older (high risk every 24 months) when used instead of sigmoidoscopy or colonoscopy	80% of approved amount after deductible	Part B deductible does not apply; 20% of approved amount
Defibrillator (implantable automatic)	Outpatient setting	80% of approved amount after deductible	Current annual deductible plus 20% of approved amount
Depression screening	One screening per year	100% of approved amount if doctor accepts assignment	Nothing for screening
Diabetes screening	Twice a year for glucose monitors, test strips, and lancets	100% of approved amount	Nothing for screening

Table 12-1	Medicare Part B: Medical Insurance—Covered Services and Preventive Care Benefits—cont'd		
SERVICES	**COVERAGE REQUIREMENTS AND LIMITATIONS**	**MEDICARE PAYS**	**PATIENT PAYS**
Diabetes self-management training	Provider must issue a written order	80% of approved amount after deductible	Current annual deductible plus 20% of approved amount
Diabetic supplies	Includes glucose testing monitors, test strips, lancet devices, lancets, glucose control solutions, and therapeutic shoes. Syringes and insulin covered if used with an insulin pump or if patient has Part D coverage	80% of approved amount after deductible	Current annual deductible plus 20% of approved amount
Doctor services	No coverage for routine physical examinations except for one-time "Welcome to Medicare" physical examination	80% of approved amount after deductible	Current annual deductible plus 20% of approved amount
Durable medical equipment (DME)	Oxygen, wheelchairs, walkers, and hospital beds for home use	80% of approved amount	20% of approved amount
Electrocardiogram screening	One-time screening	80% of approved amount	20% of approved amount
Emergency department services	Bad injury or sudden illness when patient is in serious danger	80% of approved amount after deductible	Current annual deductible plus 20% of approved amount
Eyeglasses	One pair of glasses with standard frames after cataract surgery that implants an intraocular lens	80% of approved amount after deductible	Current annual deductible plus 20% of approved amount
Flu shots	Annually to prevent influenza or flu virus	100% of approved amount	Nothing for flu shots
Foot examinations and treatment	For diabetes-related nerve damage	80% of approved amount after deductible	Current annual deductible plus 20% of approved amount
Glaucoma screening	Once every 12 months	80% of approved amount after deductible	Current annual deductible plus 20% of approved amount
Hearing and balance examination	Ordered by a doctor to determine whether medical treatment is necessary; hearing aids and examinations for fitting hearing aids are not covered	80% of approved amount after deductible	Current annual deductible plus 20% of approved amount
Hepatitis B shots	Three shots for people with high or intermediate risk	100% of approved amount	Nothing for shots
Hepatitis C	Screening test for high risk individuals	100% approved	Nothing for test
HIV screening	Once every 12 months	80% of approved amount for office visit	Nothing for test; 20% of approved amount for office visit
Home health services	Limited to reasonable and necessary part-time or intermittent skilled nursing care, home health aide services, physical therapy, and speech-language pathology; also includes DME	100% of approved amount; 80% of approved amount for DME	Nothing for services; 20% of approved amount for DME
Kidney dialysis services and supplies	In a facility or at home	80% of approved amount after deductible	Current annual deductible plus 20% of approved amount
Kidney disease education services	Six sessions of kidney disease education	80% of approved amount after deductible	Current annual deductible plus 20% of approved amount

Continued

Table 12-1   Medicare Part B: Medical Insurance—Covered Services and Preventive Care Benefits—cont'd

SERVICES	COVERAGE REQUIREMENTS AND LIMITATIONS	MEDICARE PAYS	PATIENT PAYS
Laboratory services	Certain blood tests, urinalysis, and some screening tests	100% of approved amount	Nothing for laboratory services
Mammogram screening§	Once every 12 months; also covers digital technologies	100% of approved amount	Nothing for screening
Medical nutrition therapy services	For people who have diabetes or renal disease not on dialysis or with a doctor's referral 3 years after a kidney transplantation	80% of approved amount after deductible	Current annual deductible plus 20% of approved amount
Mental health care (outpatient)	Certain limits and conditions apply	50% of approved amount after deductible	Current annual deductible plus 20% of approved amount
Obesity screening and counseling	Twenty-two face-to-face counseling sessions over 12 months	100% of approved amount if doctor accepts assignment	Nothing for counseling
Occupational therapy	To help patients return to usual activities after an illness (for example, bathing)	100% of approved amount after deductible	Current annual deductible plus 20% of approved amount
Outpatient hospital services	When received as part of a doctor's care	Medicare payment to hospital based on hospital cost	Current annual deductible plus 20% of whatever the hospital charges
Outpatient medical and surgical services and supplies	For approved procedures	80% of approved amount after deductible	Current annual deductible plus 20% of approved amount
Papanicolaou (Pap) test/pelvic§	Once every 24 months (low risk) and once every 12 months (high risk)	100% of approved amount	Nothing for test
Physical examination	One-time "Welcome to Medicare" physical examination within first 12 months patient is on Part B	80% of approved amount after deductible	Current annual deductible plus 20% of approved amount
Physical therapy	Heat, light, exercise, and massage treatment of injuries and disease	100% of approved amount after deductible	Current annual deductible plus 20% of approved amount
Pneumococcal pneumonia vaccine (PPV)	Once in a lifetime	100% of approved amount	Nothing for flu and PPV if doctor accepts assignment
Practitioner services	Clinical social worker, physician assistant, and nurse practitioner	80% of approved amount after deductible	Current annual deductible plus 20% of approved amount
Prescription drugs	Certain injectable cancer drugs; drug coverage for patients who have Part D	80% of approved amount	Current annual deductible plus 20% after deductible of approved amount
Prostate cancer screening§	Prostate-specific antigen (PSA) test and digital rectal examination once every 12 months	100% of approved amount	Nothing for test
Prosthetic/orthotic items	Arm, leg, back, and neck braces; artificial eyes; artificial limbs and replacement parts; breast prostheses after mastectomy; prosthetic devices to replace an internal body part or function (includes ostomy supplies and parenteral and enteral nutrition therapy)	80% of approved amount after deductible	Current annual deductible plus 20% of approved amount
Pulmonary rehabilitation	Referral from doctor	80% of approved amount after deductible	Current annual deductible plus 20% of approved amount
Second surgical opinions	Covered in some cases; some third surgical opinions are covered for surgery that is not an emergency	80% of approved amount after deductible	Current annual deductible plus 20% of approved amount

Table 12-1 Medicare Part B: Medical Insurance—Covered Services and Preventive Care Benefits—cont'd				
SERVICES	**COVERAGE REQUIREMENTS AND LIMITATIONS**	**MEDICARE PAYS**	**PATIENT PAYS**
Sexually transmitted infections screening and counseling	Once every 12 months or at certain times during pregnancy	100% of approved amount	Nothing for screening and counseling
Smoking cessation counseling	Eight face-to-face visits during a 12-month period if diagnosed with a smoking-related illness or if taking medicine that is affected by tobacco	100% of approved amount	Nothing for counseling sessions
Speech-language pathology services	To regain and strengthen speech skills	100% of approved amount after deductible	Current annual deductible plus 20% of approved amount
Surgical dressings	For surgical or surgically treated wound	80% of approved amount after deductible	Current annual deductible plus 20% of approved amount
Telemedicine	For some rural areas in a practitioner's office, hospital, or federally qualified health center	80% of approved amount after deductible	Current annual deductible plus 20% of approved amount
Tests	X-rays, magnetic resonance imaging, computed tomography scans, electrocardiograms, and some other diagnostic tests	80% of approved amount after deductible	Current annual deductible plus 20% of approved amount
Transplant services	Heart, lung, kidney, pancreas, intestine, and liver transplants; bone marrow and cornea transplants; immunosuppressive drugs	80% of approved amount after deductible	Current annual deductible plus 20% of approved amount
Travel	Services in United States, District of Columbia, Puerto Rico, Virgin Islands, Guam, Northern Mariana Islands, American Samoa, and Canada, or on board a ship within US territorial waters	80% of approved amount after deductible	Current annual deductible plus 20% of approved amount
Urgently needed care	Treatment for sudden illness or injury that is not a medical emergency	80% of approved amount after deductible	Current annual deductible plus 20% of approved amount

*Once the patient has incurred expenses that match the amount of the deductible for covered services in the year, the Part B deductible does not apply to any further covered services received for the rest of the year. The deductible amount for each year changes: 2012 is $140, 2013 is $147, 2014 is $147, 2015 is $147, and 2016 is $_____, 2017 is $_____.

†See Figure 12-7 for an explanation of approved amount for participating physicians and limited charges for nonparticipating physicians.

‡To the extent that the blood deductible is met under Part A of Medicare during the calendar year, it does not have to be met under Part B.

§The Patient Protection and Affordable Care Act of 2010 made this preventive test free.

examinations, and cosmetic surgery unless caused by injury or performed to improve functioning of a malformed part. However, glaucoma tests are covered once every 12 months for people at high risk (that is, those with diabetes or a family history of glaucoma). A hearing examination is covered if the physician orders it to determine whether the patient needs medical treatment. A physician may bill a patient separately for noncovered services.

Other benefits and nonbenefits are too numerous to list here. Refer to Medicare newsletters or contact the Medicare carrier to find out whether a particular procedure qualifies for payment.

Medicare Part C: Medicare Advantage Plan

The Balanced Budget Act of 1997 created **Medicare Part C,** commonly referred to as *Medicare Advantage Plan (MA plan),* formerly called *Medicare+Choice.* The program was introduced in 2004 and by 2006 replaced Medicare+Choice. This program was formed to increase the number of health care options, in addition to those that are available under Medicare Parts A and B. A Medicare beneficiary can join an MA plan if he or she has both Parts A and B and lives in the service area of the plan. Individuals who have ESRD must meet special situational requirements to join an MA plan. Individuals who sign up for MA plans are issued an insurance card and do not use the Medicare Parts A and B cards. MA plans receive a fixed amount of money from Medicare to spend on their Medicare members. Some plans may require members to pay a premium similar to the Medicare Part B premium. In 2010, national health care reform legislation froze payments to these plans with cuts in the following years. It is predicted that enrollees may lose some benefits such as free eyeglasses and hearing aids.

Plans available under this program may include the following: health maintenance organization (HMO), point-of-service (POS) plan, preferred provider organization (PPO), private fee-for-service (PFFS) plan, provider-sponsored organization (PSO), religious fraternal benefit society (RFBS), and a pilot program: Medicare medical savings account (MSA). In an MSA plan, the patient chooses an insurance policy approved by Medicare that has a high annual deductible. Medicare pays the premiums for this policy and deposits the dollar amount difference between what it pays for the average beneficiary in the patient's area and the cost of the premium into the patient's MSA. The patient uses the MSA money to pay medical expenses until the high deductible is reached. If the MSA money becomes depleted, the patient pays out of pocket until the deductible is reached. Unused funds roll over for use in the following year.

Medicare Part D

The Medicare Prescription Drug, Improvement, and Modernization Act (MMA) became effective in 2003 but drug benefits began on January 1, 2006. This legislation, known as **Medicare Part D,** provides seniors and people living with disabilities with a prescription drug benefit. It covers prescription drugs used for conditions not already covered by Medicare Parts A and B. It is a stand-alone prescription drug plan offered by insurance companies and other private companies providing drug coverage that meet standards established by Medicare. Other names for these plans are *Part D private prescription drug plans (PDPs)* and *Medicare Advantage prescription drug plans (MA-PDs).*

The two ways to get Medicare prescription drug coverage are as follows:
1. Join a Medicare prescription drug plan that adds drug coverage to the original Medicare plan, some Medicare cost plans, some Medicare PFFS plans, and Medicare MSA plans.
2. Join an MA plan, such as an HMO or PPO, that includes prescription drug coverage as part of the plan.

Individuals who enroll pay a monthly premium that varies depending on the plan. Those who decide not to enroll in a Medicare drug plan when they are first eligible may pay a penalty if they decide to join later. Enrollees pay an annual deductible that varies from plan to plan and a copayment of drug costs. Most Medicare drug plans have a coverage gap (also called the *"donut hole"*). This means that there is a temporary limit on what the drug plan will cover for drugs. The coverage gap begins after the patient and the drug plan together have spent a certain amount for covered drugs. Once the patient enters into the coverage gap, he or she pays a percentage of the plan's cost for covered brand-name drugs and a percentage of the plan's cost for covered generic drugs until he or she reaches the end of the coverage gap. This does not include the drug plan's premium. At that point, the coverage gap ends and the enrollees pay a small coinsurance (5%) or small copayment ($5 to $10) for each prescription until the end of the year. In addition, patients in the coverage gap receive a 50% discount on brand-name drugs. The federal government will close the donut hole by providing subsidies for brand-name drugs that begin at 2.5% and will increase to 25% by 2020. In 2011 it began subsidies for generic drugs at 7% of the cost.

People who are eligible for Medicaid and Medicare pay no premium or deductible and have no gap in coverage. They pay $1 per prescription for generics and $3 for brand names. Copayments are waived for those in nursing homes. In addition, several programs help people who have limited income and resources and the programs, qualifications, and copayments vary by area.

Prescription drug plans refer to the drugs in their formularies by tier numbers. A **formulary** is a list of the drugs that a plan covers. Tier one represents generic drugs and has a low copayment associated with it. Tier two covers preferred brand-name drugs and has a higher copayment than tier one. Tier three drugs are the nonpreferred drugs and could have either a copayment or a percentage of full drug cost associated with it. The fourth classification, identified as "S," represents specialty drugs and requires a percentage of total cost of the drug. The following are several classes of drugs excluded from coverage:
● Barbiturates
● Benzodiazepines
● Drugs for cosmetic purposes
● Drugs for symptomatic relief of cough and colds
● Drugs for weight loss or gain
● Erectile dysfunction drugs
● Fertility drugs
● Prescription vitamins or minerals, except prenatal

A provider who prescribes a drug that can be covered by either Part B or Part D must clarify the condition and part coverage on the prescription form (Example 12-1).

| Example 12-1 | Prescription Note Clarifying Medical Use of Drug and Coverage Determination |

Patient with psoriasis (autoimmune disorder) is prescribed methotrexate. Generally this immunosuppressive drug is prescribed for transplant patients and is covered under Medicare Part B.
Added prescription note should read: "Psoriasis for Part D."

A bonus is given to providers who electronically prescribe drugs and as of 2010, Healthcare Common Procedure Coding System (HCPCS) code G8553 should be used for reporting.

When a patient has coverage under a Medicare Part D plan, obtain a photocopy of the patient's Medicare supplement or MA plan card. Then check whether the drug that the patient needs is covered by the plan, which generic drugs are available, and whether a drug needs prior authorization. Either call the telephone number listed on the card or use a free software program—Epocrates—that is available to providers to help with these needs.

Railroad Retirement Benefits

Railroad Retirement Board offices maintain eligibility records for Medicare and provide information about the program for railroad workers and their beneficiaries. Medical insurance premiums are automatically deducted from the monthly checks of people who receive Railroad Retirement benefits. Those who do not receive a monthly check pay their premiums directly or in some cases have premiums paid on their behalf under a state assistance program. If the allowed fees differ from those allowed by the regular Medicare carrier, write or fax the Medicare railroad retiree carrier asking that fees be based on fee data from the local carrier.

Railroad Retirement beneficiaries generally are entitled to benefits for covered services received from a qualified American facility. However, under certain circumstances a Medicare beneficiary may receive care in Canada or Mexico. Benefits and deductibles under Parts A and B are the same as for other Medicare recipients.

Some railroad retirees are members of a railroad hospital association or a prepayment plan. These members pay regular premiums to the plan and then receive health services that the plan provides without additional charges. In some plans, small charges are made for certain services such as drugs or home visits. Many prepayment plans make arrangements with Medicare to receive direct payments for services they furnish that are covered under Medicare Part B. Some prepayment plans have contracts with Medicare as HMOs or competitive medical plans and can receive direct payment for services covered by either hospital or medical insurance. After a claim is transmitted to the Medicare railroad retiree carrier, which is usually to a different regional MAC, a **remittance advice (RA)** document is generated explaining the decision made on the claim and the services for which Medicare paid.

Employed Elderly Benefits

To understand various types of scenarios that may be encountered when transmitting claims for elderly individuals, one must know about several federal laws that regulate health care coverage of those age 65 and older who are employed. Such individuals may have group insurance or a Medigap (MG) policy and may fall under billing categories of Medicare first payer or **Medicare secondary payer (MSP)** (all are discussed in detail later in this chapter). The federal laws that affect employed elderly individuals are shown in Box 12-1.

ADDITIONAL INSURANCE PROGRAMS

Many Medicare recipients have Medicare in combination with other insurance plans. This section explains various coverage combinations. Guidelines for processing claims for these plans are presented later in this chapter.

Medicare/Medicaid

Patients designated as **Medicare/Medicaid (Medi-Medi)** are on both Medicare and Medicaid simultaneously. However, in the Northeast US the term *Medi-Medi* means "dual eligible" and not a patient on Medicare/Medicaid. These patients qualify for Old Age, Survivors, and Disability Insurance (OASDI) assistance benefits (older than age 65), are severely disabled, or are blind.

Medicare/Medigap

A specialized insurance policy devised for the Medicare beneficiary is called *Medigap (MG)* or *Medifill*. This type of policy is designed to supplement coverage under a fee-for-service Medicare plan. It may cover prescription costs and the deductible and copayment (for example, 20% of the Medicare allowed amount) that are typically the patient's responsibility under Medicare. These plans are offered by private third-party payers to Medicare beneficiaries who pay the monthly premiums for this supplemental insurance.

The federal government in conjunction with the insurance industry established predefined minimum benefits for 10 MG policies categorized by alpha letters A through J (Figure 12-4). Basic benefits are found in policy A. Each subsequent letter represents basic benefits

Omnibus Budget Reconciliation Act

The Omnibus Budget Reconciliation Act (OBRA) of 1981 required that in the case of a current or former employee or dependent younger than age 65 years and eligible for Medicare solely because of ESRD, the employer's group coverage is primary for up to 30 months. The Balanced Budget Act of 1997 mandated this change in the length of the coordination period. OBRA applies to all employers regardless of the number of employees. OBRA of 1986, effective in 1987, required that if an employee or dependent younger than age 65 years has Medicare coverage because of a disability other than ESRD, the group coverage is primary and Medicare is secondary. This Act applies only to large group health plans (LGHPs) having at least 100 full- or part-time employees.

Tax Equity and Fiscal Responsibility Act

The Tax Equity and Fiscal Responsibility Act (TEFRA) of 1982 established that an employee or spouse age 65 to 69 years is entitled to the same health insurance benefits offered under the same conditions to younger employees and their spouses. The group insurance is primary and Medicare is secondary. TEFRA applies to employers with at least 20 full- or part-time employees.

Deficit Reduction Act

The Deficit Reduction Act (DEFRA) of 1984, effective in 1985, was an amendment to TEFRA and stated that a spouse age 65 to 69 years or an employee of any age is entitled to the same group health plan offered to younger employees and their spouses. The group's coverage is primary and Medicare is secondary. DEFRA applies to employers with at least 20 full- or part-time employees.

Consolidated Omnibus Budget Reconciliation Act

The Consolidated Omnibus Budget Reconciliation Act (COBRA) of 1985, effective in 1986, is another amendment to TEFRA eliminating the age ceiling of 69 years. An employee or spouse age 65 or older is entitled to the same group health plan offered to younger employees and their spouses. COBRA requires that third-party payers reimburse for certain care rendered in government-run veteran and military hospitals. The group's coverage is primary and Medicare is secondary. COBRA applies to employers with at least 20 full- or part-time employees.

Tax Reform Act

The Tax Reform Act was passed in 1986 and clarified certain aspects of COBRA. A spouse and dependents may elect to receive continued coverage even if the employee does not wish insurance coverage and terminates the plan. However, the spouse and dependents must have been covered under the plan before the covered employee terminates it. Spouses who are widowed or divorced while receiving continued coverage must report such changes to the benefit plan administrator within 60 days of the employee's death to determine how many additional months of coverage are available.

ESRD, End-stage renal disease.

plus other coverage, with the most comprehensive benefits in policy J. All policies are not available in all states, so individuals in some states have fewer options than others.

A slightly different variation of the MG policy is *Medicare Select*. This policy has the same coverage as regular MG policies but there is a restriction in that the beneficiary must obtain medical care from a list of specified network doctors and providers.

Medicare Secondary Payer

In some instances, Medicare is considered secondary and classifies the situation as MSP. MSP may involve aged or disabled patients with the following qualities:

- Aged workers under group health plans with more than 20 covered employees
- Disabled individuals age 64 and younger who are covered under a group health plan with more than 100 covered employees or covered under a family member's current employment
- Medicare beneficiaries under an employer-sponsored group health plan that have ESRD during the first 18 months of the patient's eligibility for Medicare
- Cases of workers' compensation when the injury or illness occurs at work
- Individuals either currently or formerly employed with black lung disease who fall under the Federal Black Lung Program
- Individuals receiving benefits under the Department of Veterans Affairs (VA) and Medicare
- Individuals covered under a Federal Research Grant Program
- Automobile accident cases such as medical no-fault cases and third-party liability insurance cases

Follow the suggested steps in Procedure 12-1 at the end of the chapter to identify whether Medicare is primary or secondary and to determine what additional benefits the patient might have.

Managed Care and Medicare

When a patient's primary insurance is a managed care plan that requires fixed copayments, it is possible to obtain reimbursement from Medicare for those amounts. An assigned MSP claim must be filed with Medicare after the managed care organization (MCO) has paid. When Medicare's copayment reimbursement has been received, the provider must refund to the patient the copayment amount previously collected.

The practice is paid a capitated amount and there is no explanation of benefits (EOB) document. Have the patient sign a statement that explains the situation. Attach

MEDIGAP Benefits	Plans									
	A	B	C	D	F*	G	K	L	M	N**
Medicare Part A Coinsurance and hospital costs (up to an additional 365 days after Medicare benefits are used up.)	X	X	X	X	X	X	X	X	X	X
Medicare Part B Coinsurance or Copayment	X	X	X	X	X	X	50%	75%	X	X***
Blood (First 3 Pints)	X	X	X	X	X	X	50%	75%	X	X
Part A. Hospice Care Coinsurance or Copayment	X	X	X	X	X	X	50%	75%	X	X
Skilled Nursing Facility Care Coinsurance			X	X	X	X	50%	75%	X	X
Medicare Part A Deductible		X	X	X	X	X	50%	75%	50%	X
Medicare Part B Deductible			X		X					
Medicare Part B excess charges					X	X				
Foreign Travel Emergency (Up to Plan Limits)			X	X	X	X			X	X

2013 MEDIGAP PLANS

How to read the chart:
1. If an "X" appears in a column of this chart, the Medigap policy covers 100% of the described benefit.
2. If a column lists a percentage, the policy covers that percentage of the described benefit.
3. If a column is blank, the policy does not cover that benefit.
Note: The Medigap policy covers coinsurance only after the deductible has been paid unless the policy also covers the deductible.

** 2013 Out of pocket limit: $4800 $2400

* Plan F also offers a high-deductible plan. If you choose this option, you must pay for Medicare costs (coinsurance, copayments, deductibles) up to the 2013 deductible amount (not yet determined by CMS) before your policy pays anything.
** After you meet your out-of-pocket yearly limit and your yearly Part B deductible, the Medigap plan pays 100% of covered services for the rest of the calender year.
*** Plan N pays 100% of the Part B coinsurance, except for a copayment of up to $20.00 for some office visits and up to a $50.00 copayment for emergency room visits that do not result in an in-patient admission.

Note: Plans no longer for sale as of June 1, 2013, are E, H, I, and J. However, patients who are insured under these plans are recognized as insured and the plans are not canceled.

FIGURE 12-4 Medigap plans effective June 1, 2013, from a Medicare government publication.

the statement and the copayment receipts to the claim. The statement may read as shown in the following box.

Patient Name _____
Medicare Number _____
There is no Explanation of Benefits documentation available for the attached billed services. I am currently enrolled with _____ managed care plan for my health care. My physician, _____ MD, is paid on a capitated basis, and the copayment that I pay is $ _____ for each service or visit.
Patient's signature_____
Date _____

A **nonparticipating (nonpar) physician** must file an unassigned MSP claim. The patient is directly reimbursed by Medicare and no refund is necessary.

Automobile or Liability Insurance Coverage

Liability insurance is not secondary to Medicare because there is no contractual relationship between the injured party and third-party payer. A physician who treats a Medicare patient who has filed a liability claim must bill the liability insurer first unless the insurer will not pay promptly (for example, within 120 days after the liability insurance claim is filed). After 120 days have gone by without a payment from the liability insurer and if the services performed are covered Medicare benefits, a participating (par) or nonpar physician may seek conditional payment from Medicare. However, if a claim is filed with Medicare, the provider must drop the claim against the liability insurer.

If the payment made by the liability insurer is less than the physician's full charge, the physician may file an assigned claim and must accept as full payment the greater of either the Medicare-approved charge or the sum of the liability insurance primary payment and the Medicare secondary payment.

A nonpar physician may file an unassigned claim for Medicare secondary payment only if the payment by the liability insurer is less than the Medicare **limiting charge.** If the payment equals or exceeds the limiting charge, the physician must accept the disbursement as full payment.

If Medicare payments have been made but should not have been because the services are excluded under this provision or if the payments were made on a conditional basis, they are subject to recovery. A copy of the notice of payment or denial form from the other insurer should be included when sending the CMS-1500 (02-12) claim form. Medicare is secondary even if a state law or a private contract of insurance states that Medicare is primary. The physician must bill the other insurer first. A claim for secondary benefits may be transmitted to Medicare only

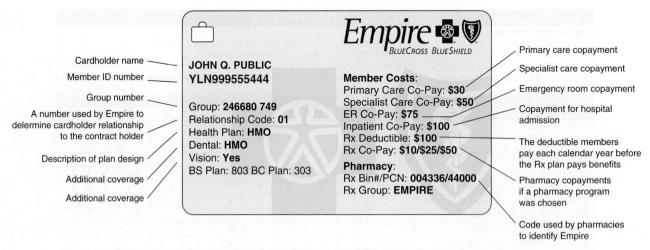

Cardholder name

Member ID number

Group number

A number used by Empire to determine cardholder relationship to the contract holder

Description of plan design

Additional coverage

Additional coverage

JOHN Q. PUBLIC
YLN999555444

Group: **246680 749**
Relationship Code: **01**
Health Plan: **HMO**
Dental: **HMO**
Vision: **Yes**
BS Plan: 803 BC Plan: 303

Member Costs:
Primary Care Co-Pay: **$30**
Specialist Care Co-Pay: **$50**
ER Co-Pay: **$75**
Inpatient Co-Pay: **$100**
Rx Deductible: **$100**
Rx Co-Pay: **$10/$25/$50**
Pharmacy:
Rx Bin#/PCN: **004336/44000**
Rx Group: **EMPIRE**

Primary care copayment

Specialist care copayment

Emergency room copayment

Copayment for hospital admission

The deductible members pay each calendar year before the Rx plan pays benefits

Pharmacy copayments if a pharmacy program was chosen

Code used by pharmacies to identify Empire

FIGURE 12-5 A senior managed care plan card.

after payment or denial has been made by the primary coverage. Liability insurance is not considered an MSP.

MEDICARE MANAGED CARE PLANS

Health Maintenance Organizations

During the spring of 1984, the Department of Health and Human Services published regulations giving Medicare enrollees the right to join and assign their Medicare benefits to HMOs. HMOs had been in operation for nearly 50 years when they became available as an option for Medicare enrollees. With a Medicare HMO (also known as a senior HMO or senior plan), the patient does not need a Medicare supplemental insurance plan. On enrollment, the Medicare beneficiary is sent an insurance card from the managed care plan (Figure 12-5). However, Medicare cards are not forfeited and an elderly patient may show two cards, leading to confusion about what the coverage is and whom to bill.

Medicare makes payments directly to the HMO on a monthly basis for Medicare enrollees who use the HMO option. Enrollees pay the HMO a monthly premium, which is an estimate of the coinsurance amounts for which the enrollee would be responsible plus the Medicare deductible. It appears that HMOs contracting to provide services for Medicare patients will be converted to an MA plan as their contract renewal dates occur.

Some HMOs provide services not usually covered by Medicare such as eyeglasses, prescription drugs, and routine physical examinations. Once a person has converted from Medicare to an HMO, he or she cannot go back to a former physician of personal choice and expect Medicare to pay the bill. The patient should receive services from a physician and hospital facility that are contracted with the HMO plan.

If a Medicare patient has switched over to a managed care plan and wishes to disenroll, the patient must do the following:
1. Notify the plan in writing of disenrollment.
2. Complete the Medicare Managed Care Disenrollment CMS-566 form, attach a copy of the disenrollment letter, and take it to the Social Security office.

Medicare Advantage plans (HMOs or PPOs) have an open enrollment period in the fall of each year. It may take the plan 30 days for disenrollment and Medicare may take as long as 60 days to reenroll a patient. Patients who disenroll may have to requalify for supplemental coverage at a higher cost.

Two types of HMO plans may have Medicare Part B contracts: HMO risk plans and HMO cost plans.

Risk Plan

As a condition of enrollment in an HMO risk plan, beneficiaries receive Medicare-covered services (except emergency, urgent need, and prior authorized services) only from providers who are contracted members of the HMO network. Enrollees of HMO risk plans are referred to as *restricted beneficiaries*. Usually services rendered by "out-of-plan" physicians are not covered when the same services are available through the organization unless a referral or prior authorization is obtained. The only exception is for emergency care. Claims for HMO risk plan beneficiaries must be sent directly to the organization.

A system of Medicare reimbursement for HMOs with risk contracts is called **diagnostic cost groups (DCGs).** The HMO enrollees are classified into various DCGs on the basis of each beneficiary's prior 12-month history of hospitalization and payments are adjusted accordingly. This payment system does not apply to disabled and hospice patients, those on renal dialysis, or those enrolled only in Medicare Part B. Patients are reclassified each year according to their previous year's use of hospital service. This is discussed further in Chapter 17.

Cost Plan

Under an HMO cost plan, beneficiaries receive Medicare-covered services from sources in or outside of the HMO network. Enrollees are referred to as *unrestricted beneficiaries.* Claims for cost plan beneficiaries may be sent to the HMO plan or the regular Medicare carrier.

If a noncontract physician treats a Medicare HMO patient, the services are considered "out-of-plan" services. The claim must be submitted to the managed care plan, which determines whether it is responsible to pay for the services. Conditions that must be met are as follows:

1. The service was an emergency and the patient was not able to get to an HMO facility or member physician (patient was out of the HMO area).
2. The service was covered by Medicare.
3. The service was medically necessary.
4. The service was authorized previously or was an approved referral.

The patient is responsible for the fee if the HMO determines that there was no emergency and denies payment. The HMO reimburses according to the Medicare Fee Schedule Allowable Amount, so the physician cannot bill the patient for the balance. If the physician does not receive 100% of the allowable amount, steps must be taken through the HMO's appeals process. If this fails, contact the Medicare Managed Care Department at the Medicare Regional CMS Operations Office. After the HMO EOB is received, denied services can be billed to the patient but no more than the Medicare fee schedule or limiting charge.

Carrier Dealing Prepayment Organization

A Carrier Dealing Prepayment Organization may be set up by a medical practice under contract to the government. Such plans are considered a service contract rather than insurance. In the past, such plans were run by HMOs but now practices of 12 to 15 physicians are opting to run their own plans. These organizations must be incorporated and have their own Medicare provider number. The organization must furnish physicians' services through employees and partners or under formal arrangement with medical groups, independent practice associations, or individual physicians. Part B services must be provided through qualified hospitals or physicians. When

operating this type of organization, the physician accepts Medicare **assignment** and agrees to deal with the Medicare carrier instead of CMS. Patients sign a contract agreeing to pay a monthly fee (usually $20 to $25). This is supposed to cover all Medicare copayments, deductibles, and nonreimbursable expenses (annual physical examinations and preventive care). The patient is not responsible for paying for noncovered services.

UTILIZATION AND QUALITY CONTROL

Quality Improvement Organizations

As explained in detail in Chapter 11, a **Quality Improvement Organization (QIO)** program (formerly known as *professional* or *peer review organization*) contracts with CMS to review **medical necessity,** reasonableness, appropriateness, and completeness and adequacy of care given in inpatient, outpatient, and emergency department hospitals, nursing facilities, home health agencies, private fee-for-service (PFFS) plans, and ambulatory surgical centers for which additional payment is sought under the outlier provisions of the **prospective payment system (PPS).**

CMS has assigned a point system for medical documentation as discussed in Chapter 4. If sufficient points are lacking, penalties can lead to fines or forfeiture of the physician's license. Therefore it is extremely important that each patient's care be well documented from the treatment standpoint as well as for justifying maximum reimbursement. A physician who receives a letter from a QIO about quality of care should consult his or her attorney before responding by letter or personal appeal. A photocopy of the patient's health record can be used to substantiate the claim if there is detailed clinical documentation.

Federal False Claims Amendment Act

Another federal law to prevent overuse of services and to spot Medicare fraud is the False Claims Amendment Act of 1986. This Act offers financial incentives of 15% to 25% of any judgment to informants **(whistleblowers)** who report physicians suspected of defrauding the federal government (this is, by overcharging or scheduling excessive visits). This is called a **qui tam action.** The laws are intended to help catch Medicare and Medicaid cheaters. The health insurance companies that process Medicare claims have a Medicare fraud unit whose job is to catch people who steal from Medicare. The Office of the Inspector General (OIG), Department of Health and Human Services, is the law enforcement agency that investigates and prosecutes people who steal from Medicare. The OIG works closely with Medicare insurance companies, the Federal Bureau of Investigation (FBI), the Postal Inspection Service, and other federal law enforcement agencies. If the physician is on an optical disk retrieval (ODR) A-1000 system, it is possible for the OIG to obtain procedure codes that show comparison billing with peers in the area. The CMS alerts the OIG of offices to investigate. To reduce the chances of a Medicare beneficiary complaining to the government, take the following actions:

● Listen to the patient's complaint and follow up.
● Publicize the provider's hotline.
● Route a beneficiary's complaint to a compliance officer or office manager.

For a detailed list of fraud and abuse issues, see Boxes 2-9 and 2-10 in Chapter 2. See Chapter 15 for information about fraud in the workers' compensation program.

Clinical Laboratory Improvement Amendments

The CLIA of 1988 established federal standards, quality control, and safety measures for all freestanding laboratories, including physician office laboratories (POLs). Various laboratory procedures fall within CLIA categories, depending on the complexity of each test. If a physician performs only tests that pose no risk to the patient, the laboratory may be eligible for a certificate of waiver that exempts it from CLIA regulations' quality control and personnel standards; however, a registration fee must still be paid for the waived category. The other two categories are moderate- or high-complexity laboratory services. Each category level requires a yearly licensing fee to be paid by the physician. A certificate is then issued and must be posted in the laboratory. Various levels of quality control measures are necessary for each CLIA level and must be performed in a timely manner (for example, daily or weekly). Fines may be levied if federal standards are not maintained. This has had an impact on office laboratories and because of the strict requirements, many physicians send patients to independent laboratories for tests (for example, blood cell counts, cytology specimens, or cultures). However, some physicians prefer to draw blood from a patient, particularly if the patient has a history of difficult venous access.

When claims to **Medicare administrative contractors (MACs)** are submitted for laboratory services performed in the physician's office, the 10-digit CLIA certificate number should be entered in Block 23 of the CMS-1500 (02-12) claim form (Figure 12-6). Physicians billing patients for outside laboratory work are not held to these standards but may charge the patient only what the laboratory charges (based on a fee schedule), plus any additional services the physician provides (for example, drawing, handling, shipping, interpretation of the blood, or office visit).

HIPAA Compliance Alert

MEDICARE BILLING COMPLIANCE ISSUES

Because Medicare is a federal program, legislation sets down the policies that must be followed. Therefore, whoever participates in the program must comply with all regulations. Billing issues about which medical practices should be aware may include but are not limited to the following:

● Release of medical information
● Reassignment of payment
● Limiting charges for nonparticipating providers
● Correct procedural code assignment and service utilization
● Accurate diagnostic code assignment
● Medical necessity of services performed
● Billing for ancillary employees (physician assistants and nurse practitioners) called "incident-to" billing
● Documentation related to selection of procedural codes for services performed
● Ancillary orders and supervision requirements
● Teaching physician and resident billing
● Routine waiver of copayments, deductibles, or professional courtesy discounts
● Stark I and II anti-referral and compensation regulations
● Credit balance refunds
● Correct Coding Initiative (CCI) edits

PAYMENT FUNDAMENTALS

Provider

Participating Physician

In a **participating (par) physician** agreement, a physician agrees to accept payment from Medicare (80% of the **approved charges**) plus payment from the patient (20% of the approved charges) after the $147 deductible (2015) has been met (Figure 12-7). The Medicare annual deductible is based on the calendar year, January 1 through December 31. This agreement is referred to as accepting assignment. The physician must complete and transmit the CMS-1500 (02-12) claim form or ASC X12 version 5010 electronic claim to the fiscal intermediary. On the CMS-1500 claim, the assignment of benefits (Block 12) is signed by the patient, the physician indicates that assignment is being accepted by checking "Yes" in Block 27, and the payment goes directly to the physician (Figure 12-8). Physicians, practitioners, and suppliers who fail to electronically transmit or manually submit claims are subject to civil monetary penalties up to $2500 for each claim.

Nonparticipating Physician

A nonpar physician does not have a signed agreement with Medicare and has an option about assignment. The physician may decline assignment for all services or accept assignment for some services and collect from the patient

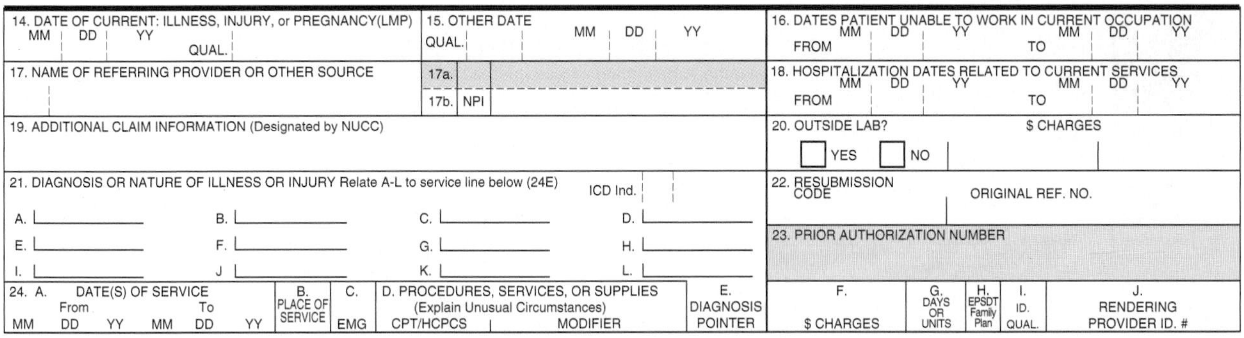

FIGURE 12-6 Section of the CMS-1500 (02-12) claim form with Block 23 emphasized, indicating where to insert a certificate number for laboratory services (CLIA No.) or a prior authorization number for a procedure when permission has been granted.

PAYMENT EXAMPLES

	Actual charge	Medicare approved amount*	Deductible	Medicare pays	Beneficiary responsible for	Medicare courtesy adjustment†
Doctor A accepts assignment.	$480	$400	$147 already satisfied	$320 (80% of approved amount)	$80 (20% of approved amount)	$80 (difference between actual charge and approved amount)
Doctor B does not accept assignment and charges the limiting amount.	$437	$380	$147 already satisfied	$304 (80% of approved amount)	$133 (20% of approved amount [$76] plus difference between limiting charge [actual charge] and approved amount [$57] = $133)	None
Doctor C accepts assignment; however, the patient has not met the deductible amount.	$480	$253 ($400 minus the deductible)	$147 has not been met	$202.40 (80% of approved amount determined after subtracting the deductible)	$197.60 (deductible plus 20% of approved amount)	$80 (difference between actual charge and approved amount)

*The Medicare approved amount is less for nonparticipating physicians than for participating physicians.
†The courtesy adjustment is the amount credited to the patient's account in the adjustment column. The word "courtesy" implies that Medicare patients are treated well and is preferred to phrases like "not allowed."

FIGURE 12-7 Payment examples for three physicians showing a physician accepting assignment versus one not accepting assignment and the amounts that the patient is responsible for paying with deductible satisfied and not met.

for other services performed at the same time and place. An exception to this policy is mandatory assignment for clinical laboratory tests and services by physician assistants. Unassigned electronic claims that are denied have no appeal rights.

Nonpar physicians receive only 95% of the Medicare-approved amount. Nonpar physicians may decide on a case-by-case basis whether to accept assignment. If the nonpar physician accepts assignment for a claim, Medicare pays 80% of the nonpar Medicare-approved amount directly to the physician and the physician collects the remaining 20% from the patient. If the nonpar physician

does not take assignment on a particular claim, he or she may "balance bill" the patient 115% of the nonpar rate because Medicare will send the payment to the patient. For example, if the nonpar rate is $100, the provider can "balance bill" the patient for $115. However, in this case, even though the physician is required to transmit the claim to Medicare, the carrier pays the patient directly and the physician therefore must collect his or her entire fee from the patient; thus physicians must "chase the money." Consequently, physicians should evaluate whether the ability to "balance bill" and collect a higher fee from the patient is worth the potential extra billing and collection costs. Furthermore, some hospitals and states, including

DRAFT - NOT FOR OFFICIAL USE

HEALTH INSURANCE CLAIM FORM

APPROVED BY NATIONAL UNIFOR MCLAIM COMMITTEE (NUCC) 02/12

☐☐ PICA   PICA ☐☐

| 1. MEDICARE ☐(Medicare#) | MEDICAID ☐(Medicaid#) | TRICARE ☐(ID#DoD#) | CHAMPVA ☐(Member ID#) | GROUP HEALTH PLAN ☐(ID#) | FECA BLK LUNG ☐(ID#) | OTHER ☐(ID#) | 1a. INSURED'S I.D. NUMBER | (For Program in Item 1) |

2. PATIENT'S NAME (Last Name, First Name, Middle Initial)

3. PATIENT'S BIRTH DATE MM DD YY   SEX M ☐ F ☐

4. INSURED'S NAME (Last Name, First Name, Middle Initial)

5. PATIENT'S ADDRESS (No., Street)

6. PATIENT RELATIONSHIP TO INSURED
Self ☐ Spouse ☐ Child ☐ Other ☐

7. INSURED'S ADDRESS (No., Street)

CITY   STATE

8. RESERVED FOR NUCC USE

CITY   STATE

ZIP CODE   TELEPHONE (Include Area Code) ( )

ZIP CODE   TELEPHONE (Include Area Code) ( )

9. OTHER INSURED'S NAME (Last Name, First Name, Middle Initial)

10. IS PATIENT'S CONDITION RELATED TO:

11. INSURED'S POLICY GROUP OR FECA NUMBER

a. OTHER INSURED'S POLICY OR GROUP NUMBER

a. EMPLOYMENT? (Current or Previous) ☐ YES ☐ NO

a. INSURED'S DATE OF BIRTH MM DD YY   SEX M ☐ F ☐

b. RESERVED FOR NUCC USE

b. AUTO ACCIDENT? ☐ YES ☐ NO   PLACE (State)

b. OTHER CLAIM ID (Designated by NUCC)

c. RESERVED FOR NUCC USE

c. OTHER ACCIDENT? ☐ YES ☐ NO

c. INSURANCE PLAN NAME OR PROGRAM NAME

d. INSURANCE PLAN NAME OR PROGRAM NAME

10d. CLAIM CODES (Designated by NUCC)

d. IS THERE ANOTHER HEALTH BENEFIT PLAN? ☐ YES ☐ NO *If yes,* complete items 9, 9a, and 9d.

READ BACK OF FORM BEFORE COMPLETING & SIGNING THIS FORM.
12. PATIENT'S OR AUTHORIZED PERSON'S SIGNATURE I authorize the release of any medical or other information necessary to process this claim. I also request payment of government benefits either to myself or to the party who accepts assignment below.

SIGNED *Signature on File*   DATE

13. INSURED'S OR AUTHORIZED PERSON'S SIGNATURE I authorize payment of medical benefits to the undersigned physician or supplier for services described below.

SIGNED

14. DATE OF CURRENT: ILLNESS, INJURY, or PREGNANCY(LMP) MM DD YY QUAL.

15. OTHER DATE QUAL. MM DD YY

16. DATES PATIENT UNABLE TO WORK IN CURRENT OCCUPATION MM DD YY FROM   TO MM DD YY

17. NAME OF REFERRING PROVIDER OR OTHER SOURCE   17a.   17b. NPI

18. HOSPITALIZATION DATES RELATED TO CURRENT SERVICES MM DD YY FROM   TO MM DD YY

19. ADDITIONAL CLAIM INFORMATION (Designated by NUCC)

20. OUTSIDE LAB? ☐ YES ☐ NO $ CHARGES

21. DIAGNOSIS OR NATURE OF ILLNESS OR INJURY Relate A-L to service line below (24E)   ICD Ind.
A. ____ B. ____ C. ____ D. ____
E. ____ F. ____ G. ____ H. ____
I. ____ J. ____ K. ____ L. ____

22. RESUBMISSION CODE   ORIGINAL REF. NO.

23. PRIOR AUTHORIZATION NUMBER

24. A. DATE(S) OF SERVICE From MM DD YY To MM DD YY	B. PLACE OF SERVICE	C. EMG	D. PROCEDURES, SERVICES, OR SUPPLIES (Explain Unusual Circumstances) CPT/HCPCS MODIFIER	E. DIAGNOSIS POINTER	F. $ CHARGES	G. DAYS OR UNITS	H. EPSDT Family Plan	I. ID. QUAL.	J. RENDERING PROVIDER ID. #
1									NPI
2									NPI
3									NPI
4									NPI
5									NPI
6									NPI

25. FEDERAL TAX I.D. NUMBER ☐ SSN ☐ EIN

26. PATIENT'S ACCOUNT NO.

27. ACCEPT ASSIGNMENT? (For govt. claims, see back) ☒ YES ☐ NO

28. TOTAL CHARGE $

29. AMOUNT PAID $

30. Rsvd for NUCC Use $

31. SIGNATURE OF PHYSICIAN OR SUPPLIER INCLUDING DEGREES OR CREDENTIALS (I certify that the statements on the reverse apply to this bill and are made a part thereof.)

SIGNED   DATE

32. SERVICE FACILITY LOCATION INFORMATION

a. NPI   b.

33. BILLING PROVIDER INFO & PH # ( )

a. NPI   b.

NUCC Instruction Manual available at: www.nucc.org   PLEASE PRINT OR TYPE   OMB APPROVAL PENDING

CARRIER — PATIENT AND INSURED INFORMATION — PHYSICIAN OR SUPPLIER INFORMATION

FIGURE 12-8 Block 12 of the CMS-1500 (02-12) claim form, where the patient signs to authorize that payment be sent to the physician, and Block 27 marked with an X, showing that the physician accepts Medicare assignment of benefits.

Minnesota, Pennsylvania, Vermont, and New York, prohibit or limit balance billing, so physicians must ascertain whether these restrictions apply before making a Medicare participation or nonparticipation decision.

Limiting charge is a percentage limit on fees, specified by legislation, that nonpar physicians may bill Medicare beneficiaries above the allowed amount. Nonpar physicians may submit usual and customary fees for assigned claims. Because of these two situations, nonpar physicians usually have a fee schedule that lists both usual fees and limiting charges. Some states have set limiting charges that are more restrictive than Medicare policies. These states are Connecticut, Massachusetts, New York, Ohio, Pennsylvania, Rhode Island, and Vermont. Inquire from the fiscal intermediary of those states for guidelines.

Prior Authorization

For Medicare patients who have additional insurance, many insurance carrier group plans and MCO senior plans require prior authorization for surgical procedures, diagnostic testing, and referrals to specialists. Some of these procedures requiring authorization are on a mandatory list, whereas others are chosen by the regional carrier. The mandatory list is composed of procedures such as the following:

- Bunionectomy
- Carotid endarterectomy
- Cataract extractions
- Cholecystectomy
- Complex peripheral revascularization
- Coronary artery bypass graft surgery
- Hysterectomy
- Inguinal hernia repair
- Joint replacements (hip, shoulder, or knee)
- Transurethral prostatectomy

Carriers may have a toll-free line to call for authorization, require the completion of a preauthorization form, or require a letter only if there is a dispute over claims payment. Check with the local carrier on its policy for preauthorization.

The prior authorization number is used when billing the Medicare carrier and is entered on the CMS-1500 (02-12) claim form in Block 23 (see Figure 12-6) or the related field of the ASC X12 version 5010 if electronically transmitted. If the procedure is not approved, the carrier sends a denial to the physician, patient, and hospital, if applicable. If the procedure is done as an emergency, notify the carrier within the time frame designated by the insurance plan so that an authorization can be arranged.

HIPAA Compliance Alert

ADVANCE BENEFICIARY NOTICE OF NONCOVERAGE

Medicare considers the appropriate use of an Advance Beneficiary Notice of Noncoverage (ABN) document as a compliance issue. Ask the patient to sign an ABN document if you know the service is not covered or if there is a possibility that a service may be denied for medical necessity or limitation of Medicare benefits. A step-by-step procedure of how to complete an ABN form is presented at the end of this chapter (see Procedure 12-2).

Waiver of Liability Provision
Limited Liability

When a patient is to receive a service from a participating physician that might be denied for medical necessity or because of *limitation of liability* by Medicare, inform the patient and have him or her agree to pay for the denied service in advance. If the Medicare guidelines or parameters are not known for a certain procedure or service, refer to *Medicare transmittals* (formerly called *program memorandums*) or call the Medicare carrier and ask. Some medical practices use a computerized method to screen for the medical necessity of a service but must have access to national coverage determinations (NCDs) and local coverage determinations (LCDs; formerly called *local medical review policies* [LMRPs]) to find out if there is limited coverage.

If you expect Medicare to deny payment (entirely or in part), instruct the patient to sign an **Advance Beneficiary Notice of Noncoverage (ABN),** also known as a *waiver of liability agreement* or *responsibility statement*, as shown in Figures 12-9 and 12-10. This form should not be given to someone who is in a medical emergency, confused, legally incompetent, or otherwise under great duress. It cannot be signed after a patient has received the service and must specifically state what service or procedure is being waived. Write the specific time frequency limitation for a particular service, such as screening colonoscopy once every 10 years. Each space on the ABN must be completed before providing the ABN to the patient. Blank or partially completed ABNs, even with the patient's signature, are not acceptable. An ABN may be mailed to a patient when presenting it face to face is not possible but the patient must have an opportunity to ask questions. When the ABN is mailed, it should be sent with a cover letter explaining that the procedure will be denied by Medicare and include contact information so that the patient can ask questions before the procedure.

To determine which services require an ABN, refer to the NCDs and the LCDs from the insurance carrier. An office policy should be in place for handling patients who refuse to sign an ABN. When sending in a claim,

A. Notifier: John Doe, MD, College Clinic, 4567 Broad Avenue, Woodland Hills, XY 12345 555-486-9002

B. Patient Name: Mary Judd   **C. Identification Number:**   0920XX7291

Advance Beneficiary Notice of Noncoverage (ABN)

NOTE: If Medicare doesn't pay for **D.** __B12 injections__ below, you may have to pay.

Medicare does not pay for everything, even some care that you or your health care provider have good reason to think you need. We expect Medicare may not pay for the **D.** __B12 injections__ below.

D.	E. Reason Medicare May Not Pay:	F. Estimated Cost
B12 injections	Medicare does not usually pay for this injection or this many injections.	$35.00

WHAT YOU NEED TO DO NOW:
- Read this notice, so you can make an informed decision about your care.
- Ask us any questions that you may have after you finish reading.
- Choose an option below about whether to receive the **D.** __B12 injections__ listed above.
  Note: If you choose Option 1 or 2, we may help you to use any other insurance that you might have, but Medicare cannot require us to do this.

G. OPTIONS: Check only one box. We cannot choose a box for you.

☑ **OPTION 1.** I want the **D.** __B12 injections__ listed above. You may ask to be paid now, but I also want Medicare billed for an official decision on payment, which is sent to me on a Medicare Summary Notice (MSN). I understand that if Medicare doesn't pay, I am responsible for payment, but **I can appeal to Medicare** by following the directions on the MSN. If Medicare does pay, you will refund any payments I made to you, less co-pays or deductibles.

☐ **OPTION 2.** I want the **D.** _____ listed above, but do not bill Medicare. You may ask to be paid now as I am responsible for payment. **I cannot appeal if Medicare is not billed**.

☐ **OPTION 3.** I don't want the **D.** _____ listed above. I understand with this choice I am **not** responsible for payment, and **I cannot appeal to see if Medicare would pay**.

H. Additional Information:

This notice gives our opinion, not an official Medicare decision. If you have other questions on this notice or Medicare billing, call **1-800-MEDICARE** (1-800-633-4227/**TTY:** 1-877-486-2048).
Signing below means that you have received and understand this notice. You also receive a copy.

I. Signature: *Mary Judd*	J. Date: *March 20, 20XX*

Form CMS-R-131 (03/11)   Form Approved OMB No. 0938-0566

FIGURE 12-9 Advance Beneficiary Notice of Noncoverage (ABN), Form CMS-R-131, which is also referred to as a *responsibility statement* or *waiver of liability agreement.*

permanently implemented when Congress enacted the Tax Relief and Health Care Act of 2006. This extended the RAC Initiative to all 50 states by 2010. Its goals are to identify Medicare underpayments and overpayments and recover overpayments using automated review and complex review. An automated review is done electronically without human review and a complex review is done using human review of the medical record. A single RAC will serve one of four geographic regions (Regions A, B, C, and D) and perform recovery audit services for all Medicare claim types in that region. RACs may identify improper payments from claims they review that may show incorrect payment amounts, noncovered services, incorrectly coded services, DRG miscoding, and duplicate services. RACs are paid a percentage of the incorrect payments they recover. When an underpayment is found, a RAC will communicate this to the MAC. If both underpayments and overpayments are found, the RAC will offset the underpayment from the overpayment. On overpayments, interest accrues from the date of the final determination. Claims identified as overpayments are subject to the Medicare appeals process.

CLAIM SUBMISSION

Local Coverage Determination

LCD, formerly known as LMRP, is a decision by the MAC whether to cover a particular service on a contractor-wide basis in accordance with the SSA (that is, a determination as to whether the service is reasonable and necessary). LCD is an educational and administrative tool to assist physicians, providers, and suppliers in transmitting correct claims for payment. Contractor medical directors and staff develop LCDs with input from the public. LCDs list covered and noncovered codes for a given Medicare policy but do not include any of the coding guidance that was found in LMRPs. LCDs outline how contractors review claims to determine whether Medicare coverage requirements have been met. CMS requires that local policies be consistent with national guidance. Use of LCDs helps to avoid situations in which claims are paid or denied without a full understanding of the basis for payment and denial. LCDs may be obtained from the Medicare carrier website at www.cms.hhs.gov/mcd.

Medicare Administrative Contractors and Fiscal Intermediaries

An organization handling claims from hospitals, NFs, **intermediate care facilities (ICFs),** long-term care facilities (LTCFs), and home health agencies is called a *fiscal intermediary.* The National Blue Cross Association holds the fiscal intermediary contract for Medicare Part A; in turn, it subcontracts it to member agencies.

Organizations handling claims from physicians and other suppliers of services covered under Medicare Part B are called *Medicare administrative contractors (MACs),* formerly called *fiscal agents.* Medicare Part B payments are handled by private insurance organizations under contract with the government. Since January 1, 1992, the rule for where to send a Medicare claim is to bill the carrier who covers the area where the service occurred or was furnished, not the carrier who services the physician's office.

Provider Identification Numbers

Another requirement of the Tax Reform Act was the establishment of several types of identification numbers for each physician and non-physician practitioner providing services paid by Medicare. Because there are so many numbers, they are easily confused and end up being the source of many errors when completing blocks on the CMS-1500 (02-12) claim form or the related fields of the ASC X12 version 5010 when electronically transmitted. The numbers defined and shown in template examples with correct placement in Chapter 7 follow:

- Unique physician identification numbers (UPINs), provider identification numbers (PINs), group, and individual. With the implementation of the National Provider Identifier (NPI) on May 23, 2007, UPINs and PINs are no longer used.
- Durable medical equipment (DME) supplier number.

Patient's Signature Authorization

Signatures for transmitting electronic claims and acceptance of financial responsibility must be obtained and retained in the office records because there are no handwritten signatures on electronic claims. A form created by the medical practice may be used or a Medicare patient's signature may be obtained in Block 12 of the CMS-1500 (02-12) claim form. This is also required for electronically transmitted claims. This block should be signed regardless of whether the physician is a participating or nonparticipating physician. The signed authorization should be kept on file in the patient's health record for an episode of care or for a designated time frame (for example, 1 year). Claims may indicate "Signature on file" or "SOF" in Block 12 of the claim form. Further information on this topic may be found in Chapters 3, 7, and 8.

SOF situations that may occur in a medical practice are as follows:

- *Illiterate or physically handicapped.* When an illiterate or physically handicapped enrollee signs by mark (X), a witness should sign his or her name and address next to the mark. If the claim is filed for the patient by another person, that person should enter the patient's name and write "By," sign his or her own name and address, indicate relationship to the patient, and state why the patient cannot sign.

- *Confinement in a facility.* Sometimes it is not possible to obtain the signature of a Medicare patient because of confinement in an NF, hospital, or home. In such cases, physicians should obtain an annual signature authorization from the patient.
- *Medigap (MG) claim.* When transmitting a **crossover claim** to an MG carrier, obtain an annual signature authorization for the MG carrier.
- *Deceased patient.* Refer to the section titled "Claims for Deceased Patients" later in this chapter for signature requirements.
- *Medi-Medi claim.* These crossover claims do not require the patient's signature.

Time Limit

The Health Care Reform of 2010 changed the filing deadline for claims. Beginning October 1, 2009, providers no longer have 15 to 24 months to file and must submit claims within 12 months of the date of service (see the box below).

For services furnished on:	The time limit for filing is:
October 1, 2015, to September 30, 2016	September 31, 2017
October 1, 2016, to September 30, 2017	September 31, 2018

On assigned claims, the provider may file without penalty up to 27 months after providing service if reasonable cause for the delay is shown to the insurance carrier. Otherwise, there is a 10% reduction in the reimbursement. On unassigned claims, the provider may be fined up to $2000 for delinquent claim submission or be dropped from Medicare. When transmitting a late claim, ask the fiscal intermediary for the guidelines that CMS considers reasonable cause for delay.

Paper Claims

The form that physicians use to submit paper claims to Medicare is CMS-1500 (02-12). Refer to Chapter 7 for instructions on how to complete the CMS-1500 (02-12) claim form for the Medicare program. The reference templates (samples of completed claim forms) for Medicare and supplemental coverage shown at the end of that chapter are as follows:

- Medicare, no secondary coverage: Figure 7-5
- Medi/Medi, crossover: Figure 7-6

- Medicare/MG, crossover: Figure 7-7
- Other insurance/Medicare MSP: Figure 7-8

Patients are not allowed to submit claims to Medicare, with four exceptions. Situations where a patient may file a claim are the following:

- Services covered by Medicare for which the patient has other insurance that should pay first, called *MSP*
- Services provided by a physician who refuses to transmit the claim
- Services provided outside the United States
- Situations in which DME is purchased from a private source

Medicare claim status is explained in detail in Chapter 7 (e.g., clean, incomplete, rejected, dirty, or other claims). To obtain the mailing address for sending Medicare claim forms in your state or county, go to the website www.cms.hhs.gov/apps/contacts/. For further information and booklets, pamphlets, and the annual *Medicare & You* handbook, contact the nearest Social Security office.

Electronic Claims

Medicare requests that all providers transmit claims electronically. All electronic transmission formats are standardized by the use of ANSI ASC X12N (837) Version 5010. Refer to Chapter 8 for information on how to transmit claims electronically to the Medicare carrier.

Medicare/Medicaid Claims

Medi-Medi patients qualify for the benefits of Medicare and Medicaid. Use the CMS-1500 (02-12) claim form or electronically transmit the claim and check "Yes" for the assignment in Block 27. If the physician does not accept assignment, then payment goes to the patient and Medicaid (in California, Medi-Cal) will not pick up the residual. The claim will be crossed over and processed automatically by Medicaid after processing is completed by Medicare. The fiscal intermediary may refer to this as a crossover claim or *claims transfer*. It is not necessary to submit another form. Claims should be sent according to the time limit designated by the Medicaid program in the state. Generally, the Medicare payment exceeds the Medicaid fee schedule and little or no payment is received except when the patient has not met his or her annual Medicare deductible.

In some states, the fiscal intermediary for a crossover claim may have a different address from that used for the processing of a patient who is on Medicare only.

Write or call the nearest Medicare fiscal intermediary for the guidelines pertinent to the state.

Medicare/Medigap Claims

Medicare has streamlined the processing of Medicare/Medigap claims in most states. Medicare carriers transmit MG claims electronically for participating physicians, thus eliminating the need to file an additional claim. This is also called a *crossover claim*. MG payments go directly to the participating physicians and a **Medicare Summary Notice (MSN)** is sent to the patient that states, "This claim has been referred to your supplemental carrier for any additional benefits."

To ensure the crossover of the Medicare/Medigap claim, for paper claims complete Blocks 9 through 9d of the CMS-1500 (02-12) claim form and list the payer identification (PAYRID) number of the MG plan in Block 9d. The PAYRID for MG plans is referred to as *Other Carrier Name and Address (OCNA)* number and a list of all OCNAs is published in the Medicare newsletter.

If automatic crossover capabilities are not offered in one's state, attach the Medicare RA to the claim form and electronically transmit or submit a claim to the MG plan separately.

Refer to Figure 7-7 for submitting claims when Medicare is primary and the patient has an MG (supplemental) policy.

Medicare/Employer Supplemental Insurance Claims

Some individuals have supplemental coverage with complementary benefits through employment plans even after retirement. In some cases, this coverage may be paid by a former employer after retirement. Usually crossover relationships exist with many insurance carriers who insure Medicare beneficiaries.

Medicare/Supplemental and Medicare Supplementary Payer Claims

Submitting a claim for a Medicare patient who has supplemental insurance can be confusing. First, decide whether the case is Medicare primary or secondary payer. The procedure for determining whether Medicare is primary or secondary is presented at the end of this chapter (see Procedure 12-1). If Medicare is primary and the secondary payer is an MG policy, follow Medi/Medi processing guidelines. After determining which insurance is primary, follow the directions on

what should be entered in each block of the CMS-1500 claim form or field of the ASC X12 version 5010 claims transmittal, depending on the primary payer, or follow MSP guidelines.

Templates (samples of completed claim forms) shown at the end of Chapter 7 make it easier to learn which blocks to complete and which to ignore, depending on the primary and secondary payer. Figure 7-8 is an example of billing other insurance primary and MSP. A copy of the front and back sides of the primary insurance's EOB document must be attached to the claim when billing Medicare.

See Chapter 7 for general instructions for completing claims in Medicare and MSP cases.

Claims for Deceased Patients

The following are two ways to submit billing for a patient who has died:
1. Participating physician accepts assignment on the claim form or electronically transmitted claim. This results in the quickest payment. No signature by a family member is necessary on the CMS-1500 (02-12) claim form or electronically transmitted claim. Insert "Patient died on (indicate date)" in Block 12 where the patient's signature is necessary.
2. The nonparticipating physician does not accept assignment, bills Medicare, and submits the following:
   a. A CMS-1500 (02-12) claim form signed by the estate representative who is responsible for the bill
   b. A statement or claim for all services provided
   c. Name and address of the responsible party
   d. Provider's statement, signed and dated, refusing to accept assignment

Nothing can be done about the open balance on the account until the estate is settled and then Medicare will pay.

Physician Substitute Coverage

Many times, special substitute coverage arrangements are made between physicians (for example, on call, vacation, or unavailable because of another commitment). These arrangements are referred to as either *reciprocal* for on-call situations or *locum tenens* for a vacation situation. Specific modifiers are used to distinguish these situations and special billing guidelines are stated as follows:
● *Reciprocal arrangement*. When transmitting Medicare claims, the regular physician must identify the service provided by the substitute doctor by listing the -Q5 modifier after the procedure code.

- *Locum tenens arrangement.* When transmitting Medicare claims, the regular physician must identify the service provided by the substitute doctor by listing the -Q6 modifier after the procedure code.

AFTER CLAIM SUBMISSION

Remittance Advice

Medicare sends a payment check and a nationally standardized document called a *Medicare remittance advice (RA)*, formerly known as an *explanation of Medicare benefits (EOMB)*, to participating physicians. The front side of the RA lists status codes that are the same nationwide, representing the reason a claim may not have been paid in full, was denied, and so forth. These codes are defined on the reverse side of the RA. If the patient has MG, supplementary, or complementary crossover coverage, the "other payer" statement states whether the claim has been transferred to the supplemental insurer.

Nonpar physicians also receive an RA with payment information about unassigned claims. The RA separates payment information about assigned claims from unassigned claims to avoid posting errors by the practice. Check the payment against the fee schedule to determine whether the benefits are for the correct amount. On each claim form, note the date on which the payment is posted for reference. Optional items to document are amount of payment, RA processing data, and batch number.

Offices transmitting claims electronically receive an electronic remittance advice (ERA) showing payment data and this may be uploaded automatically to the office computer system. The ERA electronically posts payments and the provider does not have to post them manually. Paper and electronic remittance notices have the same format.

Medicare Summary Notice

A patient is mailed a similar document called a *Medicare Summary Notice (MSN)*. This document is designed to be easier for the patient to understand but because many patients do not know what is meant by *amount charged, Medicare approved, deductible,* and *coinsurance,* it often becomes necessary for the insurance billing specialist to educate the patient. First, photocopy an RA that can be used as an example, deleting the patient's name to ensure confidentiality. Then, use the RA to illustrate to future patients what various terms mean. This will increase patient understanding and save time.

When a claim is denied, the MSN will identify the number of the LCD or NCD used in denial of the claim.

BENEFICIARY REPRESENTATIVE OR REPRESENTATIVE PAYEE

Medicare beneficiaries may have memory impairment or may be confined to a wheelchair or bed, so they have a legal right to appoint an individual to serve as their representative.

Claims assistance professionals (CAPs) act as client representatives. They have some legal standing and are recognized by Medicare to act on the beneficiary's behalf if the beneficiary completes a Beneficiary Representative Form SSA-1696. This form is available from the SSA district office. Copies of the completed form should be sent to the Medicare intermediary or carrier when appropriate.

In contrast, a representative payee is an individual or organization chosen by the SSA to receive and administer SSA benefit funds on behalf of the beneficiary. Other duties consist of assisting the beneficiary with check writing for financial obligations, such as personal care and maintenance, housing, and medical service expenses, and investing any surplus monies for the beneficiary's benefit. A representative payee is responsible for using payments received only for the benefit of the beneficiary, accounting for the benefits received on request, and contacting SSA when anything affects eligibility for SSA benefits or prevents the representative payee's ability to perform these responsibilities. Additional information on CAPs is found in Chapters 1 and 18.

Posting Payments

Usually a physician's charge is higher than the charge approved by the MAC. This does not mean that his or her charges are unreasonable. As mentioned, payments are established using a fee schedule based on an RBRVS, a **volume performance standard (VPS)** for expenditure increases, and a limiting charge for nonparticipating physicians. VPS is the desired growth rate for spending on Medicare Part B physician services that is set each year by Congress.

Because some services may be disallowed or the payments on them may be lower than those charged by the physician, know how to post payments to the patient's financial accounting record card or computerized account. Figure 12-13 illustrates how payments and contractual or courtesy adjustments are posted. The word *courtesy* implies that Medicare patients are treated well and is preferred to phrases such as "not allowed" or "write-off."

Medicare does not allow for the standardized waiving of copayments. Medicare regulations require that a patient be billed for the copayment at least three times

COLLEGE CLINIC
4567 Broad Avenue
Woodland Hills, XY 12345-0001
Telephone: 555-486-9002
Fax: 555-487-8976

Billing Date
05/24/XX

Payment Due

Responsible Party

JOHN SMITH
100 James Street
Woodland Hills, XY 12345-0001

**Please Pay
This Amount**
▼
84.99

Please Charge My:
☐ Visa/MC   ☐ Amex   ☐ Discover
Amount: _____
Card #: _____
Expiration: _____ Code: _____
Signature: _____

Patient
JOHN SMITH

Amount Enclosed

Account:
1-04140

Make Checks Payable To: COLLEGE CLINIC

Patient: JOHN SMITH   **Provider:** GASTON INPUT, MD

Date	Doc	Code	Diag	Description of Service	Charge	Payments	Balance
				The following items have been responded to by your insurance and are now due:			
03/30/XX	CI	99214		EST PT LEVEL 4	100.00		
05/04/XX	CI	-----		MEDICARE CHECK		4.24−	
05/04/XX	CI	-----		MEDICARE COURTESY ADJUSTMENT		9.71−	
05/04/XX				App. to deduct: $84.99			
05/09/XX	CI	-----		B/C #2 PMT		1.06−	
				Totals for 03/30/06 services:	**100.00**	**15.01−**	**84.99**

Billing Date	Last Payment	Paid On	Current	Over 60	Over 90	Over 120	Balance Due
05/24/XX	1.06	05/09/XX	84.99	0.00	0.00	0.00	84.99

Insurance:
Medicare - BLUE CROSS

Account:
1-04140

FIGURE 12-13 Electronically generated financial accounting record (ledger card) illustrating how payments and contractual or courtesy adjustments should be posted.

before the balance is adjusted off as uncollectable. Document this as further justification if the patient is suffering financial hardship.

When an RA is received, it may list many patients (Figure 12-14). Do not post the entire payment made in a lump sum to the daysheet. Individually post each line item paid to the patient's financial accounting record card or computerized account and to the daysheet (Figure 12-15). To prevent funds from going astray, some offices prefer to post Medicare payments to a separate daysheet and deposit each multiple reimbursement check separately. The daysheet totals will then agree with the deposit slip totals and not get confused with other monies collected.

Figure 12-16, *A*, illustrates an example of a Medicare/ Medicaid case after payment by Medicare. Medicare applied the patient's full $147 deductible amount to the

Medicare-allowed amount, reducing payment to $26.40. The Medicaid RA (Figure 12-16, *B*) shows reimbursement of the coinsurance and deductible amounts dual-billed to Medicaid.

Calculations are shown in the following box:

Medicare		Medicaid	
$180	Allowed amount	$180	Medicare allowed amount
−147	Deductible		
$ 33	Balance on which payment is	−32	Medicaid cutback
		$148	Medicaid allowed
× .80	calculated		
$26.40		26.40	Medicare paid
		$148.40	Medicaid payment

When referring to the Medicaid program, a cutback means a reduction, which is reducing Medicare's

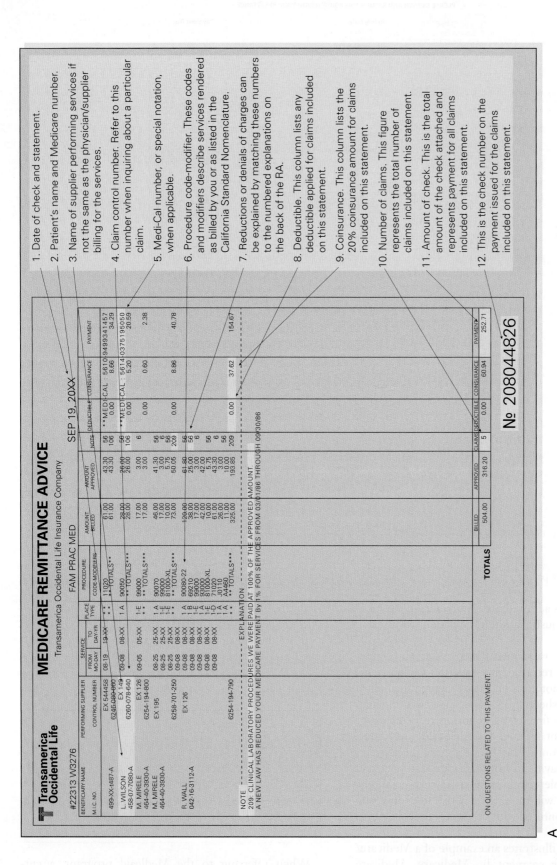

FIGURE 12-14 Medicare remittance advice (RA) document. **A,** Front. Insurance carriers are required to use Centers for Medicare and Medicaid Services (CMS) messages for Medicare RA but each carrier has its own code numbers to denote the messages.

Continued

EXPLANATION OF NOTES

Additional notes may be listed on the front of this form.

1 – See enclosed letter.

2 – Claim was filed after the time limit.

4 – These bills are handled by a special intermediary.

5 – This payment is for an adjustment of a previous claim.

6 – Charges over the maximum Medicare allowance are not covered.

7 – Services before Medicare entitlement are not covered.

8 – Services after Medicare entitlement ended are not covered.

10 – Other charges submitted with this claim may be on a separate statement which you have received or will receive soon.

12 – Routine examinations and related services are not covered.

13 – Immunizations or other routine and preventative services are not covered.

16 – We need an itemization of this charge. Please resubmit your claim with this information.

17 – Prescription drugs are not covered.

18 – Charges for this physician/supplier are not covered.

19 – We need a full description of the service or supply to consider this charge. Please resubmit your claim with this information.

23 – We need a written report for this service. Please resubmit your claim with this information.

26 – More than $312.50 annual psychiatric expense is not covered.

27 – We need from the prescribing physician the specific length of time this medical equipment is needed. Please resubmit your claim with this information.

30 – This charge was previously considered.

37 – Claims for these services will be made by a home health agency or hospital.

39 – Equipment that is not medically necessary is not covered. (See Note 89)

42 – These supplies or services are not covered.

45 – Over $62\frac{1}{2}$% of psychiatric expenses is not covered.

46 – Routine foot care is not covered.

47 – Routine eye examinations or eye refractions are not covered.

48 – Partial payment of this claim was made to the beneficiary.

49 – This service cannot be considered until the hospital makes the necessary arrangement with the carrier for its processing.

50 – The beneficiary is not responsible for this reduction/denial under the assignment agreement.

54 – Care before and/or after surgery is included in the surgery benefit. (See Note 50)

56 – This is the full charge allowed based upon the prevailing or usual and customary rate.

62 – Payment has been reduced because this test is commonly part of an automated test group. (See Note 50)

66 – This service is not covered when done by this laboratory.

70 – There were no charges or bills with your claim form. Please resubmit your claim with this information.

72 – We need a signed and dated prescription showing medical necessity and specific length of time needed. Please resubmit your claim with this information.

73 – Before another month's payment can be made, we need a new signed and dated prescription showing further necessity of the medical equipment and specific length of time needed.

80 – We need to know the place of service to consider this charge. Please resubmit your claim with this information.

83 – SSA advises us that they are unable to verify the patient's eligibility for Part B Medical Insurance Plan. For this reason, no payment can be made on this claim.

84 – The patient's HIC number shown on this claim was incorrect. Please use the correct HIC number on all future claims.

85 – The patient's name shown on this claim was incorrect. Please use the correct name on all future claims.

86 – Over $62\frac{1}{2}$% of the allowable charges for psychiatric services is not covered.

89 – If you did not know that Medicare does not pay for this medical service, you may request a review of this decision. See below paragraph entitled "Your right to review of a case."

90 – This service by a chiropractor is not covered.

93 – Over $500.00 annual expense billed by a physical therapist is not covered.

95 – These specific services by this supplier are not covered.

96 – Please verify the date of this service. Resubmit your claim with this information.

99 – We need a complete diagnosis before the claim can be considered. Please resubmit your claim with this information.

106 – The Medicare covered services on this claim have been forwarded for additional processing under Medi-Cal.

107 – This claim was not forwarded for Medi-Cal processing. Please bill Medi-Cal directly and attach a copy of this statement.

108 – The bills for these services have been transferred to Blue Shield of California Medicare Claims, Chico, CA 95976. You will hear from them.

129 – Payment for services prior to July 1 is based on the previous year's payment rate.

131 – Payment for this physician service in a hospital department is reduced since this service is commonly performed in the physician's office. (See Note 89)

138 – This amount is more than Medicare pays for maintenance treatment of renal disease.

147 – This charge is not covered because an allowance for purchase of the same equipment was previously made.

151 – Your claim was transferred to a Health Maintenance Organization for processing.

153 – These are more visits (treatments) for this diagnosis than Medicare covers unless there were unusual circumstances. (See Note 89)

154 – This service is not covered for your patient's reported condition. (See Note 89)

155 – Only one visit per month to a nursing home is covered unless special need is indicated. (See Note 89)

156 – This laboratory test for the reported condition and/or illness is not covered. (See Note 89)

158 – Procedures whose effectiveness has not been proven are not covered. (See Note 89)

161 – The frequency of services for this condition are not covered. (See Note 89)

162 – More than one visit per day for this condition are not covered. (See Note 89)

172 – This type of services billed by a psychologist are not covered.

179 – The amount for this service is included in the approved amount for the consultation/office/hospital visit.

181 – Payment for this service is included in the major surgical fee.

187 – We need the name and address of the individual doctor who performed this service. Please resubmit your claim with this information.

192 – Medicare benefits have been reduced because the patient's employer group health plan has paid some of these expenses.

198 – A claim must be sent to the patient's employer group health plan first. After the claim has been processed by that plan, resubmit this claim with the bills and the notice the other insurance company sent you.

203 – Clinical laboratory services. Blood Gas Studies and Rhythm Strips (1–3 leads) furnished in a hospital setting are reimbursed through the hospital.

205 – The date of this service is after the patient's expiration date provided to us by SSA. If service was rendered to this patient on this date, have the patient's estate contact the local Social Security Office for assistance.

206 – For payment, these services must be billed by the performing laboratory with the assignment accepted.

213 – We did not send this claim to Medicaid. Please send this statement and a copy of the claim to the agency that handles Medicaid in your area.

216 – This service or item cannot be processed until your application for a Medicare provider identification number is received and approved.

218 – Since you are Medicare participating, we have processed this claim as assigned. Future claims must be billed on assignment. If the bill was paid in full, you must immediately refund the amount due to the beneficiary.

219 – We need this charge submitted on your letterhead bill. Please resubmit your claim with this information.

221 – The name and Medicare number submitted on this claim do not match. Please verify for whom these services were rendered and provide the correct name and number on the claim and resubmit.

223 – We did not consider this for payment because you did not send the extra information we asked for. Payment can be requested again by sending us another claim form and all the information.

226 – Medicare will pay rent for the prescribed number of months or until the equipment is no longer needed, whichever occurs first. This is the first monthly rental payment.

227 – You will receive a notice each month when additional rental payments are paid.

231 – Medicare will no longer pay for rental on this item since the purchase price has been paid.

237 – The amount of this payment is the difference between the approved purchase allowance and the rental payments you have received.

YOUR RIGHT TO REVIEW OF A CASE

If you have a problem or question about the way a claim was handled or about the amount paid, please write Transamerica Occidental Life, Box 54905, Terminal Annex, Los Angeles, California 90054, within 6 months of the date of this notice. We will give your request full consideration.

Your Social Security office will help you file a request for review of a claim if it is more convenient for you.

WHERE TO SEND REFUNDS

When refunding a payment you should send a check with a letter of explanation. The letter should include your Transamerica Occidental/Medicare check number, beneficiary name and Medicare identification number (HICNo.), control number to which the payment relates, and any other information which may be pertinent to the refund. Send this information to:

Transamerica Occidental Life
C/O Check and Payment Control
Box 54905, Terminal Annex
Los Angeles, CA 90054-0905

KEY TO CODES FOR PLACE AND TYPE OF SERVICE

Place of service	Type of service
1. Office	A. Medical care
2. Home	B. Surgery (includes treatment of fractures)
3. Inpatient hospital	C. Consultation
4. Skilled nursing facility	D. Diagnostic X-ray
5. Outpatient hospital	E. Diagnostic laboratory
6. Independent laboratory	F. Radiation therapy
7. Other	G. Anesthesia
8. Independent kidney disease treatment center	H. Assistance at surgery
	I. Other medical service
	J. Whole blood or packed red cells

B

FIGURE 12-14, cont'd B, Back of Medicare RA document.

allowable charges to Medicaid's allowable charges. This would require an adjustment entry on the patient's financial accounting record. Cutbacks are common on Medicaid claims.

Medicare overpayments can occur in the following situations:
- The carrier processes the charge more than once.
- The physician receives duplicate payments from Medicare and a secondary payer.

- The physician is paid directly on an unassigned claim.
- The item is not covered but is paid.
- The payment is made on erroneous information.

If an overpayment check is received, providers have 60 days to report and return any overpayments discovered. Deposit the check and then write to Medicare notifying them of the overpayment. Include a copy of the check and the RA. Depending on the policy of the carrier, the provider can either write a check or this overpayment will be deducted from the next Medicare payment and will be shown on the RA. If the physician wishes to repay a Medicare overpayment on the installment plan, a Financial Statement of Debtor CMS-379 form may be used. This form is sent to the physician when the carrier notifies the physician that money is due back.

Refer to Chapter 9 for additional information about EOB documents from private insurance carriers.

Review and Redetermination Process

Chapter 9 outlines in detail the steps to take to have a claim reviewed and the process of appealing a claim in the Medicare program.

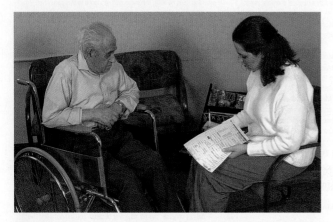

FIGURE 12-15 Insurance billing specialist explaining a Medicare remittance advice (RA) document that the physician's office has received.

MEDICARE REMITTANCE ADVICE
XYZ Insurance Company

Physician or supplier name	Dates of service From To MMDD MMDDYY	See back serv typl	Sub code (alwcode)	Billed amount	Amount allowed	See ** act cde	Beneficiary obligation Deductible Co-ins		Medicare payment to Beneficiary provider

BENEFICIARY: BILL HUTCH   HIC NUMBER: 5432-112-34
CONTROL NO.: 92106-30810-00   DE/MI: 2121D52

| John Doe MD 0310 | 0310XX | D 03 | 120101 | 245.00 | 180.00 | 101 | 147.00 | 1.00 | 0.00 | 26.40 |
| CLAIM TOTALS: | | | | 245.00 | 180.00 | 101 | 147.00 | 1.00 | 0.00 | 26.40 |

A

MEDICAID REMITTANCE ADVICE

RECIPIENT NAME	RECIPIENT MEDICAID ID NO.	CLAIM CONTROL NUMBER	SERVICE DATE MO DAY YR	PROCEDURE CODE	PATIENT ACCT. NO.	QTY.	MEDICARE ALLOWED	MEDICAID ALLOWED	PATIENT LIABILITY	COMPUTED MCR AMT.	MEDICAID PAID	EOB MESSAGE
BILL HUTCH	521345678	4006984891200	03 10 XX	49555–80		001	180.00	148.00		26.40	.00	
		4006984891200	00 00 XX			000	180.00	148.00		26.40	148.00	
BLOOD DEDUCT 00 DEDUCTIBLE 147.00 COINSUR 1.00 CUTBACK 32.00												CUTBACK 443

B

FIGURE 12-16 A, A Medicare/Medicaid case after payment by Medicare. **B,** The Medicaid remittance advice (RA) shows reimbursement of the coinsurance and deductible amounts dual billed to Medicaid.

PROCEDURE 12-1

Determine Whether Medicare Is Primary or Secondary and Determine Additional Benefits

1. Inquire whether the patient is covered under one or more of the following plans or situations:

   • *Automobile liability insurance, no-fault insurance, or self-insured liability insurance. An individual injured or ill because of an automobile accident may be covered by liability insurance or no-fault insurance.*

   • *Disability insurance. Disability insurance coverage offered through an employer-sponsored large group health plan (LGHP).*

   • *Employee group health plan (EGHP). Insurance policies for individuals 65 years of age or older who are still employed. Employers with 20 or more employees are required to offer workers and their spouses ages 65 through 69 years the same health benefits offered to younger workers. Workers may accept or reject the employer's health insurance plan. If they accept it, Medicare becomes the secondary insurance carrier.*

   • *Employer supplemental insurance. A Medicare beneficiary has this plan through a former employer. Some people are covered by employment plans even after retirement, as long as the plan allows it and the insured informs the insurance company that he or she wishes to maintain coverage. These are known as conversion policies. Complementary benefits can vary in these supplemental plans and these policies are not considered "Medigap" as defined by federal law. Note: When an employee retires and Medicare becomes the primary coverage, the company's group health plan coordinates benefits with Medicare.*

   • *Federal Black Lung Act. This Act was formed to cover employees or former coal miner employees who have illness related to black lung disorder and have acceptable diagnoses that occur on the Department of Labor's list.*

   • *Department of Veterans Affairs (VA). A Medicare beneficiary is also receiving benefits from the VA. In this situation, there must be a decision made as to where to send the claim. Medicare is not secondary to the VA and the VA is not secondary to Medicare. The claim is sent where specified by the patient. The claim can be sent to Medicare, where if the claim is processed, the patient must satisfy his or her contractual requirement to pay any deductible and copayment amounts. If the patient asks that the claim be sent to the VA instead of Medicare, the claim is processed and any payments issued are considered as payment in full. Many veterans want the claim sent to the VA.*

   • *Workers' compensation. An individual suffers a disease or injury connected with employment.*
   These plans are billed as primary (first) payer and Medicare second. Payments for these types of policies may not necessarily go to the physician but may go to the insured.

2. Ask to see the Medicare card, as well as any other insurance cards, and make photocopies of both sides of each card.

3. Inquire of the patient whether the supplemental coverage was carried over (conversion policy) from his or her employer.

4. Call both carriers if the type of plan is not clearly identified.

5. Bill the correct insurance plan.

   For Medigap (MG) cases, nonparticipating physicians may collect copayments and deductibles up to their limiting charge (unless the state forbids collection of more than the allowed amount) from patients at the time of service. Participating physicians may not collect copayments and deductibles from patients covered by MG if the patient requests that the physician submit the claim to the MG insurer. Collect copayments after receiving the Medicare/MG remittance advice (RA) document.

   For other secondary insurance, write the patient's group and policy (or certificate) numbers on the Medicare RA, attach it to either a new CMS-1500 (02-12) or a copy of the original Health Insurance Claim Form CMS-1500 (02-12), and electronically transmit or submit it to the secondary carrier. Then copy the physician's billing statement that shows date of treatment, description of service(s) rendered, fees, and diagnosis.

PROCEDURE 12-2

Complete an Advance Beneficiary Notice of Noncoverage (ABN) Form CMS-R-131

There are 10 blanks for completion labeled A through J:

A. Notifier(s): Enter the name, address, and telephone number of the provider.

B. Patient Name: Enter the first and last name and middle initial of the Medicare beneficiary.

C. Identification Number: Enter a number for the Medicare beneficiary that helps to link the notice with a related claim. However, this field is optional and choosing not to enter a number does not invalidate the ABN. The beneficiary's Medicare health insurance claim number will no longer be used.

D. Enter name of item(s), service(s), test(s), or procedure(s). If not enough space, use an attached sheet, noting it in the box.

E. Reason Medicare May Not Pay: Explain the reason why you think the service may not be covered by Medicare (for example, Medicare does not pay for

this test for the condition or Medicare does not pay for these tests as often as this [denied as too frequent]).

F. Estimated Cost: Enter a cost estimate for any item or service described in field D.

G. Options: Patient should choose and check one of the three boxes. If the beneficiary cannot make a choice, the notice should be annotated.

H. Additional Information: Insert more comments for clarification (for example, provide context on Medicare payment policy applicable to a specific benefit or other payer information).

I. Signature: Medicare beneficiary should sign the notice.

J. Date: Insert the date on which the beneficiary signed the ABN.

KEY POINTS

This is a brief chapter review, or summary, of the key issues presented. To further enhance your knowledge of the technical subject matter, review the key terms and key abbreviations for this chapter by locating the meaning for each in the Glossary at the end of this book, which appears in a section before the index.

1. Medicare is administered by the CMS.
2. Medicare is a health insurance program for people age 65 or older, people younger than age 65 with certain disabilities, and people of all ages with ESRD.
3. The patient's complete name exactly as shown on his or her insurance card and Medicare claim number, including the letter at the end, must appear on all Medicare claims.
4. Medicare Part A is for hospital insurance benefits and Medicare Part B is for medical insurance benefits.
5. Medicare Part C is referred to as *Medicare Advantage Plan (MA plan)*. This plan offers a number of health care options in addition to those available under Medicare Part A and Part B.
6. Medicare Part D Prescription Drug Plan is a standalone drug plan, presented by insurance and other private companies, that offers drug coverage that meets the standards established by Medicare.
7. Several federal acts regulate health care coverage of persons age 65 and older who are employed.
8. Medigap is a specialized Medicare supplemental insurance policy whose predefined minimum benefits are regulated by the federal government and devised for the Medicare beneficiary.
9. MSP is a primary insurance plan of a Medicare beneficiary who must pay for any medical care or services first before a Medicare fiscal intermediary is sent a claim.
10. To prevent overuse of services and spot fraud, the federal False Claims Amendments Act was enacted in 1986. It offers financial incentives to informants (whistleblowers).
11. CLIA is a federal act established in 1988 that regulates laboratory certification and accreditation standards, quality control, proficiency testing, personnel standards, program administration, and safety measures for all freestanding laboratories, including POLs.
12. Because Medicare is a federal program, providers that transmit claims to Medicare must comply with billing and coding regulations issued by CMS.
13. Participating physicians agree to accept assignment on all Medicare claims and may bill the patient only for the Medicare deductible ($147 in 2015) and coinsurance amounts.
14. An ABN is an agreement given to the patient to read and sign before rendering a service if the participating physician thinks that it may be denied for payment because of medical necessity or limitation of liability by Medicare. ABNs apply if the patient is in an original Medicare program and do not apply for patients in private fee-for-service (PFFS) or managed care plans.
15. CCI is federal legislation that attempts to eliminate unbundling or other inappropriate reporting of procedural codes for services to Medicare patients.
16. To obtain correct payment for a procedure or service, a code number must be selected from level I or II of the HCPCS coding system and transmitted to the Medicare administrative contractor (MAC).
17. The time limit for sending in Medicare claims is within 12 months from the date of service.
18. Medicare sends a payment check and a nationally standardized document to participating physicians called a *Medicare RA* and a similar document to the patient called an *MSN*.

💻 STUDENT ASSIGNMENT

✔ Study Chapter 12.
✔ Answer the fill-in-the-blank, multiple-choice, and true/false review questions in the *Workbook* to reinforce the theory learned in this chapter and to help you prepare for a future test.
✔ Complete the assignments in the *Workbook* to give you experience in computing Medicare in mathematic calculations, selecting HCPCS code numbers, abstracting from patients' health records, preparing financial accounting record cards, and completing forms pertinent to the Medicare program.
✔ Turn to the Glossary at the end of this text for a further understanding of the key terms and key abbreviations used in this chapter.

CHAPTER 13

Medicaid and Other State Programs

Marilyn Takahashi Fordney

OBJECTIVES

After reading this chapter, you should be able to:

1. Discuss the history of Medicaid.
2. Describe added benefits for Medicaid recipients afforded by the Patient Protection and Affordable Care Act and the Health Care and Education Reconciliation Act of 2010.
3. Discuss how Medicaid is administered by state governments.
4. Identify those eligible for the Medicaid Qualified Medicare Beneficiaries program.
5. Name and describe the two Medicaid eligibility classifications.
6. State eligibility requirements and claims procedures for the Maternal and Child Health Program.
7. List important information to abstract from the patient's Medicaid card.
8. Describe the Medicaid basic benefits.
9. Explain basic operations of a Medicaid-managed care system.
10. Explain basic Medicaid claim procedure guidelines.
11. File claims for patients who have Medicaid and other coverage.
12. Interpret and post a remittance advice.
13. Describe filing an appeal for a Medicaid case.

KEY TERMS

categorically needy
coinsurance
copayment
covered services
Early and Periodic Screening, Diagnosis, and Treatment

fiscal agent
Maternal and Child Health Program
Medicaid
Medi-Cal
medically needy

prior approval
recipient
share of cost
State Children's Health Insurance Program
Supplemental Security Income

KEY ABBREVIATIONS

DEFRA
EPSDT
FPL
MCHP
MN

MQMB
OBRA
OOY claims
POS machine
QI program

QMB
RA
SCHIP
SLMB
SSI

TANF
TEFRA

HISTORY

Federal participation in providing medical care to needy persons began between 1933 and 1935 when the Federal Emergency Relief Administration made funds available to pay the medical expenses of the needy unemployed. The Social Security Act of 1935 set up the public assistance programs. Although no special provision was made for medical assistance, the federal government paid a share of the monthly assistance payments, which could be used to meet the costs of medical care. However, the payment was made to the assistance recipient rather than to the provider of medical care.

In 1950, Congress passed a law mandating that all states set up a health care program of assistance, which meant that the states had to meet minimum requirements. As a result of this mandate, the states set up **Medicaid** programs. Congress authorized vendor payments for medical care—payments from the welfare agency directly to physicians, health care institutions, and other providers of medical services. By 1960, four fifths of the states had made provisions for medical vendor payments.

A new category of assistance recipient was established for the **medically needy (MN)** aged population. The incomes of these individuals were too high to qualify them for cash assistance payments but they needed help in meeting the costs of medical care. The federal government financially supports the minimum assistance level and the states must wholly support any part of the program that goes beyond the federal minimum. This is referred to as *state share.*

In 1965, Title XIX of the Social Security Act became federal law and Medicaid legally came into being. To a large extent it was the result of various attempts during the previous 30 years to provide medical care to the needy.

In 1982, the Tax Equity and Fiscal Responsibility Act (TEFRA) set down laws affecting those under the Medicare program as well as Medicaid MN recipients and those in certain other categories. See Chapter 12 for information about how TEFRA affects Medicare recipients.

Since 1983, the trend in many states has been to expand Medicaid eligibility requirements and services. Changes in Medicaid eligibility allowing more people into the program were made by many states after the passage of the Deficit Reduction Act (DEFRA) of 1984 and the Child Health Assurance Program (CHAP) by the federal government. On July 1, 2006, as part of DEFRA, a federal law became effective requiring new applicants and current beneficiaries renewing their benefits (except seniors and people with disabilities) to submit birth certificates, passports, or other documents to establish their legal right as United States (US) citizens to benefits. If no documentation of citizenship can be found, sworn affidavits from the beneficiary and at least one or two other individuals can be used.

In 2002 and 2003, states across the nation faced steep budget shortfalls. A vast majority of them made cuts of some kind in their Medicaid programs by either instituting or boosting **copayments** for certain types of services or by eliminating some services. Copayment (copay) is a required specific dollar amount that must be collected at each office visit for medical services received by an individual. Under Medicaid, different copayment amounts may be set for each patient group as listed in Box 13-1 (which appears later in this chapter) and for certain medical procedures.

Health care reform legislation, known as the *Patient Protection and Affordable Care Act (PPACA)* and the *Health Care and Education Reconciliation Act (HCERA),* was passed in 2010. These Acts affect the Medicaid program by expanding access for childless adults and nonelderly and nonpregnant individuals and include preventive services and long-term care benefits. Additional funds were allocated for maternal and child health services. Community First Choice was made available so that states could offer medical assistance for home- and community-based attendant services and support for individuals eligible for medical assistance under a state Medicaid plan. Beginning in January 2014, Medicaid eligibility limits increased so that adults earning up to 138% of the federal poverty level (FPL) are eligible. For a single person this is an annual income of $15,856 and for a two-person family this is $21,404. States were given the choice to expand and as of 2014, 18 states are not expanding, 30 states are expanding, and 3 states are expanding but using an alternative to traditional expansion. People with disabilities who qualify for Medicaid based solely on their low-income status can enroll in coverage on that basis and begin receiving benefits while waiting for disability-based Medicaid eligibility determination. People with disabilities who do not qualify for Medicaid based on their low-income status can enroll in Marketplace Qualified Health Plan coverage with advance payment of premium tax credits (APTC), if eligible, while their disability-related Medicaid eligibility is pending. They do not have to wait.

Box 13-1   Groups Eligible for Medicaid Benefits

Mandatory Eligibility Groups

- Families, pregnant women, and children
- Temporary Assistance for Needy Families (TANF)-related groups
- Non-TANF pregnant women and children
- Infants born to Medicaid-eligible pregnant women
- Children younger than age 6 and pregnant women whose family income is at or below 135% of the federal poverty level (FPL)
- Recipients of adoption assistance or foster care assistance under Title IV-E of the Social Security Act
- Aged and disabled
- Supplemental Security Income (SSI)-related groups
- Qualified Medicare beneficiaries (QMBs)
- Persons who receive institutional or other long-term care in nursing facilities (NFs) and intermediate care facilities (ICFs)
- Certain Medicaid beneficiaries
- Medicare–Medicaid beneficiaries

Optional Eligibility Groups

- Low-income persons who are losing employer health insurance coverage (Medicaid purchase if person has Consolidated Omnibus Budget Reconciliation Act [COBRA] coverage)
- Infants up to age 1 and pregnant women not covered under the mandatory rules whose family income is not more than 185% of the FPL (note that the percentage may be modified by each state)
- Children younger than age 21 who meet TANF income and resource requirements but who are otherwise not eligible for TANF
- Persons who would be eligible if institutionalized but receive care under home- and community-based service waivers
- Persons infected with tuberculosis who would be financially eligible for Medicaid at the SSI income level if they were within a Medicaid-covered category (limited coverage)
- Low-income children with the State Children's Health Insurance Program (SCHIP)
- Low-income, uninsured women who are diagnosed through the Centers for Disease Control and Prevention's (CDC's) National Breast and Cervical Cancer Early Detection Program and who are in need of treatment for breast or cervical cancer

Medically Needy Eligibility Group

- Medically indigent low-income individuals and families who have too much income to qualify under mandatory or optional eligibility Medicaid groups

MEDICAID PROGRAMS

Title XIX of the Social Security Act provides for a program of medical assistance for certain low-income individuals and families as well as for primary or supplemental coverage for people with disabilities. The program is known as Medicaid in 49 states and as **Medi-Cal** in California. In 2010, health plans were established as the result of a state mandate to transform Medi-Cal from a state-run insurance system to a locally run managed care program. Medicaid is administered by state governments with partial federal funding. Coverage and benefits vary widely from state to state because the federal government sets minimum requirements and the states are then free to enact more benefits. Thus each state designs its own Medicaid program within federal guidelines. The CMS of the Bureau of Program Operations of the US Department of Health and Human Services (DHHS) is responsible for the federal aspects of Medicaid. Medicaid is not so much an insurance program as it is an assistance program.

Arizona

Arizona is the only state without a Medicaid program similar to those that exist in other states. Since 1982, Arizona has received federal funds under a demonstration waiver for an alternative medical assistance program (prepaid care) for low-income persons called the *Arizona Health Care Cost Containment System (AHCCCS)*, pronounced as "access."

 ### Maternal and Child Health Program

Each state and certain other jurisdictions, including territories and the District of Columbia (56 programs total), operate a **State Children's Health Insurance Program (SCHIP)** with federal grant support under Title V of the Social Security Act. In some states this program may be known as **Maternal and Child Health Program (MCHP)** or *Children's Special Health Care Services (CSHCS)*. Although Title V has been amended on a number of occasions, notably between 1981 and 1987, no changes have been as sweeping as those in the Omnibus Budget Reconciliation Act (OBRA) of 1989. SCHIP insures children from families whose income is below 200% of the FPL or whose family has an income 50% higher than the state's Medicaid eligibility threshold. However, some states have expanded SCHIP eligibility beyond the 200% FPL limit and others are covering entire families and not just children. States have three options in designing their program. The state can do one of the following:

- Use SCHIP funds to expand Medicaid eligibility to children who previously did not qualify for the program.
- Design a children's health insurance program that is entirely separate from Medicaid.
- Combine both the Medicaid and the separate program options.

Federal funds are granted to states, enabling them to:

- Provide low-income mothers and children access to quality maternal and child health services.
- Reduce infant mortality and the incidence of preventable diseases and handicapping conditions among children.
- Increase the number of children immunized against disease and the number of low-income children receiving health assessments and follow-up diagnostic and treatment services.

- Promote the health of mothers and infants by providing prenatal, delivery, and postpartum care for low-income, at-risk pregnant women.
- Provide preventive and primary care services for low-income children.
- Provide rehabilitation services for the blind and disabled younger than age 16 years.
- Provide, promote, and develop family-centered, community-based, coordinated care for children with special health care needs.

The state agency tries to locate mothers, infants, and children younger than 21 years of age who may have conditions eligible for treatment under the MCHP. The conditions are diagnosed and the necessary medical and other health-related care, any hospitalization, and any continuing follow-up care are given.

After a child is examined at an MCHP clinic and a diagnosis is made, the parents are advised about the treatment that will benefit the child. The state agency then helps them to locate this care. If the parents cannot afford this care, the agency assists them with financial planning and may assume part or all of the cost of treatment, depending on the child's condition and the family's resources.

Individuals who work in a physician's office need to be aware of these services in the event that a patient needs to be referred to a state agency for assistance.

Low-Income Medicare Recipients

There are three aid programs for Medicare patients who have low incomes and have difficulty paying Medicare premiums, copayments, and deductibles. Each program addresses a different financial category and the monthly income figures are adjusted each year. The titles of the three programs are:

- Medicaid Qualified Medicare Beneficiary Program
- Specified Low-Income Medicare Beneficiary Program
- Qualifying Individual Program

The programs are usually administered through county social services departments, the same ones that administer Medicaid. One application is completed that pertains to all three programs and an individual is placed in one of the programs depending on how he or she qualifies financially.

Medicaid Qualified Medicare Beneficiary Program

The Medicaid Qualified Medicare Beneficiary (MQMB) program was introduced in the Medicare Catastrophic Coverage Act of 1988 as an amendment to the Social Security Act. In 1990, OBRA allowed for assistance to qualified Medicare beneficiaries (QMBs, pronounced "kwim-bees")

who are aged and disabled, are receiving Medicare, and have annual incomes below the FPL. Eligibility also depends on what other financial resources an individual might have.

Under this Act, states must provide limited Medicaid coverage for QMBs. They must pay Medicare Part B premiums (and Part A premiums if applicable), along with necessary Medicare deductibles and **coinsurance** amounts. Coinsurance is the portion of the Medicare allowed amount that the patient pays. When discussing Medicaid, the terms *copayment* and *coinsurance* do not have the same meaning that they do when talking about private insurance coverage issues. As discussed later in this chapter in the section titled "Copayment," there are two types of copayment for the Medicaid program depending on each state's established policy. MQMB coverage is restricted to Medicare cost sharing unless the beneficiary qualifies for Medicaid in some other way. Medicaid will not pay for the service if Medicare does not cover the service to the patient.

States are also required to pay Medicare Part A premiums but no other expenses for qualified disabled and working individuals. It is optional for states to provide full Medicaid benefits to QMBs who meet a state-established income standard.

Specified Low-Income Medicare Beneficiary Program

The Specified Low-Income Medicare Beneficiary (SLMB, pronounced "slim-bee") program was established in 1993 for elderly individuals whose income is 20% above the FPL. It pays the entire Medicare Part B premium. The patient must pay the deductible and copay and must pay for noncovered items.

Qualifying Individual Program

The Qualifying Individual (QI) program was created in 1997 for qualifying individuals whose income is at least 135% but less than 175% of the FPL. It also pays for the Medicare Part B premium.

MEDICAID ELIGIBILITY

Medicaid is available to certain needy and low-income people, such as the elderly (65 years or older), blind, disabled, and members of families with dependent children deprived of the support of at least one parent and financially eligible on the basis of income and resources. In general, Medicaid is available only to US citizens and certain "qualified immigrants." Passports and birth certificates must be submitted for proof of citizenship. If a person may be eligible for Medicaid, he or she goes to the local public service welfare office, human service, or family independence agency and applies for benefits.

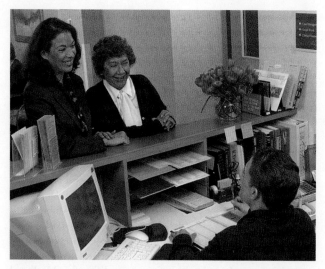

FIGURE 13-1 Medicaid patient checking in with the receptionist.

Verifying Eligibility

After acceptance into the program, the patient brings a form or card to the physician's office that verifies acceptance into the program (Figure 13-1) but this does not indicate proof of eligibility. It is the provider's responsibility to verify at each visit that the person there to receive care is eligible on the date on which the service is rendered and is the individual to whom the card was issued.

Each state decides which services are covered and what the payments are for each service. There are two classifications—categorically needy and medically needy—that contain several basic groups of needy and low-income individuals.

Categorically Needy

The first classification, the **categorically needy** group, includes all cash recipients of Temporary Assistance for Needy Families (TANF); certain other TANF-related groups; most cash recipients of the **Supplemental Security Income (SSI)** program; other SSI-related groups; QMBs; and patients in institutional, long-term care, and intermediate care facilities (see Box 13-1).

A **recipient** is an individual certified by the local welfare department to receive benefits of Medicaid under one of the specific aid categories. TANF was instituted by the *Personal Responsibility and Work Opportunity Reconciliation Act*, also known as the *Welfare Reform Act of 1996*. This federal law ended welfare as an entitlement program and requires recipients to work after receiving benefits for 2 years with a lifetime limit of 5 years of benefits paid by federal funds. This Act aims to encourage two-parent families, discourage out-of-wedlock births, and help to enforce child support. It replaced the federal program of Aid to Dependent Children (ADC), later known as Aid to Families with Dependent Children (AFDC).

Medically Needy

The second classification involves state general assistance programs for low-income people, the medically indigent, and individuals who are losing employer health insurance. This classification is sometimes referred to as the *MN class*. A Medicaid recipient in this category may or may not pay a copayment or a deductible, which must be met within the eligibility month or other specified time frame before he or she can receive state benefits (also known as **share of cost** or *spend down*). Emergency care and pregnancy services are exempt by law from copayment requirements. This may be a component of a state's general assistance program for low-income people. Another method to meet Medicaid eligibility requirements is to spend down to or below the state's MN income level by incurring medical expenses that reduce excess income. This then makes income low enough to make the individual eligible for the program. Some states have established spend down programs for aged, blind, and disabled individuals who have income that qualifies them for the program.

For those individuals who may become medically indigent as a result of high medical care expenses and inadequate health insurance coverage, a number of states have adopted a State Program of Assistance for the Medically Indigent. Box 13-1 lists the classes and basic groups for Medicaid eligibility.

Maternal and Child Health Program Eligibility

Specific conditions qualify a child for benefits under the MCHP. The state law under which each agency operates either defines the conditions to be included or directs the children's agency to define them. All state laws include children who have some kind of handicap that requires orthopedic treatment or plastic surgery; a few states add other conditions. A list of both types of conditions that qualify children for MCHP follows:
● Cerebral palsy
● Chronic conditions affecting bones and joints
● Cleft lip
● Cleft palate
● Clubfoot
● Cystic fibrosis*
● Epilepsy*
● Hearing problems*
● Mental retardation*
● Multiple handicaps*

---

*Only some states include this item in their MCHP.

Another requirement is the share of cost or *spend down* copayment. Some Medicaid recipients must meet this copayment requirement each month before Medicaid benefits can be claimed. For example, if an individual's income is too high to qualify, some states allow deduction of certain medical expenses from his or her income so that the income may fall within Medicaid guidelines. These spend down programs are available in some states for the aged, the blind, or those who have a disability. Spend down eligibility is a monthly process and patients must submit proof of medical expenses that meet the spend down amount. Expenses covered by other insurance are not eligible to be used toward the spend down amount. For example, if the income is $150 more than the limit, the excess income is equal to the spend down amount and the patient must submit $150 of acceptable medical bills or pay in the spend down amount to receive Medicaid coverage for the remainder of the month. Because the amount may change from month to month, be sure to verify the copayment each time it is collected. Obtain this copayment amount when the patient comes in for medical care and report on the claim form that it has been collected.

Prior Approval

Many times, prior approval is necessary for various goods and services, except in a bona fide emergency. **Prior approval** is the evaluation of a provider's request for a specific good or service to determine the medical necessity and appropriateness of the care requested for the patient. In some states this may be referred to as *prior authorization*. Some of these goods and services are the following:

● Durable medical equipment
● Hearing aids
● Hemodialysis
● Home health care
● Inpatient hospital care
● Long-term care facility services
● Medical supplies
● Medications
● Prosthetic or orthotic appliances
● Surgical procedures
● Transportation
● Some vision care

Usually prior authorization forms are completed to obtain permission for a specific service or hospitalization (Figure 13-4) and mailed or faxed to the Department of Health or a certain office in a region for approval. In some cases, time does not allow for a written request to be sent for prior approval, so an immediate authorization can be obtained via a telephone call to the proper department in any locale. Note the date and time that the authorization was given, the name of the person who gave authorization, and any verbal number given by the field office. Usually a treatment authorization form indicating that the service was already authorized must be sent in as follow-up to the telephone call. On July 1, 2012, under the Affordable Care Act, Medicaid implemented the provision to either make a payment adjustment or prohibit payment for any hospital-acquired condition (HAC), such as foreign object retained after surgery; air embolism; blood incompatibility; Stages III and IV pressure ulcers; vascular catheter-associated infection; mediastinitis after coronary artery bypass graft; falls and trauma resulting in fractures, dislocations, intracranial injury, crushing injury, burn, and other unspecified effects of external causes; manifestations of poor glycemic control; surgical site infection following spine, neck, shoulder, or elbow orthopedic procedures; surgical site infection following bariatric surgery for obesity; deep vein thrombosis and pulmonary embolism following a total knee or hip replacement, except for pediatric (individuals under age 21) and obstetric populations; wrong surgical procedure; correct procedure performed on the wrong patient; or correct procedure performed on the wrong body part.

Time Limit

Each state has its own time limit for the submission of a claim. The time limit can vary from 2 months to 12 or 18 months from the date that the service was rendered. A bill can be rejected if it is submitted after the time limit unless the state recognizes some valid justification. Some states have separate procedures for billing over-one-year (OOY) claims. A percentage of the claim may be reduced according to the date of a delinquent submission. Prescription drugs and dental services are often billed to a different intermediary than are services performed by a physician, depending on the state guidelines.

Reciprocity

Most states have reciprocity for Medicaid payments if a patient requires medical care while out of state. Contact the Medicaid fiscal intermediary in the patient's home state and ask for the appropriate forms. If the case was an emergency, state this on the form. File the papers with Medicaid in the patient's home state. Reimbursement will be at that state's rate.

Claim Form

As of October 1, 1986, federal law has mandated that the CMS-1500 Insurance Claim Form be adopted for the processing of Medicaid claims in all states.

STATE USE ONLY

SERVICE CATEGORY

TYPEWRITER ALIGNMENT Elite Pica

CONFIDENTIAL PATIENT INFORMATION

FOR F.I. USE ONLY

CCN

TREATMENT AUTHORIZATION REQUEST

STATE OF CALIFORNIA DEPARTMENT OF HEALTH SERVICES

F.I. USE ONLY 40 41 42 43

TYPEWRITER ALIGNMENT Elite Pica

(PLEASE TYPE) FOR PROVIDER USE (PLEASE TYPE)

VERBAL CONTROL NO.	TYPE OF SERVICE REQUESTED	REQUEST IS RETROACTIVATE?	IS PATIENT MEDICARE ELIGIBLE?	PROVIDER PHONE NO.
	DRUG [ ] OTHER [X]	YES [ ] NO [X]	YES [ ] NO [X]	(555) 555-1111 AREA

PATIENT'S AUTHORIZED REPRESENTATIVE (IF ANY) ENTER NAME AND ADDRESS

PROVIDER NAME AND ADDRESS

PROVIDER NO. HSC12345F

PLEASE TYPE YOUR NAME AND ADDRESS HERE

SMITH, SUSAN MD
727 ELM BLVD
ANYTOWN, CA 90101

30 83

NAME AND ADDRESS OF PATIENT

PATIENT NAME (LAST, FIRST, M. I.): APPLEGATE, NANCY

MEDICAL IDENTIFICATION NO.: 253971060 CHECK DIGIT

STREET ADDRESS: 1515 RIVER ROAD

SEX: F AGE: 32 DATE OF BIRTH: 06 18 70

CITY, STATE, ZIP CODE: SACRAMENTO, CA 95822

PATIENT STATUS: [X] HOME [ ] BOARD AND CARE [ ] SNF/ICF [ ] ACUTE HOSPITAL

PHONE NUMBER: (555) 545-1123

DIAGNOSIS DESCRIPTION: ENDOMETRIOSIS

ICD-9-CM DIAGNOSIS CODE: 617.9

MEDICAL JUSTIFICATION:
VISTA HOSPITAL - 1200 MAPLE ST., ANYTOWN, CA
UNCONTROLLABLE ENDOMETRIOSIS

FOR STATE USE

33 PROVIDER; YOUR REQUEST IS:

1 [X] APPROVED AS REQUESTED [ ] DENIED [ ] DEFERRED

2 [ ] APPROVED AS MODIFIED (ITEMS MARKED BELOW AS AUTHORIZED MAY BE CLAIMED) [ ] JACKSON VS RANK PARAGRAPH CODE

BY *John Doe* MEDICAL CONSULTANT

34 I.D. # 01 35 DATE 08 20 XX 44 REVIEW COMMENTS INDICATOR

COMMENTS/ EXPLANATION

RETROACTIVE AUTHORIZATION GRANTED IN ACCORDANCE WITH SECTION 51003 (B)

36 1 2 3 4 5 6

	AUTHORIZED YES	AUTHORIZED NO	APPROVED UNITS	SPECIFIC SERVICES REQUESTED	UNITS OF SERVICE	PROCEDURE OR DRUG CODE	QUANTITY	CHARGES
1	9 X		10 3	DAYS: 3 HOSPITAL DAYS REQUESTED		11	12	$
2	13 X		14 1	HYSTERECTOMY	1	15 5815070	16 1	$ $1300.00
3	17		18			19	20	$
4	21		22			23	24	$
5	25		26			27	28	$
6	29		30			31	32	$

TO THE BEST OF MY KNOWLEDGE, THE ABOVE INFORMATION IS TRUE, ACCURATE AND COMPLETE AND THE REQUESTED SERVICES ARE MEDICALLY INDICATED AND NECESSARY TO THE HEALTH OF THE PATIENT.

Susan Smith — SIGNATURE OF PHYSICIAN OR PROVIDER; *MD* — TITLE; *8-10-XX* — DATE

AUTHORIZATION IS VALID FOR SERVICES PROVIDED

37 FROM DATE 09 01 XX 38 TO DATE 09 30 XX

TAR CONTROL NUMBER

36 OFFICE 12 SEQUENCE NUMBER 61240229 PI 0

NOTE: AUTHORIZATION DOES NOT GUARANTEE PAYMENT. PAYMENT IS SUBJECT TO PATIENT'S ELIGIBILITY. BE SURE THE IDENTIFICATION CARD IS CURRENT BEFORE RENDERING SERVICE. SEND TO FIELD SERVICES (F.I. COPY)

SEE YOUR PROVIDER MANUAL FOR ASSISTANCE REGARDING THE COMPLETION OF THIS FORM. 50-1 12/87

FIGURE 13-4 Completed treatment authorization request form used in California for the Medi-Cal program.

Either physicians submit a claim form to a fiscal agent, which might be an insurance company, or the bill is sent directly to the local public service welfare office, human service, or family independence agency. These agencies have different names in each state.

Chapter 7 includes general block-by-block instructions on how to complete the CMS-1500 (02-12) claim form for the Medicaid program. Because guidelines for completing the form vary among all Medicaid intermediaries, refer to the local Medicaid intermediary for its directions. Figure 7-4 is a template emphasizing placement of basic elements on the claim form that require completion. Note that when questions about "insured" are asked on the claim form, the patient is always the insured even if a minor.

To keep up to date, always read the current bulletins or program memos on the Medicaid or Medi-Cal program at the state fiscal agent's website. Read and implement the rule changes and updates to avoid rejected claims.

Medicaid Managed Care

When filing a claim for a Medicaid managed care patient, send the bill or claim form to the managed care organization (MCO) and not to the Medicaid fiscal agent. The MCO receives payment for services rendered to eligible members via either the capitation or other managed care method.

Maternal and Child Health Program

Each state's jurisdiction operates its own MCHP with its own unique administrative characteristics. Thus each has its own system and forms for billing and related procedures. The official plans and documents are retained in the individual state offices and are not available on either a regional or a national office basis. For specific information about a state's policies, contact your local Department of Health to locate the office near you.

Medicaid and Other Plans

It is possible that a person can be eligible for Medicaid and also have group health insurance coverage through an employer. When Medicaid and a third-party payer cover the patient, Medicaid is always considered the payer of last resort. The third-party payer (other insurance) is billed first.

Third-party liability occurs if any entity is liable to pay all or part of the medical cost of injury, disease, or disability. In these cases the primary carrier is the other program or insurance carrier and it is sent the claim first. After a remittance advice (RA) or check voucher is received from the primary carrier, Medicaid (the secondary carrier) is billed. A copy of the RA or check voucher is enclosed.

Government Programs and Medicaid. When a Medicaid patient has Medicare (sometimes referred to as a *crossover case* or *dual eligible case*), TRICARE, or Veterans Health Administration (CHAMPVA), always send the insurance claim first to the federal program fiscal agent servicing the region. Usually the Medicare fiscal agent automatically forwards the claim to the secondary payer, Medicaid. If this does not occur, bill Medicaid second and attach to the claim form the RA or check voucher that has been received from the federal program. Send in a claim only if the other coverage denies payment or pays less than the Medicaid fee schedule or if Medicaid covers services not covered by the other policy.

In the past, state Medicaid programs paid the Medicare deductibles and coinsurance for dual eligible cases at the full Medicare rate. However, the Balanced Budget Act of 1997 permits states to limit payment to the amount that the Medicaid program would otherwise pay for the service. Due to the health care reform legislation in 2010, many states have lowered their cost-sharing obligations for these cases to no more than the Medicaid payment amount for the same service. If the Medicare payment amount equals or exceeds the Medicaid payment rate, the state Medicaid program does not pay the Medicare deductible or coinsurance. The result is that the reimbursement becomes that of a Medicare-only patient even though it is crossed over to the Medicaid program.

Electronic claims may be automatically crossed over from primary government programs. Chapter 12 provides additional information on crossover claim submission. Figure 7-6 is a template emphasizing placement of basic elements on the claim form that require completion for crossover claims. Chapter 14 provides further information on patients who receive benefits from TRICARE and the Veterans Health Administration (CHAMPVA).

Medicaid and Immigrants

Some immigrants may have Medicare Part A or Part B or both (see Chapter 12). If an immigrant is older than 65 years, is on Medicaid (Medi-Cal in California), and is not eligible for Medicare benefits, then bill the Medicaid processing agent and use the proper Medicaid claim form for the region. On the CMS-1500 (02-12) claim form in Block 19, indicate "Immigrant is older than 65 years and not eligible for Medicare benefits." Your *Medicaid Handbook* should provide specifics for your region or state.

AFTER CLAIM SUBMISSION

Remittance Advice

If a provider wants to receive an electronic RA, a form must be completed and submitted to the fiscal agent

(Figure 13-5). However, a provider that relies on the paper system is sent an RA or check voucher that accompanies all Medicaid payment checks. Sometimes, five categories of adjudicated claims appear on an RA—adjustments, approvals, denials, suspends, and audit/refund (A/R)

transactions—although this terminology may vary from one fiscal agent to another (Figure 13-6). *Adjudication* or *claim settlement* is the processing of an insurance claim through a series of edits for final determination of coverage (benefits) for possible payment.

ELECTRONIC EXPLANATION OF PAYMENT (EOP) AGREEMENT

GROUP/BILLING PROVIDER NUMBER: HSC 11100F

GROUP/BILLING NAME: College Clinic

ADDRESS: 4567 Broad Avenue

CITY: Woodland Hills   **STATE:** XY   **ZIP:** 12345

CONTACT: Joan Biller   **PHONE NUMBER:** 555-487-8976

SUBMITTER ID: 3664021CC

VENDOR NAME: United Billing Service

ADDRESS: 123 Main Street

CITY: Woodland Hills   **STATE:** XY   **ZIP:** 12346

VENDOR PHONE NUMBER: 555-218-4761

VENDOR CONTACT: Maria DeCortez

I (we) request to receive Electronic Explanation of Payment (EOP) information and authorize the information to be deposited in our electronic mailbox. I (we) accept financial responsibility for costs associated with receipt of Electronic EOP information.

I (we) understand that paper-formatted EOP information will continue to be sent to my (our) mailing address as maintained at EDS until I (we) submit an Electronic EOP Certification Request Form.

I (we) will continue to maintain the confidentiality of records and other information relating to recipients in accordance with applicable state and federal laws, rules, and regulations.

Authorized Signature: *Maria DeCortez*   **Date:** 1-2-XX

Title: President   **Internet Address:** DeCortez@UBS.net

Mail form to: EDS • Attn: ECS Department • P.O. Box 244035 • Montgomery, AL 36124
FAX form to: 334-215-4272 Attn: ECS Department

FOR EDS USE ONLY

BILLING MODE: _____   **EOP MODE:** _____   **PROTOCOL:** _____

CONTACT DATE: _____   **SOFTWARE MAILED:** _____

TEST DATE: _____   **AGREEMENT DATE:** _____   **APPROVAL DATE:** _____

BEGIN DATE: _____   **END DATE:** _____

NOTES: _____

FIGURE 13-5 Electronic Explanation of Payment (EOP) Agreement used by the Medicaid program in Alabama. It must be completed by a provider and authorizes the fiscal agent to transmit EOPs to the physician's electronic mail box.

MEDICAID REMITTANCE ADVICE

TO: ANYBODY, FERNANDO G.
1000 ELM STREET
ANYTOWN, XY 12345-0001

REFER TO PROVIDER MANUAL FOR DEFINITION OF RAD CODES

PROVIDER NUMBER 00AX65800	CLAIM TYPE MEDICAL	WARRANT NO 39248026	EDS SEQ NO 20000617	DATE 06/01/20XX	PAGE 1 of 1 pages

RECIPIENT NAME	RECIPIENT MEDICAID I.D. NO.	CLAIM CONTROL NUMBER	SERVICE DATES FROM MMDDYY	TO MMDDYY	PROCED CODE MODIFIER	PATIENT ACCOUNT NUMBER	QTY	BILLED AMT	PAYABLE AMT			PAID AMT	RAD CODE
APPROVES (RECONCILE TO FINANCIAL SUMMARY)													
TORRES R	559978557	5079350917901	030720XX	030720XX	Z4802		0001	20.00	16.22			16.22	0401
		5079350917901	030720XX	030720XX	Z4802		0001	20.00	16.22			16.22	0401
						TOTAL		40.00	32.44			32.44	
CHAN B	561198435	5044351314501	020320XX	020320XX	Z4800		0001	30.00	27.03			27.03	0401
		5044351314501	020320XX	020320XX	Z4800		0001	20.00	16.22			16.22	0401
						TOTAL		50.00	43.25			43.25	
		TOTALS FOR APPROVES						90.00	75.69			75.69	
												75.69	AMT PAID
DENIES (DO NOT RECONCILE TO FINANCIAL SUMMARY)													
GOMEZ M	624163192	501134031900	122720XX	122720XX	Z4800		0001	30.00					0036
		TOTAL NUMBER OF DENIES					0001						
SUSPENDS (DO NOT RECONCILE TO FINANCIAL SUMMARY)													
HERN D	562416373	5034270703001	010520XX	010520XX	Z4800		0001	20.00					0602
MART E	623105478	5034270712305	010520XX	010520XX	Z4800		0001	20.00					0602
		5034270712305	010520XX	010520XX	Z4800		0001	20.00					0602
						TOTAL		40.00					0602
LOPEZ C	560291467	5034270712502	012420XX	012420XX	Z4800		0001	20.00					0602
		PAT LIAB 932.00 OTH COVG			0.00	SALES TX		0.00					
		TOTAL NUMBER OF SUSPENDS					0004	80.00					

EXPLANATION OF DENIAL/ADJUSTMENT CODES

0401 PAYMENT ADJUSTED TO MAXIMUM ALLOWABLE
0036 RESUBMISSION TURNAROUND DOCUMENT WAS EITHER NOT RETURNED OR WAS RETURNED UNCORRECTED, THEREFORE YOUR CLAIM IS FORMALLY DENIED.
0602 PENDING ADJUDICATION
          OHC CARRIER NAME AND ADDRESS
N049 NORTHWESTERN NATIONAL LIFE   111 WASHINGTON AVE. FL 3   MINNEAPOLIS MN 55401

FIGURE 13-6 Medicaid remittance advice (RA) form showing adjustments, cutbacks, denied claims, and claims in suspense.

Adjustments occur from overpayments or underpayments by the fiscal agent. Approval is when an original claim or a previously denied claim is approved for payment. Denied claims are listed with a reason code on the RA. Claims in suspense for a certain period of time may be listed on the RA. Accounts receivable A/R transactions are miscellaneous transactions as a result of cost settlements, state audits, or refund checks received. RAs for a Medicare case and a Medicaid case are illustrated in Figure 12-16.

Appeals

The time limit to appeal a claim varies from state to state but is usually 30 to 60 days from the date listed on the RA. Most Medicaid offices consider an appeal filed when they receive it, not when it is sent. Usually appeals are sent on a special form or with a cover letter along with photocopies of documents applicable to the appeal (e.g., claim form, RA, and preauthorization forms). Appeals go first to either the regional fiscal agent or Medicaid bureau, next to the Department of Social Welfare or Human Services, and then to an appellate court that evaluates decisions by local and government agencies. At each level, an examiner looks at the case and makes a decision. If not satisfied, the physician may ask for further review at the next level.

MEDICAID FRAUD CONTROL

Each state has a Medicaid Fraud Control Unit (MFCU), which is a federally funded state law enforcement entity usually located in the state attorney general's office. The MFCU investigates and prosecutes cases of fraud and other violations, including complaints of mistreatment in long-term care facilities. The state Medicaid agency must cooperate and ensure access to records by the MFCU and agree to refer suspected cases of provider fraud to this division of the attorney general's office for investigation.

KEY POINTS

This is a brief chapter review, or summary, of the key issues presented. To further enhance your knowledge of the technical subject matter, review the key terms and key abbreviations for this chapter by locating the meaning for each in the Glossary at the end of this book, which appears in a section before the Index.

1. Medicaid was established by Title XIX of the Social Security Act, a federally aided, state-operated, and state-administered program that provides medical benefits for certain low-income persons in need of health and medical care.

2. Medicaid is administered by each state's government with partial federal funding.

3. The Patient Protection and Affordable Care Act (PPACA) and the Health Care and Education Reconciliation Act (HCERA) passed in 2010 affect the Medicaid program by expanding access for childless adults and nonelderly and nonpregnant individuals and including preventive services and long-term care benefits.

4. Coverage and benefits vary widely from state to state.

5. Each state operates a children's health insurance program with federal support under Title V of the Social Security Act.

6. Some federal acts allow assistance to qualified Medicare beneficiaries (QMBs) and Specified Low-Income Medicare Beneficiaries (SLMBs) who are aged and/or disabled and receiving Medicare but have annual incomes below the federal poverty level (FPL).

7. A medically needy (MN) Medicaid classification may or may not pay a deductible, copayment, or share of cost (spend down) within a specific time frame before receiving state benefits.

8. Providers must enroll for participation in the Medicaid program with the fiscal agent or local public service welfare office.

9. Medicaid benefits identification cards are issued monthly to recipients.

10. Medicaid eligibility must be verified before providing medical services to patients. Some patients may have retroactive eligibility.

11. Sometimes prior approval is required for medical services and procedures.

12. Each state may have a different time limit for submitting a claim for reimbursement.

13. The CMS-1500 (02-12) insurance claim form has been adopted for processing Medicaid claims in all states to a regional fiscal agent.

14. A remittance advice (RA) or check voucher accompanies all Medicaid payment checks sent by the fiscal agent to the provider of services.

15. Each state has a Medicaid Fraud Control Unit (MFCU) that investigates and prosecutes cases of fraud and other violations, including complaints of mistreatment in long-term care facilities.

STUDENT ASSIGNMENT

✔ Study Chapter 13.
✔ Answer the fill-in-the-blank, multiple-choice, and true/false review questions in the *Workbook* to reinforce the theory learned in this chapter and to help you prepare for a future test.
✔ Complete the assignments in the *Workbook* to give you hands-on experience in abstracting from case histories,

posting to financial accounting record cards, and completing forms pertinent to the Medicaid program in your state. As an option, obtain Medicaid forms for your locale to use for your assignments.
✔ Turn to the Glossary at the end of this text for a further understanding of the key terms and key abbreviations used in this chapter.

TRICARE and Veterans' Health Care

Marilyn Takahashi Fordney

OBJECTIVES

After reading this chapter, you should be able to:

1. Discuss the history of TRICARE.
2. State who is eligible for TRICARE.
3. List the circumstances when a nonavailability statement is necessary.
4. Explain the benefits of the TRICARE Standard government program.
5. State the TRICARE fiscal year.
6. Name authorized providers who may treat a TRICARE Standard patient and discuss preauthorization and payments.
7. List the managed care features of TRICARE Extra and discuss enrollment, preauthorization, and payments.
8. State the managed care features of TRICARE Prime and discuss enrollment, Primary Care Managers, preauthorization, and payments.
9. Discuss the TRICARE Reserve Select, TRICARE Retired Reserve, and TRICARE Young Adult programs.
10. Explain TRICARE for Life benefits and those who are eligible individuals.
11. Name individuals eligible for TRICARE Plus and discuss enrollment, preauthorization, and payments.
12. Define individuals who may enroll in the TRICARE Prime Remote program and discuss enrollment, preauthorization, and payments.
13. Discuss the Supplemental Health Care Program, including enrollment and payments.
14. Discuss the TRICARE Hospice Program and TRICARE and HMO coverage.
15. Identify individuals who are eligible for the Veterans Health Administration program (CHAMPVA) and discuss enrollments and preauthorization.
16. Describe how to process a claim for an individual who is covered by various types of TRICARE programs.
17. State the components of a TRICARE Summary Payment Voucher.
18. List the components of a Veterans Health Administration (CHAMPVA) Explanation of Benefits document.
19. Discuss quality assurance programs and the appeal process in relation to TRICARE-managed care programs.

KEY TERMS

active duty service member
allowable charge
authorized provider
beneficiary
catastrophic cap
catchment area
cooperative care
coordination of benefits
cost share

Defense Enrollment Eligibility
 Reporting System
Department of Veterans Affairs
emergency
health benefits advisor
health care finder
medically (or psychologically)
 necessary
Military Treatment Facility

nonparticipating physician or
 provider
other health insurance
participating physician or
 provider
partnership program
point-of-service option
preauthorization
primary care manager

quality assurance program
regional contractor
service benefit program
service-connected injury
service retiree (military retiree)
sponsor

summary payment voucher
total, permanent service-
    connected disability
TRICARE Extra
TRICARE for Life
TRICARE Prime

TRICARE service center
urgent care
veteran
Veterans Health Administration

KEY ABBREVIATIONS

ADSM	HCF	par	TPR
CHAMPVA	MHS	PCM	TPRADFM
DEERS	MTF	POS option	TSC
FTM	NAS	SHCP	USFHP
HAC	nonpar	TFL	VA
HBA	OHI	TMA	

Service to Patients

Know what types of health care services require prior approval from the TRICARE health contractor so that you can promptly assist patients by obtaining necessary permissions for scheduling procedures or hospital admission.

HISTORY OF TRICARE

The United States (US) Congress created Civilian Health and Medical Program of the Uniformed Services (CHAMPUS) in 1966 under Public Law 89-614 because individuals in the military were finding it increasingly difficult to pay for the medical care required by their families. CHAMPUS is a federally funded comprehensive health benefits program. Beginning in 1988, CHAMPUS beneficiaries had a choice of retaining their benefits under CHAMPUS or enrolling in a regional managed care plan called *CHAMPUS Prime*, a plan to control escalating medical costs and standardize benefits. Enrollees may be dependents of personnel who are actively serving in the armed services and military retirees and their dependents. In January 1994, TRICARE became the new title for CHAMPUS. TRICARE Management Activity (TMA) is the current name of the administrative office that was formerly known as the Office of Civilian Health and Medical Programs of the Uniformed Services (OCHAMPUS). Individuals have the following three choices to obtain health care under TRICARE:
- TRICARE Standard (fee-for-service cost-sharing type of option)
- **TRICARE Extra** (preferred provider organization–type option)
- **TRICARE Prime** (health maintenance organization–type option)

In 2005, the former 11 TRICARE regions in the US consolidated and merged to form the following: Region West, Region North, and Region South. Figure 14-1 shows the locations of the states merged into these regions. In addition, there is TRICARE Europe, Canada/Latin America, and Puerto Rico/Virgin Islands.

The TRICARE programs meet standards set by the 2010 health care reform federal legislation.

TRICARE PROGRAMS

Eligibility

The following individuals are entitled to medical benefits under TRICARE:
- Active duty uniformed service members in a program called *TRICARE Prime Remote* for members of Army, Navy, Air Force, Marines, Coast Guard, Public Health Service, and National Oceanic and Atmospheric Administration
- Eligible family members of active duty service members
- Military retirees and their eligible family members
- Surviving eligible family members of deceased, active, or retired service members
- Wards and preadoptive children
- Former spouses of active or retired service members who meet certain length-of-marriage rules and other requirements
- Family members of active duty service members who were court-martialed and separated from their families for spouse or child abuse
- Abused spouses, former spouses, or dependent children of service members who were eligible for retirement but lost that eligibility as a result of abuse of the spouse or child

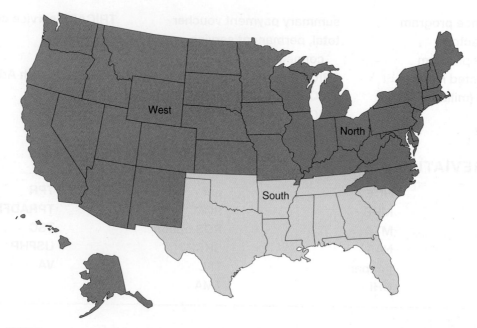

FIGURE 14-1 Map of TRICARE West Region, North Region, and South Region, which shows states that have been merged into each of the regions.

• Spouses and children of North Atlantic Treaty Organization (NATO) nation representatives, under certain circumstances
• Families of activated Reserve and National Guard members if the military sponsor's active duty orders are for 30 consecutive days or an indefinite period
• Disabled beneficiaries younger than 65 years of age who have Medicare Parts A and B and who qualify under one of the aforementioned categories
• Medicare-eligible beneficiaries in a program called *TRICARE for Life (TFL)*

An individual who qualifies for TRICARE is known as a **beneficiary**; the **active duty service member (ADSM)** is called the **sponsor**. A person who is retired from a career in the armed forces is known as a **service retiree (military retiree)** and remains in a TRICARE program until age 65, at which time the individual becomes eligible for the Medicare program. No further family benefits are provided in the event that an active duty military person served from 4 to 6 years and then chose to leave the armed services, thereby giving up a military career. Veterans Health Administration (also known as CHAMPVA) beneficiaries are not eligible for TRICARE.

Defense Enrollment Eligibility Reporting System

All TRICARE-eligible persons must be enrolled in the **Defense Enrollment Eligibility Reporting System (DEERS)** computerized database. TRICARE claims processors check DEERS before processing claims to verify beneficiary eligibility. A TRICARE beneficiary

may check his or her status by contacting the nearest personnel office of any branch of the service or by calling the toll-free number of the DEERS center.

Nonavailability Statement

A Nonavailability Statement (NAS) is a certification from a military hospital stating that it cannot provide the care needed. As of December 2003, this type of certification is no longer necessary for TRICARE and Veterans Health Administration beneficiaries for outpatient procedures or for those who wish to receive treatment as inpatients at a civilian hospital and who live within a **catchment area** (specific geographic region) surrounding a **Military Treatment Facility (MTF)**. An MTF is a uniformed services hospital sometimes referred to as a *military hospital*, formerly called a *US Public Health Service (USPHS) hospital*. The only exception is that an NAS is still required for nonemergency inpatient mental health care services.

Catchment Area

The catchment area is a specific geographic region defined by zip codes and is based on an area of approximately 40 miles in radius surrounding each MTF in the US. Individuals whose home address zip code falls outside the local military hospital's service area do not need an NAS before seeking civilian health care under TRICARE.

TRICARE STANDARD

TRICARE Standard is a health care program offered to spouses and dependents of service personnel with

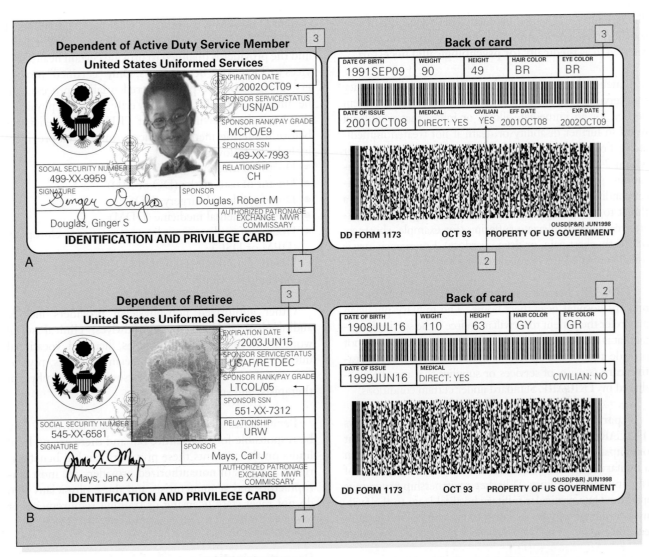

FIGURE 14-2 A, TRICARE Standard active duty dependent's identification card (DD Form 1173) from which essential information must be abstracted. **B,** Sample identification card (DD Form 1173) for a retiree's widowed spouse. Cards indicate: *1,* sponsor's status and rank; *2,* authorization status for treatment by a civilian provider; and *3,* expiration date.

uniform benefits and fees implemented nationwide by the federal government.

Enrollment

Those entitled to medical benefits under TRICARE are automatically enrolled in the TRICARE Standard program.

Identification Card

All dependents 10 years of age or older are required to have a uniformed services (military) identification and privilege card for TRICARE Standard. Dependents and survivors of active duty personnel and retirees carry a military identification card, DD Form 1173 (Figure 14-2). Dependents younger than 10 years of age are not normally issued uniformed services identification cards;

information for their claims should be provided from either parent's card. Refer to the back of the card under "medical" to ensure that the card authorizes civilian medical benefits. Essential information must be abstracted from the front and back of the card; therefore photocopy both sides to retain in the patient's medical record.

Benefits

In the TRICARE Standard program, beneficiaries may receive a wide range of civilian health care services with a significant portion of the cost paid by the federal government. Patients are not limited to using network providers and benefits include medical or psychological services or supplies that are considered appropriate care. Such services are generally accepted by qualified professionals to be reasonable and adequate for the diagnosis and treatment of illness, injury, pregnancy, and mental disorders or to be reasonable and adequate for well-baby care. These services are referred to as **medically (or psychologically) necessary.**

Beneficiaries also may receive urgent care and emergency care services. **Urgent care** is medically necessary treatment needed for an immediate illness or injury that would not result in further disability or death if not treated immediately. Treatment should not be delayed but should occur within 24 hours to avoid development of further complications. An **emergency** is a sudden and unexpected medical condition, or the worsening of a condition, that poses a threat to life, losing a limb, or sight and requires immediate treatment to alleviate suffering (for example, shortness of breath, chest pain, or drug overdose). Emergency care is usually obtained at a hospital emergency department.

TRICARE Standard patients usually seek care from a military hospital near their home. The military physician may refer the patient to a civilian source if the service hospital that is managing the TRICARE Standard patient cannot provide a particular service or medical supplies. **Cooperative care** consists of services or supplies that may be cost-shared by TRICARE Standard under certain conditions.

A **partnership program** is another option that allows TRICARE Standard–eligible persons to receive inpatient or outpatient treatment from civilian providers of care in a military hospital or from uniformed services providers of care in civilian facilities. Whether a partnership program is instituted at a particular military hospital is up to the facility's commander, who makes the decision on the basis of economics.

In addition, there are times when there is no service hospital in the catchment area and a TRICARE Standard beneficiary may seek care through a private physician's office or hospital. Delivery of care through the private physician is emphasized in this chapter.

Read carefully through Figures 14-3 and 14-4 to see the overall picture of TRICARE benefits, which includes cost sharing (deductibles and copayments).

Fiscal Year

The TRICARE fiscal year begins October 1 and ends September 30. It is different from most programs; therefore office staff should be alert when collecting deductibles.

Authorized Providers of Health Care

An **authorized provider** is a physician or other individual authorized provider of care or a hospital or supplier approved by TRICARE to provide medical care and supplies. These providers may treat a TRICARE Standard patient. This means that the provider can be reimbursed by TRICARE for its share of costs for medical benefits and the provider is qualified to provide certain health services to TRICARE beneficiaries. Only "certified" providers, those who have passed a credentialing process, can be authorized by TRICARE. Verify with the physician that he or she is certified to treat TRICARE beneficiaries before rendering medical services. Authorized providers include the following:

- Doctor of medicine (MD)
- Doctor of osteopathy (DO or MD)
- Doctor of dental surgery (DDS)
- Doctor of dental medicine (DDM)
- Doctor of podiatric medicine or surgical chiropody (DPM or DSC)
- Doctor of optometry (OD)
- Psychologist (PhD)

Other authorized non-physician providers include audiologists, certified nurse midwives, clinical social workers, licensed practical nurses, licensed vocational nurses, nurse practitioners, physician assistants, psychiatric social workers, registered nurses, registered physical therapists, and speech therapists.

Beneficiaries who use nonauthorized providers may be responsible for their entire bill and there are no legal limits on the amounts these providers can bill beneficiaries. Examples of nonauthorized providers are most chiropractors and acupuncturists and those physicians who do not meet state licensing or training requirements or who were rejected for authorization by TRICARE.

Preauthorization

There are certain referral and **preauthorization** requirements for TRICARE Standard patients. When specialty care or hospitalization is necessary, the MTF must be used if services are available. If services are not available, the **health care finder (HCF)** can assist with the referral or preauthorization process. A TRICARE referral/authorization form is shown in Figure 14-5. An HCF is a health care professional, usually a registered nurse, who helps the patient to work with his or her primary care physician (PCP) to locate a specialist or obtain a preauthorization for care. HCFs are found at a **TRICARE service center (TSC)**, which is an office staffed by HCFs and beneficiary service representatives. All admissions, ambulatory surgical procedures, and other selected procedures require preauthorization. Certain types of health care services requiring prior approval from the TRICARE health contractor follow:

- Arthroscopy
- Breast mass or tumor removal
- Cardiac catheterization
- Cataract removal
- Cystoscopy

TRICARE Costs for Active Duty Family Members

Deductibles	TRICARE Prime	TRICARE Standard/Extra	
	No deductibles (Unless Point of Service is used)	E4 and Below: $50/person, $100/family E5 and Above: $150/person, $300/family	

Outpatient Services	TRICARE Prime	TRICARE Extra	TRICARE Standard
■ Ambulance Services ■ Durable Medical Equipment (DME) ■ Emergency Room Services ■ Enhanced Clinical Preventive Services ■ Laboratory and X-ray Services ■ Medical Supplies ■ Medication Management ■ Mental Health (Behavioral Health) ■ Occupational Therapy ■ Office Visits ■ Physical Therapy ■ Prosthetic Devices ■ Radiology/Pathology/Cardio Studies ■ Urgent Care	No copay	15%	20%
■ Ambulatory Surgery (Same Day)	No copay	$25*	$25*

■ Clinical Preventive Services:
   (Effective 10/01/2008 no cost for Standard beneficiaries)
   ■ Breast MRIs[†]
   ■ Clinical Preventive Exams[†] (Except School Physicals)
   ■ Colonoscopies/Other Colon Cancer Screening[†]
   ■ Immunizations[†]
   ■ Mammograms[†]
   ■ Pap Smears[†]
   ■ Well Child Care Visits[†]
■ Home Health Care
■ Hospice Care
■ Outpatient Maternity Office Visits
	No copay	No cost share	No cost share

Inpatient Services	TRICARE Prime	TRICARE Extra	TRICARE Standard
■ Hospitalization for Medical/Surgical Care ■ Inpatient Maternity ■ Skilled Nursing Facility (SNF) Care	No copay	$17.65/day ($25 min. charge)	$17.65/day ($25 min. charge)
■ Hospitalization for Mental Illness ■ Substance Use Treatment ■ Partial Hospitalization Program (PHP) - Mental Health ■ Residential Treatment Center (RTC)	No copay	$20/day ($25 min. charge)	$20/day ($25 min. charge)

Pharmacy	Generic (Tier 1)	Brand Name[‡] (Tier 2)	Non-Formulary (Tier 3)
Military Pharmacy (up to 90-day supply)	$0	$0	Not Applicable
Mail Order (up to 90-day supply)	$3	$9	$22
Network Retail (up to 30-day supply)	$3	$9	$22
Non-Network Retail (up to 30-day supply)	Prime: POS fees apply Standard: Greater of $9 or 20%		Prime: POS fees apply Standard: Greater of $22 or 20%

*The copay is for facility fees; there is no separate copay for professional fees, and deductibles are not applied to the facility or professional claims.
[†]Clinical Preventive Services are screenings or treatment with no symptoms. Diagnostic services due to a symptom will have outpatient office visit or ancillary service copay/cost shares.
[‡]Prescription for a brand name needs to document one or more of the following: Patient must experience, or would likely experience, significant adverse effects from the generic medicine; generic medicine has resulted in, or is likely to result in, therapeutic failure; patient previously responded to the brand name medicine and a change to a generic medicine would incur unacceptable clinical risk.

FIGURE 14-3 TRICARE Prime, Extra, and Standard benefits and costs for active duty family members.

TRICARE Costs for Retirees, Their Family, and Others

- Cost-shares for TRICARE Standard and Extra are applied after the deductible has been satisfied.
- TRICARE Extra is when a TRICARE Standard beneficiary uses a network provider.
- TRICARE Standard beneficiaries may be required to pay up to 15% above the TRICARE allowed amount when using a provider that does not participate in TRICARE.
- Cost-shares are subject to change at the beginning of each fiscal year (October 1).
- Copayments below are per occurrence or per visit.
- Percentage cost shares are based on the TRICARE allowed amount or negotiated rate.

Deductibles	TRICARE Prime	TRICARE Standard/Extra
	No deductibles (Unless Point of Service is used)	$150/person, $300/family

Deductibles are applied each fiscal year, which begins October 1.

Outpatient Services	TRICARE Prime	TRICARE Extra	TRICARE Standard
■ Laboratory and X-ray Services ■ Medication Management Visits ■ Occupational Therapy ■ Office Visits/Consultations ■ Physical Therapy ■ Urgent Care	$12	20%	25%
■ Ambulatory Surgery (Same Day)	$25*	20%	25%
■ Ambulance Services	$20	20%	25%
■ Home Health Care ■ Hospice Care	No copay	No cost	No cost
■ Radiology/Pathology/Cardio Studies ■ Maternity Care Office Visits	No copay	20%	25%
■ Durable Medical Equipment (DME) ■ Medical Supplies ■ Prosthetic Devices	20%	20%	25%
■ Emergency Room Services	$30*	20%	25%
■ Mental Health (Behavioral Health)	Individual/Family Therapy $25 Group Therapy $17	20%	25%

*The copay is for the facility fees, there is no separate copay for professional fees.

Inpatient Services	TRICARE Prime	TRICARE Extra	TRICARE Standard
■ Hospitalization for Medical/Surgical Care ■ Inpatient Maternity	$11/day ($25 min. charge)**	Lesser of $250/day or 25%; plus 20% of professional fees**	Lesser of $535/day or 25%; plus 25% of professional fees**
■ Skilled Nursing Facility (SNF) Care	$11/day ($25 min. charge)**	Lesser of $250/day or 20%; plus 20% of professional fees**	25%**
■ Hospitalization for Mental Illness ■ Substance Use Treatment	$40/day	20%	High Volume Hospital: 25% Low Volume Hospital: lesser of $197/day or 25%; plus 25% of professional fees
■ Partial Hospitalization Program (PHP)-Mental Health ■ Residential Treatment Center (RTC)	$40/day	20%	25%

**Inpatient care at a Military Treatment Facility (MTF) has a copay of $14.80 per day.

Pharmacy	Generic (Tier 1)	Brand Name (Tier 2)	Non-Formulary (Tier 3)
Military Pharmacy (up to 90-day supply)	$0	$0	Not Applicable
Mail Order (up to 90-day supply)	$3	$9	$22
Network Retail (up to 30-day supply)	$3	$9	$22
Non-Network Retail (up to 30-day supply)	Prime: POS fees apply Standard: Greater of $9 or 20%		Prime: POS fees apply Standard: Greater of $22 or 20%

FIGURE 14-4 TRICARE Prime, Extra, and Standard benefits and costs for retirees, their families, and others.

TRICARE PATIENT REFERRAL/AUTHORIZATION FORM

TRICARE West

Patient Name _Mary Smith_   Patient SSN _123-45-6798_

Address _4444 Doghouse Lane_   Date of Birth _09/02/47_

City, State, ZIP _Death Valley, CA 88888_

Home Telephone _(111) 555-2222_

Sponsor Name _John Smith_   Sponsor SSN _123-54-9876_

Patient's Relationship to Sponsor _Wife_

Requesting Provider/Specialty _John Adams, MD, Internal Medicine_   TIN _999999999_

Contact Name/Direct Telephone _Nancy Chong - (111) 555-2323_

Address _222 Prairie Vale Dr., Mohave, CA 81818_

Telephone _(111) 555-9898_   Fax _(999) 000-1111_

Diagnosis _Abdominal pain, pancreatitis & bloating_   ICD-9 _789.0, 577.0, 787.3_

Requested Service _colonoscopy, colon cancer screen_

Date of Service _09/05/XX_   # of Visits _1_

CPT4/HCPCS Code(s) (List all) _45380-45392_

| ☐ Inpatient | ☒ Outpatient Facility | ☐ Office | ☐ Home | (Select One) |

| ☐ Emergency | ☒ Urgent | ☐ Routine | (Select One) |

Servicing Provider/Specialty _Joe Hangnail, MD, Gastroenterologist_   TIN _11111111_

Address _1010101 E. Overpass, Desert Sunrise, CA 88990_

Telephone _(111) 555-5555_   Fax _(999) 010-0101_

Facility _Prickly Pear Memorial Hospital_   TIN _010101010_

Telephone _(111) 555-0101_   Fax _(999) 000-0000_

FIGURE 14-5 TRICARE Patient Referral/Authorization Form.

- Dental care
- Dilatation and curettage
- Durable medical equipment (DME) purchases
- Gastrointestinal endoscopy
- Gynecologic laparoscopy
- Hernia repairs
- Laparoscopic cholecystectomy
- Ligation or transection of fallopian tubes
- Magnetic resonance imaging (MRI)
- Mental health care
- Myringotomy or tympanostomy

- Neuroplasty
- Nose repair (rhinoplasty and septoplasty)
- Strabismus repair
- Tonsillectomy or adenoidectomy

Payment

Deductible and Copayment

Deductibles and copayments are determined according to two groups: (1) active duty family members and (2) retirees, their family members, and survivors.

Spouses and Children of Active Duty Members. For inpatient (hospitalized) care, the beneficiary pays the first $25 of the hospital charge or a small fee for each day, whichever is greater, and TRICARE pays the remainder of the allowable charges for authorized care. **Allowable charge** is the amount that TRICARE calculates to be the patient's cost share for covered care. This is based on 75% to 80% of the allowable charge.

For outpatient (nonhospitalized) care, the beneficiary pays the first $150 (deductible) plus a 20% coinsurance (on charges more than the $150 deductible). A family with two or more eligible beneficiaries pays a maximum of $300 (deductible) plus a 20% coinsurance (on charges in excess of $300). TRICARE pays the remainder of the allowable charges, which is 80%.

All Other Eligible Beneficiaries. The "all other eligible beneficiaries" category consists of retired members, dependents of retired members, dependents of deceased members who died in active duty, and so forth.

For inpatient (hospitalized) care, the beneficiary pays 25% of the hospital charges and fees of professional personnel. TRICARE pays the remaining allowable charges for authorized care, or 75%.

For outpatient (nonhospitalized) care, the beneficiary pays $150 (deductible) plus a 25% coinsurance (on charges more than the $150 deductible). A family with two or more eligible beneficiaries pays a maximum of $300 (deductible) plus a 25% coinsurance (on charges in excess of $300). TRICARE pays the remainder of the allowable charges for authorized care, which is 75%.

Refer to Figures 14-3 and 14-4 for further clarification and to see the differences in benefits between the three TRICARE program options.

Participating Provider

A **participating (par) physician or provider** is a physician who has signed a participating provider contractual agreement with TRICARE to give medical care to TRICARE beneficiaries. Some provisions of the participating provider agreement are that the provider agrees to accept assignment, agrees to accept the TRICARE-determined allowable charge as payment in full, and transmits claims to the regional contractor directly. Assignment status (yes or no) is indicated when the CMS-1500 (02-12) claim form is transmitted to the regional contractor. The provider may bill the patient for his or her **cost share** or coinsurance (20% to 25% of the allowable charge after the deductible has been met) and for any uncovered services or supplies. The provider may not bill for the difference between the provider's usual charge and the allowable charge.

Beneficiaries pay only a certain amount each year for the cost share and annual deductible. This amount is known as the **catastrophic cap.** After this cap is reached, TRICARE pays 100% of the allowable charges for the rest of the year. A note should be attached to the claim when the patient has met the catastrophic cap; this may help to expedite claims processing and payment. After the claim is completed and sent to the regional contractor, the payment goes directly to the physician.

Nonparticipating Provider

A health care provider who chooses not to participate in TRICARE is called a **nonparticipating (nonpar) physician or provider** and as of November 1, 1993, may not bill the patient more than 115% of the TRICARE allowable charge, which is referred to as the *limiting charge.*

For example, if the TRICARE allowable charge for a procedure is $100, providers who decide not to participate in TRICARE may charge TRICARE patients no more than $115 for that procedure. The patient pays the deductible (20% or 25% of the charges determined to be allowable) and any amount more than the allowable charge up to 115% when the physician does not accept assignment. Nonpar providers may choose to accept TRICARE assignment on a case-by-case basis. Assignment should always be accepted when the service member is transferring within 6 months, because this avoids collection problems.

TRICARE EXTRA

Enrollment

TRICARE Extra is a preferred provider organization type of option in which the individual does not have to enroll or pay an annual fee. On a visit-by-visit basis, the individual may seek care from an authorized network provider and receive a discount on services and reduced cost share (copayment). An unenrolled beneficiary automatically becomes a TRICARE Extra beneficiary when care is rendered by a network provider. If an unenrolled beneficiary receives care from a non-network provider, the services received are covered under TRICARE Standard. Providers receive a contract rate for giving care.

Identification Card

A TRICARE Extra beneficiary must present the military identification card as proof of eligibility when receiving care. The military identification card indicates a "Yes" in Box 15B (back of card) if the beneficiary is eligible. Children younger than 10 years of age may use the sponsor's identification card (attach a copy of the child's card to the claim). Individuals older than 10 years must have their own identification card.

Contact the local HCF to verify eligibility. Active duty and retiree dependents and survivors carry an orange or brown military identification card (see Figure 14-2). Retirees carry a blue-gray military identification card.

Benefits

With TRICARE Extra, patients choose providers within the TRICARE network, where available, and pay lower cost shares compared to TRICARE Standard, in which the patient chooses TRICARE-authorized providers outside of the TRICARE Network and pays higher cost shares. TRICARE Extra is available to non–active duty beneficiaries who are not able to, or choose not to, enroll in a TRICARE Prime option. There are no enrollment forms or fees except for an annual deductible for outpatient services and cost shares for most services.

See Figures 14-3 and 14-4 for outpatient and inpatient benefits and deductible and copayment amounts.

Network Provider

The network provider is the physician who has a contract with a regional contractor to provide services and is authorized by TRICARE. A network provider provides medical care to TRICARE beneficiaries under the TRICARE Extra program at contracted rates. He or she has discount agreements with the TRICARE program.

Preauthorization

Referrals from other network providers are coordinated through the HCF. The network provider refers the beneficiary for additional services, when necessary, after precertification requirements and completing a referral form.

Payments
Deductible and Copayment

Deductibles and copayments are determined by group: (1) active duty family members and (2) retirees, their family members, and survivors.

Spouses and Children of Active Duty Members. No copayment is required for inpatient (hospitalized) care.

For outpatient (nonhospitalized) care, the beneficiary pays the first $150 (deductible) plus a 15% coinsurance (on charges more than the $150 deductible). A family with two or more eligible beneficiaries pays a maximum of $300 (deductible) plus a 15% coinsurance (on charges in excess of $300). TRICARE pays the remainder of the allowable charges (85%).

All Other Eligible Beneficiaries. For inpatient (hospitalized) care, the copayment is $250 per day or 25% of the plan's allowable charges, whichever is less, plus 20% of separately billed professional charges at the plan's allowable rate.

For outpatient (nonhospitalized) care, the beneficiary pays $150 (deductible) plus a 20% coinsurance (on charges more than the $150 deductible). A family with two or more eligible beneficiaries pays a maximum of $300 (deductible) plus a 20% coinsurance (on charges in excess of $300). TRICARE pays the remainder of the allowable charges for authorized care (80%).

See Figures 14-3 and 14-4 for further clarification of deductibles and copayments.

TRICARE PRIME

TRICARE Prime is a voluntary health maintenance organization (HMO)–type option. Participation in TRICARE Prime is optional. Beneficiaries who are not enrolled as members in TRICARE Prime may continue to receive services through TRICARE Extra from network providers or through TRICARE Standard using non-network providers. The beneficiary may no longer use the TRICARE Standard program once enrolled in TRICARE Prime.

Enrollment

An individual must complete an application and enroll for a minimum of 12 months to become a TRICARE Prime member. An annual enrollment fee is charged per person or family except for active duty families, who may enroll free. ADSMs are enrolled automatically in TRICARE Prime and are not eligible for benefits under TRICARE Standard or TRICARE Extra. These members are able to use the local military and civilian provider network with necessary authorization.

Enrollees normally receive care from within the Prime network of civilian and military providers. The beneficiary has the option of choosing or being assigned a **primary care manager (PCM)** for each family member. The PCM manages all aspects of the patient's health care (except emergencies), including referrals to specialists. Enrolled beneficiaries may not use a non-network provider, except in emergencies or for pharmaceuticals, without a specific referral from an HCF.

Identification Card

Individuals who enroll are issued a TRICARE Prime identification card, as shown in Figure 14-6. This card does not guarantee TRICARE eligibility; therefore providers must check the TRICARE Uniformed Services

TRICARE Prime Enrollment Card

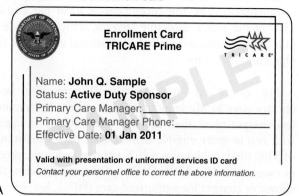

A

*TRICARE Prime Remote
Enrollment Card*

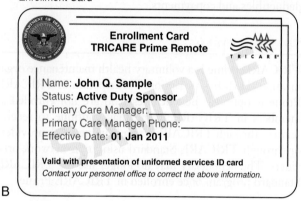

B

*TRICARE Prime Remote for
Active Duty Family Members
Enrollment Card*

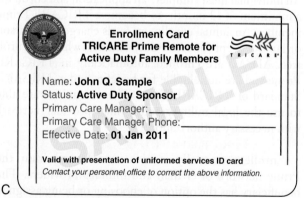

C

FIGURE 14-6 TRICARE Prime identification cards. **A,** TRICARE Prime enrollment card. **B,** TRICARE Prime Remote enrollment card. **C,** TRICARE Prime Remote for Active Duty Family Members enrollment card. When one of these cards is presented, it is only valid if accompanied by a uniformed services ID card, a sample of which is shown in Figure 14-7.

military identification card for the effective and expiration dates or call the local HCF. Copies of the military identification card and the TRICARE Prime card should always be made and retained in the patient's file. For TRICARE Prime patients, both cards should be checked at every visit.

Benefits

Covered services are the same as those for TRICARE Standard patients plus there are additional preventive and primary care services. For example, periodic physical examinations are covered at no charge under TRICARE Prime but are not covered under TRICARE Extra or TRICARE Standard. Prime also covers certain immunizations and annual eye examinations for dependent children of retirees that are not a benefit under Extra or Standard. A dental plan is available for an additional monthly premium. An NAS is necessary only for nonemergency inpatient mental health care services if the beneficiary resides within the designated MTF catchment area. See Figures 14-3 and 14-4 for outpatient and inpatient benefits and deductible and copayment amounts.

Primary Care Manager

The PCM is a physician who is responsible for coordinating and managing the beneficiary's entire health care unless there is an emergency. A provider who decides to participate in a managed care program goes through a credentialing process. This is done approximately every 2 years for all physicians who participate as providers. The PCM may refer the beneficiary for additional services, when necessary, but specific referral and preauthorization requirements must be carried out. Referral patterns are evaluated to determine excessive or inappropriate referrals to specialists. A pattern of such referrals could result in termination of participation in TRICARE Prime.

Preauthorization

All admissions, ambulatory surgical procedures, and other selected procedures require preauthorization. Outpatient or ambulatory surgery must be on the approved procedure list before it is performed. The list is in the *TRICARE Handbook* available at www.tricare.osd.mil.

The **health benefits advisor (HBA)** at the nearest military medical facility should be called to determine whether an NAS statement is necessary for the procedure before the surgery is scheduled in the approved facility. An HBA is a person at a military hospital or clinic who is there to help beneficiaries obtain medical care needed through the military and TRICARE. A **point-of-service (POS) option** is available if no authorization is obtained. This means that the individual can choose to get TRICARE-covered nonemergency services outside the Prime network of providers without a referral from the PCM and without authorization from the HCF. There is an annual deductible and 50% cost share if the POS option is used.

Payments

Copayment

TRICARE Prime copayments for inpatient hospital services vary for active duty family members and for retirees and their family members and survivors. For outpatient services, copayments are the same for active duty family members and for retirees and their family members and survivors but vary in amounts depending on the type of service received. Copayments should be collected at the time services are rendered. Refer to Figures 14-3 and 14-4 for further clarification of copayments.

TRICARE RESERVE SELECT

TRICARE Reserve Select (TRS) is a premium-based health plan available for purchase by qualified members of the Selected Reserve and their families who are not eligible for or enrolled in the Federal Employee Health Benefits (FEHB) program or currently covered under FEHB, either under their own eligibility or through a family member. These can include the Army National Guard, Army Reserve, Navy Reserve, Marine Corps Reserve, Air National Guard, Air Force Reserve, and Coast Guard Reserve. TRS health care benefits are similar to TRICARE Standard and Extra.

TRICARE RETIRED RESERVE

TRICARE Retired Reserve (TRR) is a premium-based health plan that qualified retired Reserve members and survivors may purchase. TRR offers coverage similar to TRICARE Standard and Extra. Retired National Guard and Reserve personnel may qualify to purchase TRR coverage if they are members of the retired Reserve of a Reserve component of the armed forces, under the age of 60, and not eligible for or enrolled in the Federal Employees Health Benefits (FEHB) program. At age 60, TRR coverage is automatically terminated and the retiree becomes eligible for TRICARE Prime/Standard/Extra and may enroll in one of those programs.

TRICARE YOUNG ADULT

The TRICARE Young Adult (TYA) program is a premium-based health care plan available for purchase by qualified dependents. TYA offers TRICARE Standard or TRICARE Prime coverage based on the sponsor's status. It has medical and pharmacy benefits but no dental coverage. To join this program, the enrollee must be a dependent of an eligible uniformed service sponsor, unmarried, at least age 21, and not eligible to enroll in an employer-sponsored health plan. He or she can also enroll if under the age of 26 and enrolled in a full-time course of study at an approved institution of higher learning and if the sponsor provides at least 50% of his or her financial support.

TRICARE FOR LIFE

In October 2001, **TRICARE for Life (TFL)** was enacted. It offers additional TRICARE benefits as a supplementary payer to Medicare for uniformed service retirees, their spouses, and survivors age 65 or older. This plan was originally introduced as TRICARE Senior Prime. When beneficiaries become entitled to receive Medicare Part A and Medicare Part B at age 65, they experience no break in TRICARE coverage. The only change is that TRICARE will pay secondary to Medicare beginning on the first day of the month in which they turn 65.

TFL is provided to the following beneficiaries:

- Medicare-eligible uniformed service retirees, including retired National Guard and Reservists
- Medicare-eligible family members, including widows and widowers
- Certain former spouses if they were eligible for TRICARE before age 65

Dependent parents and parents-in-law are not eligible for TRICARE benefits. They may continue to receive services within an MTF on a space-available basis.

Enrollment

Most beneficiaries must be eligible for Medicare Part A and enrolled in Medicare Part B to qualify for TFL. An exception is Uniformed Services Family Health Plan (USFHP) members. Prospective TFL beneficiaries do not have to sign up or enroll for the program; however, they should be enrolled in DEERS. TFL has no enrollment fees. The member is required to enroll in Medicare Part B but without surcharge.

The DEERS notifies a beneficiary within 90 days before his or her 65th birthday that the medical benefits are about to change. It asks the beneficiary to contact the nearest Social Security Administration office about enrollment in Medicare. The beneficiary must elect to enroll in Medicare Part B to be eligible for TFL benefits. If the beneficiary is age 65 or older and has only Medicare Part A, he or she can enroll in Medicare Part B during the annual general enrollment period, which runs from January 1 to March 31 every year. Medicare Part B coverage then begins on July 1 of the year in which the beneficiary enrolls.

Identification Card

Beneficiaries who qualify for TFL do not need a TRICARE enrollment card.

Benefits

Each beneficiary receives a matrix comparing Medicare benefits to TRICARE benefits. Certain benefits (for example, prescription medications) are covered under the TRICARE Senior Pharmacy Program. Pharmacy benefits provide Medicare-eligible retirees of the uniformed services, their family members, and survivors the same pharmacy benefit as retirees who are younger than age 65. This includes access to prescription drugs at MTFs, retail pharmacies, and through the National Mail Order Pharmacy. Medicare Part B enrollment is not mandatory to receive TRICARE Senior Pharmacy Program benefits.

Referral and Preauthorization

There are no preauthorization requirements for the TFL program. All services and supplies must be benefits of the Medicare or TRICARE programs to be covered.

Payment

The following four scenarios represent most cases and explain the payment mechanism:
1. Services covered under both Medicare and TRICARE: Medicare pays first at the Medicare rate and the remaining amount is paid by TRICARE, which covers the beneficiary's cost share and deductible. No copayment, cost share, or deductible is paid by the TFL beneficiary.
2. Services covered under Medicare but not TRICARE: Medicare pays the Medicare rate and the beneficiary pays the Medicare cost share and deductible amounts. TRICARE pays nothing.
3. Services covered under TRICARE but not Medicare: TRICARE pays the allowed amount and Medicare pays nothing. The beneficiary is responsible for the TRICARE cost share and deductible amounts.
4. Services not payable by TRICARE or Medicare: The beneficiary is entirely responsible for the medical bill.

TRICARE PLUS

Enrollment

TRICARE Plus is open to persons eligible for care in military facilities and not enrolled in TRICARE Prime or a commercial HMO. TRICARE Plus allows some Military Health System (MHS) beneficiaries to enroll with a military primary care provider. TRICARE Plus has no enrollment fee.

Identification Card

Persons enrolled in TRICARE Plus are issued an identification card and identified in the DEERS.

Benefits

The TRICARE Plus program is designed to function in the following ways:
- Enrollees use the MTF as their source of primary care; it is not a comprehensive health plan.
- Enrollees may seek care from a civilian provider but are discouraged from obtaining nonemergency primary care from sources outside the MTF.
- Enrollees are not guaranteed access to specialty providers at the MTF.
- Enrollees may not use their enrollment at another facility.
- The MTF's commander determines the enrollment capacity at each MTF.

Payment

TRICARE Plus offers the same benefits as TRICARE Prime when using an MTF. It has no effect on the enrollees' use or payment of civilian health care benefits; therefore TRICARE Standard, TRICARE Extra, or Medicare may pay for civilian health care services obtained by a TRICARE Plus enrollee.

TRICARE PRIME REMOTE PROGRAM

Enrollment

TRICARE Prime Remote (TPR) is a program designed for ADSMs who work and live more than 50 miles or 1 hour from MTFs (military hospitals and clinics). An ADSM is an active member of the US government military services (for example, Army, Navy, Air Force, Marines, or Coast Guard). ADSMs must enroll for this program, which enables them to receive care from any civilian provider. TRICARE Prime Remote for Active Duty Family Members (TPRADFM) is the TPR benefit for family members with similar benefits and program requirements. TPR and TPRADFM are offered in the 50 United States only and both require enrollment.

Identification Card

ADSMs must present their military identification card to receive care from providers (Figure 14-7). Photocopy the front and reverse sides of the card so that information is available for reference when completing the insurance claim form.

Benefits

TPR program benefits are similar to TRICARE Prime. Services may be received from an MTF when available or from any civilian provider. Primary routine care does not require prior authorization (for example, office visits, preventive

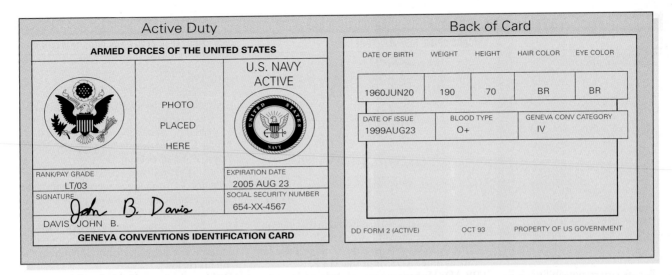

FIGURE 14-7 Military identification card for an active duty individual in the armed forces. It is used as the identification card for the TRICARE Prime and Prime Remote programs and is considered a sponsor identification card.

health care). The HCF must be contacted to receive authorization for referrals, inpatient admissions, maternity, physical therapy, orthotics, hearing appliances, family planning (tubal ligation or vasectomy), outpatient and inpatient behavioral health services, and transplants. Table 14-1 provides a summary of the unique aspects of TPR.

Referral and Preauthorization

Routine primary care (for example, office visits, preventive health care) does not require prior authorization. The PCM must initiate all specialty referrals and coordinate requests through the HBA for certain outpatient services, all inpatient surgical or medical services, maternity services, physical therapy, orthotics, hearing appliances, family planning, transplants, and inpatient or outpatient behavioral health services. The HBA is a government employee who is responsible for helping all MHS beneficiaries to obtain medical care.

Payments

Those persons covered and receiving benefits under TPR are not responsible for any out-of-pocket costs. ADSM claims for services provided by a TRICARE network provider are paid at the same contracted rate as other TRICARE beneficiary claims.

SUPPLEMENTAL HEALTH CARE PROGRAM

Enrollment

The Supplemental Health Care Program (SHCP) covers both MTF-referred care and civilian health care

provided to ADSMs. The MTF always administers routine care (for example, routine office visits, preventive health care).

Identification Card

ADSMs must present their military identification card to receive care from providers (see Figure 14-7). The front and reverse sides of the card should be photocopied so that information is available for reference when the insurance claim form is completed.

Benefits

See Table 14-1 for a summary of the unique aspects of SHCP. SHCP enables beneficiaries to be referred to a civilian provider for care. The MTF must initiate all referrals to civilian providers and use a DD Form 2161 signed by the facility commander. There is no deductible, copayment, or cost share for services provided by a civilian provider.

Referral and Preauthorization

The MTF initiates all referrals for ADSMs and other designated patients to civilian specialists when needed.

Payments

Those covered and receiving benefits under SHCP are not responsible for any out-of-pocket costs. ADSMs claims for services provided by a TRICARE network provider are paid at the same contracted rate as other TRICARE beneficiary claims.

Table 14-1	Summary of Unique Aspects of TRICARE Prime Remote Program and Supplemental Health Care Program	
	TRICARE PRIME REMOTE (TPR)	**SUPPLEMENTAL HEALTH CARE PROGRAM (SHCP)**
Plan description	TPR is a program for ADSMs who live and work more than 50 miles or 1 hour from an MTF. ADSMs must enroll.	SHCP is a program for • ADSMs • Inpatients at military treatment facilities who are not TRICARE eligible (for example, eligible parents, parents-in-law) referred by an MTF to a civilian provider for care (usually for a specific test, procedure, or consultation) • Non-MTF-referred ADSMs (for example, ROTC students, cadets/midshipmen, eligible foreign military)
Provider type	Any civilian provider	Any civilian provider
Beneficiary access to care	TPR ADSMs receive care from any civilian provider or from an MTF when available. Under TPR, ADSMs will have the same priority to care as other ADSMs at the MTF.	The beneficiary may receive services from any civilian provider in accordance with referral and preauthorization requirements (below).
Beneficiary responsibility	TPR ADSMs have no annual deductible, cost shares, or copayments. The TPR ADSM must present his or her military ID card at the time care is received.	ADSMs and others eligible for SHCP referred to civilian providers have no copayment, deductible, or cost share. Beneficiary must present his or her military ID card at the time care is received.
Point-of-Service (POS)	POS does not apply. If the ADSM receives care without a referral or preauthorization, the claim will be processed if it meets all other TRICARE requirements on a case-by-case basis.	The POS option does not apply.
Program benefits	Offers benefits similar to TRICARE Prime. Some benefits (including all behavioral health care) require preauthorization.	Offers benefits similar to TRICARE Prime. Some benefits (including all behavioral health care) require preauthorization.
Referrals and preauthorizations	*Primary care:* ADSMs can receive primary care from a provider without a referral or preauthorization. ADSMs with an assigned PCM will receive primary care from their PCM. ADSMs with no PCM can use any TRICARE-certified provider. Or, he or she can contact an HCF for assistance in locating a provider. *Specialty and inpatient care:* The SPOC will review requests for specialty and inpatient care.	*Specialty and inpatient care:* The MTF will review all requests for specialty and inpatient care for ADSMs. The MTF Commander or designee signature on a DD Form 2161 is required for designated patients referred for civilian care. Preauthorization for nonreferred ADSMs for specialty, inpatient, and behavioral health care must be obtained from the SPOC or the HCF.

ADSMs, Active duty service members; *HCF,* health care finder; *MTF,* Military Treatment Facility; *PCM,* primary care manager; *ROTC,* Reserve Officers' Training Corps; *SPOC,* service point of contact.

TRICARE HOSPICE PROGRAM

The TRICARE hospice program is based on Medicare's hospice program. It is designed to provide care and comfort to patients who are expected to live less than 6 months if the terminal illness runs its normal course. Those persons who receive care under the hospice program cannot receive other services under the TRICARE basic programs (treatments aimed at a cure) unless the hospice care has been formally revoked. Many additional rules and limits apply to the hospice program; therefore the HBA at the nearest military medical facility should be called and a copy of the guidelines requested.

TRICARE AND HMO COVERAGE

TRICARE considers HMO coverage to be the same as any other primary health insurance coverage.

TRICARE shares the cost of covered care received from an HMO (including the HMO's user fees), after the HMO has paid all it is going to pay, under the following conditions:

• The provider must meet TRICARE provider certification standards.
• The type of care must be a TRICARE benefit and medically necessary.
• TRICARE does not pay for emergency services received outside the HMO's normal service area.

TRICARE does not cost-share services that an individual obtains outside the HMO if the services are available through the HMO. For example, if an HMO provides psychiatric services but the patient does not like the HMO's psychiatrist and obtains services outside the HMO, TRICARE will not pay anything on the claim.

VETERANS HEALTH ADMINISTRATION PROGRAM

The Veterans Health Care Expansion Act of 1973 (PL93-82) authorized a CHAMPUS-like program called the Civilian Health and Medical Program of the Department of Veterans Affairs (CHAMPVA) (now known as the **Veterans Health Administration**), which became effective on September 1, 1973. The Veterans Health Administration (or CHAMPVA) plan is not an insurance program in that it does not involve a contract guaranteeing the indemnification of an insured party against a specified loss in return for a premium paid. It is considered a **service benefit program;** therefore there are no premiums.

This program is for the spouse and children of a veteran with a **total, permanent service-connected disability** or for the surviving spouse and children of a veteran who died as a result of a service-connected disability. A **veteran** is any person who has served in the armed forces of the United States, is no longer in the service, and has received an honorable discharge. Just as in the TRICARE program, individuals who qualify for the Veterans Health Administration (or CHAMPVA) program are known as *beneficiaries* and the veteran is called the *sponsor.*

Examples of total, permanent service-connected disabilities are an injury with paraplegic results, a bullet wound with neurologic damage, and loss of a limb. These contrast with a chronic or temporary service-connected disability, which might exist if an individual improperly lifts a heavy object while in the Navy, suffers a back injury with ongoing sporadic symptoms, and requires continuing medical care after leaving the service. Both scenarios involve service-connected disabilities; however, the first example illustrates a person permanently disabled, whereas the second illustrates what may be a chronic or temporary disability.

Eligibility

The following persons are eligible for Veterans Health Administration (or CHAMPVA) program benefits as long as they are not eligible for TRICARE Standard and not eligible for Medicare Part A as a result of reaching age 65:

- The husband, wife, or unmarried child of a veteran with a total disability, permanent in nature, resulting from a **service-connected injury**
- The husband, wife, or unmarried child of a veteran who died as the result of a service-connected disability or who, at the time of death, had a total disability, permanent in nature, resulting from a service-connected injury
- The husband, wife, or unmarried child of an individual who died in the line of duty while in active service

Qualifying children are those unmarried and younger than age 18, regardless of whether dependent or not, or those up to age 23 who are enrolled in a course of instruction at an approved educational institution.

Determination of eligibility is the responsibility of the **Department of Veterans Affairs (VA).** The prospective beneficiary visits the nearest VA medical center and receives a VA identification card if eligible.

Enrollment

Dependents of veterans must have a Social Security number and must have contacted the local VA regional office to establish dependency on the veteran sponsor. The individual obtains and completes an application by telephone, fax, or downloading from the VA's website.

Identification Card

The issuing station's number appears on the identification card to identify the home station where the beneficiary's case file is kept. The identification card number is the veteran's VA file number with an alpha suffix. The suffix is different for each beneficiary of a sponsor. All dependents 10 years of age or older are required to have a uniformed services (military) identification and privilege card for Veterans Health Administration, as shown in Figure 14-8.

Benefits

The VA elected to provide these beneficiaries with benefits and cost-sharing plans similar to those received by dependents of retired and deceased uniformed services personnel under TRICARE Standard. An overall picture of Veterans Health Administration benefits, which includes cost sharing (deductibles and copayments), can be seen in Table 14-2.

Provider

The beneficiaries of the Veterans Health Administration (CHAMPVA) program have complete freedom of choice in selecting their civilian health care providers.

Preauthorization

Preauthorization is necessary for organ and bone marrow transplantation, hospice services, most mental health or substance abuse services, all dental care, and all DME with a purchase price or total rental cost of $300 or more. Preauthorization requests are made directly to Veterans Health Administration (at 800-733-8387) or by mail to VA Health Administration Center CHAMPVA, Attn: Preauthorization, PO Box 65023, Denver, CO 80206-9023.

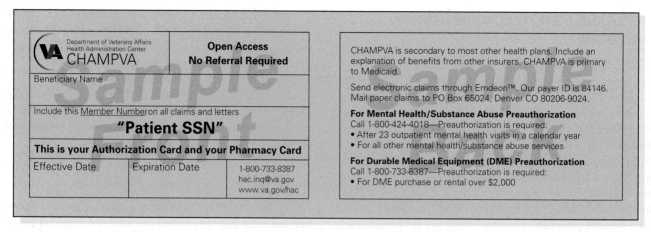

FIGURE 14-8 CHAMPVA card.

Table 14-2	Veterans Health Administration (CHAMPVA) Service Benefits and Cost Share Summary Chart		
	Beneficiary Pays*		
BENEFIT (COVERED SERVICES)	**DEDUCTIBLE ($50/INDIVIDUAL OR $100/FAMILY PER CALENDAR YEAR)**	**COST SHARE†**	**VETERANS HEALTH ADMINISTRATION PAYS**
Outpatient Services			
Ambulatory			
Family services	No	25% of allowable	75% of allowable
Professional services	Yes	25% of allowable	75% of allowable
Pharmacy services	Yes	25% of allowable	75% of allowable
DME			
Non-VA source	Yes	25% of allowable	75% of allowable
VA source	No	None	100% of VA cost
Inpatient Services			
Facility Services			
DRG based	No	Lesser of (1) per day amount × number of inpatient days, (2) 25% of billed amount, or (3) DRG rate	DRG rate less beneficiary cost share
Non-DRG based	No	25% of allowable	75% of allowable
Mental Health Services			
High-volume/RTC	No	Lesser of (1) per day amount × number of inpatient days or (2) 25% of billed amount	Balance of allowable *after* beneficiary cost share
Low-volume	No		
Professional services	No	25% of allowable	75% of allowable

DME, Durable medical equipment; *DRG,* diagnosis-related group; *RTC,* residential treatment center; *VA,* Department of Veterans Affairs.
*Services received at VA health care facilities under the CHAMPVA In-house Treatment Initiative (CITI) program are exempt from beneficiary cost sharing.
†Under catastrophic protection plan (Cat Cap), annual beneficiary cost sharing is limited to $7500.

CLAIMS PROCEDURE

Regional Contractor

TRICARE Standard is governed by the Department of Defense (DoD). As such, it is not subject to those state regulatory bodies or agencies that control the insurance business. The DoD and the VA have agreed to use the Office of the Assistant Secretary of Defense and the TRICARE Standard system of fiscal intermediaries and hospital contractors to receive, process, and pay Veterans Health

Administration (CHAMPVA) claims, following the same procedures currently used for TRICARE Standard.

A **regional contractor,** also known as a *fiscal intermediary (FI)* or *claims processor,* is an organization under contract to the government that handles insurance claims for care received under the TRICARE Standard and Veterans Health Administration (CHAMPVA) programs.

TRICARE Standard and Veterans Health Administration (CHAMPVA)

The most efficient way to file claims for TRICARE Standard and Veterans Health Administration (CHAMPVA) is electronic transmission of ASC X12 Version 5010 (Professional) Health Insurance Portability and Accountability Act (HIPAA) claim transaction and format to the Health Administration Center (HAC). Paper claims on the CMS-1500 (02-12) claim form are also accepted but the turnaround time to payment is, on average, an additional 20 days. Remember to abstract the correct information from the front and back of the patient's identification card. Service members move often and it

is common for providers to have an old or temporary address on file. Always ask beneficiaries to update their information during each office visit. Refer to Chapter 7 and follow the TRICARE or Veterans Health Administration (CHAMPVA) instructions for completing the CMS-1500 (02-12) claim form. Refer to Figure 7-9 for an example of a completed TRICARE case with no other insurance and to Figure 7-10 for an example of a completed Veterans Health Administration (CHAMPVA) case. If electing to complete the VA Form 10-1759A for a Veterans Health Administration (CHAMPVA) case, refer to the instructions presented later in this chapter.

If the physician is nonparticipating and does not accept assignment, the patient completes the top portion of the CMS-1500 (02-12) claim form, attaches the physician's itemized statement, and submits the claim. Alternatively, the patient may submit the claim on the white TRICARE claim DD Form 2642 Patient's Request for Medical Payment. Patients and providers of care for health services in foreign countries must use DD Form 2520. The Uniform Bill (UB-04) form is used for inpatient hospital billing.

HIPAA Compliance Alert — MEDICAL RECORD ACCESS

Privacy Act of 1974: The Privacy Act of 1974 became effective on September 27, 1975, and established an individual's right to review his or her medical records maintained by a federal medical care facility, such as a VA medical center or US Public Health Service facility, and to contest inaccuracies in such records. The Act directs each agency to make its own rules establishing access procedures. Agencies are allowed to adopt special procedures when it is believed that direct access could be harmful to a person. The Act requires that an individual from whom personal information is requested be informed of (1) the authority for the request, (2) the principal purpose of the information requested, (3) routine use of the information, and (4) the effect on an individual who does not provide the information.

Some federal agencies or federally funded institutions may be regulated by both the Privacy Act and HIPAA standards. Such entities are required to comply with both sets of regulations. Although HIPAA standards generally provide more restrictive regulations, entities are advised to revise their policies and procedures to comply with both HIPAA standards and the Privacy Act. Under certain situations, HIPAA standards are likely to prevail and require regulated entities to obtain individual authorization for some disclosures that they now make without authorization under the

"routine uses" exception. HIPAA compliance managers should make a determination of the effects of the interplay between the federal laws and HIPAA standards, consult with legal counsel, and plan an entity's compliance initiatives accordingly.

Computer Matching and Privacy Protection Act of 1988: The Computer Matching and Privacy Protection Act of 1988 is specific to TRICARE. It permits the government to verify information by way of computer matches. By law, the provider must tell a TRICARE member that he or she is calling TRICARE, which is governed by the DoD, and only information to determine eligibility and to learn what services are covered is to be obtained.

Both of these Acts are mentioned on the back of the CMS-1500 (02-12) claim form. TRICARE patients must be made aware of this information by physicians who treat them so that they are knowledgeable about routine use and disclosure of medical data. Providers must follow both HIPAA and the Computer Matching and Privacy Protection Act of 1988. Patients may make a Privacy Protection Act request in writing, in person, or by telephone. Individuals should call the facility to determine the required procedures to obtain access to the records and what to include in making a written request.

Time Limit

Effective January 1, 1993, claims must be filed within 1 year from the date a service is provided or (for inpatient care) within 1 year from the patient's date of discharge from the inpatient facility.

Claims Office

The TRICARE program is administered by the DoD, TRICARE Management Activity, 16401 East Centretech Parkway, Aurora, CO 80011-9043 but claims are not processed in Colorado. The insurance billing specialist must understand that when transmitting or sending the claim to TRICARE, the claim goes to the TRICARE claims office nearest to the residence of the military sponsor. For example, if the patient is a child who was treated in California but the sponsor is an ADSM stationed in Florida, the claim should be transmitted to the TRICARE claims office in the south region and not a claims office in the west region. Refer to the TRICARE website to locate the address of the regional claims processor for submitting a TRICARE Standard claim in each state. Write to the TRICARE Support Office or contact the HBA at the nearest MTF to obtain a current *TRICARE Standard Handbook* or for answers to any questions about the name of the regional claims processor, benefits, nonbenefits, the need for an NAS, and so on.

Because of the September 11, 2001, attacks and the activation of the US National Guard and Reserve components to the Middle East, the provider's office may come in contact with members of the National Guard or Reserve component. The members of these two organizations normally join a unit located near their place of residence. The National Guard and Reserve are only called to active duty in certain circumstances. Otherwise, they are required to perform their duties once in "drill status" and to participate in "annual training." Drill status occurs on a Saturday and a Sunday. Annual training occurs for 2 weeks, normally during the summer. While these service members are on drill status or in annual training, they are entitled to medical care at government expense. The government pays for an illness or injury incurred while on the way to drill status, during drill status, and on the way home from drill status. If the service member stops anywhere on the way to or from drill (for example, to put gas in the car), any injury received is not paid for by the government. Sometimes, when a service member is injured or becomes ill, he or she may have medical personnel available within the unit to provide medical care. If not, the service member is sent to a clinic or hospital near the drill center. This injury or illness is not covered by workers' compensation. The military unit must be contacted to be compensated for the medical care. Each unit has a staff member called a *full-time manager (FTM)*. This person is assigned to the unit and works full-time during the week and attends drills with the unit on weekends. He or she processes all medical claims for unit members. Medical records must accompany the claim for it to be paid. The unit also may require the physician to prepare additional forms that must accompany the claim. The payment is not paid by the unit. The claim is sent to a higher command, where the illness or injury is investigated. This is a time-consuming procedure and it could take months for the claim to be paid. It is better to bill the service member for payment if payment is not received within 60 to 90 days.

The Veterans Health Administration (CHAMPVA) program is administered by the VA, Health Administration Center, PO Box 65023, Denver, CO 80206-9023.

TRICARE Extra and TRICARE Prime

The beneficiary does not file any claim forms under TRICARE Extra or TRICARE Prime programs when using network providers. Providers must electronically transmit 5010 claims to TRICARE subcontractors for services given to beneficiaries. Referral and preauthorization numbers are required when applicable.

Time Limit

For outpatient care, a claim must be transmitted to the state or region's TRICARE contractor within 1 year of the date that the provider rendered the service to the patient. For inpatient care, a claim must be received by the contractor within 1 year from the date that the patient was discharged from the facility. If a claim covers several different medical services or supplies that were provided at different times, the 1-year deadline applies to each item on the claim.

When a claim is electronically transmitted on time but the contractor returns it for more information, the claim should be retransmitted with the requested information so that it is received by the contractor no later than 1 year after the medical services or supplies were provided or 90 days from the date the claim was returned to the provider, whichever is later.

A contractor may grant exemptions from the filing deadlines for several reasons. A request that includes a complete explanation of the circumstances of the late filing, all available documentation supporting the request, and the claim denied for late filing should be transmitted electronically to the contractor.

Claims Office

See the TRICARE website to determine where claims should be transmitted electronically and to obtain more information about this program.

TRICARE Prime Remote and Supplemental Health Care Program

Outpatient professional services are electronically transmitted using a 5010 HIPAA transaction and format, or paper claims may be submitted using a CMS-1500 (02-12) claim form. Primary care service claims are processed and paid without a referral or preauthorization from a network or non-network provider. A referral number provided by the HCF must be included for specialty medical or surgical care and for behavioral health counseling and therapy sessions. The POS option and NAS requirements do not apply to TPR and SHCP claims.

Time Limit

A claim must be transmitted electronically within 1 year from the date on which a service is provided or (for inpatient care) within 1 year from the patient's date of discharge from the inpatient facility.

Claims Office

Claims of ADSM patients should not be transmitted electronically to TRICARE. Claims for patients on active duty must be received by the specific branch of service (that is, Army, Navy, Air Force, or Marines). Claims are submitted to Palmetto Government Benefits Administrators (PGBAs) for processing and payment.

TRICARE for Life

If the beneficiary receives care from a civilian provider, the provider electronically transmits claims to Medicare. Medicare pays its portion and then electronically forwards the claim to TRICARE for the remaining amount. TRICARE sends its payment directly to the provider. The beneficiary receives a TRICARE **summary payment voucher** that indicates the amount paid to the provider.

TRICARE/Veterans Health Administration and Other Insurance

By law, TRICARE/Veterans Health Administration (CHAMPVA) is usually the second payer when a beneficiary is enrolled in **other health insurance (OHI)** or a civilian health plan or belongs to an HMO or preferred provider organization. OHI may be coverage through an employer, an association, or a private insurer. However, two exceptions are as follows:

- When a plan is administered under Title XIX of the Social Security Act (Medicaid), electronically transmit TRICARE or Veterans Health Administration (CHAMPVA) claims first if the beneficiary is a recipient of the Medicaid program.

- When coverage is specifically designed to supplement TRICARE benefits (for example, Medigap [MG] health plan), electronically transmit TRICARE or CHAMPVA claims first.

When the patient has other health insurance that is primary (meaning that it pays before TRICARE Standard or the Veterans Health Administration [CHAMPVA]), electronically transmit or send a paper claim using the CMS-1500 (02-12) insurance claim form. Attach the explanation of benefits (EOB) from the primary carrier. If the patient is submitting his or her claim to the other insurance, take these steps:

1. Bill the other insurance carrier with the form it has supplied.
2. Bill TRICARE or Veterans Health Administration (CHAMPVA) by completing the top section of the CMS-1500 (02-12) after receiving payment and an EOB from the other third-party payer. Submit the physician's itemized statement, which must contain the following:
   a. Provider's name
   b. Date on which the services or supplies were provided
   c. Description of each service or supply
   d. Place of treatment
   e. Number or frequency of each service
   f. Fee for each item of service or supply
   g. Procedure code number(s)
   h. Diagnostic code number(s) or description of condition(s) for which treatment is being received
   i. Billing statements showing only total charges, canceled checks, or cash register receipts (or similar-type receipts) are not acceptable as itemized statements.
3. Attach a photocopy of the EOB from the other third-party payer.
4. Electronically transmit the TRICARE or Veterans Health Administration (CHAMPVA) claim to the local contractor (claims processor/regional contractor).

Medicare and TRICARE

TRICARE is considered secondary to Medicare for persons younger than age 65 who have Medicare Part A as a result of a disability and who have enrolled in Medicare Part B. Those eligible for Medicare Part A are not covered by TRICARE unless disabled. Claims should be electronically transmitted to Medicare, then to TRICARE with a copy of the Medicare remittance advice. Services covered by TRICARE but not covered by Medicare (for example, prescriptions) are paid by TRICARE. Participating providers may obtain a TRICARE fee schedule by contacting their regional contractor.

Medicare and Veterans Health Administration (CHAMPVA)

Effective December 5, 1991, CHAMPVA became secondary payer to Medicare for persons younger than age 65 who are enrolled in Medicare Parts A and B and who are otherwise eligible for the Veterans Health Administration (CHAMPVA) program. Claims first must be transmitted electronically to Medicare because the Veterans Health Administration (CHAMPVA) is a secondary payer.

Dual or Double Coverage

A claim must be filed if a patient has an additional private insurance policy that provides double coverage. Refusal by the beneficiary to claim benefits from other health insurance coverage results in a denial of TRICARE benefits. In double coverage situations, TRICARE pays the lower of the following:

- The amount of TRICARE-allowable charges remaining after the double coverage plan has paid its benefits
- The amount TRICARE would have paid as primary payer

There must be **coordination of benefits (COB)** so that there is no duplication of benefits paid between the double coverage plan and TRICARE.

Third-Party Liability

If the patient is in an automobile accident or receives an injury that may have third-party involvement, the following two options are available for reimbursement:

1. **Option 1:** TRICARE Form DD 2527 (Statement of Personal Injury, Possible Third-Party Liability) must be sent with the regular claim form for cost sharing of the civilian medical care. All five sections of the form should be completed by the patient. This form allows TRICARE to evaluate the circumstances of the accident and the possibility that the government may recover money for medical care from the person who injured the patient. If a CMS-1500 (02-12) claim form is submitted without TRICARE Form DD 2527, a request is made to complete it. This form must be returned within 35 days of the request or the claims processor will deny the original and all related claims. Then the regional contractor submits a claim to the third party for reimbursement or files a lien for reimbursement with the liability insurance carrier, the liable party, or the attorneys or court involved.

2. **Option 2:** The provider can submit claims exclusively to the third-party liability carrier for reimbursement. Claims submitted with ICD-10-CM diagnostic codes between S00 and T88 (Injuries, Poisonings, and External Causes) trigger the fact that there might be third-party litigation and the claims processor may request the completion of DD Form 2527.

Workers' Compensation

If a TRICARE or Veterans Health Administration (CHAMPVA) beneficiary is injured on the job or becomes ill because of his or her work, a workers' compensation claim must be filed with the compensation insurance carrier. TRICARE or the Veterans Health Administration (CHAMPVA) can be billed when all workers' compensation benefits have been exhausted.

In some situations it must be decided whether a case that involves an accident or illness is work related and the claim might be transmitted electronically to the TRICARE or Veterans Health Administration (CHAMPVA) claims regional contractor. In those instances, the claims processor files a lien with the workers' compensation carrier for recovery when the case is settled.

AFTER CLAIM SUBMISSION

TRICARE Summary Payment Voucher

For each TRICARE claim, the claims processor issues a summary payment voucher (Figure 14-9) that details the payment of the claim (that is, service or supplies received, allowable charges, amount billed, amount TRICARE paid, how much deductible has been paid, and patient's cost share amount). When the provider participates (accepts assignment), the voucher is sent to him or her with the check. The patient always receives a copy of the voucher, even if the provider receives payment directly from the regional contractor.

Veterans Health Administration (CHAMPVA) Explanation of Benefits Document

On completion of the processing of a claim, a payment check is generated and an EOB document is sent to the beneficiary (including the provider if the claim is filed by the provider). The EOB summarizes the action taken on the claim and contains information as illustrated and explained in Figure 14-10. Beneficiaries who receive durable medical equipment or VA services from a CHAMPVA In-house Treatment Initiative (CITI, pronounced "city") do not receive an EOB.

Quality Assurance

A **quality assurance program** continually assesses the effectiveness of inpatient and outpatient care. The quality assurance department reviews providers' outpatient

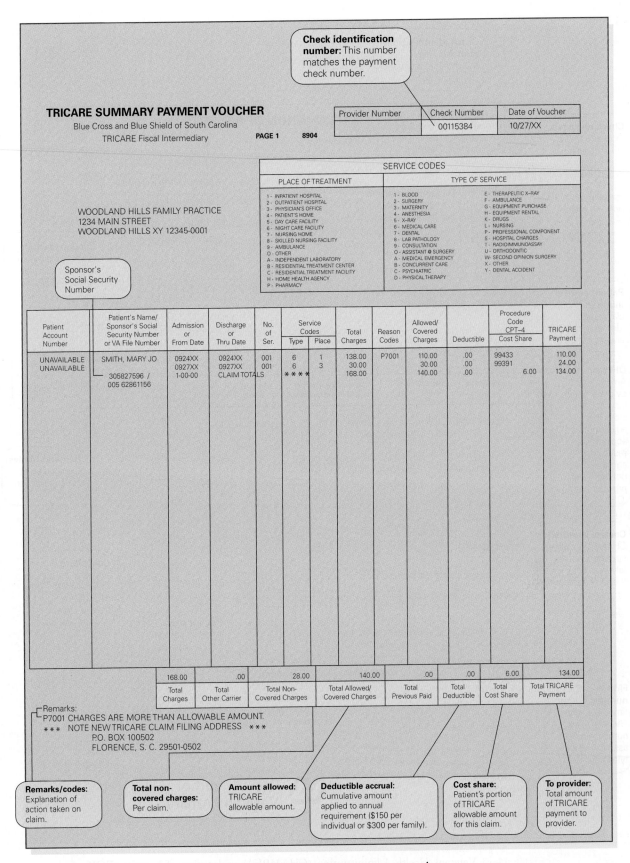

FIGURE 14-9 TRICARE summary payment voucher.

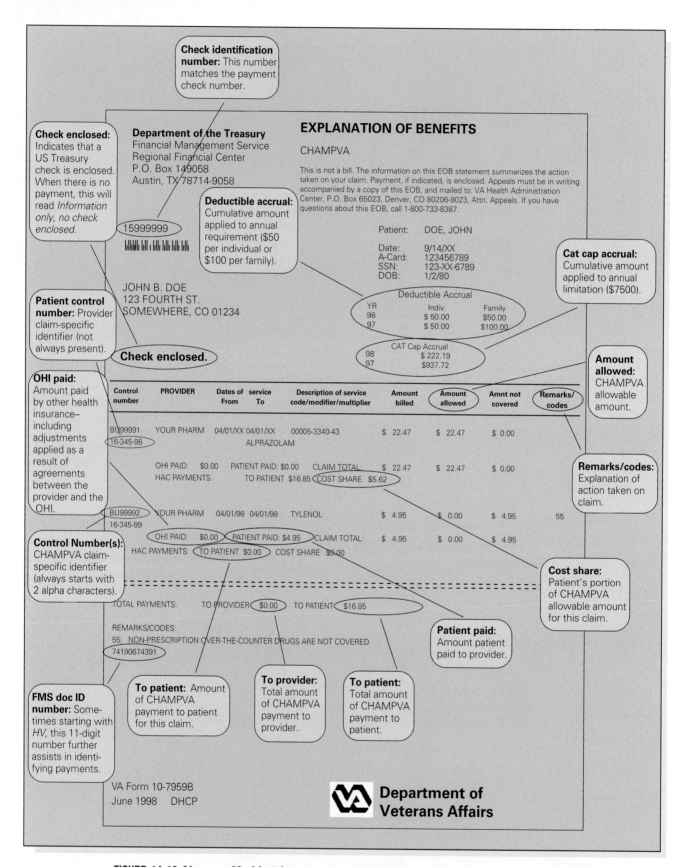

FIGURE 14-10 Veterans Health Administration (CHAMPVA) explanation of benefits (EOB) document.

records on a random basis for clinical and administrative quality. Grievance procedures have been established for members and providers if any complaint arises from an administrative process, a service provided by a physician, or an issue involving quality of care.

TRICARE–managed care programs have a quality assurance program to continually assess the effectiveness of care and services rendered by providers. This includes inpatient and outpatient hospital care, mental health services, long-term care, home health care, and programs for people with disabilities. Providers are notified in writing when a potential quality issue has been confirmed as a breach of quality standards. Recommended corrective action plans are given and noncompliance may lead to suspension or termination of a provider.

Claims Inquiries and Appeals

Through the appeal process, providers may request reconsideration of a denial of certification for coverage or of the amount paid for a submitted claim. See Chapter 9 for inquiring about the status of a claim and to learn the procedures for how to file reviews and appeals.

KEY POINTS

This is a brief chapter review, or summary, of the key issues presented. To further enhance your knowledge of the technical subject matter, review the key terms and key abbreviations for this chapter by locating the meaning for each in the Glossary at the end of this book, which appears in a section before the Index.

1. TRICARE is a three-option managed health care program offered to spouses and dependents of service personnel with uniform benefits and fees implemented nationwide by the federal government. It also covers retirees, reservists on active duty after 30 days, widows, and widowers.

2. An electronic database called Defense Enrollment Eligibility Reporting System (DEERS) is used to verify beneficiary eligibility for those individuals in the TRICARE programs.

3. The TRICARE fiscal year begins October 1 and ends September 30.

4. Under the TRICARE Standard program, the annual fiscal year deductible is $150 per person and $300 per family.

5. There are certain referral and preauthorization requirements for TRICARE Standard patients.

6. If the physician agrees to accept assignment in a TRICARE Standard case, the participating provider agrees to accept the TRICARE-determined allowable charge as payment in full. The provider may bill the patient for his or her cost share or coinsurance (20% to 25% of the allowable charge after the deductible has been met) and for any noncovered services or supplies.

7. TRICARE Extra is a preferred provider organization–type option in which the individual does not have to enroll or pay an annual fee.

8. TRICARE Prime is a voluntary health maintenance organization (HMO)–type option.

9. TRICARE for Life (TFL) is a health care program that offers additional TRICARE benefits as a supplementary payer to Medicare for uniformed service retirees, their spouses and survivors age 65 or older, and certain former spouses.

10. TRICARE Prime Remote (TPR) is a program designed for active duty service members who work and live more than 50 miles or 1 hour from military treatment facilities (military hospitals and clinics).

11. The Veterans Health Administration (CHAMPVA) program is a service benefit program similar to TRICARE and is for veterans with total, permanent service-connected disabilities or surviving spouses and dependents of veterans who died of service-connected disabilities.

12. TRICARE Standard and Veterans Health Administration (CHAMPVA) claims must be billed on the CMS-1500 (02-12) claim form and submitted to the regional contractor for processing within 1 year from the date a service is provided or (for inpatient care) within 1 year from the patient's date of discharge from a facility.

13. The Computer Matching and Privacy Protection Act of 1988 permits the government to verify TRICARE patients' information by way of computer matches.

14. For each TRICARE claim, the claims processor issues a summary payment voucher that details the payment of the claim to the provider and sends a copy to the patient.

🖥 STUDENT ASSIGNMENT

✔ Study Chapter 14.

✔ Answer the fill-in-the-blank, multiple-choice, and true/false review questions in the *Workbook* to reinforce the theory learned in this chapter and help you prepare for a future test.

✔ Complete the assignments in the *Workbook* for computing mathematic calculations and giving you hands-on experience in completing TRICARE and Veterans Health Administration (CHAMPVA) insurance claim forms and proficiency in procedural and diagnostic coding.

✔ Turn to the Glossary at the end of this text for a further understanding of the key terms and key abbreviations used in this chapter.

OBJECTIVES

After reading this chapter, you should be able to:

1. Discuss the history of workers' compensation, including statutes and reform.
2. State the purposes of workers' compensation laws.
3. Discuss self-insurance and managed care when it comes to workers' compensation insurance.
4. Specify who is eligible for insurance coverage under federal workers' compensation laws.
5. Name persons entitled to be insured under state workers' compensation laws.
6. Define and discuss *second-injury fund.*
7. Determine the waiting period in each state before benefits begin.
8. Describe the types of compensation benefits.
9. Define *nondisability, temporary disability,* and *permanent disability claims.*
10. List signs of fraud and abuse involving employees, employers, insurers, medical providers, and lawyers.
11. State when to report fraud or abuse involving a workers' compensation claim.
12. Explain OSHA's role in protecting employees.
13. Explain two ways in which depositions are used.
14. Explain the advantages of filing a lien.
15. Define and discuss third-party subrogation.
16. Describe workers' compensation health and financial record keeping in a medical practice.
17. Explain the procedure of completing the doctor's first report of occupational injury or illness.
18. Name the contents of a progress or supplemental medical report.
19. Complete workers' compensation forms properly and discuss fee schedules.
20. Discuss electronic claims submission and explain how to handle out-of-state claims.
21. Describe actions to take in following up on delinquent workers' compensation claims.

KEY TERMS

accident
adjudication
by report
claims examiner
compromise and release
deposition
ergonomic
extraterritorial
Federal Employees' Compensation Act
fee schedule
injury

insurance adjuster
lien
medical service order
nondisability claim
occupational illness or disease
Occupational Safety and Health Administration
permanent and stationary
permanent disability
petition
reexamination report
second-injury fund

sequelae
sub rosa films
subsequent-injury fund
temporary disability
third-party liability
third-party subrogation
waiting period
work hardening
Workers' Compensation Appeals Board
workers' compensation insurance

KEY ABBREVIATIONS

AME	IAIABC	OSHA	SIF
BR	IME	P and S	TD
C and R	LHWCA	PD	WCAB
ERISA	MSDS	QME	WP
FECA	ND claim	ROM	

Service to Patients

If a patient who has a work-related injury or illness arrives for an appointment without the employer's signed permission for treatment, telephone the employer and ask to have the employer representative fax the authorization. This will expedite the medical care and necessary documents and forms that must be completed for the patient in a workers' compensation case.

Always educate the patient on the medical practice's billing policies for workers' compensation cases by having him or her complete a patient agreement form to pay the physician's fees if the case is declared non–work related or an illness is discovered that is not work related.

Always ask the patient for the date of injury to confirm it is indeed a workers' compensation claim. If the patient is covered under workers' compensation, it is a violation of medical coding ethics to bill his or her personal health insurance plan.

HISTORY

Before the establishment of a workers' compensation program in the United States (US), either the employer was responsible for any injury or death to his or her employees resulting from administrative negligence or employees paid for medical expenses. Employees are individuals employed by another, generally for wages, in exchange for labor or services. A physician whose practice is incorporated is also considered an employee under workers' compensation laws.

Originally the worker had to prove legally that injury was caused by negligence on the part of the employer. By the close of the nineteenth century, the number of accidents had increased and legal processes were uncertain; therefore federal and state legal provisions were required. In the early 1900s, employers' liability laws were adopted by many states but there was still a great need for improvement. In 1911, the first workers' compensation laws that allowed injured employees to receive medical care without first taking employers to court were enacted. All states currently have workers' compensation laws.

Workers' compensation insurance is the most important coverage written to insure industrial accidents. Previously, this form of insurance was known as "workmens' compensation." The term *workmen* was changed to *workers* for a more generic title and to avoid sexual bias in language. Employers use employers' liability coverage occasionally to protect themselves when their employees do not come within the scope of a compensation law.

Workers' Compensation Statutes

There are two kinds of statutes under workers' compensation: federal compensation laws and state compensation laws. Federal laws apply to miners, maritime workers, and those who work for the government; they do not apply to state and private business employees. State compensation laws apply to employers and employees within each state but the laws vary for each state.

The workers' compensation statutes relieve the employer of liability for injury received or illness contracted by an employee in a work situation, except in gross negligence cases. They also enable the employee to be more easily and quickly compensated for loss of wages, medical expenses, and **permanent disability (PD)**. Before these statutes were passed, the employer could be found legally responsible for the employees' injuries or illnesses and frequently there were delays in the employee's attempt to recover damages.

Workers' Compensation Reform

By 1994, dysfunctional workers' compensation systems were costing companies more than $65 billion annually in many US cities, driving insurers to deny insurance to businesses and causing companies to close their doors. Some employers began moving their businesses to states requiring lower premiums. Widespread legal and medical corruption and abuse had evolved throughout the system in the form of record-high medical treatment and legal expenses. Reforms of the compensation of health care workers became necessary because of these problems. Reform laws have been introduced in a number of states that deal with the following issues:
- Antifraud legislation and increased penalties for workers' compensation fraud
  - Anti-referral provisions (for example, restrictions of physicians referring patients for diagnostic studies to sites where the physician has a financial interest).

- Proof of the medical necessity for treatment (or tests) as well as appropriate documentation. If guidelines are not adhered to, the carrier may refuse to pay the entire fee (for example, utilization review of inpatient and outpatient claims and treatment plans).
- Preauthorization for major operations and expensive tests (for example, computed tomography and magnetic resonance imaging)
- Caps on vocational rehabilitation
- Use of a disabled worker in another division of the company where he or she was employed so that the worker may be gainfully employed while not using the injured part of the body
- Increase in occupational safety measures
- Employers offering a variety of managed care plans from which employees can choose, with some of these restricting their choice of provider (for example, health maintenance organizations [HMOs] and preferred provider organizations [PPOs])
- Development of **fee schedules**
- Medical bill review (mandatory review by law or payers' voluntary review identifying duplicate claims and billing errors)
- Use of mediators instead of lawyers to reach agreement between employers and the injured employee
- Prosecuting of physicians, lawyers, and employees who abuse the system

Although the system is far from perfect or complete, much progress has been made toward reducing high costs by trimming reimbursement for medical services and minimizing abuses of the system.

WORKERS' COMPENSATION LAWS AND INSURANCE

Purposes of Workers' Compensation Laws

Workers' compensation laws have been developed for a variety of reasons and accomplish much, including the following:

1. Provide the best available medical care necessary to ensure a prompt return to work of any injured or ill employee as well as achieving maximum recovery.
2. Provide income to the injured or ill worker or to his or her dependents, regardless of fault.
3. Provide a single remedy and reduce court delays, costs, and workloads arising out of personal injury litigation.
4. Relieve public and private charities of financial drains resulting from uncompensated industrial accidents.
5. Eliminate payment of fees to attorneys and witnesses as well as time-consuming trials and appeals.
6. Encourage maximum employer interest in safety and rehabilitation through an appropriate experience-rating mechanism.

7. Promote the study of causes of accidents and reduce preventable accidents and human suffering rather than concealing fault.

Self-Insurance

Self-insurance is another way that employers can fight high medical costs after an accident. A large employer can save money by insuring employees for a predetermined amount of money and then purchasing policies with large deductibles to cover catastrophic problems. A self-insuring company pays for medical expenses instead of insurance premiums. Benefits are variable from plan to plan and precertification for certain services may be required. Because of health reform in 2010, companies that offer health plans must allow their employees to keep their children on their plans until the children are 26 years old. Employers are prohibited from putting lifetime caps and some annual caps on benefits for their employees. Employers that have existing plans for their employees at the time of the passing of this legislation may be able to change medical benefits, such as copayments and deductibles, or reduce what their plans cover.

Self-insured employers are covered by the Employee Retirement Income Security Act (ERISA). This federal law mandates reporting and disclosure requirements for group life and health plans with guidelines for administration, servicing of plans, some claims processing, and appeals; therefore the state insurance commissioner does not have jurisdiction over such plans. Because they are not state regulated, they often overlook timely payment. ERISA regulations state that a claim must be paid or denied within 90 days of receipt or submission; however, this regulation is not helpful because there is no penalty for violation of the 90-day deadline. Thus physicians who care for individuals under such plans may wish to negotiate payment terms to be 60 days or less.

Sometimes a self-insured plan may have stop-loss or reinsurance that becomes active on large claims, or a set dollar limit per policy year or employee, depending on how it is structured. Such provisions give the insurer an excuse to delay claims until the reinsurer decides to fund the claim. In such cases, it may be necessary to become aggressive and ask for the name, address, and telephone number of the reinsurer to learn the claim status. Prompt processing and payment should be demanded because delaying claims is a violation of federal laws and ERISA regulations.

With the passing of the federal legislation known as the *Patient Protection and Affordable Care Act (Affordable Care Act)* and *H.R. 4872, the Health Care and Education*

Reconciliation Act of 2010 (Reconciliation Act) beginning in 2014, almost everyone is required to be insured or they will pay a fine. Large employers with more than 50 employees must pay a $2000-per-employee fee excluding the first 30 employees from the assessment if the government subsidizes their workers' coverage. Refer to Figure 10-2 for more details on patient benefits under the Affordable Care Act.

At the time of the printing of this edition, the health care reform legislation and its impact on ERISA is not completely known. To keep you up to date, information will be placed on the Evolve website as it is released (see the ERISA section in Chapter 11 for additional information).

A form of self-insurance designed to serve a small manufacturing company is known as *captive insurance*. This is best for companies that have good safety records and those willing to implement worker safety programs to keep claims to a minimum. Members of captive self-insurance programs may hire an outside firm to process claims and purchase extra insurance for major claims. They share overhead expenses and investment income if any remains after paying expenses and claims. Most captive programs are based in Bermuda or the Cayman Islands to take advantage of favorable tax benefits.

Managed Care

Increasing numbers of employers are seeking managed care contracts with PPOs and HMOs to insure their workers against industrial accidents and illnesses. Some states have adopted laws authorizing managed care programs and other states are conducting pilot programs to test the effectiveness of managed care networks. Managed care contracts are not uniform and may limit the choice of providers, use fee schedule–based payments, require precertification for certain procedures, implement hospital and medical bill review, and incorporate utilization review of medical services.

ELIGIBILITY

Individuals entitled to workers' compensation insurance coverage are private business employees, state employees, and federal employees (for example, postal workers, Internal Revenue Service [IRS] employees, coal miners, and maritime workers). **Workers' compensation insurance** coverage provides cash benefits to employees and their dependents if employees suffer work-related injury, illness, or death.

Industrial Accident

An **accident** is an unplanned and unexpected happening traceable to a definite time and place and causing **injury** (damage or loss).

Workers' compensation (industrial) accidents do not necessarily occur at the customary work site. For example, an individual may be asked to obtain cash for the petty cash reserve during the lunch hour. He or she may misstep off the curb while walking to the bank and suffer a fractured ankle. This person is considered to be working, although not at the customary work site, and the injury is covered under workers' compensation insurance.

Occupational Illness

Occupational illness or disease is any abnormal condition or disorder caused by exposure to environmental factors associated with employment, including acute and chronic illnesses or diseases that may be caused by inhalation, absorption, ingestion, or direct contact. Occupational diseases usually become apparent soon after exposure. However, some diseases may be latent for a considerable amount of time. Therefore some states have extended periods during which claims may be filed for certain slowly developing occupational diseases. These diseases include silicosis, asbestosis, pneumoconiosis, berylliosis, anthracosilicosis, radiation disability, loss of hearing, cumulative trauma, and repetitive motion illnesses (for example, carpal tunnel syndrome).

COVERAGE

Federal Laws

Employees who work for federal agencies are covered by a number of federal workers' compensation laws.

● *Workmen's Compensation Law of the District of Columbia.* This law became effective on May 17, 1928, and provides benefits for those working in Washington, DC.

● *Federal Coal Mine Health and Safety Act.* This Act, also referred to as the *Black Lung Benefits Act*, became effective on May 7, 1941. The Act provides benefits to coal miners and is administered through the national headquarters in Washington, DC.

● *Federal Employees' Compensation Act.* The **Federal Employees' Compensation Act (FECA)** was instituted on May 30, 1908, to provide benefits for on-the-job injuries to all federal employees. The insurance is provided through an exclusive fund system. Many different claim forms are used depending on the type of injury. Payment is based on a schedule of maximum allowable charges. The time limit for submitting a bill is December 31 of the year after the year in which services were rendered (or December 31 of the year after the year the condition was accepted as work compensable, whichever is later).

● *Longshore and Harbor Workers' Compensation Act (LHWCA).* This Act became effective on March 4, 1927, and provides benefits for private or public employees engaged in maritime work nationwide. It is administered through regional offices in Boston, Chicago, Cleveland, Denver, Honolulu, Jacksonville, Kansas City, New Orleans, New York City, Philadelphia, San Francisco, Seattle, and Washington, DC. This type of insurance corresponds to that available through the private insurance system.

State Laws

State compensation laws cover those workers not protected by the previously mentioned federal statutes. Federal law mandates that states set up laws to meet minimum requirements. If an employer does not purchase workers' compensation insurance from a private insurance company, the employer must self-insure and have enough cash in reserve to cover the cost of medical care for all workers who suffer work-related injuries. An employer may be reluctant to file a workers' compensation report with the state in some instances, preferring to pay medical expenses out of pocket rather than have premium rates increase. It is illegal for an employer to fail to report a work-related accident when reporting is required by state law and some states consider it a misdemeanor. Different penalties can be imposed, depending on state law, such as imprisonment or assessment of fines of $50 to $2500 or more.

Statutes require that employers have employers' liability insurance in addition to workers' compensation protection. The difference between workers' compensation insurance and employers' liability insurance is that the latter is coverage that protects against claims arising out of bodily injury to others (nonemployees) or damage to their property when someone is on business premises. It is not considered insurance coverage for someone who is working at a business site.

State compensation laws are compulsory or elective, which may be defined as follows:
1. **Compulsory law.** Each employer is required to accept its provisions and provide for specified benefits.
2. **Elective law.** The employer may accept or reject the law. If the statute of the law is rejected, the employer loses the three common-law defenses, which are the following:
   a. Assumption of risk
   b. Negligence of fellow employees
   c. Contributory negligence

Coverage is elective in only one state, New Jersey. This means that, in effect, all laws are "compulsory."

Minors

Minors are covered by workers' compensation; in some states, double compensation or added penalties are provided. Minors also receive special legal benefit provisions in many states.

Interstate Laws

Questions may arise as to which state's law determines payment of compensation benefits if a worker's occupation takes him or her into another state (for example, truck drivers). Most compensation laws are **extraterritorial** (effective outside of the state) by either specific provisions or court decisions. When billing, follow the rules and fee schedule of the state in which the workers' compensation claim was originally filed. This may or may not be the same as the patient's current state of residence. The only exception is workers' compensation for federal employees, which has nationwide rules. For railroad workers, most states abide by nationwide rules but some states have their own. Claims submission for out-of-state claims is discussed later in this chapter.

Volunteer Workers

Several states have laws to compensate civil defense and other volunteer workers, such as firefighters who are injured in the line of duty.

Program Funding

Six states (Nevada, North Dakota, Ohio, Washington, West Virginia, and Wyoming), two US territories, and most provinces require employers to insure through a state-specific fund. Puerto Rico and the Virgin Islands require employers to insure through a fund specific to their local government regulations. Employers may qualify as self-insurers in 48 states and territories. A number of states permit employers to purchase insurance from either a competitive state fund or a private insurance company.

The employer pays the premiums for workers' compensation insurance; the amount depends on the employee's job and the risk involved in job performance. The physician usually must supply comprehensive information and the reporting requirements vary from state to state (Table 15-1). The state bureau or individual insurance carrier should be contacted to obtain instructions and proper forms.

Second-Injury Fund (Subsequent-Injury Fund)

The **second-injury fund,** also known as the **subsequent-injury fund (SIF),** was established to meet problems arising when an employee has a preexisting injury or condition and is subsequently injured at work. The preexisting injury combines with the second injury to produce disability that is greater than that caused by the latter alone.

Table 15-1 Employers' or Physicians' Report of Accident[1]

JURISDICTION	TIME LIMIT	INJURIES COVERED
Alabama	Within 15 days	Death or disability exceeding 3 days
Alaska	Within 10 days	Death, injury, disease, or infection
American Samoa	Within 10 days of employer notification	Death, injury, or disease
Arizona	Within 10 days	All injuries
Arkansas	Within 10 days from notice of injury	Indemnity, injuries, or death[2]
		Controverted, medical only
California	Immediately (employer)	Death or serious injuries
	As prescribed	Disability of 1 day or more, other than first aid
	Within 5 days	Occupational diseases or pesticide poisoning
Colorado	Immediately 10 days[3]	Death
		Injuries causing lost time of 3 days or more or 3 shifts
		Any accident in which three or more employees are injured
		Occupational disease cases
		Cases of permanent physical impairment
Connecticut	Within 7 days or as directed	Disability of 1 day or more
Delaware	Within 48 hours[4]	Death or injuries requiring hospitalization
	Within 10 days	Other injuries
District of Columbia	Within 10 days	All injuries
Florida	Within 24 hours[5]	Death
	Within 7 days to carrier	All injuries requiring medical treatment
Georgia	Within 21 days[6]	All injuries requiring medical or surgical treatment or causing more than 7 days of absence
Hawaii	Within 48 hours	Death
	Within 7 working days	All injuries
Idaho	As soon as practicable but not later than 10 days after the accident[7]	All injuries requiring treatment by a physician or absence from work for one (1) or more days
Illinois	Within 2 working days	Death or serious injuries
	Between the 15th and 25th of the month	Disability of more than 3 days
	As soon as determinable	Permanent disability (PD)
Indiana	Within 7 working days[8]	Disability of more than 1 day
Iowa	Within 4 days	Disability of more than 3 days, PP disability, or death
Kansas	Within 28 days of knowledge[9]	Death cases or disability of more than remainder of day or shift.
Kentucky	Within 7 days[10]	Disability of more than 1 day
Louisiana	Within 10 days of employer's actual knowledge of injury[11]	Lost time over 1 week or death
Maine	Within 7 days of ER's knowledge lost time	Only injuries causing 1 day or more of lost time[13]
Maryland	Within 10 days	Disability of more than 3 days
Massachusetts	Within 7 days, except Sundays and holidays[12]	Disability of 5 or more calendar days
Michigan	Immediately	Death, disability of 7 days or more, and specific losses
Minnesota	Within 48 hours	Death or serious injury
	Within 14 days	Disability of 3 days or more
Mississippi	Within 10 days[13]	Death or disability of more than 5 days[14]
Missouri	Within 30 days[14]	Death or injury
Montana	Within 6 days	All injuries
Nebraska	Within 10 days[15]	All injuries or diagnosed occupational diseases that result in death, time away from work, restricted work, or termination of employment; loss of consciousness; or medical treatment other than first aid
Nevada	Within 6 working days after report from physician[16]	All injuries requiring medical treatment
New Hampshire	Within 5 calendar days	All injuries involving lost time or medical expenses
New Jersey	Within 3 weeks of learning of occupational disease	All injuries, other than those requiring first aid
New Mexico	Within 10 days of employer notification[17]	Any injury or illness resulting in 7 or more days of lost time
New York	Within 10 days[18]	Disability of 1 day beyond working day or shift on which accident occurred or requiring medical care beyond two first aid treatments
North Carolina	Within 5 days of knowledge of injury or allegation	Disability of more than 1 day or charges for medical compensation exceeding the amount set by the commission
North Dakota	Within 7 days	All injuries
Ohio	Within 1 week	Injuries causing total disability of 7 days or more
Oklahoma	Within 10 days of knowledge of death or injury	Fatalities; all injuries causing lost time or requiring treatment away from worksite

JURISDICTION	TIME LIMIT	INJURIES COVERED
Oregon	Within 5 days after employer knowledge[19]	All claims or injuries that may result in compensable inquiry claims injuries
Pennsylvania	Within 48 hours	Death
	After 7 days but not later than 10 days	Disability of 1 day or more
Rhode Island	Within 48 hours	Death
	Within 10 days	Disability of 3 days or more and all injuries requiring medical treatment
		Any claim resulting in medical expense
South Carolina	Within 10 days	All injuries requiring medical attention costing more than $500, more than 1 day disability, or permanency
South Dakota	Within 7 days	Disability of 7 days or more, other than first aid or injuries requiring medical treatment
Tennessee	Within 14 days	Report of Injury must be filed when employee receives medical care outside of employer's premises
Texas	Within 8 days[20]	Lost time of more than 1 day or death/an occupational disease
Utah	Within 7 days	All injuries requiring medical attention
Vermont	Within 72 hours; Sundays and legal holidays excluded	Disability of 1 day or more requiring medical care
Virgin Islands	Within 8 days	Injury or disease
Virginia	Within 10 days[21]	All injuries
Washington	Immediately	Deaths and accidents resulting in workers' hospitalizations or inability to work
West Virginia	Within 5 days	All injuries
Wisconsin	Within 14 days	Disability beyond 3-day waiting period (WP)
Wyoming	Within 10 days	All injuries
Federal Employees' Compensation Act (FECA)	Within 10 working days	All injuries involving medical expenses, disability, or death
Longshore and Harbor Workers' Compensation Act (LHWCA)	10 days	Injuries that cause loss of one or more shifts of work or death

[1]Federal Occupational Safety and Health Act of 1970 established uniform requirements and forms to meet its criteria for all businesses affecting interstate commerce to be used for statistical purposes and compliance with the Act. 12 U.S.C. §651.

[2]Arkansas. Medical only claims reported monthly.

[3]Colorado. Failure to report tolls time limit for claims. Disability of 3 days or less must be reported to insurer. The insurer then reports this information by monthly summary to the Division.

[4]Delaware. Supplemental report on termination of disability.

[5]Florida. Death cases—by telephone to workers' compensation division within 24 hours. All injuries—carrier to send first report form to division, if injury involved lost time.

[6]Georgia. Supplemental report on first payment and suspension of payment and within 30 days after final payment. Case progress reports must be filed within one year of the first date of disability, within 30 days from last payment for closure, upon request of the Board, every 12 months from the date of the last filing on all open cases, to re-open a case, within 40 days of final payment made pursuant to an approved settlement and within 90 days of receipt of an open case by the new third party administrator.

[7]Idaho. Supplemental report required after 60 days or upon termination of disability.

[8]Indiana. Supplemental report within 10 days after termination of compensation period.

[9]Kansas. Failure to report tolls time limit for claims. *Childress v. Childress Painting Co.,* 1979.

[10]Kentucky. Supplemental report required after 60 days or on termination of disability.

[11]Louisiana. Employers with more than 10 employees must also report within 90 days death, any nonfatal occupational illness or injury causing loss of consciousness, restriction of work or motion, job transfer, or medical treatment other than first aid. Report within 90 days any occupational death, non-fatal.

[12]Massachusetts - After third violation.

[13]Mississippi. Permanent disability (PD), serious head or facial disfigurement also covered.

[14]Missouri. Every employer or his insurer shall, within 30 days after knowledge of the injury, file with the division a report of every injury or death to any employee for which the employer would be liable to furnish medical aid, other than immediate first aid. Employers shall report all injuries to their insurance carrier (or third-party administrator) within 5 days of the date of the injury or within 5 days of the date of the injury or within 5 days of the date on which the injury was reported to the employer by the employee, whichever is later. Where an employer reports injuries covered by the Missouri Workers' Compensation Law to his insurer or third-party administrator shall be responsible for filing the report with the Division of Workers' Compensation. If medical treatment or temporary benefits will continue past 30 days, a status report including estimated dates of completion of medical treatment and temporary benefits shall be provided to the division at that time. A final report shall be filed on conclusion or termination of medical treatment and medical benefits. A final medical report shall be filed with the final report.

[15]Nebraska. Report may be made by insurance carrier or employer. Failure to report tolls time limits.

[16]Nevada. For minor injuries not requiring medical treatment, the employee may file a "Notice of Injury," which must be retained by the employer for 3 years. A claim for compensation is filed with the insurer for lost time and claims requiring medical care.

[17]New Mexico. For electronic data interchange (EDI) filings all injuries having more than $300 of expenses must be reported to the administration. A subsequent report from the claims administrator is required on payment of any claim.

[18]New York. Carrier or employer, if self-insured, is required to provide a written statement of rights under the law to injured employee or dependent if worker deceased.

[19]Oregon. Insurers to send initial disabling claims acceptance, aggravation claims acceptance, and claim denial to Workers' Compensation Division within 14 days of action.

[20]Texas. Supplemental report required on termination of disability or change in postinjury earnings.

[21]Virginia. Beginning 7/1/09, all accident reports to the commission must be submitted electronically either through EDI transmission or WebFile.

Two functions of the fund are (1) to encourage hiring of the physically disabled and (2) to allocate more equitably the costs of providing benefits to such employees. Second-injury employers pay compensation related primarily to the disability caused by the second injury, even though the employee receives benefits relating to the combined disability. The difference is made up from the SIF.

Scenario: Second-Injury Fund

Bob Evans lost his left thumb while operating machinery. Then, 2 years later, Bob lost his left index finger in a second work-related accident. A question could arise of whether the second injury added to a preexisting condition or was related to the prior injury. This case illustrates that the existence of the former injury or disability substantially increased (added to) the disability caused by the latter injury. The employer would pay compensation related to the second injury and funds would come from a second-injury fund to pay for the difference between the first and second injuries.

Minimum Number of Employees

Each state requires a minimum number of employees at one business before the state workers' compensation law comes into effect. The majority of the states require at least one employee but the exceptions are American Samoa (two employees); Arkansas, Georgia, Michigan, New Mexico, North Carolina, and Virginia (three employees); Florida and South Carolina (four employees); and Alabama, Mississippi, Missouri, and Tennessee (five employees). Many states have exemptions for certain occupations, such as domestic or casual employees, laborers, babysitters, newspaper vendors or distributors, charity workers, and gardeners. Some states do not require compensation insurance for farm employees or may specify a larger number of farm employees than the standard number of regular employees.

Waiting Periods

The laws state that a **waiting period (WP)** must pass before income benefits are payable. WP affects only wage compensation because medical and hospital care are provided immediately. See Table 15-2 for the WP in each state.

State Disability and Workers' Compensation

Five states and one US territory have state disability insurance (also known as *unemployment compensation disability insurance*): California, Hawaii, New Jersey, New York, Rhode Island, and Puerto Rico. If a recipient is collecting benefits from a workers' compensation insurance carrier and the amount that the compensation carrier pays is less than that allowed by the state disability insurance program, the latter pays the balance. See Chapter 16 for further information on state disability insurance.

BENEFITS

Five principal types of state compensation benefits that may apply in ordinary cases are the following:
1. *Medical treatment.* This includes hospital, medical and surgical services, medications, and prosthetic devices. Treatment may be rendered by a medical doctor, osteopath, dentist, or chiropractor.
2. *Temporary disability indemnity.* This is in the form of weekly cash payments made directly to the injured or ill person.
3. *Permanent disability indemnity.* This may consist of either weekly or monthly cash payments based on a rating system that determines the percentage of PD or a lump sum award. California has a unique system of PD evaluation that requires a separate determination by the disability rating bureau in San Francisco. No other state has this system.
4. *Death benefits for survivors.* This consists of cash payments to dependents of employees who are fatally injured. A burial allowance is also given in some states.
5. *Rehabilitation benefits.* This can be medical or vocational rehabilitation in cases of severe disabilities.

TYPES OF STATE CLAIMS

There are three types of state workers' compensation claims: nondisability (ND) claims, temporary disability (TD) claims, and PD claims. Each type is discussed in detail to provide a clear definition and understanding of the determination process.

Nondisability Claim

The simplest type of claim is a **nondisability (ND) claim,** which generally involves a minor injury in which the patient is seen by the physician but is able to continue working (Figure 15-1). This type of case does not require weekly TD payments.

Temporary Disability Claim

Temporary disability occurs when a worker has a work-related injury or illness and is unable to perform the duties of his or her occupation for a specific time or range of time. The time period of TD can extend from the date of injury until the worker returns to full duty without residual ratable disability (discussed later), returns to modified work, or has ratable residual disability that the physician states is **permanent and stationary (P and S).**

An **insurance adjuster** is the person at the workers' compensation insurance carrier who oversees the industrial case. He or she is responsible for keeping in contact with the physician's office about the patient's ongoing progress. The insurance adjuster's most important

Table 15-2	Waiting Period for Income and Medical Benefits*		
JURISDICTION	**WAITING PERIOD (DAYS)**	**JURISDICTION**	**WAITING PERIOD (DAYS)**
Alabama	3	Nebraska	7
Alaska	3	Nevada	5
Arizona	7	New Hampshire	3
Arkansas	7	New Jersey	7
California	3	New Mexico	7
Colorado	3	New York	7
Connecticut	3	North Carolina	7
Delaware	3	North Dakota	5
District of Columbia	3	Ohio	7
Florida	7	Oklahoma	3
Georgia	7	Oregon	3
Hawaii	3	Pennsylvania	7
Idaho	5	Rhode Island	3
Illinois	3	South Carolina	7
Indiana	7	South Dakota	7
Iowa	3	Tennessee	7
Kansas	7	Texas	7
Kentucky	7	Utah	3
Louisiana	7	Vermont	3
Maine	7	Virgin Islands	0
Maryland	3	Virginia	7
Massachusetts	5	Washington	3
Michigan	7	West Virginia	3
Minnesota	3	Wisconsin	3
Mississippi	5	Wyoming	3
Missouri	3	FECA	3
Montana	4 days or 32 hours, whichever is less	LHWCA	3

FECA, Federal Employees' Compensation Act; *LHWCA*, Longshore and Harbor Workers' Compensation Act.
*These are statutory provisions for waiting periods (WPs). Statutes provide that a WP must elapse, during which income benefits are not payable. This WP affects only compensation because medical and hospital care are provided immediately.

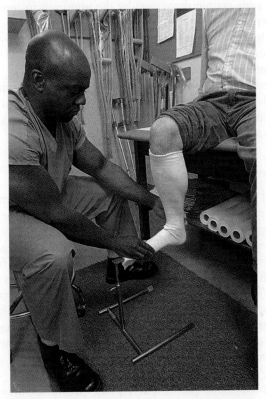

FIGURE 15-1 Physician interacting with an injured worker in the examination room.

function is adjusting an industrial claim. This means that the insurance adjuster must evaluate the injury or illness, predict in advance the amount of money reserves needed to cover medical expenses, and calculate as accurate a reserve as possible for weekly TD payments to the injured. This is frequently a difficult task because a seemingly minor back strain ultimately may require fusion or a small cut may become gangrenous and lead to an amputation. The insurance carrier wants to provide the best possible medical care for the patient. The patient is immediately referred to the specialist if a specialist is necessary.

Usually workers' compensation weekly TD payments are based on a percentage of the employee's earnings at the time of the injury. Compensation benefits are not subject to income tax.

Sometimes a patient is released to modified work to effect a transition between the period of inactivity caused by disability and a return to full duty, especially when heavy work is involved. Other times an employee is returned to the company and placed in a different department or division so that he or she is gainfully employed while not using the injured body part. This topic is further detailed in the next section.

Vocational Rehabilitation

Many states provide vocational rehabilitation in the form of retraining, education, job guidance, and placement to assist an injured individual in finding work before TD compensation benefits expire. In any successful rehabilitation program, the insurance carrier, physician, physical therapist, employer supervisor, and personnel department must act as a team with the common goal of getting an injured employee back to light duty or regular work as soon as possible. It is believed that the longer a person remains out of work, the less chance there is that he or she will return to the workplace. The employer and insurance adjuster must remain in communication with rehabilitation center therapists to determine when the injured person will be able to resume some form of work. The physician may suggest a rehabilitation center that provides good care or the employer may have an in-house program.

Work Hardening

Sports medicine therapy and physical medicine rehabilitation are often used to strengthen the injured worker. Physical medicine/therapy Current Procedural Terminology (CPT) codes 97001 to 97542 are used to report these services. Another type of therapy, called **work hardening,** is an individualized program using simulated or real work tasks to build up strength and improve the worker's endurance toward a full day's work. CPT codes 97545 and 97546 are used to report work hardening conditioning.

Ergonomics

In some cases, an **ergonomic** evaluation of the work site is performed and modifications may be instituted to the job or work site to lessen the possibility of future injury and to get the employee back to gainful employment. CPT code 97537 may be used to report a work site modification analysis. Injured individuals may also be retrained into another career field if their disability prevents them from returning to their former occupation.

Permanent Disability Claim

In this type of claim, the patient or injured party is usually on TD benefits for a time and then concludes that he or she is unable to return to his or her former occupation. The physician states in the report that the patient has residual disability that will hamper his or her opportunity to compete in the open job market. Examples of residual disability include loss of a hand, an eye, or a leg and neurologic problems. Each patient who has PD is rated according to the severity of the injury, the age of the injured person, and the patient's occupation at the time of the injury. The older the person, the greater the PD benefit. One might think that a younger person deserves higher compensation because he or she will be disabled for a longer portion of his or her working career. However, the workers' compensation laws assume that a young person has a better chance of being rehabilitated into another occupation.

In a PD claim, the physician's final report must include the words "permanent and stationary" (P and S). This phrase means that damage from the injury or illness is permanent, the patient has recovered to the fullest extent possible, the physician is unable to do anything more for the patient, and the patient will be hampered by the disability to some extent for the rest of his or her life. The P and S examination is usually comprehensive and a Level 5 CPT code may be appropriate. Depending on the fee schedule, a modifier indicating that the evaluation and management (E/M) service is a P and S examination may also be used. The case is rated for PD and a settlement, called a **compromise and release (C and R),** is made. This is an agreement between the injured party and the insurance company on a total sum. The case can then be closed.

Reasons that may delay closing a workers' compensation case include the following:
1. Unanswered questions or incomplete answers to data required on workers' compensation forms by the employee, employer, or physician
2. Vague terminology used by the physician in medical reports
3. Omitted signatures on forms or written reports by the employee, employer, or physician
4. Incorrect billing by the physician's office
5. Inadequate progress reports (for example, the physician fails to send in a medical report routinely to update the insurance carrier when the injured employee is seen in subsequent visits)

Rating

Final determination of the issues involving settlement of an industrial accident is known as **adjudication,** or the rating of a case. A physician does not rate disability but renders a professional opinion on whether the injured individual has TD or PD that prevents him or her from gainful employment. Rating itself is carried out by the state's industrial accident commission or workers' compensation board. Wage loss, earning capacity, and physical impairment are three categories that may be taken into consideration to rate temporary partial, permanent partial, or total disabilities.

In addition, permanent partial disabilities may be rated by using a scheduled or nonscheduled injury award system. This system is based on a set number of weeks of compensation for a specific loss, such as 288 weeks for the loss of a leg. Scheduled injuries may be loss of a body part, disfigurement, permanent hearing loss, and so on. Nonscheduled injuries are more general, such as disability caused by injury to the back or neck.

If an injured person is dissatisfied with the rating after the case has been declared P and S, he or she may appeal the case (by **petition**—formal written request) to the **Workers' Compensation Appeals Board (WCAB)** or the Industrial Accident Commission.

Surveillance

Sub rosa films are provided occasionally when rating a case to document the extent of a patient's PD. Videotapes are made over a period of 2 to 3 days without the patient's knowledge. This surveillance is expensive and is used as a last resort, especially in a case in which a person receiving workers' compensation benefits is suspected of making exaggerated complaints. It is also used in cases when a worker has been off work for a long time and supposedly is unable to perform any work activity, even light duty.

Investigators have been known to carry a camera in a gym bag and videotape a supposedly disabled claimant bench pressing at the gym. Patients also have been videotaped going into the physician's office for an appointment wearing a neck brace and removing the brace after returning to their car.

FRAUD AND ABUSE

Increases in the number of fraudulent workers' compensation claims were noted throughout many large metropolitan cities in the 1990s. These problems involved employers, employees, insurers, medical providers, and lawyers. An increasing number of states have enacted some kind of antifraud legislation and stiffened penalties for workers' compensation fraud, making it a felony. Some states require reporting suspected insurance fraud and have forms to incorporate wording in regard to fraudulent statements. An example is shown in Figure 15-2.

Physicians are responsible for determining the legitimacy of work injuries and reporting findings accurately. If a report is prepared with the intent to use it in support of a fraudulent claim or if a fraudulent claim is knowingly submitted for payment under an insurance contract, the physician may be subject to fines or imprisonment and the revocation or suspension of his or her medical license. Some physicians sign and send a disclosure statement with the medical report certifying that they personally performed an evaluation. The physician may list the total time spent in reviewing records, face-to-face time

with the patient, preparing a report, and other relevant activities.

It is the responsibility of all individuals who deal with workers' compensation cases to notify the insurance carrier of any suspicious situation. By doing so, action can be taken to have the case investigated further by personnel from the fraud divisions or referred to the district attorney's office. Perpetrators and signs of workers' compensation fraud and abuse are listed in Box 15-1.

See Chapters 2, 12, and 13 for further information on fraud and abuse in the medical setting.

OCCUPATIONAL SAFETY AND HEALTH ADMINISTRATION ACT OF 1970

Background

Congress established an office known as the **Occupational Safety and Health Administration (OSHA)** to protect employees against on-the-job health and safety hazards. This program includes strict health and safety standards and a sensible complaint procedure that enables individual workers to trigger enforcement measures.

Work standards are designed to minimize exposure to on-the-job hazards, such as faulty machinery, noise, dust, and toxic chemical fumes. Employers are required by law to meet these health and safety standards. Failure to do so can result in fines against the employer that could run into thousands of dollars.

Coverage

The Act provides that if a state submits an OSHA plan and it is approved by the government, the state may assume responsibility for carrying out OSHA policies and procedures and is excluded from federal jurisdiction.

The Act applies to almost all businesses, large or small. It applies to heavy, light, and service industries; nonprofit and charitable institutions; churches' secular activities in hospitals; farmers; and retailers. Employees of state and local governments are also covered. Federal employees, a farmer's immediate family, church employees engaged in religious activities, independent contractors, and household domestic workers are not covered.

Regulations

Specific regulations that affect the medical setting are those aimed at minimizing exposure to hepatitis B virus (HBV), human immunodeficiency virus (HIV), and other bloodborne pathogens. Any worker who comes in contact with human blood and infectious materials must receive

State of California
Department of Industrial Relations
DIVISION OF WORKERS' COMPENSATION

WORKERS' COMPENSATION CLAIM FORM (DWC 1)

Estado de California
Departamento de Relaciones Industriales
DIVISION DE COMPENSACIÓN AL TRABAJADOR

PETITION DEL EMPLEADO PARA DE COMPENSACIÓN DEL
TRABAJADOR (DWC 1)

Employee: Complete the **"Employee"** section and give the form to your employer. Keep a copy and mark it **"Employee's Temporary Receipt"** until you receive the signed and dated copy from your employer. You may call the Division of Workers' Compensation and hear recorded information at **(800) 736-7401**. An explanation of workers' compensation benefits is included as the cover sheet of this form.

You should also have received a pamphlet from your employer describing workers' compensation benefits and the procedures to obtain them.

Empleado: Complete la sección *"Empleado"* y entregue la forma a su empleador. Quédese con la copia designada *"Recibo Temporal del Empleado"* hasta que Ud. reciba la copia firmada y fechada de su empleador. Ud. puede llamar a la Division de Compensación al Trabajador al *(800) 736-7401* para oir información gravada. En la hoja cubierta de esta forma esta la explicatión de los beneficios de compensación al trabajador.

Ud. también debería haber recibido de su empleador un folleto describiendo los benficios de compensación al trabajador lesionado y los procedimientos para obtenerlos.

Any person who makes or causes to be made any knowingly false or fraudulent material statement or material representation for the purpose of obtaining or denying workers' compensation benefits or payments is guilty of a felony.

Toda aquella persona que a propósito haga o cause que se produzca cualquier declaración o representación material falsa o fraudulenta con el fin de obtener o negar beneficios o pagos de compensación a trabajadores lesionados es culpable de un crimen mayor "felonia".

Employee—complete this section and see note above *Empleado—complete esta sección y note la notación arriba.*

1. Name. *Nombre.* Ima B. Hurt   Today's Date. *Fecha de Hoy.* 4-3-20XX
2. Home Address. *Dirección Residencial.* 300 East Central Avenue
3. City. *Ciudad.* Woodland Hills   State. *Estado.* XY   Zip. *Código Postal.* 12345-0001
4. Date of Injury. *Fecha de la lesión (accidente).* 4-3-20XX   Time of Injury. *Hora en que ocurrió.* _____ a.m. 2:00 p.m.
5. Address and description of where injury happened. *Dirección/lugar dónde occurió el accidente.* The Conk Out Company
   45 South Gorman Street, Woodland Hills, XY 12345   Injured in Stock Room
6. Describe injury and part of body affected. *Describa la lesión y parte del cuerpo afectada.* Fell off ladder in stock room.
   Injured left ankle.
7. Social Security Number. *Número de Seguro Social del Empleado.* 120-XX-6542
8. Signature of employee. *Firma del empleado.* Ima B. Hurt

Employer—complete this section and see note below. *Empleador—complete esta sección y note la notación abajo.*

9. Name of employer. *Nombre del empleador.* The Conk Out Company
10. Address. *Dirección.* 45 South Gorman Street, Woodland Hills, XY 12345
11. Date employer first knew of injury. *Fecha en que el empleador supo por primera vez de la lesión o accidente.* 4-3-20XX
12. Date claim form was provided to employee. *Fecha en que se le entregó al empleado la petición.* 4-3-20XX
13. Date employer received claim form. *Fecha en que el empleador devolvió la petición al empleador.* 4-3-20XX
14. Name and address of insurance carrier or adjusting agency. *Nombre y dirección de la compañía de seguros o agencia adminstradora de seguros.*
    XYZ Insurance Company, P.O. Box 5, Woodland Hills, XY 12345
15. Insurance Policy Number. *El número de la póliza de Seguro.* B 12345
16. Signature of employer representative. *Firma del representante del empleador.* J.D. Hawkins
17. Title. *Título.* Owner   18. Telephone. *Teléfono.* 555-430-3488

Employer: You are required to date this form and provide copies to your insurer or claims administrator and to the employee, dependent or representative who filed the claim within **one working day** of receipt of the form from the employee.

SIGNING THIS FORM IS NOT AN ADMISSION OF LIABILITY

Empleador: Se requiere que Ud. feche esta forma y que provéa copias a su compañía de seguros, administrador de reclamos, o dependiente/representante de reclamos y al empleado que hayan presentado esta petición dentro del plazo de *un día hábil* desde el momento de haber sido recibida la forma del empleado.
EL FIRMAR ESTA FORMA NO SIGNIFICA ADMISION DE RESPONSABILIDAD

❏ Employer copy/*Copia del Empleador*   ❏ Employee copy/ *Copia del Empleado*   ❏ Claims Administrator/*Administrador de Reclamos*   ❏ Temporary Receipt/*Recibo del Empleado*

6/10 Rev.

FIGURE 15-2 Employee's claim form for workers' compensation benefits. Note the insert about fraudulent material.

Box 15-1   Perpetrators and Signs of Workers' Compensation Fraud and Abuse

Employee

- Symptoms are all subjective.
- Misses the first physician's visit or cancels or repeatedly reschedules appointments.
- Cannot describe the pain or is overly dramatic, such as an employee who comes to the physician's office limping on the left leg, suddenly starts limping on the right leg, and then goes back to limping on the left leg.
- Delays in reporting the injury.
- Does not report Friday's injury until Monday morning.
- First reports an injury to a legal or regulatory agency.
- Reports an injury after missing several days of work.
- Changes physicians frequently.
- Is a short-term worker.
- Has a curious claim history.
- Fabricates an injury.
- Exaggerates a work-related injury to obtain larger benefits, such as an injured employee who has a back pain and claims inability to bend over or lift. Surveillance cameras capture the individual at work on weekends repairing cars in the driveway at home—a task he is supposedly unable to perform.
- Blames an injury that occurred off the job on the employer.
- Adds symptoms in response to efforts to return the person to work.

Employer

- Misrepresents the annual payroll to get lower premium rates.
- Misrepresents the number of workers employed.
- Gives a false address with the least expensive premium rates.
- Falsely classifies the job duties of workers (as not hazardous), such as stating the job title as a clerical worker when in fact the employee is using a lathe every day.
- Conspires with the employee to defraud.
- Insurer.
- Refuses to pay valid medical claims.
- Forces the injured worker to settle by using unethical tactics. For example, an insurance agent tells an employee that he has a back sprain. Relying on that information, the worker settles the case. Later, a myelogram reveals a

herniated intervertebral disk. The patient is left with a permanent partial disability.

Medical Provider

- Makes immediate referral for psychiatric care despite the worker's report of a trauma injury.
- Orders or performs unnecessary tests.
- Treatment dates fall on weekends and holidays.
- Renders unnecessary treatment.
- Lists a diagnosis that is not consistent with the course of treatment.
- Charges the insurance carrier for services never rendered.
- Prolongs treatment for what appears to be a minor injury.
- Participates in a provider mill scheme (see explanation under "Lawyer").
- Makes multiple referrals from a clinic practice regardless of type of injury.
- Sends medical reports that look photocopied with the same information typed in (for example, employer's address, description of injury) or that read almost identical to other reports.
- Sends in many claims in which injuries are of a subjective nature, such as stress, emotional distress, headaches, and inability to sleep.
- Sends in claims from one employer showing several employees with similar injuries, using the same physicians and/or attorneys.
- Bills both the workers' compensation carrier and the health insurer for the same service.

Lawyer

- Overbills clients.
- Participates in a medical provider mill scheme. For example, an individual is solicited while in the unemployment line by a recruiter known as a "capper." The capper tells the worker it is possible to obtain more money on disability than through unemployment. The worker is referred to an attorney and a "provider mill" clinic, which help the individual to fabricate a claim by claiming stress or an on-the-job injury. In some states, such acts may be considered a public offense and are punishable as a misdemeanor or felony.

proper information and training and use universal precautions (protective safety measures) to avoid infection. Vaccinations must be provided for those who are at risk for exposure to hepatitis B and comprehensive records must be maintained. For fact sheets, booklets, and guidelines on bloodborne pathogens, contact the nearest OSHA office or write to OSHA Publications Office, 200 Constitution Avenue NW, Room N3101, Washington, DC 20210.

Chemicals and hazardous substances that impose dangers in many work settings are used. Businesses are required to obtain material safety data sheets (MSDSs) for each hazardous chemical used on site. Employers that produce a hazardous chemical must develop MSDSs. A compliance kit is available from the Superintendent of

Documents, US Government Printing Office, Washington, DC 20402.

Filing a Complaint

To file a complaint, the proper form is obtained from the federal Division of Industrial Safety or a state OSHA office and completed by the employee. It is against the law for an employer to take any adverse action against an employee who files such a complaint.

Inspection

A compliance officer (inspector) may call for an appointment or may be sent unannounced to the place of employment. If an officer arrives unannounced, the office manager must be notified so that an appointment may be arranged for the inspection to take place. A court warrant may be required to search a company's premises if the employer does not consent to OSHA entry. A business may be cited and, depending on the violation, fines or criminal penalties may be imposed.

Record Keeping and Reporting

Employers must keep records of their employees' work-related injuries and illnesses on OSHA Form No. 200. Forms may be obtained from the OSHA office or from any office of the US Department of Labor. This document must be on file at the workplace and available to employees and OSHA compliance officers on request. Form 200 must be retained in the file for 5 years. After 6 days, a case recorded on Form 200 must have a supplementary record (OSHA Form 101) completed and kept in the files. Some states have modified their workers' compensation forms so that they may be used as substitutes for Form 101. Certain low-hazard industries are exempt from having to complete and retain Forms 200 and 101.

Companies with fewer than 11 employees must complete safety survey OSHA Form 200-S. Companies are also required to display OSHA posters to inform employees of their job safety rights. Federal law states that an accident that results in the death or hospitalization of five or more employees must be reported to OSHA.

LEGAL SITUATIONS

Medical Evaluator

Physicians who conduct medical–legal (ML) evaluations of injured workers must pass a complex medical examination. They are then certified by the Industrial Medical Council (IMC) and may be referred to as one of the following titles:
- Agreed medical evaluator (AME)
- Independent medical evaluator (IME)
- Qualified medical evaluator (QME)

The medical evaluator is hired by the insurance company or appointed by the referee or appeals board to examine an individual, independent from the attending physician, and render an unbiased opinion about the degree of disability of an injured worker. When the physician performs an evaluation on an injured worker, the workers' compensation fee schedule may have specific procedure codes to bill for the examination. E/M consultation codes or the CPT code for work-related evaluation by "other" physician (99456) may be used. Some state fee schedules may have specific ML procedure codes to bill for various levels of examination. When a case involves

a medical evaluation, a deposition may be taken of the medical evaluator's testimony.

Depositions

A **deposition** is a proceeding in which an attorney asks a witness questions about a case and the witness answers under oath but not in open court. It may take place in the attorney's office or often in the physician's office. In PD workers' compensation cases, depositions are usually taken from the physician and the injured party by the attorney representing the workers' compensation insurance company. The injured party's attorney is also present if the witness is the defendant. Direct questioning and cross-examination may be done by both attorneys.

The session may be recorded on a stenotype machine, in shorthand, or by audiotape or videotape. Video depositions are used in several instances. For example, if a plaintiff in a case is terminally ill and the plaintiff's attorney wishes to preserve the plaintiff's testimony, a video deposition may be used as substantive (essential) evidence. A video deposition may also be taken if a witness cannot be present at the trial. In a case in which a witness may be in Arizona and cannot appear in Pennsylvania, the attorney takes the deposition in Arizona and proves to the court that the witness is beyond its jurisdiction. The same is true for a physician defendant who is not available for some reason.

Exhibits may be entered into evidence. The witness is allowed to read the transcript and make corrections or changes. The witness may be asked to sign the transcript but can waive a signature if his or her attorney recommends against signing it. The deposition is used when the case comes to trial.

Depositions may be taken to find out additional information, the physician's version of the facts, the patient's version of the facts, what kind of witnesses the physician and patient will be, and so on. Another use for a deposition is to impeach (challenge the credibility or validity of) a witness on cross-examination. If the witness takes the stand and the testimony is inconsistent with the deposition, the attorney will make this known to the jury.

Medical Testimony

In the instance of an accident case with **third-party liability,** the physician may have to testify as an expert witness, take time to give a deposition, or attend a pretrial conference. There should be a clear understanding of the terms of testimony and payment to eliminate future misunderstandings. A written agreement from the patient's lawyer should be obtained stating exactly what compensation the physician will receive for research (preparation), time spent waiting to testify (if appointments must be canceled), and actual testimony time (Figure 15-3). In some cases, the physician may want to ask for partial payment in advance. If the physician is subpoenaed, he or she must appear in court regardless of whether an agreement exists. The correct CPT code for medical testimony is 99075. This agreement should be signed by the physician and sent to the attorney. The attorney should return the original to the physician, retaining a copy for his or her files.

Liens

The word **lien** derives from the same origin as the word *liable* and the right of lien expresses legal claim on the property of another for the payment of a debt. To file a lien, the physician must obtain permission from the patient (Figure 15-4). An example of a complete lien can be found in Figure 15-5. Liens sometimes are called *encumbrances* and may be filed for a number of reasons.

The advantages of filing a lien are as follows:

- It is a written agreement and is recognized in court.
- It is a source of protection in the event of litigation.
- It ensures that payment for previously rendered medical services are received when the attorney and patient have reached a settlement with the insurance company in an accident case.
- It is an inexpensive method of collecting the fee. The physician can file suit and try to get a judgment against the patient but this is relatively expensive when compared to filing a lien.
- The physician will collect the full fee. If the physician assigns such a delinquent account to a collection agency, he or she may lose as much as 50% of the fee when it is collected.
- If the physician wishes to bill more than what is allowed for a given service or services, a lien can be filed and the judge will determine whether it is reasonable.
- It avoids harassment in trying to collect the bill.

MEDICAL TESTIMONY AGREEMENT

AGREEMENT made this _____day of _____20XX, between_____
herein referred to as attorney, and _____,
of _____ , _____ , _____ _____ , a licensed _____.
     (street address)   (city)   (state)   (ZIP code)

In consideration of their mutual covenants set forth herein, the parties agree as follows:

1. The doctor will give medical testimony in the case of:
_____
as a treating physician or as an expert witness (delete the unwanted phrase).

2. The doctor agrees to appear promptly when called and to present his or her medical testimony in a well-prepared professional manner.

3. The doctor will be compensated for time away from the practice of his or her medical duties in accordance with the following:
    (a) $_____ per hour for reports and preparation of medical testimony.
    (b) $_____ per hour for pretrial conferences.
    (c) $_____ per hour for court appearance, including travel time to and from the office.
    (d) $_____ per hour for deposition.
    (e) $_____ per hour for being on call with cancellation of appointments but not appearing in court.

4. The doctor will appear in court on_____ hour's notice from the attorney, unless prior arrangements have been made for the exact time of appearance.

5. The doctor will be compensated on completion of his or her medical testimony, and payment will not be contingent upon the outcome of the case. However, if the case is settled before reaching the court, the doctor will be compensated for being on call as noted above.

This contract shall be binding upon the parties.

IN WITNESS WHEREOF, the said parties hereto have subscribed their respective signatures.

_____
    (physician)

_____
    (attorney)

Date:_____

FIGURE 15-3 Example of a medical testimony agreement between physician and attorney. This is signed by the physician and sent to the attorney for signature. A copy is retained by the attorney and the original is kept by the physician.

**REQUEST FOR ALLOWANCE OF LIEN
ASSIGNMENT AND AUTHORIZATION**

WHEREAS, I have a right or cause of action arising out of personal injury, to wit:

I, _____ hereby authorize _____ ,
    patient's name   physician's name

to furnish, upon request, to my attorney, _____ ,
any and all medical records, or reports of examination, diagnosis, treatment, or prognosis but not necessarily limited to those items as set forth herein, in addition to an itemized statement of account for services rendered therefore or in connection therewith, which my attorney may from time to time request in connection with the injuries described above and sustained by me on the _____ day of _____ , 20XX.

I, hereby irrevocably authorize and direct my said attorney set forth herein to pay to_____ all charges for attendance in court,
                 physician's name

if required as an expert witness whether he testifies or not; reports or other data supplied by him; depositions given by said doctor; medical services rendered or drugs supplied; and any other reasonable and customary charges incurred by my attorney as submitted by_____ and in
                                    physician's name

connection with said injury. Said payment or payments are to be made from any money or monies received by my attorney whether by judgment, decree, or settlement of this case, prior to disbursement to me and payment of the amount as herein directed shall be the same as if paid by me. This authorization to pay the aforementioned doctor shall constitute and be deemed as assignment of so much of my recovery I receive. It is agreed that nothing herein relieves me of the primary responsibility and obligation of paying my doctor for services rendered, and I shall at all times remain personally liable for such indebtedness unless released by the aforementioned doctor or by payment disbursed by my attorney.
I accept the above assignment:
Dated: _____ Patient:_____

As the attorney of record for the above-named patient, I hereby agree to observe the terms of this agreement, and to withhold from any award in this case such sums as are required for the adequate protection of Dr._____
_____ .

Date: _____ Attorney:_____

FIGURE 15-4 Patient's authorization to release information to an attorney and grant lien to the physician against proceeds of settlement in connection with accident, industrial, or third-party litigation cases.

The chief disadvantage of not filing a lien is that there is no legal documentation if the case goes to court as far as collecting monies owed to the physician. A case could be settled, the attorney would get his or her fee, and the physician's fee may be placed last on the list for payment or remain unpaid.

A time limit should be specified when a lien form is completed; reaching a settlement may involve several years of litigation. Some patients may be persuaded to pay before a legal settlement is made or at least make payments until a settlement is reached. The lien becomes null and void at the end of the time limit. If the patient's financial status has changed, one might be able to collect because the patient can then be billed. If not, an amended or subsequent lien should be filed that states the actual balance of the patient's account.

The word "amended" should be typed on the new lien below the Workers' Compensation Appeals Board (WCAB) case number.

The physician's fee should be protected by having the attorney sign the lien, thereby indicating that he or she will pay the physician directly from any money received in a settlement. This makes the attorney responsible for the fee. The patient's file must be placed in a Hold for Settlement category until the case comes up in court. In some states, the physician's fee owed by the patient constitutes a first lien against any such money settlement and the attorney must first satisfy the lien of the physician before the patient or attorney receives any money from the settlement. State laws should be checked. The office of the patient's attorney should be called at least quarterly for an update.

**STATE OF CALIFORNIA
DIVISION OF WORKERS' COMPENSATION
WORKERS' COMPENSATION APPEALS BOARD
NOTICE AND REQUEST FOR ALLOWANCE OF LIEN**

Date Of Original Lien: 6-5-XX
MM/DD/YYYY   ☑ Original Lien   ☐ Amended Lien

CA-46739-04
Case No.
(Choose only one)
☑ a specific injury on 4-3-XX
(DATE OF INJURY: MM/DD/YYYY)

1. Must include case number and date of injury. Determine if the injury occurred on a specific date or over a period of time.

☐ a cumulative injury which began on _____ and ended on _____
(START DATE: MM/DD/YYYY)   (END DATE: MM/DD/YYYY)

120XX6542   8-14-19XX
SSN (Numbers Only)   (DATE OF BIRTH: MM/DD/YYYY)

Injured Worker:

IMA   B
First Name   MI

2. Patient demographic information.

HURT
Last Name

300 EAST CENTRAL AVENUE
Address/PO Box (Please leave blank spaces between numbers, names or words)

WOODLAND HILLS   CA   12345
City   State   Zip Code

Attorney/Representative for Injured Worker:

3. Information for patient's attorney.

I'M HERE FOR THE PATIENT LAWYERS FIRM
Name

232 NORTH RIVERSIDE DRIVE
Address/PO Box (Please leave blank spaces between numbers, names or words)

CALABASSAS   CA   12345
City   State   Zip Code

Lien Claimant (Completion of this section is required):

4. The physician is the lien claimant.

RAYMOND SKELETON, MD
Name of Organization filing lien (for individual lien claimants, leave blank)

RAYMOND
First Name of Individual filing lien (organizational lien claimants, leave blank)

SKELETON, MD
Last Name of Individual filing lien (organizational lien claimants, leave blank)

4567 BROAD AVE
Address/PO Box (Please leave blank spaces between numbers, names or words)

WOODLAND HILLS   CA   12345
City   State   Zip Code

(555) 486-9002
Phone
DWC/ WCAB Form 6 (Page 1) Rev(11/2008)

FIGURE 15-5 Notice and request for lien. This form is used to file a lien on behalf of a physician who is providing services to a workers' compensation patient and has not been paid.

Continued

Lien Claimant's Attorney/Representative, if any

☑ Law Firm/Attorney ☐ Non-Attorney Representative ☐ Lien Claimant not represented

CORPORATE REPRESENTATIVE LAWYERS FIRM
Lien Claimant Law Firm/Representative

5. Attorney for the physician.

DANIEL
First Name

DIAMOND
Last Name

P.O. BOX 34285
Address/PO Box (Please leave blank spaces between numbers, names or words)

SIMI VALLEY   CA   17394
City   State   Zip Code

(555) 938-4930
Phone

Employer

6. Injured patient employer.

THE CONK OUT COMPANY
Name

45 SOUTH GORMAN ST.
Address/PO Box (Please leave blank spaces between numbers, names or words)

WOODLAND HILLS   CA   12345
City   State   Zip Code

Insurance Carrier or Claims Administrator

7. Workers' comp insurance company.

STATE COMPENSATION INSURANCE FUND
Name

P.O. BOX 28918
Address/PO Box (Please leave blank spaces between numbers, names or words)

FRESNO   CA   93729
City   State   Zip Code

Employer or Claims Administrator Attorney/Representative (if known)

8. Attorney for employer.

NONE
Name

Address/PO Box (Please leave blank spaces between numbers, names or words)

City   State   Zip Code

FIGURE 15-5, cont'd

The lien claimant hereby requests the Workers' Compensation Appeals Board to determine and allow as a lien the sum

of $ _____45,362.90_____ against any amount now due or which may hereafter become payable as

Total Lien Amount

compensation to the above-named employee on account of the above-claimed injury.

> 9. *Amount of outstanding medical claims by this physician. If additional fees are incurred, an amended lien is filed with an updated amount.*

This request and claim for lien is for (mark appropriate box):

☑ A reasonable attorney's fee for legal services pertaining to any claim for compensation either before the appeals board or before any of the appellate courts, and the reasonable disbursements in connection therewith. (Labor Code § 4903 (a).)

☐ The reasonable expense incurred by or on behalf of the injured employee, as provided by Labor Code § 4600. (Labor Code § 4903 (b).)

☐ Reasonable expense incurred by or on behalf of the injured employee for medical-legal expenses. (Labor Code § 4903 (b).)

☐ The reasonable value of the living expenses of an injured employee or of his or her dependents, subsequent to the injury. (Labor Code § 4903 (c).)

☐ The reasonable burial expenses of the deceased employee. (Labor Code § 4903 (d).)

> 10. *Various requests depending on the facts of the case.*

☐ The reasonable living expenses of the spouse or minor children of the injured employee, or both, subsequent to the date of the injury, where the employee has deserted or is neglecting his or her family. (Labor Code § 4903 (e).)

☐ The reasonable fee for interpreter's services performed on _____ 20 ___ . (Labor Code § 4600 (f).)

☐ The amount of indemnification granted by the California Victims of Crime Program. (Labor Code § 4903 (i).)

☐ The amount of compensation, including expenses of medical treatment, and recoverable costs that have been paid by the Asbestos Workers' Account. (Labor Code § 4903 (j).)

☐ Other Lien(s): Specify nature and statutory basis.

NOTE: ITEMIZED STATEMENT JUSTIFYING THE LIEN MUST BE ATTACHED

> 11. *This box should always be checked.*

☑ A copy of the lien claim and supporting documents was served by mail or delivered to each of the above-named parties.

Daniel Diamond	*Raymond Skeleton, MD*	6-5-XX
(Signature of Attorney/Representative for Lien Claimant)	(Signature of Lien Claimant)	Date (MM/DD/YYYY)

Physician's attorney	Physician's signature

DWC/ WCAB Form 6 (Page 3) Rev(11/2008)

FIGURE 15-5, cont'd

Scenario: Filing a Lien

Problem 1: Suppose Attorney Blake advises client Roger Reed not to pay the physician until after the trial. Or what happens if payment is not made for Dr. Practon's courtroom testimony and the case is lost? Suppose that medical reports are ordered and Attorney Blake neglects to pay for them. What happens if Roger Reed forgets about the physician's bill?

Solution: If a lien had been signed, then once the case has been settled the money would be paid to the physician; otherwise, the settlement would belong to the patient, Roger Reed, and he could take any action with the money that he wanted.

Problem 2: Suppose that Dr. Practon had an oral agreement covering his fee. The patient, Katie Crest, was unable to pay for medical treatment except on legal monetary recovery. When Katie Crest settled her case, the proceeds went almost entirely to welfare agencies because she received retroactive Medicaid. Dr. Practon sued the patient's attorney and lost.

Solution: If Dr. Practon had gotten a written assignment of the proceeds, the lawyer could have been held liable for the fee.

If there is a third-party litigation involved in an industrial case or a decision has not been reached as to whether an accident is caused by industrial or nonindustrial causes, both a regular lien and a workers' compensation lien should be filed. In most states a special lien form for workers' compensation filing is available and should be used. A copy of the lien should be completed and sent to all concerned parties, including the following:

- Appeals board
- Employer of the patient
- Employee (the patient)
- Insurance carrier
- Physician's files (lien claimant or one who is filing for the lien)

The patient/employee consents to the lien by his or her signature. Do not accept a lien form unless it is also signed by the patient's attorney. Check with the local Division of Industrial Accidents for forms pertinent to filing a lien and instructions on the formalities, number of copies required, and where they are to be sent.

Third-Party Subrogation

The legal term *subrogation* is the process of initiating a legal claim against either another individual, an individual's insurer, or, in the case of a car accident, one's own automobile insurance company to pay health insurance bills. **Third-party subrogation** means "to substitute" one party for another. When applied to workers' compensation cases, it means a transfer of the claims and rights from the original creditor (workers' compensation insurance carrier) to the third-party liability carrier. In a compensation case, the insurance

carrier that is "subrogated" to the legal claims has a right to be paid all of the monies it paid out for the injuries. That reimbursement is obtained from any money the injured collects from a legal claim, directly from the individual who caused the injury, or from another insurer.

Scenario: Third-Party Subrogation

Scenario: As Monica Valdez, a secretary, went to the bank to deposit some money for her employer, her car was rear-ended by another automobile and she was injured.

Subrogation solution: In such a case, there is no question of fault and no question of cause. Monica was hurt during the performance of her work and the workers' compensation insurance carrier is liable. The carrier must adjust the claim, provide all medical treatment, and pay all TD and PD benefits.

However, the insurance carrier does have legal recourse. It may send a representative to visit with Monica, explain to her that she has a good subrogation case, encourage her to seek the advice of an attorney and sue the third party (other automobile driver) in civil court. This is sometimes referred to as *litigation*, which is the process of carrying on a lawsuit. If Monica agrees to sue, the insurance carrier files a demand with the court for repayment of all money it has paid out. This is called a *lien*, which is discussed earlier in the chapter. When the case is settled, if an award is made to Monica, the insurance carrier is reimbursed for all that it has paid and Monica receives the balance. In some states, such as California, the patient is legally prevented from collecting twice.

MEDICAL REPORTS

Health Information Record Keeping

If a private patient comes to the office with an industrial injury, a separate health record (chart) and financial record (ledger) should be set up for the work-related injury. A private health record should never be combined with an industrial case record because separate disclosure laws apply to each and the workers' compensation case may go to court. Some medical practices use a colored file folder or tabs for the industrial health record, which makes filing of all private and workers' compensation documents easier for the insurance billing specialist. If two charts are maintained, it is easy to pull the industrial health record and financial accounting record quickly without having to go through the patient's previously unrelated private health records.

It is preferable that a patient not be scheduled to see a physician for a workers' compensation follow-up examination and an unrelated complaint during the same appointment. Separate appointments (back to back, if necessary) should be arranged. This allows for separate dictation without intermixing the required documentation for each chart.

WORKERS' COMPENSATION AND HIPAA COMPLIANCE

It is important to note that workers' compensation programs are not included under the definition of a "health plan" as identified in the Health Insurance Portability and Accountability Act (HIPAA). Therefore workers' compensation programs are not required to comply with HIPAA standards; however, it is beneficial to workers' compensation insurance payers and health care providers to use the adopted HIPAA Transaction and Code Set (TCS) to work harmoniously within the claims processing activities used throughout the industry.

PRIVACY AND CONFIDENTIALITY

The HIPAA Privacy Rule allows for the disclosure of protected health information (PHI) to workers' compensation insurers, state administrators, and employers to the extent necessary to comply with laws relating to workers' compensation. The HIPAA Privacy Rule recognizes the legitimate need of insurers and other entities involved in the workers' compensation systems to have access to individuals' health information as authorized by state or other law. Because of the significant variability among such laws, the HIPAA Privacy Rule permits disclosures of health information for workers' compensation purposes in a number of different ways.

1. *Disclosures without Individual Authorization.* The HIPAA Privacy Rule permits covered entities to disclose PHI to workers' compensation insurers, state administrators, employers, and other persons or entities involved in workers' compensation systems without the individual's authorization. This relates to workers' compensation injuries or illnesses and federal programs, such as Black Lung Benefits Act, FECA, the Longshore and Harbor Workers' Compensation Act (LHWCA), and Energy Employees Occupational Illness Compensation Program Act. The disclosure must comply with and be limited to what the state law requires. Disclosure is allowed for purposes of obtaining payment for any health care provided to the injured or ill worker.
2. *Disclosures with Individual Authorization.* Covered entities may disclose PHI to workers' compensation insurers and others involved in workers' compensation systems to which the individual has provided his or her authorization for the release of the information to the entity. For example, if a patient's attorney calls the physician's office for information, it is only ethical and legal to get a signed authorization from the patient and to ask permission from the insurance carrier before giving out any medical information. The contract exists between the physician and insurance carrier, not the physician and patient.
3. *Minimum Necessary.* Covered entities are required to limit the amount of PHI disclosed to the minimum necessary to accomplish the workers' compensation purpose. Under this requirement, PHI may be shared for such purposes to the full extent authorized by state or other law.

If you get the patient's authorization to disclose the information, you do not need to include it or track it for accounting because the disclosures that are made following somebody's authorization do not need to be accounted for.

Documentation

Documentation must show the necessity for the procedures performed. If there is no accurate diagnostic code to explain the patient's condition, a report that describes the details of the diagnosis should be sent.

As discussed in Chapter 5, the ICD-10-CM code book has a section that lists External Causes of Morbidity, which are categorized by external causes of injuries, poisonings, and adverse effects. These codes (V01-Y99) describe how injuries occur. In workers' compensation cases, it is important to use these codes because they indicate the external cause of injury, such as W19 (accidental fall not otherwise specified). Some cases may need two of these codes, one for the circumstance of the event and one for its location. External Causes of Morbidity codes are never used as a primary diagnosis but they give supplemental information to the insurance carrier. This may help the insurance carrier to differentiate between the claims and get a claim paid quicker.

As of the printing of this edition, some workers' compensation insurers have announced plans to adopt the ICD-10-CM and have moved to accept electronic claims using the 5010 electronic format and EHR attachments, such as the Ohio Bureau of Workers' Compensation (OBWC) and Anthem Workers' Compensation. More insurers are expected to adopt the ICD-10-CM in the future.

CPT code 99080 may be used to bill for workers' compensation reports. The monetary value assigned to the code is usually determined by the number of pages in the report. If health records are reviewed before consulting or treating a workers' compensation patient, a bill should be submitted for this service. Refer to Chapter 4 for comprehensive information on the topic of documentation.

Terminology

Most workers' compensation cases involve accidents causing bodily injuries. Therefore one should become familiar with anatomic terms, directional and range-of-motion words, types of fractures, body activity terms, and words that describe pain and symptoms (Box 15-2). This terminology appears in progress chart notes and industrial injury reports. The more knowledgeable one becomes about the meaning of the documentation, the more proficient one will be in knowing whether the procedure and diagnostic codes assigned are substantiated or if code selection is deficient and should be enhanced for better payment. One should learn how to spell the words and find the definitions of the words in the dictionary.

Directional terms are commonly used when a case is being rated for PD. A range-of-motion (ROM) test determines whether the body part is able to move to the full extent possible. Often, after an injury to an extremity or joint, there is restriction of motion and loss of strength (for example, grip). ROM can be improved with activity and therapy. It is measured with special measurement devices and documented each time a patient is examined. Fractures can occur from falling, blows, impact hits, a disease process, or direct violence, such as in an automobile accident. Healing may take months and depends on the location and severity of the injured part, associated injury, and complications or infections.

REPORTING REQUIREMENTS

Employer's Report

The laws clearly state that the injured person must promptly report the industrial injury or illness to his or her employer or immediate supervisor, which may be a safety officer in some businesses. By law in most states, the employer must send an Employer's Report of Occupational Injury or Illness form (Figure 15-6) to the insurance company. The time limit for submission of this form varies from immediately to as long as 30 days in different states (see Table 15-1). Many states have adopted the form shown in Figure 15-6 to meet the requirements of the federal OSHA Act of 1970 and for state statistical purposes.

Medical Service Order

In addition to the employer's report, the employer may complete and sign a **medical service order,** giving this to the injured employee to take to the physician's office (Figure 15-7). This authorizes the physician to treat the injured employee. The form should be photocopied and the copy retained for the physician's files. The original should be attached to the Doctor's First Report of Occupational Injury or Illness (preliminary report). An employer may prefer to write the service order on his or her business letterhead, on billhead, or simply on a piece of scratch paper.

Authorizations may also be obtained over the telephone. However, if a patient arrives for an appointment without written authorization, some offices prefer that the employer be telephoned and asked to have the authorized person e-mail or fax the permission for treatment. Subsequently, if payment is not received or the claim is disputed, it may be easier to collect if a copy of the written authorization is included when sending collection follow-up correspondence.

A copayment is not collected for a workers' compensation patient who submits a completed Employer's Report of Occupational Injury or Illness form (Figure 15-8). If a patient was injured on the job but does not have this form, standard protocol is to bill the patient's primary health insurance and collect the appropriate copayment. The patient may decide to bring in the Employer's Report of Occupational Injury or Illness at a later time. The physician has the right to reevaluate the patient under the workers' compensation policy and submit a medical service order (Figure 15-9).

A charge can be made if an appointment was arranged by the employer or insurance company for a workers' compensation patient and was not canceled 72 hours before the appointment time.

If outside testing or treatment is necessary, authorization should be obtained from the employer or the adjuster for the insurance company. When this is done by telephone, the name of the procedure or test and the medical necessity for it should be stated. The name and title of

---

Box 15-2　Terms that Describe Intensity of Pain and Frequency of Occurrence of Symptoms

Definitions that describe intensity of pain and frequency of symptoms were developed to assist the physician when documenting subjective complaints.

- A *severe* pain would preclude the activity causing the pain.
- A *moderate* pain could be tolerated but would cause marked handicap in the performance of the activity precipitating the pain.
- A *slight* pain could be tolerated but would cause some handicap in the performance of the activity precipitating the pain.
- A *minimal (mild)* pain would constitute an annoyance but would cause no handicap in the performance of the particular activity. It would be considered a nonratable permanent disability (PD).
- *Occasional* means approximately 25% of the time.
- *Intermittent* means approximately 50% of the time.
- *Frequent* means approximately 75% of the time.
- *Constant* means 90% to 100% of the time.

State of California **EMPLOYER'S REPORT OF OCCUPATIONAL INJURY OR ILLNESS**	**Please complete in triplicate (type if possible) Mail two copies to:** XYZ Insurance Company P.O. Box 5 Woodland Hills XY 12345	**OSHA CASE NO.** # 18 **FATALITY** ☐

Any person who makes or causes to be made any knowingly false or fraudulent material statement or material representation for the purpose of obtaining or denying workers compensation benefits or payments is guilty of a felony.	California law requires employers to report within **five days** of knowledge every occupational injury or illness which results in lost time beyond the date of the incident **OR** requires medical treatment beyond first aid. If an employee subsequently dies as a result of a previously reported injury or illness, the employer must file within **five days** of knowledge an amended report indicating death. In addition, every serious injury, illness, or death must be **reported immediately** by telephone or telegraph to the nearest office of the California Division of Occupational Safety and Health.

EMPLOYER

1. FIRM NAME The Conk Out Company	Ia. Policy Number B12345	**Please do not use this column**
2. MAILING ADDRESS: (Number, Street, City, Zip) 45 South Gorman St. Woodland Hills, XY 12345	2a. Phone Number (555) 430-3488	**CASE NUMBER**
3. LOCATION if different from Mailing Address (Number, Street, City and Zip)	3a. Location Code	**OWNERSHIP**
4. NATURE OF BUSINESS; e.g.. Painting contractor, wholesale grocer, sawmill, hotel, etc. Plumbing Repair	5. State unemployment insurance acct.no	

6. TYPE OF EMPLOYER: ☑ Private ☐ State ☐ County ☐ City ☐ School District ☐ Other Gov't, Specify: _____	**INDUSTRY**

7. DATE OF INJURY / ONSET OF ILLNESS (mm/dd/yy) 04/03/20	8. TIME INJURY/ILLNESS OCCURRED AM ___ 2:00 PM	9. TIME EMPLOYEE BEGAN WORK 8:00 AM ___ PM	10. IF EMPLOYEE DIED, DATE OF DEATH (mm/dd/yy)	**OCCUPATION**
11. UNABLE TO WORK FOR AT LEAST ONE FULL DAY AFTER DATE OF INJURY? ☑ Yes ☐ No	12. DATE LAST WORKED (mm/dd/yy) 04/03/20	13. DATE RETURNED TO WORK (mm/dd/yy)	14. IF STILL OFF WORK, CHECK THIS BOX: ☑	
15. PAID FULL DAYS WAGES FOR DATE OF INJURY OR LAST DAY WORKED? ☑ Yes ☐ No	16. SALARY BEING CONTINUED? ☐ Yes ☑ No	17. DATE OF EMPLOYER'S KNOWLEDGE /NOTICE OF INJURY/ILLNESS (mm/dd/yy) 04/03/20	18. DATE EMPLOYEE WAS PROVIDED CLAIM FORM (mm/dd/yy) 04/03/20	**SEX**

INJURY OR ILLNESS

19. SPECIFIC INJURY/ILLNESS AND PART OF BODY AFFECTED, MEDICAL DIAGNOSIS if available, e.g., Second degree burns on right arm, tendonitis on left elbow, lead poisoning Ankle Injury. Swelling, possible fracture.	**AGE**
20. LOCATION WHERE EVENT OR EXPOSURE OCCURRED (Number, Street, City, Zip) 45 Gorman St. Woodland Hills, XY 12345	20a. COUNTY	21. ON EMPLOYER'S PREMISES? ☑ Yes ☐ No	**DAILY HOURS**
22. DEPARTMENT WHERE EVENT OR EXPOSURE OCCURRED, e.g.. Shipping department, machine shop. Stock Room	23. Other Workers injured or ill in this event? ☐ Yes ☑ No	**DAYS PER WEEK**
24. EQUIPMENT, MATERIALS AND CHEMICALS THE EMPLOYEE WAS USING WHEN EVENT OR EXPOSURE OCCURRED, e.g.. Acetylene, welding torch, farm tractor, scaffold 6 Foot Ladder	**WEEKLY HOURS**
25. SPECIFIC ACTIVITY THE EMPLOYEE WAS PERFORMING WHEN EVENT OR EXPOSURE OCCURRED, e.g.. Welding seams of metal forms, loading boxes onto truck. Climbed ladder to remove a ream of paper from top shelf; Fell	**WEEKLY WAGE**
26. HOW INJURY/ILLNESS OCCURRED. DESCRIBE SEQUENCE OF EVENTS. SPECIFY OBJECT OR EXPOSURE WHICH DIRECTLY PRODUCED THE INJURY/ILLNESS, e.g., Worker stepped back to inspect work and slipped on scrap material. As he fell, he brushed against fresh weld, and burned right hand. USE SEPARATE SHEET IF NECESSARY Worker climbed ladder to remove a ream of paper from the top shelf in stock room. She was descending and mis-stepped falling to the floor. She tried to land upright and her leg took the brunt of the fall.	**COUNTY**
27. Name and address of physician (number, street, city, zip) Raymond Skeleton, MD 4567 Broad Ave., Woodland Hills, XY 12345	27a. Phone Number	**NATURE OF INJURY**
28. Hospitalized as an inpatient overnight? ☐ No ☐ Yes If yes then, name and address of hospital (number, street, city, zip)	28a. Phone Number	**PART OF BODY**
	29. Employee treated in emergency room? ☑ Yes ☐ No	**SOURCE**

ATTENTION This form contains information relating to employee health and must be used in a manner that protects the confidentiality of employees to the extent possible while the information is being used for occupational safety and health purposes. See CCR Title 8 14300.29 (b)(6)–(10) & 14300.35(b)(2)(E)2.
Note: Shaded boxes indicate confidential employee information as listed in CCR Title 8 14300.35(b)(2)(E)2*.

EMPLOYEE

30. EMPLOYEE NAME Ima B. Hurt	31. SOCIAL SECURITY NUMBER	32. DATE OF BIRTH (mm/dd/yy)	**EVENT**
33. HOME ADDRESS (Number, Street, City, Zip)	33a. PHONE NUMBER	**SECONDARY SOURCE**
34. SEX ☐ Male ☒ Female	35. OCCUPATION (Regular job title, NO initials, abbreviations or numbers)	36. DATE OF HIRE (mm/dd/yy)	
37. EMPLOYEE USUALLY WORKS ___ hours per day, ___ days per week, ___ total weekly hours	37a. EMPLOYMENT STATUS ☐ regular, full-time ☐ part-time ☐ temporary ☐ seasonal	37b. UNDER WHAT CLASS CODE OF YOUR POLICY WHERE WAGES ASSIGNED	**EXTENT OF INJURY**
38. GROSS WAGES/SALARY $ ___ per ___	39. OTHER PAYMENTS NOT REPORTED AS WAGES/SALARY (e.g. tips, meals, overtime, bonuses, etc.)? ☐ Yes ☐ No	
Completed By (type or print)	Signature & Title	Date (mm/dd/yy)

• Confidential information may be disclosed only to the employee, former employee, or their personal representative (CCR Title 8 14300.35), to others for the purpose of processing a workers' compensation or other insurance claim; and under certain circumstances to a public health or law enforcement agency or to a consultant hired by the employer (CCR Title 8 14300.30). CCR Title 8 14300.40 requires provision upon request to certain state and federal workplace safety agencies.

FORM 5020 (Rev7) June 2002   FILING OF THIS FORM IS NOT AN ADMISSION OF LIABILITY

FIGURE 15-6 Employer's Report of Occupational Injury or Illness. This form complies with OSHA requirements and California State Workers' Compensation laws.

**WORKERS' COMPENSATION
MEDICAL SERVICE ORDER**

To: Dr./Clinic _____ Martin Feelgood, MD _____

Address _____ 4567 Broad Avenue, Woodland Hills, XY 12345 _____

We are sending _____ Mrs. Ima Hurt _____

Address _____ 300 East Central Ave., Woodland Hills, XY 12345 _____

Social Security No. _ 120-XX-6542 _ Date of birth 3-4-1966 _____
         to you for treatment in accordance with the terms of the Workers'
         Compensation Laws. Please submit your report to the
         _____ XYZ Insurance Company _____
         at once. Compensation cannot be paid without complete medical
         information.
Insurance carrier _ XYZ Insurance Company _____

Address P.O. Box 5, Woodland Hills, XY 12345 Telephone 555-271-0562

Employer _____ The Conk Out Company _____

Address 45 S. Gorman St. Woodland Hills, XY 12345 Telephone 555-430-3488

Signature _____ *J.D. HAWKINS, MD* _____ Date _____ 4-3-20XX _____
         If patient is able to return to work today or tomorrow, please
         show date and time below — sign and give to patient to return to
         employer. If there are any work restrictions indicate on the back
         of this form. Please submit your usual first report in any case.

Date/Time _____ By _____

FIGURE 15-7 Medical service order.

the person giving authorization should be obtained and written in the patient's chart and on the order form along with the date. No authorization numbers are issued in workers' compensation cases.

The insurance adjuster handling the case should be contacted if a translator is necessary for a workers' compensation patient. He or she should make arrangements for an official translator to be present for all appointments. A member of the patient's family or the patient's friend should not be allowed to serve as a translator because there may be no legal recourse for the physician if miscommunicated information leads to a bad outcome.

Scenario: Multiple Injuries and Dates of Injury

Problem: A patient has a workers' compensation claim for the left wrist and the right big toe. The patient needed to address pain in the left wrist on 10/4/20YY for carpel tunnel syndrome and was injured on 6/8/20YY when a steel bar crushed the patient's big toe.

Solution: Be sure to keep accurate records and file the medical claims for both injuries separately. If by chance the big toe injury was billed with the date of injury for the wrist, the claim will automatically be rejected. The insurance billing specialist should be accurate in posting the correct reimbursed amounts for the correct corresponding injury.

Physician's First Report

After the physician sees the injured person, he or she completes a medical evaluation of the patient and sends this medical report detailing the injury together with a CMS-1500 (02-12) claim form (Figure 15-10) and the Doctor's First Report of Occupational Injury or Illness form (used in California) (see Figure 15-16) within 5 days of seeing the patient. Some states either have modified the CMS-1500 (02-12) claim form, which allows for additional data so that an accompanying medical report may not be required, or have created a first treatment medical report form.

When coding for the office visit, patient injury or illness evaluation, and creating a report, use CPT codes 99455, 99466, or 99080. CPT codes 99455 and 99456 are both designated to cover work-related or medical disability exams. The first covers an exam provided by the treating physician and the second covers an exam provided by someone other than the treating physician. According to CPT, both codes should be used to report "evaluations performed to establish baseline information," when "no active management of the problem(s) is undertaken during the encounter." If other evaluation and management (E/M) services or procedures are performed for the patient on the same date, you should also

| State of California

EMPLOYER'S REPORT OF OCCUPATIONAL INJURY OR ILLNESS | Please complete in triplicate (type, if possible). Mail two copies to:

XYZ Insurance Company
PO Box 5
Woodland Hills, XY 12345 | OSHA
Case No.
 # 18
☐ Fatality |

| Any person who makes or causes to be made any knowingly false or fraudulent material statement or material representation for the purpose of obtaining or denying workers' compensation benefits or payments is guilty of a felony. | NOTICE: California law requires employers to report within **five days** of knowledge every occupational injury or illness which results in lost time beyond the date of the incident **OR** requires medical treatment beyond first aid. If an employee subsequently dies as a result of a previously reported injury or illness, the employer must file within **five days** of knowledge an amended report indicating death. In addition, every serious injury/illness, or death must be reported **immediately** by telephone or telegraph to the nearest office of the California Division of Occupational Safety and Health. |

EMPLOYER

1. FIRM NAME *The Conk Out Company*	1A. POLICY NUMBER *B12345*	DO NOT USE THIS COLUMN
2. MAILING ADDRESS (Number and Street, City, ZIP) *45 South Gorman St. Woodland Hills, XY 12345*	2A. PHONE NUMBER *555-430-3488*	Case No.
3. LOCATION, IF DIFFERENT FROM MAILING ADDRESS (Number and Street, City, ZIP)	3A. LOCATION CODE	Ownership
4. NATURE OF BUSINESS, e.g., painting contractor, wholesale grocer, sawmill, hotel, etc. *Plumbing Repair*	5. STATE UNEMPLOYMENT INSURANCE ACCT. NO.	Industry
6. TYPE OF EMPLOYER ☒ PRIVATE ☐ STATE ☐ CITY ☐ COUNTY ☐ SCHOOL DIST. ☐ OTHER GOVERNMENT - SPECIFY _____		Occupation

EMPLOYEE

7. EMPLOYEE NAME *Ima B. Hurt*	8. SOCIAL SECURITY NUMBER *120-XX-6542*	9. DATE OF BIRTH (mm/dd/yy) *3-4-66*	Sex
10. HOME ADDRESS (Number and Street, City, ZIP) *300 E. Central Ave. Woodland Hills, XY 12345*		10A. PHONE NUMBER *555-476-9899*	Age
11. SEX ☐ MALE ☒ FEMALE	12. OCCUPATION (Regular job title — NO initials, abbreviations or numbers) *Clerk Typist*	13. DATE OF HIRE (mm/dd/yy) *1-20-86*	Daily Hours
14. EMPLOYEE USUALLY WORKS *8* hours per day *5* days per week *40* total weekly hours	14A. EMPLOYMENT STATUS (check applicable status at time of injury) X regular full-time ___ part-time ___ temporary ___ seasonal	14B. Under what class code of your policy were wages assigned? *7219*	Days per week
15. GROSS WAGES/SALARY $ *700.00* per *week*	16. OTHER PAYMENTS NOT REPORTED AS WAGES/SALARY (e.g. tips, meals, lodging, overtime, bonuses, etc.)? ☐ YES $ ____ PER ____ ☒ NO	Weekly hours

INJURY OR ILLNESS

17. DATE OF INJURY OR ONSET OF ILLNESS (mm/dd/yy) *4-3-XX*	18. TIME INJURY/ILLNESS OCCURRED ___ A.M. *2:00* P.M.	19. TIME EMPLOYEE BEGAN WORK *8:00* A.M. ___ P.M.	20. IF EMPLOYEE DIED, DATE OF DEATH (mm/dd/yy)	Weekly wage
21. UNABLE TO WORK AT LEAST ONE FULL DAY AFTER DATE OF INJURY? ☒ YES ☐ NO	22. DATE LAST WORKED (mm/dd/yy) *4-3-XX*	23. DATE RETURNED TO WORK (mm/dd/yy)	24. IF STILL OFF WORK, CHECK THIS BOX ☒	County
25. PAID FULL WAGES FOR DAY OF INJURY OR LAST DAY WORKED? ☒ YES ☐ NO	26. SALARY BEING CONTINUED? ☐ YES ☒ NO	27. DATE OF EMPLOYER'S KNOWLEDGE/NOTICE OF INJURY/ILLNESS (mm/dd/yy) *4-3-XX*	28. DATE EMPLOYEE WAS PROVIDED *4-3-XX*	Nature of injury
29. SPECIFIC INJURY/ILLNESS AND PART OF BODY AFFECTED, MEDICAL DIAGNOSIS, if available, e.g., second degree burns on right arm, tendonitis of left elbow, lead poisoning. *ankle injury swelling, possible fracture*				Part of body
30. LOCATION WHERE EVENT OR EXPOSURE OCCURRED (Number, Street, City) *45 South Gorman St. Woodland Hills, XY 12345*		30B. ON EMPLOYERS PREMISES? ☒ YES ☐ NO	Source
31. DEPARTMENT WHERE EVENT OR EXPOSURE OCCURRED, e.g., shipping department, machine shop. *stock room*	32. OTHER WORKERS INJURED/ILL IN THIS EVENT? ☐ YES ☒ NO	Event
33. EQUIPMENT, MATERIALS AND CHEMICALS THE EMPLOYEE WAS USING WHEN EVENT OR EXPOSURE OCCURRED, e.g., acetylene, welding torch, farm tractor, scaffold. *6 foot ladder*		Sec. Source
34. SPECIFY THE ACTIVITY THE EMPLOYEE WAS PERFORMING WHEN EVENT OR EXPOSURE OCCURRED, e.g., welding seams of metal forms, loading boxes onto truck. *climbed ladder to remove a ream of paper from shelf; fell*		Extent of injury

35. HOW INJURY/ILLNESS OCCURRED. DESCRIBE SEQUENCE OF EVENTS. SPECIFY OBJECT OR EXPOSURE WHICH DIRECTLY PRODUCED THE INJURY/ILLNESS, e.g., worker stepped back to inspect work and slipped on scrap material. As he fell, he brushed against fresh weld, and burned right hand. USE SEPARATE SHEET IF NECESSARY.

Worker climbed ladder to remove a ream of paper from top shelf in stock room. She was descending and mis-stepped falling to the floor. She tried to land upright, and her left leg took the brunt of the fall.

| 36. NAME AND ADDRESS OF PHYSICIAN (Number and Street, City, ZIP) *Raymond Skeleton, MD*   *4567 Broad Ave., Woodland Hills, XY 12345* | 36A. PHONE NUMBER *555-486-9002* |
| 37. IF HOSPITALIZED AS AN INPATIENT, NAME AND ADDRESS OF HOSPITAL (Number and Street, City, ZIP) | 37A. PHONE NUMBER |

| Completed by (type or print) J.D. Hawkins | Signature *J. D. Hawkins* | Title *owner* | Date *4-3-XX* |

FILING THIS REPORT IS NOT AN ADMISSION OF LIABILITY

FIGURE 15-8 Employer's Report of Occupational Injury or Illness. This form complies with OSHA requirements and California State Workers' Compensation laws.

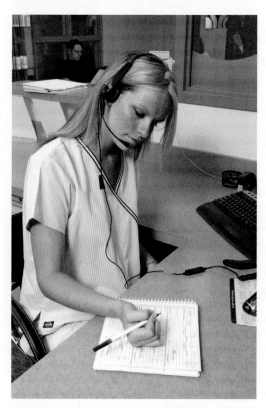

FIGURE 15-9 Receptionist receiving a medical service order via telephone for the worker to receive medical services.

report the appropriate E/M or procedure code. Attaching a -25 modifier might help to ensure that both services are reimbursed. The CPT code 99080 is used to get reimbursed for the report submitted with the CMS-1500 (02/12); include the number of pages in the units column on the CMS-1500 (02/12) form.

If the physician prefers to submit a narrative letter, the medical report should include the components, if relevant, shown in Table 15-3. The time limit for filing this report varies; state requirements are provided in Table 15-1. Failure to file the report can be a misdemeanor. Copies of the report form go to the insurance carrier and the state. Because the report is a legal document, each copy *must be signed in ink* by the physician. The insurance company waits for the physician's report and bill, then issues payment to the physician. The case can be closed if there is no further treatment or disability.

Progress or Supplemental Report

In a TD case, a supplemental report is sent to the insurance carrier after 2 to 4 weeks of treatment to give information on the current status of the patient. If there is a significant change in the prognosis, a detailed progress report (sometimes called a **reexamination report**) is sent to the insurance carrier. Subsequent progress or supplemental

reports should be sent to the insurance carrier after each hospitalization and office visit to update the progress of a case (Figure 15-11). Every evaluation and report submitted must be mailed promptly to the insurance company along with a CMS-1500 (02/12) form. If the disability is ongoing over a period of time, monthly progress reports should be submitted. A follow-up report must contain the following information:

1. Date of most recent examination
2. Present condition and progress since last report
3. Measurements of function
4. X-ray or laboratory report since last examination
5. Treatment (give type and duration)
6. Work status (patient working or estimated date of return to work if patient is still temporarily disabled)
7. PD to be anticipated

Final Report

TD ends when the physician tells the insurance carrier that the patient is able to return to work or if the disability is longer than 24 months. When the TD case is closing, the physician will submit a final evaluation report that provides an overview of the care provided and the patient's progress with the disability. When the patient resumes work, the insurance carrier closes the case and the TD benefits cease.

A physician's final report indicating any impairment or PD should be submitted with a CMS 1500 (02/12) claim form.

CLAIM SUBMISSION

Financial Responsibility

As discussed in Chapter 3, the contract for treatment in a personal illness or injury case is between the physician and patient, who is responsible for the entire bill. However, when a business is self-insured, a person is under a state program for care, or an individual is being treated as a workers' compensation case, the financial responsibility exists between the physician and insurance company or state program. As long as treatment is authorized by the insurance carrier, the insurance company is responsible for payment. A physician who agrees to treat a workers' compensation case must agree to accept payment in full according to the workers' compensation fee schedule. For workers' compensation cases, patients are not financially responsible so copayments or coinsurances cannot be collected.

An injured worker is under obligation to be evaluated by the employer's physician. However, the patient has the right to choose a different physician to seek care, but this request needs to be approved by the employer.

DRAFT - NOT FOR OFFICIAL USE

HEALTH INSURANCE CLAIM FORM

APPROVED BY NATIONAL UNIFOR MCLAIM COMMITTEE (NUCC) 02/12

PICA

1. MEDICARE	MEDICAID	TRICARE	CHAMPVA	GROUP HEALTH PLAN	FECA BLK LUNG	OTHER	1a. INSURED'S I.D. NUMBER	(For Program in Item 1)
☐ (Medicare#)	☐ (Medicaid#)	☐ (ID#DoD#)	☐ (Member ID#)	☐ (ID#)	☐ (ID#)	☒ (ID#)	B785700	

2. PATIENT'S NAME (Last Name, First Name, Middle Initial)	3. PATIENT'S BIRTH DATE	SEX	4. INSURED'S NAME (Last Name, First Name, Middle Initial)
Task, Lester, M	MM 05 DD 06 YY 1990	M ☒ F ☐	Jonas Construction Company

5. PATIENT'S ADDRESS (No., Street)	6. PATIENT RELATIONSHIP TO INSURED	7. INSURED'S ADDRESS (No., Street)
5400 Holly Street	Self ☐ Spouse ☐ Child ☐ Other ☒	300 Main Street

CITY	STATE	8. RESERVED FOR NUCC USE	CITY	STATE
Woodland Hills	XY		Woodland Hills	XY

ZIP CODE	TELEPHONE (Include Area Code)	ZIP CODE	TELEPHONE (Include Area Code)
12345-0000	(555) 7833200	12345-0000	(555) 3099800

9. OTHER INSURED'S NAME (Last Name, First Name, Middle Initial)	10. IS PATIENT'S CONDITION RELATED TO:	11. INSURED'S POLICY GROUP OR FECA NUMBER

a. OTHER INSURED'S POLICY OR GROUP NUMBER	a. EMPLOYMENT? (Current or Previous)	a. INSURED'S DATE OF BIRTH	SEX
	☒ YES ☐ NO	MM DD YY	M ☐ F ☐

b. RESERVED FOR NUCC USE	b. AUTO ACCIDENT? PLACE (State)	b. OTHER CLAIM ID (Designated by NUCC)
	☐ YES ☒ NO	

c. RESERVED FOR NUCC USE	c. OTHER ACCIDENT?	c. INSURANCE PLAN NAME OR PROGRAM NAME
	☐ YES ☒ NO	

d. INSURANCE PLAN NAME OR PROGRAM NAME	10d. CLAIM CODES (Designated by NUCC)	d. IS THERE ANOTHER HEALTH BENEFIT PLAN?
		☐ YES ☐ NO *If yes*, complete items 9, 9a, and 9d.

READ BACK OF FORM BEFORE COMPLETING & SIGNING THIS FORM.

12. PATIENT'S OR AUTHORIZED PERSON'S SIGNATURE I authorize the release of any medical or other information necessary to process this claim. I also request payment of government benefits either to myself or to the party who accepts assignment below.

SIGNED _____ DATE _____

13. INSURED'S OR AUTHORIZED PERSON'S SIGNATURE I authorize payment of medical benefits to the undersigned physician or supplier for services described below.

SIGNED _____

14. DATE OF CURRENT: ILLNESS, INJURY, or PREGNANCY(LMP)	15. OTHER DATE	16. DATES PATIENT UNABLE TO WORK IN CURRENT OCCUPATION
MM 08 DD 11 YY 20XX QUAL.	QUAL. MM DD YY	FROM MM 11 DD 08 YY 20XX TO MM 12 DD 08 YY 20XX

17. NAME OF REFERRING PROVIDER OR OTHER SOURCE	17a.	18. HOSPITALIZATION DATES RELATED TO CURRENT SERVICES
	17b. NPI	FROM MM 11 DD 08 YY 20XX TO MM 11 DD 10 YY 20XX

19. ADDITIONAL CLAIM INFORMATION (Designated by NUCC)	20. OUTSIDE LAB? $ CHARGES
	☐ YES ☒ NO

21. DIAGNOSIS OR NATURE OF ILLNESS OR INJURY Relate A-L to service line below (24E) ICD Ind. 0	22. RESUBMISSION CODE ORIGINAL REF. NO.
A. S82.001B B. _____ C. _____ D. _____	
E. _____ F. _____ G. _____ H. _____	23. PRIOR AUTHORIZATION NUMBER
I. _____ J. _____ K. _____ L. _____	

24. A. DATE(S) OF SERVICE From				To		B. PLACE OF SERVICE	C. EMG	D. PROCEDURES, SERVICES, OR SUPPLIES (Explain Unusual Circumstances) CPT/HCPCS	MODIFIER	E. DIAGNOSIS POINTER	F. $ CHARGES	G. DAYS OR UNITS	H. EPSDT Family Plan	I. ID. QUAL.	J. RENDERING PROVIDER ID. #
MM	DD	YY	MM	DD	YY										
1	11	08	20XX				21		99222		A	125 00	1		NPI	46789377XX
2	11	08	20XX				21		27524		A	600 00	1		NPI	46789377XX
3															NPI	
4															NPI	
5															NPI	
6															NPI	

25. FEDERAL TAX I.D. NUMBER	SSN EIN	26. PATIENT'S ACCOUNT NO.	27. ACCEPT ASSIGNMENT? (For govt. claims, see back)	28. TOTAL CHARGE	29. AMOUNT PAID	30. Rsvd for NUCC Use
7544530XX	☐ ☒	1577	☐ YES ☐ NO	$ 725 00	$	$

31. SIGNATURE OF PHYSICIAN OR SUPPLIER INCLUDING DEGREES OR CREDENTIALS (I certify that the statements on the reverse apply to this bill and are made a part thereof.)	32. SERVICE FACILITY LOCATION INFORMATION	33. BILLING PROVIDER INFO & PH # (555)4590087
Gregory Getwell MD 110820XX	College Hospital 4500 Broad Ave Woodland Hills XY 12345-0001	Gregory T Getwell MD 60 North State Street Woodland Hills XY 12345-0001
SIGNED *Gregory Getwell MD* DATE	a. X950731067 b.	a. 36644021CC b.

NUCC Instruction Manual available at: www.nucc.org   *PLEASE PRINT OR TYPE*   OMB APPROVAL PENDING

FIGURE 15-10 Example of a completed CMS-1500 (02-12) Health Insurance Claim Form for a workers' compensation case.

CARRIER

PATIENT AND INSURED INFORMATION

PHYSICIAN OR SUPPLIER INFORMATION

Table 15-3   Narrative Medical Report Issues, If Relevant

History	• Outline all specific details of accident, injury, or illness. • Physician should state whether there is a causal connection between the accident and conditions that may appear subsequently but are not obvious **sequelae** (diseased conditions following and usually resulting from a previous disease). If facts were obtained by reviewing prior records or x-ray films, the source should be mentioned. When a history is obtained through an interpreter, include that person's name.
Present complaints	Usually given as subjective complaints. Subjective refers to statements made by the patient about symptoms and how he or she feels. Subjective disability is evaluated by: • A description of the activity that produces the disability • The duration of the disability • The activities that are precluded by and those that can be performed with the disability • The means necessary for relief
Past history	Description of any previous, current, or subsequent medical information relevant to this injury or illness and whether there is a preexisting defect that might entitle the injured person to benefits from the subsequent injury fund or represent the actual cause of the present condition.
Examination findings	Usually given as objective findings. State all significant physical or psychiatric examination, testing, laboratory, or imaging findings.
Diagnostic impression	State all diagnostic findings and opinion as to relationship, if any, between the injury or disease and the condition diagnosed. Use diagnostic terminology that corresponds to the diagnostic code book.
Disability and prognosis	• Period during which the patient has been unable to work because of the injury or illness. • Opinion as to probable further temporary disability (TD) and a statement as to when the patient will be able to return to work or has returned to work. • Statement indicating whether the condition is currently permanent and stationary (P and S) as well as the probability of future permanent disability (PD). • Statement indicating, "All objective tests for organic pathology are negative. There is obviously a strong functional or emotional overlay," when a patient has multiple complaints but no clinical objective findings.
Work limitations	Description of any limitations to all activities.
Causation	Description of how the PD is related to the patient's occupation and the specific injury or cumulative events causing the illness.

Some states have a medical program wherein employers can reduce their workers' compensation rates by paying the first $1000 in medical bills. This is similar to a deductible for the employer's policy. The physician will first file the insurance claim with the workers' compensation insurance plan. The explanation of benefits will then direct the physician to bill the employer for the deductible amount. The statement should be sent to the employer for payment in this situation.

When billing a workers' compensation case for the initial visit, always check your state regulations about how to bill for the physician's service. If a physician sees an established patient who comes in with an injury sustained while working, some states do not issue payment based on new or established patient criteria but ask for the correct level of E/M service verified by the documentation. Other states require physicians to bill a patient as new for each new injury, even when the patient is an established patient.

Health insurance information should always be obtained in case services provided are not work related or should be billed for or the injury or illness is declared nonindustrial. To assist in informing patients of financial responsibility for nonrelated illness, the worker should sign an agreement for nonrelated medical expenses, as shown in Figure 15-12. If the workers' compensation carrier declares that the case is nonindustrial, bill the patient's health insurance, attaching a copy of the refusal by the workers' compensation carrier.

Sometimes a physician discovers a problem unrelated to the industrial injury or illness (for example, high blood pressure) while examining an injured worker. The physician may bill the workers' compensation carrier for the examination but should code the claim carefully with regard to treatment of the injury. If treatment is initiated for the patient's high blood pressure, that portion of the examination becomes the financial obligation of the patient (or his or her private insurance plan) and not of the workers' compensation carrier.

Fee Schedules

Some states have developed and adopted a workers' compensation fee schedule, while other states pay medical claims on the basis of the Medicare fee schedule plus a certain percentage. All claims are sent to the workers' compensation insurance and no billing statements are sent to the patient. Fee schedules assist with the following:
1. They limit the amount that providers will be paid.
2. They make the allowable charges and procedures more consistent.
3. They provide follow-up procedures in case of a fee dispute.

ATTENDING PHYSICIAN'S REPORT

Employee: __Mrs. Ima B. Hurt__   Claim number: __120 XX 6542__

Employer: __The Conk Out Company__   Date of injury(ies): __4-3-20XX__   Date of next exam: __4-24-20XX__

Date of this exam: __4-10-XX__   Patient Social Security No: __120 XX 6542__

Current diagnosis: __824.6 closed fracture; L. trimalleolar ankle__
(include ICD•9 code)

PATIENT STATUS

Since the last exam, this patient's condition has:

☒ improved as expected.   ☐ improved, but slower than expected.   ☐ not improved significantly.

☐ worsened.   ☐ plateaued, no further improvement is expected.   ☐ has been determined to be non-work related.

Briefly, describe any change in objective or subjective complaint: _____

TREATMENT

Treatment plan: (only list changes from prior status)   ☐ No change   ☐ Patient is/was discharged from care on_____

Est. discharge date: __5-18-20XX__   Medications: __Tylenol for pain__

Therapy: Type _____ Times per week _____ Estimated date of completion_____

Diagnostic studies: __X-ray, L. ankle 3 views__

Hospitalization/surgery: _____

Consult/other service: _____

WORK STATUS

The patient has been instructed to:

☐ return to full duty with no limitations or restrictions.

☐ remain off the rest of the day and return to work tomorrow:

_____ with no limits or restrictions. _____ with limits listed below.

☐ return to work on_____

   work limitations: _____

☒ remain off work until __5-17-20XX — discharge exam scheduled__

Estimated date patient can return full duty: __5-18-20XX__

DISABILITY STATUS

☐ Patient discharged as cured.

Please supply a brief narrative report if any of the below apply:

☐ Patient will be permanently precluded from engaging in his/her usual and customary occupation.

☐ Patient's condition is permanent and stationary.

☐ Patient will have permanent residuals   ☐ Patient will require future medical care.

Physician name: __Martin Feelgood, MD__   Address: __4567 Broad Avenue, Woodland Hills, XY 12345__

Date: __April 10, 20XX__   Telephone: __(555)__ __482-9002__

Signature: __Martin Feelgood, MD__

reference initials

FIGURE 15-11 Physician's supplemental report form.

PATIENT AGREEMENT

Patient's Name_____ James Doland _____ Soc. Sec. # 431-XX-1942

Address 67 Blyth Dr., Woodland Hills, XY 12345 ____ Tel. No. 555-372-0101

WC Insurance Carrier ____ Industrial Indemnity Company ____

Address____ 30 North Dr., Woodland Hills ____ Telephone No. 555-731-7707

Date of illness____ 2-13-20XX _____ Date of first visit____ 2-13-20XX

Emergency Yes ___ X ___No_____

Is this condition related to employment Yes X ____ No_____

If accident: Auto_____Other_____

Where did injury occur?____ Construction site ____

How did injury happen?____ fell 8 ft from scaffold suffering fractured right tibia ____

Employee/employer who verified this information____ Scott McPherson ____

Employer's name and address____ Willow Construction Company ____

Employer's telephone no.____ 555-526-0611 ____

In the event the claim for workers' compensation is declared fraudulent for this illness or condition or it is determined by the Workers' Compensation Board that the illness or injury is not a compensable workers' compensation case, I____ James Doland ____, hereby agree to pay the physician's fee for services rendered.

I have been informed that I am responsible to pay any services rendered by Dr.____ Raymond Skeleton ____ with regard to the discovery and treatment of any condition not related to the workers' compensation injury or illness. I agree to pay for all services not covered by workers' compensation and all charges for treatment and personal items unrelated to my workers' compensation illness or injury.

Signed ____ *James Doland* ____ Date____ 2-13-20XX ____

FIGURE 15-12 Patient agreement to pay the physician's fees if the case is declared not work related or an illness is discovered and treated that is not work related.

Some workers' compensation fee schedules list maximum reimbursement levels for physicians and other non-hospital providers. However, the physician is generally expected to accept payment by the insurance company as payment in full when reimbursement is based on a fee schedule. If the fee charged is more than the amount listed, the following factors may be considered:

- Provider's medical training, qualifications, and time in practice
- Nature of services provided
- Fees usually charged by the provider
- Fees usually charged by others in the region where services were given
- Other relevant economic factors of the provider's practice
- Any unusual circumstances in the case

The insurance carrier may pay the additional amount if documentation is sent validating the fee and noting the aforementioned facts.

Types of Fee Schedules

Types of fee schedules include the following:

- *Percentile of charge schedule*, which is designed to set fees at a percentile of the providers' usual and customary fee.
- *Relative value scale schedule*, which takes into account the time, skills, and extent of the service provided by the physician. Each procedure is rated on how difficult it is, how long it takes, the training a physician must have to perform it, and expenses the physician incurs, including the cost of malpractice insurance. Many of the fee schedules are similar to the CPT format in regard to sections (for example, E/M; anesthesia; surgery; radiology, nuclear medicine, and diagnostic ultrasound; pathology and laboratory; and medicine).

A *conversion factor* that uses a specific dollar amount is used for each of the sections of the fee schedule. Conversion factors may be adjusted to reflect regional differences and in some states are recalculated annually

Box 15-3	2013 Conversion Factors of the Utah Labor Commission Industrial Accident Division Medical Fee Standards
$50/unit	Anesthesia
$58/unit	Surgery
$53/unit	Radiology
$52/unit	Pathology
$46/unit	Medicine
$46/unit	Restorative Services
$46/unit	Evaluation and Management (E/M)

(Box 15-3). The amount of work, the location of the practice, and malpractice rates affect conversion rates.

Actual covered procedures, descriptions, modifiers, global periods, and other elements of a fee guideline may significantly differ from those used for other plans or programs. Sometimes a schedule includes modifiers and code numbers not listed in the CPT code book. The workers' compensation codes should be used regardless of what is done for other insurance plans. Some states have their fee schedules posted on their state website. If the fee schedules are not available online, telephone your state's program to obtain a copy.

Reviews or audits may be performed by the following entities to enforce fee schedules:
- The state agency or state fund responsible for overseeing workers' compensation (bill review)
- The payer, employer, or insurance carrier (bill review)
- The payer (bill review) and state agency (compliance audit)

Helpful Billing Tips

The following are helpful hints for billing workers' compensation claims.
1. Ask whether the injury occurred within the scope of employment and verify insurance information with the benefits coordinator for the employer. This will promote filing initial claims with the correct insurance carrier.
2. Obtain the date of injury. This date will be associated with the patient's care for the duration of patient care for the specific episode.
3. Either ask the employer the name of the claims adjuster or request that the patient obtain the claim number of his or her case when he or she comes in for the initial visit.
4. Ask the workers' compensation carrier who is going to review the claim. Sometimes independent third-party billing vendors work for the insurance carriers. Get the name and contact information.

5. Educate the patient on the medical practice's billing policies for workers' compensation cases by having him or her complete the patient agreement form shown in Figure 15-12.
6. Verify whether prior authorization is necessary before a surgical procedure is performed.
7. Document in the patient's record all data for authorization of examination, diagnostic studies, or surgery (for example, date, name of individual who authorizes, response).
8. Obtain the workers' compensation fee schedule for the relevant state.
9. Use appropriate CPT codes and modifiers to ensure prompt and accurate payment for services rendered.
10. Include a diagnostic E code as secondary to the primary diagnosis to report the cause of the injury.
11. Complete the Doctor's First Report of Occupational Injury or Illness form for the relevant state. Refer to the instructions in Procedure 15-1 at the end of this chapter. Submit the form within the time limit shown in Table 15-1. Some states (for example, California) allow a late fee if payment is not received within 30 to 45 days.
12. Ask whether there is a state-specific insurance form or if the CMS-1500 (02-12) form is acceptable.
13. Ask what year CPT and ICD-9-CM code books the insurance carrier uses. Some carriers use 2009 or earlier books, which do not reflect the deletion or addition of some procedure and diagnostic codes.
14. Clearly define any charges in excess of the fee schedule. Attach any x-ray reports, operative reports, discharge summaries, pathology reports, and so on to clarify such excess charges or when **by report (BR)** is shown for a code selected from the workers' compensation procedure code book.
15. Itemize in detail and send invoices for drugs and dressings furnished by the physician. Bill medical supplies on a separate claim or statement and do not bill with services because this may be routed to a different claims processing department.
16. Call the insurance carrier and talk with the **claims examiner** (also known as the *claims adjuster* or *claims representative*) who is familiar with the patient's case if there is a question about the fee.
17. Search the internet for a website or write to the workers' compensation state plan office in each state for booklets, bulletins, forms, and legislation information.
18. Find out if the insurance carrier uses "usual and customary" payments tied to the physician's zip code. Most carriers use fee schedules.
19. Follow up and track the date on which the claim was filed. If no payment has been received or payment has been received beyond the 30- to 45-day deadline, determine whether it meets eligibility requirements for interest.

Billing Claims

Electronic Claims Submission and Reports

Uniform data processing codes and universal electronic injury report forms have been developed by the American National Standards Institute (ANSI) and the International Association of Industrial Accident Boards and Commissions (IAIABC). ANSI is a national organization founded in 1918 to coordinate the development of voluntary business standards in the US. Texas is one of the first states to establish an insurance regulation requiring workers' compensation carriers to use universal electronic transmission for first report of injury forms and subsequent reports developed by IAIABC.

Electronic Data Systems, Inc. (EDS) in Dallas and Insurance Value Added Network Services (IVANS) in Greenwich, Connecticut, introduced the nation's first coast-to-coast electronic claims processing and report filing network, called *Workers' Compensation Reporting Service.* EDS processes all claims and follow-up reports. IVANS provides the network service and marketing of software to employers. This system is operational in many states.

Some workers' compensation insurance companies are using telephone reporting of claims. Employers report injuries occurring on the job by calling a toll-free number. Calls go to a regional center where service representatives document the first report of injury and electronically transmit it to the local claims office handling workers' compensation insurance. Employers avoid tardiness of reporting when using this system. Employers neglecting prompt reporting of injuries could delay payments to physicians.

Because workers' compensation is operated under state laws, each state is required to report financial data, statistics on injuries and illnesses, and other information to state insurance regulators. In the states that use telephone reporting service, workers' compensation payers use the system to reduce the paper processing costs that have escalated out of proportion and to improve administrative efficiency.

Out-of-State Claims

When billing for an out-of-state claim, insurance billing specialists must follow all workers' compensation regulations from the jurisdiction (state) in which the injured person's claim was originally filed.

However, companies that have employees who travel to other states are required to obtain workers' compensation insurance in those states unless they have a policy that covers out-of-state employees. Sometimes a patient may seek care from a physician in an adjacent state because he or she feels that the physician provides a higher quality of care or the patient needs a specialized type of surgery, expensive diagnostic tests, or treatment. Referral requirements should be met before the patient is seen (for example, letter of referral or preauthorization from the managing doctor with a copy to the workers' compensation carrier). Nine states hold the injured employee responsible for unauthorized care (Alabama, Alaska, Arkansas, New Jersey, North Dakota, Ohio, Washington, West Virginia, and Wisconsin). When a patient crosses a state line for treatment, he or she may be liable for some balance billing and the patient should be informed of this fact. The date on which the employer subcontracts with another company to have the work performed must be researched. Many times the injured employee states that he or she works for ABC Company. The claim is denied because the employee is actually working for XYZ Company, which has subcontracted with ABC Company.

This also happens with hospitals. One may think that a hospital employee is being treated, when an employee working for a company hired by the hospital is actually being treated. In these cases, extra time is spent identifying the subcontractor and it may be discovered that the subcontractor does not have workers' compensation insurance and expected the hiring company to provide the coverage. In another scenario, a cruise ship employee injured at sea does not fall under state workers' compensation laws and is not required to have insurance in the state. Many cruise ships have maritime companies that settle these types of claims. Normally the claim should be paid in full but many of these companies try to negotiate a much lower rate. This rate can be accepted in lieu of futile attempts to collect from the patient.

When the claim is billed, the out-of-state fee schedule should be obtained to determine the proper procedure codes, modifiers, and amounts. It should be determined whether the claimant's jurisdiction accepts electronic submission of the CMS-1500 (02-12) claim form or another form and whether other documents (for example, the operative report) are required to be submitted with the bill.

Delinquent or Slow Pay Claims

If payment of a workers' compensation claim is slow or the claim becomes delinquent (no payment for more than 45 days after the date of service), the insurance billing specialist should use an organized standard follow-up procedure.

1. Telephone the human resources department at the patient's employer. Note the name of the person with whom you speak; the name, address, and telephone number of the workers' compensation carrier; and the claim number. Verify the employer's address.
2. Send a copy of the claim form and the Doctor's First Report of Occupational Illness or Injury form. Send a letter and include details of the accident if necessary (Figure 15-13). For problem claims, it may be wise to obtain and complete a Certificate of Mailing form from the US Postal Service. The form is initialed and

postmarked at the post office and returned to the insurance biller for the office file. Because the post office does not keep a record of the mailing, this certificate costs less than certified mail. It shows proof that a special communication was mailed or sent on a certain date if a deadline is in question.

3. Telephone the insurance carrier after 45 working days, and request the expected date of payment.

4. Be reminded of that payment date by using a computer-automated reminder or a note on the desk calendar. If payment is not received on or before that day, call the carrier again and ask for payment on a day determined by the facility's expectations.

5. Telephone the patient's employer and explain that there is difficulty with the carrier. Ask the employer to contact the carrier and have the carrier send payment immediately. You also might talk to the patient and suggest that he or she discuss the problem with his or her employer to see if this will bring positive action.

6. Send the employer a copy of the financial account statement showing the outstanding balance. If the carrier is not paying, ask the employer for payment. An employer's legal obligation to pay may vary from case to case.

7. Contact the patient only if given information by the carrier or employer that the injury is not work related.

8. Develop office policies that address when an outstanding account should be reviewed (perhaps after 90 or 120 days), whether to continue collection efforts internally, and at which point the account should be turned over to a collection agency.

It may be necessary to send subsequent letters to the employer after receiving a response from the insurance carrier. For example, a letter should be sent to the employer (Figure 15-14) if the insurance company notifies the physician's office that the employer's preliminary report of injury has not been received.

If 30 days have elapsed from the date on which the letter was sent requesting the Employer's Report of Work Injury and the employer has not responded, a letter should be sent to the state Workers' Compensation Board or Industrial Accidents Commission (Figure 15-15).

Refer to Chapter 9 for additional information and helpful suggestions on following up on delinquent claims.

FIGURE 15-13 Letter sent to the insurance carrier when a workers' compensation claim becomes 45 days delinquent.

FIGURE 15-14 Letter sent to the employer when the insurance company notifies the physician's office that the employer's preliminary report of injury has not been received.

Martin Feelgood, MD
4567 Broad Avenue
Woodland Hills, XY 12345
555-486-9002

July 15, 20XX

Division of Industrial Accidents
State Office Building
107 South Broadway, Room 4107
Woodland Hills, XY 12345

Dear Madam or Sir:

Re: Failure of employer to follow Section No. 3760

Your office is being solicited to help secure an Employer's
Report of Work Injury from the employer listed below.

Case No.:	120 XX 6542
Name of Employer:	The Conk Out Company
Address:	45 South Gorman Street
	Woodland Hills, XY 12345
Name of Injured:	Mrs. Ima B. Hurt
Address:	300 East Central Avenue
	Woodland Hills, XY 12345
Date of Injury:	April 3, 20XX
Name of Insurance Carrier:	XYZ Insurance Company
Amount of Unpaid Bill:	$148.92

Your cooperation in this matter will be greatly appreciated. If you
need further information, please feel free to contact my office.

Sincerely yours,

Martin Feelgood , MD

ref initials

FIGURE 15-15 Letter sent to the Workers' Compensation Board or Industrial Accident Commission in your state if the employer does not respond to your letter requesting the Employer's Report of Work Injury after 30 days have elapsed from the date of the letter.

PROCEDURE 15-1

Completing the Doctor's First Report of Occupational Injury or Illness

The submission of this form (Figure 15-16) has a deadline, from immediately to within 5 days after the patient has been seen by the physician, depending on each state's law. An original and three or four copies should be distributed as follows:

- Original to the insurance carrier (unless more copies are required)
- One copy to the state agency
- One copy to the patient's employer
- One copy retained for the physician's files in the patient's workers' compensation file folder

In some states, attending physicians may file a single report directly to the insurer or self-insured employer within a specified number of days from initial treatment. The insurer or self-insured employer, in turn, is required to send a report to the state agency. This reduces paperwork and postage. Table 15-1 provides the time limit in each state during which the physician must submit the initial report.

1. Enter the insurance carrier's complete name, street address, city, state, and zip code.
2. Enter the employer's full name and policy number if known. Some insurance carriers file by employer and then by policy number. Sometimes the employer's telephone number is necessary on this line.
3. Enter the employer's street address, city, state, and zip code.
4. Enter the type of business (for example, repairing shoes, building construction, retailing men's clothes).
5. Enter the patient's complete first name, middle initial, and last name.
6. Enter a check mark in the appropriate box to indicate the patient's gender.
7. Enter the patient's birth date and list the year as four digits.
8. Enter the patient's street address, city, state, and zip code.
9. Enter the patient's home telephone number.
10. Enter the patient's specific job title. Be accurate in listing the occupation with the job title so that the insurance carrier may be certain the patient was doing the job for which he or she was insured.
11. Enter the patient's Social Security number. Some insurance carriers use the Social Security number as the industrial case number.
12. Enter the exact location where the patient was injured. Many times the injury may occur off the premises of the company or factory, depending on the type of job on which the employee was working. List the county where the patient was injured.
13. Enter the date the patient was injured and time of the injury. List the year as four digits.
14. Enter the date the patient last worked. This date should coincide with the date the patient reported to work and worked any portion of his or her shift (workday). This may be the same date of injury. This item is important because it informs the insurance carrier of the working status of the patient or whether the patient has been disabled and cannot return to work. List the year as four digits.
15. Enter the date and hour of the physician's first examination. The insurance carrier should know how soon after the accident the patient sought medical attention. List the year as four digits.
16. Enter a check mark in the appropriate box indicating whether the physician or an associate treated the patient previously.
17. Have the patient complete this section if possible in his or her own words, stating how the illness or injury occurred. The physician also may dictate this information after obtaining it from the patient.
18. Enter the answers to these questions about the patient's complaints and medical findings, which may be found in the patient's health record. List all of the patient's subjective complaints.
19A. Enter all objective findings from physical examination.
19B. Enter all x-ray and laboratory results. If none, state "none" or "pending."
20. Enter a check mark in "yes" or "no" to indicate if chemical or toxic compounds are involved. Enter the diagnosis and diagnostic code number. Specify etiologic agent and duration of exposure if occupational illness.
21. Enter a check mark in "yes" or "no" to indicate if the findings and diagnosis are consistent with the history of injury or onset of illness. Insert an explanation if "yes."
22. Enter a check mark in "yes" or "no" to indicate if there is any other current condition that will impede or delay the patient's recovery. Insert an explanation if "yes."
23. Enter a full description of what treatment was rendered.
24. Enter an explanation if further treatment is necessary and, if so, specify the treatment plan. Indicate if physical therapy is necessary and its frequency and duration.
25. Enter the name and location of the hospital, admission date, and estimated stay if the patient is to be hospitalized.
26. Enter a check mark in "yes" or "no" to indicate whether the patient is able to work as usual. If the answer is "no," give the date when it is estimated

Continued

STATE OF CALIFORNIA

DOCTOR'S FIRST REPORT OF OCCUPATIONAL INJURY OR ILLNESS

Within 5 days of your initial examination, for every occupational injury or illness, send two copies of this report to the employer's workers' compensation insurance carrier or the insured employer. Failure to file a timely doctor's report may result in assessment of a civil penalty. In the case of diagnosed or suspected pesticide poisoning, send a copy of the report to Division of Labor Statistics and Research, P.O. Box 420603, San Francisco, CA 94142-0603, and notify your local health officer by telephone within 24 hours.

	PLEASE DO NOT USE THIS COLUMN
1. INSURER NAME AND ADDRESS XYZ Insurance Company, P.O. Box 5, Woodland Hills, XY 12345	Case No.
2. EMPLOYER NAME The Conk Out Company Policy #B12345	
3. Address No. and Street City Zip 45 So. Gorman St Woodland Hills, XY 12345	Industry
4. Nature of business (e.g., food manufacturing, building construction, retailer of women's clothes.) Plumbing Repair	County

5. PATIENT NAME (first name, middle initial, last name) Ima B. Hurt	**6. Sex** ☐ Male ☒ Female	**7. Date of** Mo. Day Yr. **Birth** 3-4-1966	Age
8. Address: No. and Street City Zip 300 East Central Ave., Woodland Hills, XY 12345		**9.** Telephone number (555) 476-9899	Hazard
10. Occupation (Specific job title) Clerk Typist		**11.** Social Security Number 120-XX-6542	Disease
12. Injured at: No. and Street City County 45 So. Gorman St. Woodland Hills, XY 12345 Humbolt			Hospitalization
13. Date and hour of injury Mo. Day Yr. or onset of illness 4-3-20XX Hour __ a.m. 2:00 p.m.		**14.** Date last worked Mo. Day Yr. 4-3-20XX	Occupation
15. Date and hour of first Mo. Day Yr. examination or treatment 4-3-20XX Hour __ a.m. 4:00 p.m.		**16.** Have you (or your office) previously treated patient? ☐ Yes ☒ No	Return Date/Code

Patient please complete this portion, if able to do so. Otherwise, doctor please complete immediately, inability or failure of a patient to complete this portion shall not affect his/her rights to workers' compensation under the California Labor Code.

17. DESCRIBE HOW THE ACCIDENT OR EXPOSURE HAPPENED. (Give specific object, machinery or chemical. Use reverse side if more space is required.) I climbed a ladder in the stock room and while I was coming down I missed a step, lost my balance, and fell hurting my left ankle.

18. SUBJECTIVE COMPLAINTS (Describe fully. Use reverse side if more space is required.)

Pain in left ankle

19. OBJECTIVE FINDINGS (Use reverse side if more space is required.)
A. Physical examination

Pain, swelling and discoloration of L. ankle

B. X-ray and laboratory results (State if non or pending.)   Ankle x-ray (left) 3 views

20. DIAGNOSIS (if occupational illness specify etiologic agent and duration of exposure.) Chemical or toxic compounds involved? ☒ Yes ☐ No
Trimalleolar ankle fracture (left)   ICD-9 Code __ __ __ - __ __

21. Are your findings and diagnosis consistent with patient's account of injury or onset of illness? ☒ Yes ☐ No If "no", please explain.

22. Is there any other current condition that will impede or delay patient's recovery? ☐ Yes ☒ No If "yes", please explain.

23. TREATMENT RENDERED (Use reverse side if more space is required.)
Examination, x-rays, closed treatment of trimalleolar ankle fracture (left) without manipulation.
Return in one week for recheck.

24. If further treatment required, specify treatment plan/estimated duration.

25. If hospitalized as inpatient, give hospital name and location   Date admitted   Mo. Day Yr.   Estimated stay

26. WORK STATUS -- Is patient able to perform usual work? ☐ Yes ☐ No
If "no", date when patient can return to: Regular work 05 / 17 /20XX
Modified work ___/___/___   Specify restrictions _____

Doctor's Signature _Martin Feelgood MD_   CA License Number A 12345

Doctor Name and Degree (please type) Martin Feelgood, MD   IRS Number 95-36640XX

Address 4567 Broad Avenue, Woodland Hills,XY 12345   Telephone Number (555) 486-9002

FORM 5021 (Rev. 4)
1992

Any person who makes or causes to be made any knowingly false or fraudulent material statement or material representation for the purpose of obtaining or denying workers' compensation benefits or payments is guilty of a felony.

FIGURE 15-16 Doctor's First Report of Occupational Injury or Illness form, used in California.

PROCEDURE 15-1—cont'd

that the patient will be able to return to regular or modified work. List the year as four digits. Specify any work restrictions. It is very important for the insurance company to anticipate how long the patient will be off work so that money may be set aside for TD benefits, medical benefits, and, if necessary, PD benefits. If the estimated date of return to work should change after the form is submitted, a supplemental report or progress note should be sent to the insurance carrier to change the date of the disability.
Bottom of Form: If not preprinted, enter the physician's name and degree (for example, MD, DC), complete

address, state license number, federal tax identification number, and telephone number. Indicate the date the report is submitted. The insurance billing specialist should type reference initials in the lower left-hand corner of the form. This form must be signed in ink by the physician. Any carbon copies or photocopies must be signed in ink, too. A stamped signature will not be accepted because sometimes these cases go into litigation or are presented for a PD rating. Only those documents considered original health records are acceptable; this means that a handwritten signature by the attending physician is necessary.

KEY POINTS

This is a brief chapter review, or summary, of the key issues presented. To further enhance your knowledge of the technical subject matter, review the key terms and key abbreviations for this chapter by locating the meaning for each in the Glossary at the end of this book, which appears in a section before the Index.

1. Federal and state regulations require that employers have workers' compensation insurance coverage against on-the-job injury or illness and pay the premium for each of their employees.

2. Workers' compensation programs are not included under the definition of a health plan as identified in the HIPAA statutes.

3. Employees who work for federal agencies are covered by a number of federal workers' compensation laws.

4. The second-injury fund, also known as the *subsequent-injury fund*, was established to meet problems arising when an employee has a preexisting injury or condition and is subsequently injured at work.

5. Each state's legislation lists a waiting period (WP) that must elapse before income benefits are paid. However, medical and hospital care for industrial injuries is provided immediately.

6. Workers' compensation benefits consist of medical treatment, temporary disability (TD) indemnity, permanent disability (PD) indemnity, death benefits for survivors, and rehabilitation benefits.

7. A nondisability (ND) claim involves a minor injury in which the patient is seen by the physician but is able to continue to work.

8. A TD claim occurs when a worker has a work-related injury or illness and is unable to perform the duties of his or her occupation for a specific time.

9. A PD consists of an illness or injury (impairment of the normal use of a body part) that is expected to continue for the lifetime of the injured worker and prevents the person from performing the functions of his or her occupation, therefore impairing his or her earning capacity.

10. In a PD case, the physician's final report must contain the words "permanent and stationary" (P and S) so that the case can be adjudicated or rated, settlement can be reached (called a *compromise and release [C and R]*), and the case can be closed.

11. It is the responsibility of all individuals who handle workers' compensation cases to notify the insurance carrier of any fraudulent or suspicious situation.

12. Occupational Safety and Health Administration (OSHA) is the federal agency that regulates and investigates safety and health standards at work sites for the protection of employees.

13. Depositions from the physician and the injured individual by the attorney representing the workers' compensation insurance company are usually taken in PD cases.

14. The physician should file a lien in a workers' compensation case that has gone into third-party litigation or if there is a question whether the case is compensable.

15. A private health record should never be combined with an industrial case record because separate disclosure laws apply to each and the workers' compensation case may go to court.

16. The first report of an industrial injury must be completed by the employer and the physician and is required by law in most states.

17. A medical service order given to the employee by the employer authorizes the physician to treat the injured worker.

18. In industrial cases, all medical reports and forms are legal documents and must be signed in ink by the physician.

💻 **STUDENT ASSIGNMENT**

✔ Study Chapter 15.

✔ Answer the fill-in-the-blank, multiple-choice, and true/false review questions in the *Workbook* to reinforce the theory learned in this chapter and to help you prepare for a future test.

✔ Complete the assignments in the *Workbook* for hands-on experience in completing workers' compensation

insurance claim forms and reports as well as enhanced proficiency in procedural and diagnostic coding.

✔ Turn to the Glossary at the end of this text for a further understanding of the key terms and key abbreviations used in this chapter.

Disability Income Insurance and Disability Benefit Programs

Marilyn Takahashi Fordney and Karen Levein

OBJECTIVES

After reading this chapter, you should be able to:

1. Discuss the history of disability income insurance.
2. Describe benefits and exclusions contained in individual and group disability income insurance.
3. Name and describe federal disability benefit programs.
4. Differentiate between SSDI and SSI.
5. State eligibility requirements, benefits, and limitations of SSDI and SSI.
6. Explain disability benefit programs for disabled active military personnel, veterans, and their dependents.
7. Name states that have state disability insurance plans.
8. State eligibility requirements, benefits, and limitations of state disability plans.
9. Explain voluntary disability insurance plans.
10. Describe topics and contents of a medical report.
11. List guidelines for federal disability claims.
12. Explain procedures for state disability claims.
13. Recognize forms used for processing state disability plans.

KEY TERMS*

accidental death and dismemberment
Armed Services Disability
benefit period
Civil Service Retirement System
consultative examiner
cost-of-living adjustment
Disability Determination Services
disability income insurance
double indemnity
exclusions
Federal Employees Retirement System
future purchase option

guaranteed renewable
hearing
long-term disability insurance
noncancelable clause
partial disability
reconsideration
regional office
residual benefits
residual disability
short-term disability insurance
Social Security Administration
Social Security Disability Insurance program
State Disability Insurance
supplemental benefits

Supplemental Security Income
temporary disability
temporary disability insurance
total disability
Unemployment Compensation Disability
Veterans Affairs disability program
Veterans Affairs outpatient clinic card
voluntary disability insurance
waiting period
waiver of premium

---

*Some of the insurance terms presented in this list are italicized and may seem familiar from previous chapters. However, their meanings may have a slightly different connotation when referring to disability income insurance.

KEY ABBREVIATIONS

AIDS	FERS	SDI	TDI
CE	HIV	SSA	UCD
CSRS	OASDI	SSDI program	VA
DDS	RO	SSI	

> **Service to Patients**
>
> Efficiently and quickly completing the attending physician's portion of the disability insurance form assists the patient in obtaining disability income when he or she is unable to work because of a non–work-related illness or injury.

DISABILITY CLAIMS

Not everyone has disability insurance but when working with patients who do have it, one may encounter some interesting and unique accidents, injuries, or illnesses. After reading these extracts or direct quotations from disability insurance claim applications, one may ask, "How in the world could something like this happen?" The following gems show just how funny some situations can appear.

> **Describe How Your Disability Occurred**
>
> "A hernia from pulling cork out of bottle."
>
> "Put tire patch on Playtex girdle and it caused infection on right thigh."
>
> "While waving goodnight to friends, fell out a two-story window."
>
> "Back injury received from jumping off a ladder to escape being hit by a train."
>
> One victim graphically described an experience most of us have had: "Getting on a bus, the driver started before I was all on." Can you hear them asking at the hospital: "Was this your assigned seat?"
>
> Another victim stated: "I dislocated my shoulder swatting a fly." When asked, "Have you ever dislocated a shoulder at this sport?" he stated, "I have—I knocked over two table lamps, several high-balls, and skinned an elbow."
>
> Because this is near the end of the course on insurance billing and a great deal of information has been covered, one may feel a bit overwhelmed by the many rules and regulations and their ever-changing nature. This introduction was intended to add a bit of levity before one delves into the world of disability insurance.

This chapter introduces various types of **disability income insurance** plans as well as a number of disability benefit programs. The first topic, disability income insurance, is a form of insurance that provides periodic payments under certain conditions when the insured is unable to work because of illness, disease, or injury—not as a result of a work-related accident or condition.

The second section describes major programs administered by the United States (US) government related to industrial accidents and other disability benefit programs unrelated to work injuries.

The third part of the chapter deals with nonindustrial state disability programs administered in five states and Puerto Rico as well as **voluntary disability insurance** plans.

Guidelines for federal, state, individual, and group disability claim procedures are presented at the end of the chapter.

HISTORY

Before the late 1800s, disability income insurance provided only accident protection. Some life insurance contracts had disability income riders attached to them that offered limited benefits. In the early 1880s, insurance companies began selling disability income policies that offered coverage for accident and illness. The Paul Revere Life Insurance Company introduced the first "noncancelable" disability income policy in the early 1900s. The **noncancelable clause** guaranteed that the contract would be in force for a certain period of time and the premium would not be increased. By 1956, Congress had enacted legislation under the Social Security program that provided disability income protection to disabled individuals older than 50 years of age. This program was expanded in 1965 to cover workers without regard to age as long as certain eligibility standards were met.

Today, disability income insurance is available from private insurance companies (individual policies) and employer-sponsored plans (group policies). Government-funded and state benefit programs are also available for disabled persons. All of these plans and programs are discussed in this chapter, along with the role of the insurance billing specialist in dealing with this type of insurance.

DISABILITY INCOME INSURANCE

Individual

Individual disability income insurance is coverage that provides a specific monthly or weekly income when a person becomes unable to work, temporarily or totally, because of an illness or injury. Disability income policies do not provide medical expense benefits. The disability cannot be work related. As explained in Chapter 15, an illness or accident that is work related is covered by workers' compensation insurance.

For individuals who are self-employed, this insurance is particularly important because a business could not meet its financial obligations if the owner became injured or too ill to work. For example, if an individual is self-employed with a home-based business, repetitive stress injuries (RSIs) would not allow that individual to use the computer for several months. The main purpose of these policies is to provide some benefits while the person is unable to work. To collect benefits, the individual must meet the policy's criteria of what constitutes partial, temporary, or **total disability.** These policies terminate when the individual retires or reaches a certain age, usually 65 years.

Waiting Period

The period from the beginning of disability to receiving the first payment of benefits is called an *elimination period* or **waiting period (WP).** During this initial period, a disabled individual is not eligible to receive benefits even though he or she is unable to work.

Benefit Period

A **benefit period** is the maximum amount of time that benefits will be paid to the injured or ill person for the disability (for example, 2 years, 5 years, to age 65, or lifetime).

Benefits

Compensation paid to the insured disabled person is called *indemnity benefits* and can be received daily, weekly, monthly, or semiannually, depending on the policy. Premiums and benefits depend on several risk factors, such as age, gender, health history and physical state, income, and occupational duties. Some policies include residual or **partial disability** income benefits. Benefits are not taxable if premiums are paid by the individual.

Residual benefits pay a partial benefit when the insured is not totally disabled. If one becomes partially disabled or can work only part time or in a limited capacity, the residual benefits make up the difference between what an individual can earn at present and what he or she would have earned working full time.

Supplemental benefits may consist of insurance provisions that will increase monthly indemnity, such as

a **future purchase option** or a **cost-of-living adjustment.** Cost-of-living adjustment (COLA) means to increase monthly benefits in disability income benefit, pension benefit, or life income benefit to make up for a change in the cost of living. This is also known as future purchase option or cost-of-living rider. Provisions also distribute a percentage of the policy premiums if an individual keeps a policy in force for 5 or 10 years or does not file any claims.

An **accidental death and dismemberment** benefit is written into some contracts. This offers the insured person protection when loss of sight or loss of limb occurs. In some policies (for example, life insurance), a special provision known as **double indemnity** applies if an unintended, unexpected, and unforeseeable accident results in death. This feature provides for twice the face amount of the policy to be paid if death results from accidental causes.

Types of Disability

A disability may be partial, temporary, or total. There is no standard definition for total disability and the definition stated in each disability income policy varies. For example, a liberal definition might read as follows: "The insured must be unable to perform the major duties of his or her specific occupation." Social Security has a restrictive definition presented later in this chapter.

The terms **residual disability** and *partial disability* are defined as occurring "when an illness or injury prevents an insured person from performing one or more of the functions of his or her regular job"—in other words, when a person cannot perform all of his or her job duties.

Temporary disability (TD) exists when a person cannot perform all of the functions of his or her regular job for a limited period of time.

Clauses

With a **guaranteed renewable** policy, the insurer is required to renew the policy as long as premium payments are made for a specified number of years or to a specified age, such as 60, 65, or 70 years, or for life. However, the premium may be increased when it is renewed. When the policy has a noncancelable clause, the premium cannot be increased.

If a **waiver of premium** is included in the insurance contract, the policy pays all premiums while the employee is disabled; the employee does not have to pay. Usually, this provision is used as a total and permanent disability benefit and may be available in certain other cases.

Exclusions

Exclusions are provisions written into the insurance contract denying coverage or limiting the scope of coverage. Examples are preexisting conditions; disability because of war, riot, self-inflicted injury, or attempted suicide; mental or nervous conditions; disability while legally intoxicated or under the influence of narcotics (unless prescribed by a licensed physician); conditions arising from normal pregnancy; conditions arising during the act of committing a felony; or if benefits are being received under workers' compensation or a government program. The phrase "legally intoxicated" means intoxication in an individual whose blood alcohol level, when tested, exceeds limits set by state law.

Acquired Immunodeficiency Syndrome and Human Immunodeficiency Virus Infection

States have statutes governing questions that can and cannot be asked on insurance application forms about acquired immunodeficiency syndrome (AIDS) and human immunodeficiency virus (HIV) testing; therefore each state has developed its own forms. If a private insurance company wishes to test an applicant, a consent or notice form, including acceptance of pretest and posttest counseling, must be signed.

Group

Some employers elect to offer group disability income insurance as a fringe benefit. These contracts are drawn up between the insurer and employer. Premiums may be paid by the employer with or without contributions from the employee. Employees hold certificates of insurance and are covered under the employer's policy; therefore they are not called policyholders. When the employee leaves the company, the insurance terminates unless the employee is disabled. A few group policies allow conversion to a limited benefit individual policy.

Benefits

Benefits vary from one plan to another but are usually for **short-term disability insurance** (13 weeks to 24 months) or **long-term disability insurance** (to age 65). To qualify for benefits, an individual must be unable to perform the major duties of his or her occupation during the initial period of disability (for example, the first 2 years). Benefits cease when the employee returns to work, even part time. However, some of these policies offer the worker partial disability income benefits to motivate a disabled individual to return to work on a part-time basis. Monthly benefits are usually paid directly to the employee and are taxable if the employee is not making any contribution toward the premiums.

Exclusions

Disabilities commonly excluded from coverage include those seen in individual disability income insurance policies, as previously described.

FEDERAL DISABILITY PROGRAMS

Workers' Compensation

The federal government has a number of programs that cover workers from loss of income because of work-related disability. These programs are mentioned in Chapter 15 because work-related disabilities fall under workers' compensation laws. When an individual is eligible under more than one program, coordination of benefits is used so that a worker cannot receive benefits that result in an amount greater than what the person receives when working. Coordination of benefits is a provision preventing double payment for expenses by making one of the programs the primary payer and ensuring that no more than 100% of the costs are covered.

Disability Benefit Programs

The government's major disability programs are as follows:
- **Social Security Disability Insurance (SSDI) program**
- **Supplemental Security Income (SSI)**
- **Civil Service Retirement System (CSRS)**
- **Federal Employees Retirement System (FERS)**
- **Armed Services Disability**
- **Veterans Affairs (VA) disability program**

The **Social Security Administration (SSA)** manages two programs that pay monthly disability benefits to people younger than age 65 who cannot work for at least 1 year because of a severe disability: SSDI and SSI. Medical requirements are the same for both programs.

Social Security Disability Insurance Program

Background. In 1935, the Social Security Act, the Old Age, Survivors, Health and Disability Insurance (OASHDI) Program, was enacted. It is now referred to as OASDI. It provided benefits for death, retirement, disability, and medical care. In 1956, Congress established a program for long-term disability known as *Social Security Disability Insurance (SSDI)* under Title II of the Social Security Act. This is an entitlement (not welfare) program that provides monthly benefits to workers and those self-employed who meet certain conditions.

Disability Definition. *Disability* under Social Security has a strict definition: "inability to engage in any substantial gainful activity by reason of any medically determinable physical or mental impairment which can be expected to result in death or which has lasted or can be expected to last for a continuous period of not less than 12 months."

Eligibility. The following is a list of individuals who meet eligibility requirements for SSDI:

- Disabled workers younger than age 65 years and their families
- Individuals who become disabled before age 22 years, if a parent (or in certain cases, a grandparent) who is covered under Social Security retires, becomes disabled, or dies
- Disabled widows or widowers, age 50 years or older, if the deceased spouse worked at least 10 years under Social Security
- Disabled surviving divorced spouses older than age 50 years, if the ex-spouse was married to the disabled person for at least 10 years
- Blind workers whose vision in the better eye cannot be corrected to better than 20/200 or whose visual field in the better eye, even with corrective lenses, is 20 degrees or less

Workers must be fully insured in accordance with standards set by the SSA in terms of age, number of quarters worked, and amount of wages earned per quarter. The processing of eligibility application forms may take up to 2 months.

Benefits. Monthly benefits are paid to qualified individuals. After 24 months of disability payments, the disabled individual also becomes eligible for Medicare. The benefits convert to retirement benefits when an individual reaches age 65.

Supplemental Security Income

Eligibility. The Supplemental Security Income (SSI) program is under Title XVI of the Social Security Act and provides disability payments to people (adults and children) with limited income and few resources. No prior employment is necessary. Many SSI recipients also qualify for Medicaid, a state assistance program. The following individuals may qualify for SSI disability payments:

- Disabled persons younger than 65 years who have limited income and resources
- Disabled children younger than age 18 years, if the disability compares in severity with one that would prevent an adult from working and has lasted or is expected to last at least 12 months or result in death
- Blind adults or children who have a visual acuity no better than 20/100 or have a visual field of 20 degrees or less in the better eye, with the use of corrective lenses

Disability Determination Process. To establish disability under SSDI or SSI, an individual calls or visits any Social Security office and completes application forms with the help of a social worker. This triggers a determination process. A physician may be involved in the determination process in one of three ways: (1) as a treating source who provides medical evidence on behalf of his or her patient, (2) as a **consultative examiner (CE)** who is paid a fee and examines or tests the applicant, or (3) as a full- or part-time medical or psychologic consultant reviewing claims for a state or **regional office (RO).**

In addition to a medical report from one of these sources, other criteria taken into consideration are the individual's age and vocational and educational factors that may contribute to the person's ability to work. It is possible that a person may be eligible for disability payments under one government program and not be eligible under Social Security because the rules differ. The SSA may use reports that an applicant has from another agency to determine whether the person is eligible for Social Security disability payments. Many SSA state agencies have a division known as **Disability Determination Services (DDS).** Determination of disability is made by a DDS team composed of a physician or psychologist and disability examiner (DE), not by the applicant's physician.

Appeals Evaluation Process. If a claimant does not agree with the determination of disability, the following four-level appeals process is available:

1. A **reconsideration,** which is a complete review of the claim by a medical or psychologic consultant or disability examiner team that did not take part in the original disability determination.
2. A **hearing** before an administrative law judge who had no part in the initial or reconsideration determinations of the claim. The hearing is held within 75 miles of the claimant's home. The claimant and his or her representative are permitted to present their case in person and present a written statement. They are also permitted to review information the judge will use to make a decision and question any witnesses.
3. A review by the Appeals Council, which considers all requests for review but may deny a request if it believes that the decision by the administrative law judge was correct. If the Appeals Council decides that the case should be reviewed, it will make a decision on the case or return it to an administrative law judge for further review.
4. A review by the federal court for which the claimant may file an action where he or she resides.

Disability cases are reviewed from time to time to be sure that the individuals are still disabled. The frequency depends on the nature and severity of the impairment, the likelihood of improvement, rehabilitation, ability to work, and so on.

Benefits. Social Security disability programs are designed to give long-term protection and benefits to individuals totally disabled who are unable to do any type of work in the national economy. In contrast, short-term disability may be provided through workers' compensation, insurance, savings, and investments.

Work Incentives. Special rules allow disabled or blind people presently receiving Social Security or SSI to work and still receive monthly benefits as well as Medicare or Medicaid (for example, an SSDI recipient who is given a 90-day trial of work and at the end of that time either continues to work and loses SSDI coverage or leaves the temporary employment and remains on SSDI). A limit exists as to how much the person can earn in a calendar year. These are referred to as "work incentives"; the rules are different for Social Security beneficiaries and SSI recipients. Occasionally a person may be working and receiving SSDI benefits, as illustrated by the earlier example.

Civil Service and Federal Employees Retirement Systems

Background. There are two types of federal retirement, Civil Service Retirement System (CSRS) and Federal Employees Retirement System (FERS). CSRS began in 1920, until a second system, FERS, was introduced in 1984. People who began working for the federal government in 1984 or later are covered by FERS instead of CSRS. Some workers who had been covered by the CSRS program changed to the FERS program when it became available.

Eligibility. Federal employees who work in civil service fall under the CSRS. This system has provisions for those who become totally disabled. This program is a combination of federal disability and Social Security disability. Both portions of the program must be applied for by the worker. The disability cannot be work related and 5 years of service is necessary before benefits are payable. Eighteen months of service is necessary under the FERS.

Benefits. Those who qualify are entitled to benefits that are payable for life. For example, an individual who works for the Internal Revenue Service (IRS) performing clerical and filing job duties is involved in an automobile accident on the weekend. The head injuries are so severe that the person is unable to return to gainful employment at any job. He or she could apply for benefits under either CSRS or FERS, depending on his or her eligibility status.

Armed Services Disability

Eligibility. Individuals covered under this program must be members of the armed services on active duty who suffer a disability or illness.

Benefits. Monthly benefits are payable for life if a disability occurs or is aggravated while the individual is serving in the military service. Benefit amounts are based on years of service, base pay, and severity of disability. This is also subject to review.

Veterans Affairs Disability

Eligibility. The VA is authorized by law to provide a wide range of benefits to both those who have served their country in the armed forces and those individuals' dependents. If a veteran who is honorably discharged files a claim for a service-connected disability within 1 year of sustaining that injury, he or she is eligible for outpatient treatment. Veterans with non–service-connected disabilities who are in receipt of housebound or aid-in-attendance benefits are eligible for treatment from a private physician if they are unable to travel to a VA facility because of geographic inaccessibility. Their identification card, benefits, and claims procedures are identical to those of veterans with service-connected disabilities who receive outpatient medical care.

Benefits. A general list of veterans' medical benefits follows below. Each benefit requires that certain criteria be met. These criteria are ever-changing and are not mentioned here. A complete up-to-date booklet listing all benefits is available.*

- Hospital care in a VA hospital
- Nursing home care in a VA facility
- Domiciliary care
- Outpatient medical treatment at a VA facility or by a private physician
- Emergency treatment in a hospital for a service-connected condition
- Prescription drugs and medications issued by a VA pharmacy or other participating pharmacy (only bona fide emergency prescriptions can be filled by a private pharmacy)
- Certain medical equipment, such as oxygen and prosthetics
- Travel expenses when receiving VA medical care
- Outpatient dental treatment (if the veteran files a claim within 90 days from the date that he or she was discharged from the service)
- Treatment for Agent Orange or nuclear radiation exposure
- Alcohol and drug dependence outpatient care
- Readjustment counseling services

---

*The annually published booklet, *Federal Benefits for Veterans, Dependents and Survivors,* may be obtained for a small fee from the US Government Printing Office: http://bookstore.gpo.gov.

The physician must accept what the VA pays as payment in full for treatment of a service-connected disability and cannot bill the patient for any additional charges, even if there is a balance after the VA pays the claim. If the treatment is likely to cost more than $40 per month, the physician must obtain prior authorization from the nearest VA facility. A separate financial accounting record card must be prepared for VA benefits if the physician is also treating the patient for ailments other than a service-connected disability. Any professional service that is not related to a service-connected disability must be paid for by the veteran out of his or her own pocket. For example, a Vietnam veteran who has a long history of stump pain at the site of an amputation or suffers from old shrapnel wounds as the result of stepping on a land mine during active duty is seen and treated for acute gastroenteritis. The VA disability benefits do not apply to the episode of acute gastroenteritis and the veteran must personally pay for professional services related to that diagnosis.

Veterans with non–service-connected disabilities may have copayments when they seek treatment. For example, individuals on Medicare may be responsible for the deductible for the first 90 days of care during any 365-day period. For each additional 90 days of hospital care, the patient is charged half of the Medicare deductible, $10 a day for hospital care, and $5 a day for VA nursing home care. For outpatient care, the copayment is 20% of the cost of an average outpatient visit.

Outpatient Treatment. Veterans eligible for outpatient treatment may obtain outpatient medical care by checking in with the **Veterans Affairs outpatient clinic card** (Figure 16-1) issued since May 2014. Usually a veteran seeks care at the nearest VA outpatient clinic. However, when a VA facility is not within reasonable distance, when the veteran is too ill to travel to the nearest

location, or when the condition needs prompt attention, the veteran can apply for and be granted medical care by a private physician through the Non-VA Medical Care Program formerly called Home Town Care Program. This program permits medical care provided in the community that is paid by the Department of Veterans Affairs. The VA outpatient clinic must be notified within 15 days of the treatment rendered. In such cases, the treating physician must submit evidence of medical necessity (for example, detailed justification on the invoice) to the VA outpatient clinic. Form 10-583, Claim for Payment of Cost of Unauthorized Medical Services (Figure 16-2), generally used for hospital emergency care, can also be used for professional care if the doctor is billing after the 15-day period has elapsed. Some patients have both Medicare and medical coverage from the VA. In such cases, Medicare is not secondary to the VA and the VA is not secondary to Medicare. The claim is to be sent where specified by the patient. The claim can be sent to Medicare, where, if the claim is processed, the patient must satisfy his or her contractual requirement to pay any deductible and copayment amounts. If the patient asks that the claim be sent to the VA instead of Medicare, the claim is processed and any payments issued are considered as payment in full. Many veterans prefer to have the claim sent to the VA.

Veterans Affairs Installations. For information on veterans' benefits or assistance in locating VA installations, go to the Evolve website http://evolve.elsevier.com/Fordney/handbook for a link to the VA home website.

STATE DISABILITY INSURANCE

Background

In 1944, Rhode Island began a **State Disability Insurance (SDI)** program that proved successful. This form

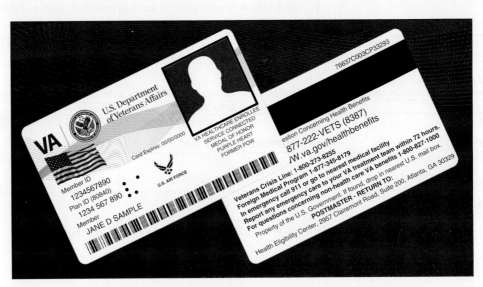

FIGURE 16-1 Veterans Health Identification Card (VHIC).

NOTE: Instructions are written for a multi-part form. Print additional copies as necessary.

OMB No: 2900-0080
Estimated Burden: 15 min.

 Department of Veterans Affairs

CLAIM FOR PAYMENT OF COST OF UNAUTHORIZED MEDICAL SERVICES

The Paperwork Reduction Act of 1995 requires us to notify you that this information collection is in accordance with the clearance requirements of section 3507 of the Paperwork Reduction Act of 1995. We may not conduct or sponsor, and you are not required to respond to, a collection of information unless it displays a valid OMB number. We anticipate that the time expended by all individuals who must complete this form will average 15 minutes. This includes the time it will take to read instructions, gather the necessary facts and fill out the form. Comments regarding this burden estimate or any other aspect of this collection, including suggestions for reducing the burden, may be addressed by calling the Health Benefits Contact Center at 1-877-222-8387.

PRIVACY ACT INFORMATION: The information requested on this form is solicited under authority of Title 38, United States Code, "Veterans Benefits," and will be used to assist us in determining your entitlement to reimbursement for services rendered. It will not be used for any other purpose. Disclosure is voluntary. However, failure to furnish the information will result in our inability to process your claim. Failure to furnish this information will have no adverse effect on any other benefit to which you may be entitled. This form and relevant documents need to be sent to the VA Medical Facility where the Veteran is enrolled for medical care

PART I

1A. VETERAN'S NAME (Last, first, middle initial) (This is a mandatory field.)	1B. CLAIM NUMBER	1C. SOCIAL SECURITY NUMBER (Mandatory field.)
Thornberg, Joey T.	C-	421xx4182

1D. VETERAN'S ADDRESS (Include complete ZIP Code)
4628 Image St., Woodland Hills, XY 12345-0001

2A. NAME AND ADDRESS OF PERSON, FIRM OR INSTITUTION MAKING CLAIM (Leave blank if same as above) Gerald Practon, MD 4567 Broad Ave., Woodland Hills, XY 12345-1290	2B. SOCIAL SECURITY NO. OR EMPLOYEE IDENTIFICATION NO.

3. STATEMENT OF CIRCUMSTANCES UNDER WHICH THE SERVICES WERE RENDERED (Include diagnosis, symptoms, whether emergency existed, and reason VA facilities were not used)

Patient fell on sidewalk of home and suffered traumatic injury to right arm.
Symptoms: Localized pain, swelling and bruising of right arm near elbow.
AP and lateral x-rays of right elbow show anterior dislocation of right radius. Negative for fracture.
Medical care rendered in Emergency Dept. at College Hospital (99282)
Pt. unable to go to VA facility as this was 60 miles from patient's residence.
Treatment of closed elbow dislocation without anesthesia (23400)
Diagnosis: Anterior closed dislocation right radius (S32.014A)

4. AMOUNT CLAIMED $237.02	Attach bills or receipts showing services furnished, dates and charges

5. COMPLETE A OR B AS APPROPRIATE

A. Amount charged does not exceed that charged the general public for similar services. Payment has not been received.	B. I certify that the amount claimed has been paid and reimbursement has not been received.

Gerald Practon, M.D. SIGNATURE AND TITLE OF PROVIDER OF SERVICE AND DATE	05/XX/20XX (mm/dd/yyyy)	 SIGNATURE OF VETERAN OR REPRESENTATIVE AND DATE	(mm/dd/yyyy)

PART II - FOR VETERANS AFFAIRS USE ONLY

6. ACTION ☐ APPROVED $ ☐ DISAPPROVED	CLAIM MEETS THE REQUIREMENT OF VA REGULATION ☐ 6080 ☐ 6081

7. SIGNATURE OF CHIEF, MEDICAL ADMINISTRATION SERVICE	8. DATE	9. ADMINISTRATIVE VOUCHER NUMBER

VA FORM
DEC 2010 **10-583**

FIGURE 16-2 Veterans Affairs Form 10-583, Claim for Payment of Cost of Unauthorized Medical Services.

of insurance is part of an employment security program that provides temporary cash benefits for workers suffering a wage loss because of off-the-job illness or injury. It can be referred to as **Unemployment Compensation Disability (UCD)** or **temporary disability insurance (TDI)**. California became the second state to add nonindustrial disability coverage to the Social Security protection afforded to its citizens by appending Article 10 to the Unemployment Insurance Act. This became law on May 21, 1946; when the legislation took effect on December 1, 1946, this article diverted the 1% tax formerly paid by workers for unemployment insurance to a disability insurance fund. New York and New Jersey soon followed with similar programs. Two decades later, in 1969, Puerto Rico and Hawaii passed nonindustrial disability insurance laws.

Some accidents that occur are quite serious at the time but can appear rather humorous on review.

Unique Accident

The patient was under the kitchen sink repairing a leak when the family cat came along, watched for a while, then playfully—but painfully—reached up and clawed him. Startled, the man threw his head back, cracked it on the bottom of the sink, and was knocked out cold. He came to as he was being carried out on a stretcher and explained to the attendants what had happened. One stretcher bearer laughed so hard that he relaxed his hold and the patient fell to the ground and broke his arm.

State Programs

Nonindustrial disability insurance programs existed in only five states and Puerto Rico as of 2010. The law is known by a different name in each area.

Funding

To fund SDI, a small percentage of wages is deducted from employees' paychecks each month, or the employer may elect to pay all or part of the cost of the plan as a fringe benefit for employees. The money is then sent in quarterly installments to the state and put in a special fund.

Eligibility

To receive SDI benefits, an employee must meet the following criteria:
- Employed full or part time or actively looking for work when disability begins
- Suffering a loss of wages because of disability
- Eligible for benefits, depending on the amount withheld during a previous period before disability began

- Under the care and treatment of a physician who certifies that the employee is disabled
- Disabled at least 7 calendar days
- Filing a claim within the time limit

If the worker was employed at the time of disability, benefits are not subject to federal income tax. An employee who retires is no longer eligible for the insurance. A worker may file a claim with the state seeking exemption from program participation on religious grounds.

Types of workers not covered are employees of school districts, community college districts, and churches; state workers; federal employees; interstate railroad workers; employees of nonprofit organizations; and domestic workers.

Benefits

Weekly benefits are determined by the wages earned in a base period or based on a percentage of average weekly wages (Table 16-1). Benefits begin after the seventh consecutive day of disability. There is no provision under the law for hospital or other medical benefits.

Limited Benefits

In some states, a patient may qualify for benefits if he or she is a resident of an approved alcoholic recovery facility or an approved drug-free residential facility.

Reduced Benefits

An individual may be entitled to partial benefits if he or she is receiving certain types of income, such as the following:
- Sick leave
- Vacation
- Wages paid by employer
- Insurance settlement for the disability
- Workers' compensation benefits
- Unemployment benefits

Time Limits

A claim for SDI should be filed within the time limit of the state laws (see Table 16-1). There is usually a grace period of 7 or 8 days after the deadline. After the claim is approved, basic benefits become payable after the seventh day of disability. A person may continue to draw disability insurance for a maximum of 26 weeks in Hawaii, New Jersey, New York, and Puerto Rico; 30 weeks in Rhode Island; and 52 weeks in California on the same illness or injury or overlapping disabilities. An employee is also

| | | **MAXIMUM BENEFIT** | **TIME LIMIT FOR** | **2014 DEDUCTIONS FROM** | |
STATE	**NAME OF STATE LAW**	**PERIOD (WEEKS)**	**FILING CLAIMS**	**SALARY (%)**	**BENEFITS**
California	California Unemployment Insurance Code	52	49 days from disability	1.0 of first $100,880 ($1008.80)	55% of average weekly earnings in highest quarter of base period
Hawaii	Temporary Disability Insurance Law	26	90 days from disability	0.5 paid by the employee. Up to half of plan costs paid by the employer.	Based on 58% of average weekly wage
New Jersey	Temporary Disability Benefits Law	26	30 days from disability	0.38 of first $31.500 of annual earnings paid by employee. Employer pays 0.1 to 0.75 of the first $31.500 of annual earnings.	66.67% based on average weekly wage (max $595/week)
New York	Disability Benefits Law	26	30 days from disability	0.5 of the first $120 (max 60 cents/week). Employer pays balance of plan costs.	Based on 50% of average weekly wage (max $170/week)
Puerto Rico	Disability Benefits Act	26	3 months from disability	0.6 of first $9000 of annual earnings shared by employer and employee	Based on 65% of weekly earnings
Rhode Island	Temporary Disability Insurance Act	30	1 year from disability	1.2 of first $62,700 of annual earnings	4.62% of total high base period quarter wages

Table 16-1   State Disability Information Summary

entitled to disability benefits 15 days after recovery from a previous disability or illness. For example, if a patient is discharged by the physician to return to work and is on the job 15 calendar days and then becomes ill with the same ailment, he or she may file a new claim.

Medical Examinations

The claimant may be required to submit to an examination or examinations by an independent medical examiner to determine any mental or physical disability. Fees for such examinations are paid by the state department that handles disability insurance. Code 99450 for billing these medical examinations may be found in the Special Evaluation and Management Services section of Current Procedural Terminology (CPT).

Restrictions

Disability insurance has many restrictions. A few of the major situations in which a claim could be denied are listed here.

1. Conditions covered by workers' compensation unless the rate is less than the disability insurance rate. In that case, the state pays the difference between the two rates.
2. Applicants receiving unemployment insurance benefits that are more than a certain specified amount. *Exception:* If the applicant is on unemployment insurance and then becomes ill or injured, he or she is put on TDI until able to go on a job interview.

3. Disabilities beginning during a trade dispute. If an employee is on strike and is injured while walking a picket line, he or she is considered to still be employed. If injured while picketing, it may be considered workers' compensation. However, if the union is on strike and an individual member remains at home and then becomes ill or injured, he or she can claim disability and will receive benefits.
4. Confinement by court order or certification in a public or private institution as an alcoholic, drug addict, or sexual psychopath.
5. When the pursuit of legal custody of a child is the cause of inability to work.
6. When the employing company has a voluntary disability plan and is not paying into a state fund.
7. Religious exemption certificate on file by employee or company with no payment being made into a state fund.
8. Pregnancy-related disability, unless the pregnancy is complicated (for example, cases in which the patient has diabetes, varicose veins, ectopic pregnancy, or cesarean section). *Exceptions:* California, Hawaii, New Jersey, and Rhode Island have maternity benefits that may be applied for at the time the physician tells the patient to stop working.

VOLUNTARY DISABILITY INSURANCE

Persons residing and working in states that do not have SDI programs may elect to contact a local private insurance carrier to arrange for coverage under a voluntary disability insurance plan. If these persons become ill or disabled, they receive a fixed weekly or monthly income, usually for approximately 6 months. If the disability or illness is permanent and the individual is unable to return to work, there is sometimes a small monthly income for the duration of the person's life. Some of the state laws provide that a "voluntary plan" may be adopted instead of the "state plan" if a majority of company employees consent to private coverage.

CLAIMS SUBMISSION GUIDELINES

Disability Income Claims

When the insurance billing specialist is handling disability income claim forms, he or she should note that the insured (claimant) is responsible for notifying the insurance company of the disability. A proof of loss form is completed to establish disability.

The necessary facts are as follows:
- Date on which the disability occurred
- Date on which the disabled person is expected to be well enough to return to work
- Description of how the disability occurred
- Name of treating physician
- Explanation of how the disability prevents the insured person from working

The report must show that the patient's disability meets the policy's definition of disability or benefits will be denied. Because the definition of disability varies among policies, the critical issues are the content and wording on the claim form.

A portion of this form is usually completed by the attending physician. The following data are necessary:
- Medical history
- Date on which patient became disabled
- Subjective symptoms (patient's own words about his or her chief complaints)
- Objective findings on physical examination (for example, rashes, lacerations, abrasions, or contusions)
- Severity of the illness or injury (range-of-motion [ROM] tests)
- Photocopies of laboratory tests, x-ray studies, or hospital discharge report
- Medication
- Treatment dates
- Diagnosis
- Prognosis (outcome of the disease or injury)
- Names of any other treating physician
- Date on which the patient is expected to return to work
- Description of job duties and patient's ability to perform work

Providing this information helps to verify the disability. In some cases, the physician may wish to dictate a medical report and attach it to the claim form instead of completing a portion of the form. The insurance billing specialist must be prepared to extract data from source documents, such as medical and financial records, to complete the claim form. In such situations, the physician should be asked to read the information carefully before signing the document. The patient should always be asked to sign an authorization form to release medical information. Reasons for denial of benefits often include improper choice of words or inadequate medical information.

The insurance company may request information from other places, such as employer's records, employee's wage statements or tax forms, or the patient's health records from the attending physician, to justify payment of benefits. A company representative may interview the insured if conflicting information exists.

If disability continues, additional claim forms should be completed monthly or more frequently by the insured and attending physician. Other sources of information may be requested; for example, records from medical specialists or Social Security records.

If the validity of the case is in question, an independent medical examiner may be asked by the insurance company to examine the disabled individual. If the claimant neglects to return claim forms, refuses telephone calls, misses appointments, or engages in questionable activities, the insurance company will discreetly engage in surveillance of the insured through the services of a professional investigation firm.

Federal Disability Claims

The SSA division called *Disability Determination Services (DDS)* has a teledictation service so that the physician or psychologist can dictate the medical report over the telephone instead of completing a medical report form. The service is available at any time, including nights and weekends. A typed transcript is sent to the physician to review, sign, and return to the SSA state agency or a report may be typed on the physician's stationery. The physician may photocopy relevant portions of the patient's chart and submit that information but it should be legible. An authorization signed by the patient to release information should be on file. Copies of consultation reports and hospital summaries are also helpful. By law, only data no more than 1 year old are allowed.

A medical report must include the following:
- Relevant medical history, past history, social history, and family history.
- Subjective complaints (patient's symptoms).

- Objective findings on physical examination (for example, results of physical or mental status examination, blood pressure).
- Laboratory and x-ray findings.
- Diagnostic studies (for example, treadmill tests, pulmonary function tests, and electrocardiogram [ECG] tracings).
- Diagnosis (statement of disease or injury based on signs and symptoms).
- Treatment prescribed, with patient's response and prognosis.
- Medical prognosis about disability based on medical findings. A description of the individual's ability to perform work-related activities, such as standing, sitting, lifting, carrying, walking, handling objects, hearing, speaking, and traveling, is necessary. For cases of mental impairment, the statement should present the individual's capacity for understanding and remembering, sustained concentration and persistence, social interaction, and adaptation.

Veterans Affairs Disability Outpatient Clinic Claims

The processing of invoices from private physicians is a somewhat lengthy procedure as required by VA regulations and involves several steps. To keep the delay in payment to a minimum, private physicians are urged to bill the VA monthly. To ensure prompt processing, invoices should contain the following information:

- Patient's name as shown on the ID card, VA Form 10-1174 (see Figure 16-1).
- Patient's Social Security number.
- Condition treated, shown on every invoice, because this is the basis for approval of payment.
- Diagnosis being treated must be listed on the ID card or authorized by the statement "for any condition." Abstract the diagnosis exactly as it is stated on the ID card.
- Treatment given and dates rendered.
- Physician's usual and customary fee for services rendered.
- Name and address of private physician and his or her Social Security or Federal Taxpayer ID number. If the ID number is assigned to a group and the physician wants to be paid individually, the VA outpatient clinic must be so advised.

Private physicians as well as veterans are urged to read the instructions on the ID card carefully. This is sometimes neglected and can lead to misunderstanding.

If the physician does not wish to bill the VA outpatient clinic, the patient can pay the physician and then be reimbursed but the veteran must carefully follow the instructions on the back of the VA outpatient clinic card.

State Disability Claims

Residents of a state that provides state disability benefits may call or write to the nearest office that handles SDI to obtain a claim form and insurance pamphlet. See the state disability websites for detailed information about each state's benefits, claim procedures, and claim forms.

In some states, the claim form is in three parts and must be completed by the claimant, employer, and physician. In other states, the form is in two parts and is completed by the claimant and physician (Figures 16-3 and 16-4). In either instance, the case must be substantiated by a physician before the applicant may begin receiving benefits. All information from the SDI office should be read carefully and the directions followed precisely. The data requested should be provided and the physician and patient should sign the forms. The form should be submitted within the stated time limits.

After the claim has been completed by all parties concerned, it is submitted to the nearest local office for processing. The most important items on the claim form are the following:

- The claimant's Social Security number; without it the claim cannot be researched properly to establish wages earned in the base period.
- The first day on which the patient was too sick to perform all of his or her regular work duties (item 3). This cannot be the same day the patient worked, even if the patient went home sick.
- The last day the patient worked (item 4). List the last day on which the patient worked even if for only part of the day.

NOTE: The two dates listed in items 3 and 4 cannot be the same; for example, if the patient went home sick on October 4, that would be considered the last day worked; October 5 would be the first day the patient was unable to work.

California has been selected as the model state for examples of the different forms used in the processing of disability insurance. To establish a claim, the Claim for Disability Insurance Benefits, Form DE 2501, must be completed by both the patient (see Figure 16-3) and the attending physician (see Figure 16-4). If an extension of disability is necessary, the Physician/Practitioner's Supplementary Certificate, Form DE 2525XX, must be completed by the physician (Figure 16-5). This accompanies the last check issued to the patient. For additional medical information that might be necessary, Forms DE 2547 and DE 2547A are sometimes sent to the attending physician for completion (Figures 16-6 and 16-7).

EDD Employment
Development
Department
State of California

Claim for Disability Insurance (DI) Benefits

250104121

Health Insurance Portability and Accountability Act (HIPAA) Authorization

Claimant Social Security Number

Claimant Name   (First)   (MI)   (Last)

I authorize

(Person/Organization providing the information) to furnish and disclose all my health information and to allow inspection of and provide copies of any medical, vocational rehabilitation, and billing records concerning my disability for which this claim is filed that are within their knowledge to the following employees of the California Employment Development Department (EDD): Disability Insurance Branch examiners, their direct supervisors/managers and any other EDD employee who may have a need to access this information in order to process my claim and/or determine eligibility for State Disability Insurance benefits.

I understand that EDD is not a health plan or health care provider, so the information released to EDD may no longer be protected by federal privacy regulations. (45 CFR Section 164.508(c)(2)(iii)). EDD may disclose information as authorized by the California Unemployment Insurance Code.

I agree that photocopies of this authorization shall be as valid as the original.

I understand I have the right to revoke this authorization by sending written notification stopping this authorization to EDD, DI Branch MIC 29, PO Box 826880, Sacramento, CA 94280. The authorization will stop on the date my request is received. I understand that the consequences for my revoking this authorization may result in denial of further State Disability Insurance benefits.

I understand that, unless revoked by me in writing, this authorization is valid for fifteen years from the date received by EDD or the effective date of the claim, whichever is later. I understand that I may not revoke this authorization to avoid prosecution or to prevent EDD's recovery of monies to which it is legally entitled.

I understand that I am signing this authorization voluntarily and that payment or eligibility for my benefits will be affected if I do not sign this authorization. The consequences for my refusal to sign this authorization may result in an incomplete claim form that cannot be processed for payment of State Disability Insurance benefits.

I understand I have the right to receive a copy of this authorization.

Claimant Signature (Do Not Print)

Date Signed
M M D D Y Y Y Y

DE 2501 Rev. 78 (4-12)

CU

FIGURE 16-3 Form DE 2501, Claim for Disability Insurance (DI) Benefits. The first four pages of this seven-page form are completed by the claimant.

Continued

Your disability claim can also be filed online at www.edd.ca.gov/
PLEASE PRINT WITH BLACK INK.

250104122

PART A - CLAIMANT'S STATEMENT

A1. YOUR SOCIAL SECURITY NUMBER
5 4 0 X X 9 8 8 1

A2. IF YOU HAVE PREVIOUSLY BEEN ASSIGNED AN EDD CUSTOMER ACCOUNT NUMBER, ENTER THAT NUMBER HERE

A3. CALIFORNIA DRIVER LICENSE OR ID NUMBER
A 0 8 7 6 6 1 3

A4. GENDER
MALE FEMALE   X

A5. IF YOU EVER USED OTHER SOCIAL SECURITY NUMBERS, ENTER THOSE NUMBERS BELOW

A6. STATE GOVERNMENT EMPLOYEE (IF "YES" INDICATE BARGAINING UNIT#)
YES X NO   UNIT#

A7. YOUR DATE OF BIRTH
0 3 0 4 1 9 7 2

A8. YOUR LEGAL NAME (FIRST) (MI) (LAST) SUFFIX
M A R C I A   M M O N R O E

A9. OTHER NAMES, IF ANY, UNDER WHICH YOU HAVE WORKED
(FIRST) (MI) (LAST) SUFFIX

(FIRST) (MI) (LAST) SUFFIX

A10. YOUR HOME AREA CODE AND TELEPHONE NUMBER
5 5 5   4 1 2 0 7 3 1

A11. YOUR CELL AREA CODE AND TELEPHONE NUMBER
5 5 5   2 7 4 1 3 0 0

A12. LANGUAGE YOU PREFER TO USE
ENGLISH SPANISH CANTONESE VIETNAMESE ARMENIAN PUNJABI TAGALOG OTHER
X

A13. YOUR MAILING ADDRESS, PO BOX OR NUMBER/STREET/APARTMENT, SUITE, SPACE#, OR PMB# (PRIVATE MAIL BOX)
3 5 0 1   M A P L E   S T
CITY   STATE ZIP OR POSTAL CODE   COUNTRY (IF NOT U.S.A.)
W O O D L A N D   H I L L S   X Y   1 2 3 4 5

A14. YOUR RESIDENCE ADDRESS, REQUIRED IF DIFFERENT FROM YOUR MAILING ADDRESS NUMBER/STREET/APARTMENT OR SPACE#
CITY   STATE ZIP OR POSTAL CODE   COUNTRY (IF NOT U.S.A.)

A15. YOUR LAST OR CURRENT EMPLOYER - IF YOUR LAST OR CURRENT EMPLOYMENT WAS SELF-EMPLOYMENT, ENTER "SELF" AND FILL-IN THIS OPTION.
NAME OF YOUR EMPLOYER [STATE GOVERNMENT EMPLOYEES: PROVIDE THE AGENCY NAME (FOR EXAMPLE: CALTRANS)] ☐ SELF
A   A N D   B   C O M P A N Y
NUMBER/STREET/SUITE# (STATE GOVERNMENT EMPLOYEES: PLEASE PROVIDE THE ADDRESS OF YOUR PERSONNEL OFFICE)
4 0 1   S T A T E   S T
CITY   STATE ZIP OR POSTAL CODE   COUNTRY (IF NOT U.S.A.)
W O O D L A N D   H I L L S   X Y   1 2 3 4 5
EMPLOYER'S TELEPHONE NUMBER
5 5 5   4 8 7 9 9 8 0

A16. AT ANY TIME DURING YOUR DISABILITY, WERE YOU IN THE CUSTODY OF LAW ENFORCEMENT AUTHORITIES BECAUSE YOU WERE CONVICTED OF VIOLATING A LAW OR ORDINANCE?
YES X NO

A17. BEFORE YOUR DISABILITY BEGAN, WHAT WAS THE LAST DAY YOU WORKED?
1 0 0 9 2 0 X X

A18. WHEN DID YOUR DISABILITY BEGIN?
1 0 1 0 2 0 X X

A19. DATE YOU WANT YOUR CLAIM TO BEGIN IF DIFFERENT THAN THE DATE ENTERED IN A18
M M D D Y Y Y Y

A20. SINCE YOUR DISABILITY BEGAN, HAVE YOU WORKED OR ARE YOU WORKING ANY FULL OR PARTIAL DAYS?
YES X NO

A21 A. IF YOU RECOVERED, ENTER DATE:
M M D D Y Y Y Y

A21 B. IF YOU RETURNED TO WORK, ENTER DATE:
M M D D Y Y Y Y

DE 2501 Rev. 78 (4-12)

FIGURE 16-3, cont'd

250104123

PART A - CLAIMANT'S STATEMENT - CONTINUED

A22. PLEASE RE-ENTER YOUR SOCIAL SECURITY NUMBER   5 4 0 X X 9 8 8 1

A23. WHAT IS YOUR REGULAR OR CUSTOMARY OCCUPATION?   S E C R E T A R Y

A24. WHY DID YOU STOP WORKING? (SELECT ONLY ONE BOX)   [X] ILLNESS, INJURY, OR PREGNANCY
[ ] LAYOFF   [ ] UNPAID LEAVE OF ABSENCE   [ ] VOLUNTARILY QUIT OR RETIRED   [ ] TERMINATED   [ ] OTHER REASON

A25. HOW WOULD YOU DESCRIBE OR CLASSIFY YOUR JOB?
[X] Mostly sit; occasionally stand or walk; occasionally lift, carry, push, pull, or otherwise move objects that weigh 10 lbs. or less.

[ ] Mostly walk/stand; occasionally lift, carry, push, pull, or otherwise move objects that weigh up to 20 lbs.

[ ] Constantly lift, carry, push, pull, or otherwise move objects that weigh up to 10 lbs.; frequently up to 20 lbs.; occasionally up to 50 lbs.

[ ] Constantly lift, carry, push, pull, or otherwise move objects that weigh up to 20 lbs.; frequently up to 50 lbs.; occasionally up to 100 lbs.

[ ] Constantly lift, carry, push, pull, or otherwise move objects that weigh over 20 lbs.; frequently over 50 lbs.; occasionally over 100 lbs.

A26. IF YOUR EMPLOYER(S) CONTINUED OR WILL CONTINUE TO PAY YOU DURING YOUR DISABILITY, INDICATE TYPE OF PAY:
SICK   VACATION   Paid Time Off (PTO)   ANNUAL   OTHER (EXPLAIN)

A27. MAY WE DISCLOSE BENEFIT PAYMENT INFORMATION TO YOUR EMPLOYER(S)?
YES [X]   NO

A28. SECOND EMPLOYER NAME (IF YOU HAVE MORE THAN ONE EMPLOYER)

NUMBER/STREET/SUITE#

CITY   STATE   ZIP OR POSTAL CODE   COUNTRY (IF NOT U.S.A.)

BEFORE YOUR DISABILITY BEGAN, WHAT WAS THE LAST DAY YOU WORKED FOR THIS EMPLOYER?   EMPLOYER'S TELEPHONE NUMBER
M M D D Y Y Y Y

A29. IF YOU HAVE MORE THAN 2 EMPLOYERS CHECK HERE.

A30. IF YOU ARE A RESIDENT OF AN ALCOHOLIC RECOVERY HOME OR A DRUG-FREE RESIDENTIAL FACILITY, PROVIDE THE FOLLOWING:
NAME OF FACILITY

NUMBER/STREET/SUITE#

CITY   STATE   ZIP OR POSTAL CODE   AREA CODE AND TELEPHONE NUMBER

A31. HAVE YOU FILED OR DO YOU INTEND TO FILE FOR WORKERS' COMPENSATION BENEFITS?
[ ] YES - COMPLETE ITEMS A32 THROUGH A38   [X] NO - SKIP ITEMS A33 THROUGH A38

A32. WAS THIS DISABILITY CAUSED BY YOUR JOB?
[ ] YES   [X] NO

A33. DATE(S) OF INJURY SHOWN ON YOUR WORKERS' COMPENSATION CLAIM
M M D D Y Y Y Y   M M D D Y Y Y Y   M M D D Y Y Y Y   M M D D Y Y Y Y

A34. WORKERS' COMPENSATION INSURANCE COMPANY NAME   AREA CODE AND TELEPHONE NUMBER   EXTENSION (IF ANY)

NUMBER/STREET/SUITE#

CITY   STATE   ZIP CODE   WORKERS' COMPENSATION CLAIM NUMBER

DE 2501 Rev. 78 (4-12)

FIGURE 16-3, cont'd

Continued

250104124

PART A - CLAIMANT'S STATEMENT - CONTINUED

A35. PLEASE RE-ENTER YOUR SOCIAL SECURITY NUMBER

A36. WORKERS' COMPENSATION ADJUSTER'S NAME   AREA CODE AND TELEPHONE NUMBER   EXTENSION (IF ANY)

A37. EMPLOYER'S NAME SHOWN ON YOUR WORKERS' COMPENSATION CLAIM   AREA CODE AND TELEPHONE NUMBER   EXTENSION (IF ANY)

A38. YOUR ATTORNEY'S NAME (IF ANY) **FOR YOUR WORKERS' COMPENSATION CASE**   AREA CODE AND TELEPHONE NUMBER   EXTENSION (IF ANY)

ATTORNEY'S ADDRESS NUMBER/STREET/SUITE#

CITY   STATE   ZIP CODE   WORKERS' COMPENSATION APPEALS BOARD/ADJ CASE NUMBER

PLEASE REVIEW, SIGN, AND DATE ITEM A39, AND IF APPLICABLE, ITEMS A40 AND A41

A39. Declaration and Signature. By my signature on this claim statement, I claim benefits and certify that for the period covered by this claim I was unemployed and disabled. I understand that willfully making a false statement or concealing a material fact in order to obtain payment of benefits is a violation of California law and that such violation is punishable by imprisonment or fine or both. I declare under penalty of perjury that the foregoing statement, including any accompanying statements, is to the best of my knowledge and belief true, correct, and complete. By my signature on this claim statement, I authorize the California Department of Industrial Relations and my employer to furnish and disclose to State Disability Insurance all facts concerning my disability, wages or earnings, and benefit payments that are within their knowledge. By my signature on this claim statement, I authorize release and use of information as stated in the "Information Collection and Access" portion of this form (see Informational Instructions, page D). I agree that photocopies of this authorization shall be as valid as the original, and I understand that authorizations contained in this claim statement are granted for a period of fifteen years from the date of my signature or the effective date of the claim, whichever is later.

CLAIMANT'S SIGNATURE (DO NOT PRINT) OR SIGNATURE MADE BY MARK (X)   DATE SIGNED

Marcia M. Monroe   `1 0 1 2 2 0 X X`

A40. IF YOUR SIGNATURE IS MADE BY MARK (X), CHECK THE BOX AND IT MUST BE ATTESTED BY TWO WITNESSES WITH THEIR ADDRESSES. ☐

1st WITNESS SIGNATURE (PRINT AND SIGN)   DATE SIGNED   M M D D Y Y Y Y

NUMBER/STREET/APARTMENT OR SPACE#, PO BOX OR PRIVATE MAIL BOX ADDRESSES NOT ACCEPTABLE.

CITY   STATE   ZIP CODE

2nd WITNESS SIGNATURE (PRINT AND SIGN)   DATE SIGNED   M M D D Y Y Y Y

NUMBER/STREET/APARTMENT OR SPACE#, PO BOX OR PRIVATE MAIL BOX ADDRESSES NOT ACCEPTABLE.

CITY   STATE   ZIP CODE

A41. ☐ CHECK THIS BOX IF YOU ARE THE PERSONAL REPRESENTATIVE SIGNING ON BEHALF OF CLAIMANT AND COMPLETE THE FOLLOWING:

(FIRST)   (MI)   (LAST)

I,   , REPRESENT THE CLAIMANT IN

THIS MATTER AS AUTHORIZED BY ☐ DECLARATION OF INDIVIDUAL CLAIMING DISABILITY INSURANCE BENEFITS DUE AN INCAPACITATED OR DECEASED CLAIMANT, DE 2522 (SEE INSTRUCTION & INFORMATION A, UNDER HOW TO APPLY #4) ☐ POWER OF ATTORNEY (ATTACH COPY)

PERSONAL REPRESENTATIVE'S SIGNATURE (DO NOT PRINT)   DATE SIGNED   M M D D Y Y Y Y

DE 2501 Rev. 78 (4-12)

FIGURE 16-3, cont'd

Claim for Disability Insurance (DI) Benefits -
Physician/Practitioner's Certificate
PLEASE PRINT WITH BLACK INK.

250104125

PART B - PHYSICIAN/PRACTITIONER'S CERTIFICATE

B1. PATIENT'S SOCIAL SECURITY NUMBER 5 4 0 X X 9 8 8 1

B2. PATIENT'S FILE NUMBER M 3 7 6 2

B3. IF YOU KNOW THE PATIENT'S ELECTRONIC RECEIPT NUMBER, ENTER IT HERE: R

B4. PATIENT'S DATE OF BIRTH 0 3 0 4 1 9 7 2

B5. PATIENT'S NAME (FIRST) M A R C I A (MI) M (LAST) M O N R O E

B6. PHYSICIAN/PRACTITIONER'S LICENSE NUMBER C 1 4 0 2 0

B7. STATE **OR** COUNTRY (IF NOT U.S.A.) THAT ISSUED LICENSE NUMBER ENTERED IN B6 STATE X Y COUNTRY

B8. PHYSICIAN/PRACTITIONER LICENSE TYPE M D

B9. SPECIALTY (IF ANY)

B10. PHYSICIAN/PRACTITIONER'S NAME AS SHOWN ON LICENSE
(FIRST) D A V I D (MI) W (LAST) S M I T H SUFFIX

B11. PHYSICIAN/PRACTITIONER'S ADDRESS
MAILING ADDRESS, PO BOX OR NUMBER/STREET/SUITE# 4 5 6 7 B R O A D A V E
CITY W O O D L A N D H I L L S STATE X Y ZIP OR POSTAL CODE 1 2 3 4 5 COUNTRY (IF NOT U.S.A.)

COUNTY HOSPITAL/GOVERNMENT FACILITY ADDRESS
FACILITY NAME (IF APPLICABLE)

FACILITY ADDRESS, NUMBER/STREET/SUITE#

CITY STATE ZIP OR POSTAL CODE COUNTRY (IF NOT U.S.A.)

B12. THIS PATIENT HAS BEEN UNDER MY CARE AND TREATMENT FOR THIS MEDICAL PROBLEM
FROM 1 0 1 2 2 0 X X TO 1 0 1 9 2 0 X X [X] CHECK HERE TO INDICATE YOU ARE STILL TREATING THE PATIENT
AT INTERVALS OF: [ ] DAILY [ ] WEEKLY [ ] MONTHLY [X] AS NEEDED [ ] OTHER

B13. AT ANY TIME DURING YOUR ATTENDANCE FOR THIS MEDICAL PROBLEM, HAS THE PATIENT BEEN INCAPABLE OF PERFORMING HIS/HER REGULAR OR CUSTOMARY WORK?
YES - ENTER DATE DISABILITY BEGAN 1 0 1 0 2 0 X X NO - SKIP TO B33
WAS THE DISABILITY CAUSED BY AN ACCIDENT OR TRAUMA? [ ] YES [X] NO
M M D D Y Y Y Y IF YES, INDICATE THE DATE THE ACCIDENT OR TRAUMA OCCURRED.

B14. DATE YOU RELEASED OR ANTICIPATE RELEASING PATIENT TO RETURN TO HIS/HER REGULAR OR CUSTOMARY WORK
("UNKNOWN", "INDEFINITE", ETC., NOT ACCEPTABLE.) 1 0 3 0 2 0 X X
[ ] CHECK HERE TO INDICATE PATIENT'S DISABILITY IS PERMANENT AND YOU NEVER ANTICIPATE RELEASING PATIENT TO RETURN TO HIS/HER REGULAR OR CUSTOMARY WORK

B15. IF PATIENT IS NOW PREGNANT OR HAS BEEN PREGNANT, PLEASE CHECK THE APPROPRIATE BOX AND ENTER THE FOLLOWING:
ESTIMATED DELIVERY DATE: M M D D Y Y Y Y DATE PREGNANCY ENDED: M M D D Y Y Y Y
TYPE OF DELIVERY, IF PATIENT HAS DELIVERED: [ ] VAGINAL [ ] CESAREAN

DE 2501 Rev. 78 (4-12)

FIGURE 16-4 Form DE 2501, Physician/Practitioner's Certificate. These pages of the form are completed by the attending physician. It is submitted within a set time period, determined by the beginning date of disability, to initiate benefits.

Continued

250104126

PART B - PHYSICIAN/PRACTITIONER'S CERTIFICATE - CONTINUED

B16. PLEASE RE-ENTER PATIENT'S SOCIAL SECURITY NUMBER   5 4 0 X X 9 8 8 1

B17. IF THE PATIENT HAS NOT DELIVERED AND YOU DO NOT ANTICIPATE RELEASING THE PATIENT TO RETURN TO REGULAR OR CUSTOMARY WORK PRIOR TO THE ESTIMATED DELIVERY DATE, ENTER THE **NUMBER OF DAYS** THAT THE PATIENT WILL BE DISABLED POSTPARTUM, FOR EACH DELIVERY TYPE:

VAGINAL DELIVERY [ ]   CESAREAN DELIVERY [ ]

B18. IN CASE OF AN ABNORMAL PREGNANCY AND/OR DELIVERY, STATE THE COMPLICATION(S) CAUSING MATERNAL DISABILITY

B19. ICD DIAGNOSIS CODE(S) FOR DISABLING CONDITION THAT PREVENT THE PATIENT FROM PERFORMING HIS/HER REGULAR OR CUSTOMARY WORK (REQUIRED)

(Check only one box)

PRIMARY   J 1 8 ▪ 9

EXAMPLE OF HOW TO COMPLETE ICD CODES

ICD-9   3 2 0 ▪ 1   [ ] ICD-9

ICD-10   G 0 0 ▪ 1   [X] ICD-10

SECONDARY   ▪

SECONDARY   ▪

SECONDARY   ▪

B20. DIAGNOSIS (REQUIRED) - IF NO DIAGNOSIS HAS BEEN DETERMINED, ENTER A DETAILED STATEMENT OF SYMPTOMS

B I L A T E R A L   P N E U M O N I T I S

B21. FINDINGS - STATE NATURE, SEVERITY, AND EXTENT OF THE INCAPACITATING DISEASE OR INJURY, INCLUDE ANY OTHER DISABLING CONDITIONS

B I L A T E R A L   P N E U M O N I T I S   C O N F I R M E D   B Y   A P

A N D   L A T E R A L   C H E S T   X - R A Y S

B22. TYPE OF TREATMENT/MEDICATION RENDERED TO PATIENT

B E D   R E S T   A N D   A N T I B I O T I C S

B23. IF PATIENT WAS HOSPITALIZED, PROVIDE DATES OF ENTRY AND DISCHARGE   M M D D Y Y Y Y   TO   M M D D Y Y Y Y

[ ] CHECK HERE TO INDICATE THE PATIENT IS STILL HOSPITALIZED

B24. [ ] CHECK HERE IF PATIENT IS DECEASED, PLEASE PROVIDE DATE OF DEATH   M M D D Y Y Y Y

CITY   COUNTY   STATE

DE 2501 Rev. 78 (4-12)

FIGURE 16-4, cont'd

250104127

PART B - PHYSICIAN/PRACTITIONER'S CERTIFICATE - CONTINUED

B25. PLEASE RE-ENTER PATIENT'S SOCIAL SECURITY NUMBER   5 4 0 X X 9 8 8 1

B26. WAS THE PATIENT SEEN PREVIOUSLY BY ANOTHER PHYSICIAN/PRACTITIONER OR MEDICAL FACILITY FOR THE CURRENT DISABILITY/ILLNESS/INJURY?

☐ YES   ☒ NO   ☐ UNKNOWN   IF YES, WHAT WAS THE DATE OF FIRST TREATMENT?   M M D D Y Y Y Y

B27. DATE AND TYPE OF SURGERY/PROCEDURE MOST RECENTLY PERFORMED OR TO BE PERFORMED

M M D D Y Y Y Y

WAS THE PATIENT UNABLE TO WORK IMMEDIATELY PRIOR TO THE SURGERY OR PROCEDURE?   ☐ YES   ☐ NO

M M D D Y Y Y Y   IF YES, PLEASE PROVIDE THE FIRST DATE THE PATIENT WAS UNABLE TO WORK BEFORE THE SURGERY OR PROCEDURE

B28. ICD PROCEDURE CODE(S)   ☐ ICD-9   ☐ ICD-10

CPT CODE(S) (DO NOT INCLUDE MODIFIERS)
9 9 2 1 3   7 1 0 2 0

B29. WAS THIS DISABLING CONDITION CAUSED AND/OR AGGRAVATED BY THE PATIENT'S REGULAR OR CUSTOMARY WORK?   ☐ YES   ☒ NO

B30. ARE YOU COMPLETING THIS FORM FOR THE SOLE PURPOSE OF REFERRAL/RECOMMENDATION TO AN ALCOHOLIC RECOVERY HOME OR DRUG-FREE RESIDENTIAL FACILITY AS INDICATED BY THE PATIENT IN QUESTION A30?   ☐ YES   ☒ NO

B31. DATE YOUR PATIENT BECAME A RESIDENT OF A DRUG OR ALCOHOL FACILITY (IF KNOWN)   M M D D Y Y Y Y

B32. WOULD DISCLOSURE OF THE INFORMATION ON THIS FORM BE MEDICALLY OR PSYCHOLOGICALLY DETRIMENTAL TO YOUR PATIENT?   ☐ YES   ☒ NO

B33. **ALL PERSONS AUTHORIZED TO CERTIFY (REQUIRED)**
(CHECK ONE)

☒ **ALL PHYSICIANS** (MEDICAL OR OSTEOPATHIC PHYSICIAN, SURGEON, CHIROPRACTOR, DENTIST, PODIATRIST, OPTOMETRIST OR PSYCHOLOGIST)

I CERTIFY UNDER PENALTY OF PERJURY THAT THE PATIENT IS UNABLE TO PERFORM HIS/HER REGULAR OR CUSTOMARY WORK BECAUSE OF THE DISABLING CONDITION(S) LISTED ABOVE AND I HAVE TREATED THE PATIENT WITHIN MY SCOPE OF PRACTICE.

☐ **NURSE PRACTITIONER**

I CERTIFY UNDER PENALTY OF PERJURY THAT THE PATIENT IS UNABLE TO PERFORM HIS/HER REGULAR OR CUSTOMARY WORK BECAUSE OF THE DISABLING CONDITION(S) LISTED ABOVE AND I HAVE TREATED THE PATIENT WITHIN MY SCOPE OF PRACTICE. IF FOR A CONDITION OTHER THAN A NORMAL PREGNANCY OR DELIVERY, I CERTIFY THAT I HAVE PERFORMED A PHYSICAL EXAMINATION AND HAVE COLLABORATED WITH A PHYSICIAN OR SURGEON.

☐ **REGISTRAR OF A COUNTY HOSPITAL IN CALIFORNIA OR MEDICAL OFFICER OF A US GOVERNMENT MEDICAL FACILITY**

I CERTIFY UNDER PENALTY OF PERJURY THAT THE PATIENT IS UNABLE TO PERFORM HIS/HER REGULAR OR CUSTOMARY WORK BECAUSE OF THE DISABLING CONDITION(S) LISTED ABOVE AND THESE CONDITIONS ARE SHOWN BY THE PATIENT'S HOSPITAL CHART.

☐ **OTHER:** TITLE OF PERSON IF NOT COVERED ABOVE:
(MUST BE ABLE TO LEGALLY CERTIFY TO A DISABILITY)

PHYSICIAN/PRACTITIONER'S ORIGINAL SIGNATURE - **RUBBER STAMP IS NOT ACCEPTABLE**   DATE SIGNED   AREA CODE/PHONE NUMBER

David W. Smith, M.D.   1 0 1 9 2 0 X X   5 5 5   4 8 6 9 0 0 2

UNDER SECTIONS 2116 AND 2122 OF THE CALIFORNIA UNEMPLOYMENT INSURANCE CODE, IT IS A VIOLATION FOR ANY INDIVIDUAL WHO, WITH INTENT TO DEFRAUD, FALSELY CERTIFIES THE MEDICAL CONDITION OF ANY PERSON IN ORDER TO OBTAIN DISABILITY INSURANCE BENEFITS, WHETHER FOR THE MAKER OR FOR ANY OTHER PERSON, AND IS PUNISHABLE BY IMPRISONMENT AND/OR A FINE NOT EXCEEDING $20,000. SECTION 1143 REQUIRES ADDITIONAL ADMINISTRATIVE PENALTIES.

DE 2501 Rev. 78 (4-12)   OSP 12 127141

FIGURE 16-4, cont'd

2525XX03121

Mailing Date

RETURN TO: →

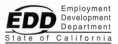

Employment
Development
Department
State of California

PHYSICIAN/PRACTITIONER'S SUPPLEMENTARY CERTIFICATE

EDD Customer Account Number (EDDCAN)	CLAIM ID	SSN/ECN	CED

Claimant Instructions: If you are still disabled, contact your physician/practitioner immediately for completion of the Physician/Practitioner's Supplementary Certificate which must be submitted within twenty (20) days of the mailing date shown above or you may lose additional benefits.

Instrucciones al Solicitante de Beneficios: Si Ud. aun sigue incapacitado. comuniquese con su Médico/Profesional (Medico) lo más pronto posible para completar el documento titlado en inglés "Physician/Practitioner Supplementary Certificats" el cual debe ser presentado dentro de un plazo de veinte (20) días de la fecha de envio indicada arriba o de lo contrario es posible que pueda perder beneficios adicionales.

Physician/ Practitioner Instructions: For faster processing, the physician/practitioner may complete and submit this form online at www.edd.ca.gov. If this form is submitted online, you do not have to mail this form back to EDD. When completing this form, **PLEASE PRINT WITH BLACK INK.**

1. ARE YOU STILL TREATING THE PATIENT?   YES   NO   DATE OF LAST TREATMENT

2. WHAT CURRENT CONDITION(S) CONTINUES TO MAKE THE PATIENT DISABLED? (DIAGNOSIS REQUIRED, IF MADE)

3. DAT OF NEXT APPOINTMENT

4. ICD DIAGNOSIS CODE(S) FOR DISABLING CONDITION THAT PREVENT THE PATIENT FROM PERFORMING HIS/HER REGULAR OR CUSTOMARY WORK (REQUIRED)

EXAMPLE OF HOW TO COMPLETE ICD CODES

ICD-9   3 2 0 • 1

ICD-10   G 0 0 • 1

(Check only on box)

☐ ICD-9

☐ ICD-10

PRIMARY

SECONDARY

SECONDARY

SECONDARY

ADDITIONAL QUESTIONS ON FOLLOWING PAGES

FIGURE 16-5 Notice of Final Payment and Physician/Practitioner's Supplementary Certificate, Form DE 2525XX. This form indicates that the period of disability is "closed" or terminated with the accompanying check on the basis of the information in the claim records. Benefits will cease unless the reverse side of the form is completed by the claimant's physician, extending the duration of disability. This form is pink. One side of the form is in English and the other is in Spanish.

2525XX03121

5. DESCRIBE HOW THE PATIENT'S PRESENT CONDITION/IMPAIRMENT PREVENTS HIM/HER FROM RETURNING TO HIS/HER REGULAR OR CUSTOMARY WORK.

6. WHAT FACTORS OR COMPLICATIONS ARE DISABLING THE PATIENT LONGER THAN PREVIOUSLY ESTIMATED?

7. IF PATIENT WAS HOSPITALIZED, PROVIDE DATES OF ENTRY AND DISCHARGE   M M D D Y Y Y Y   TO   M M D D Y Y Y Y
   ☐ CHECK HERE TO INDICATE THE PATIENT IS STILL HOSPITALIZED

8. DATE AND TYPE OF SURGERY/PROCEDURE PERFORMED OR TO BE PERFORMED
   M M D D Y Y Y Y

9A. ICD PROCEDURE CODE(S)   ☐ ICD-9   ☐ ICD-10

9B. CPT CODE(S) (DO NOT INCLUDE MODIFIERS)

10. CURRENT ESTIMATED DATE PATIENT (EVEN IF STILL UNDER TREATMENT) WILL BE ABLE TO PERFORM HIS/HER REGULAR OR CUSTOMARY WORK)"UNKNOWN," "INDEFINITE," ETC., NOT ACCEPTABLE)
    M M D D Y Y Y Y

    ☐ CHECK HERE TO INDICATE PATIENT'S DISABILITY IS PERMANENT AND YOU NEVER ANTICIPATE RELEASING PATIENT TO RETURN TO HIS/HER REGULAR OR CUSTOMARY WORK

11. WOULD DISCLOSURE OF THE INFORMATION ON THIS FORM BE MEDICALLY OR PSYCHOLOGICALLY DETRIMENTAL TO YOUR PATIENT? | YES | NO |

ADDITIONAL QUESTIONS ON FOLLOWING PAGES

FIGURE 16-5, cont'd

Continued

2525XX03121

12. PHYSICIAN/PRACTITIONER'S LICENSE NUMBER

13. STATE OR COUNTRY (IF NOT U.S.A.) THAT ISSUED THE LICENSE NUMBER ENTERED IN QUESTION 12

STATE   COUNTRY

14. PHYSICIAN/PRACTITIONER'S NAME

(FIRST)   (MI)   (LAST)   (SUFFIX)

15. PHYSICIAN/PRACTITIONER LICENSE TYPE   **16. SPECIALTY, IF ANY**

17. PHYSICIAN/PRACTITIONER'S ADDRESS
MAILING ADDRESS, PO BOX, OR NUMBER/STREET/SUITE#

CITY   STATE   ZIP OR POSTAL CODE   COUNTRY (IF NOT U.S.A.)

18. COUNTY HOSPITAL/GOVERNMENT FACILITY ADDRESS
FACILITY NAME (IF APPLICABLE)

FACILITY ADDRESS, NUMBER/STREET/SUITE#

CITY   STATE   ZIP OR POSTAL CODE   COUNTRY (IF NOT U.S.A.)

ALL PERSONS AUTHORIZED TO CERTIFY (REQUIRED)

☐ **All Physicians** (Medical or Osteopathic Physician, Surgeon, Chiropractor, Dentist, Podiatrist, Optometrist or Psychologist)
I certify under penalty of perjury that the patient is unable to perform his/her regular or customary work because of the disabling condition(s) listed above and I have treated the patient within my scope of practice.

☐ **Nurse Practitioner**
I certify under penalty of perjury that the patient is unable to perform his/her regular or customary work because of the disabling condition(s) listed above and I have treated the patient within my scope of practice. If for a condition other than a normal pregnancy or delivery, I certify that I have performed a physical examination and have collaborated with a physician or surgeon.

☐ **Registrar of a County Hospital in California or Medical Officer of a U.S. Government Medical Facility**
I certify under penalty of perjury that the patient is unable to perform his/her regular or customary work because of the disabling condition(s) listed above and these conditions are shown by the patient's hospital chart.

☐ **Other**: Title of person if not covered above:
(must be able to legally certify to a disability)

19. PHYSICIAN/PRACTITIONER'S ORIGINAL SIGNATURE – RUBBER STAMP IS NOT ACCEPTABLE

SIGNATURE   DATE SIGNED   AREA CODE/PHONE NUMBER
M M D D Y Y Y Y

Under sections 2116 and 2122 of the California Unemployment Insurance Code, it is a violation for any individual who, with intent to defraud, falsely certifies the medical condition of any person in order to obtain Disability Insurance benefits, whether for the maker or for any other person, and is punishable by imprisonment and/or a fine not exceeding $20,000. Section 1143 requires additional administrative penalties.

DE 2525XX Rev. 3 (3-12)   Page 3 of 3

FIGURE 16-5, cont'd

STATE OF CALIFORNIA
EMPLOYMENT DEVELOPMENT DEPARTMENT

FOR DEPT. USE ONLY

REFER TO

4920 – Our File No.
Marcia M. Monroe – Your Patient
Secretary – Regular or Customary Work

REQUEST FOR ADDITIONAL
MEDICAL INFORMATION

David W. Smith, MD
4567 Broad Avenue
Woodland Hills, XY 12345

The original basic information and estimate of duration of your patient's disability have been carefully evaluated. At the present time, the following additional information based upon the progress and present condition of this patient is requested. This will assist the Department in determining eligibility for further disability insurance benefits. Return of the completed form as soon as possible will be appreciated.

WM. C. SCHMIDT, M.D., MEDICAL DIRECTOR

CLAIMS EXAMINER   **DOCTOR: Please complete either Part A or B, date and sign.**

PART A   IF YOUR PATIENT HAS RECOVERED SUFFICIENTLY TO BE ABLE TO RETURN TO HIS/HER REGULAR OR CUSTOMARY WORK LISTED ABOVE, PLEASE GIVE THE DATE, _____ 20_____ .

PART B   THIS PART REFERS TO PATIENT WHO IS STILL DISABLED.

Are you still treating the patient?   YES ☒   NO ☐   November   15 , 20 xx
DATE OF LAST TREATMENT

What are the medical circumstances which continue to make your patient disabled?
Bilateral pneumonitis. Patient has had continual fever 100°F to 102°F, productive cough, chest pains, and lethargy.

What is your present estimate of the date your patient will be able to perform his/her regular or customary work listed above? Date   November   30 20   xx   .

Further Comments: _____

Would the disclosure of this information to your patient be medically or psychologically detrimental to the patient?   YES ☐   NO ☒

Date   November   17 20____ xx

David W. Smith M.D.
DOCTOR'S SIGNATURE

David W. Smith, MD

SE
ENCLOSED IS A STAMPED PREADDRESSED ENVELOPE FOR YOUR CONVENIENCE.

DE 2547 R v. 18 (8-84)

FIGURE 16-6 Request for Additional Medical Information, Form DE 2547. This form is mailed to the physician when the normal expectancy date of the disability is reached, provided that the physician has requested a longer than normal duration without complications as indicated.

STATE OF CALIFORNIA

EMPLOYMENT DEVELOPMENT DEPARTMENT
P.O. Box 1529, Santa Barbara, CA 93102
(555) 963-9611

For Dept. Use Only

REFER TO

MEDICAL INQUIRY

4920
Marcia M. Monroe
Secretary

- Our File No.
- Your Patient
- Regular Work

David W. Smith, MD
4567 Broad Avenue
Woodland Hills, XY 12345

A review of the medical certificate received in conjunction with a claim for disability insurance benefits filed by your patient, named above, reveals that some additional information is needed in order to evaluate the claim properly. Your cooperation in answering the question or questions below and returning the form in the enclosed stamped and addressed envelope will be appreciated.

WM. C. SCHMIDT, MD, MEDICAL DIRECTOR

CLAIMS EXAMINER

What is the name and address of the facility that took the x-rays on this patient?

Speedy Radiology Service
4598 Main Street
Woodland Hills, XY 12345

Would the disclosure of this information to your patient be medically or psychologically detrimental to the patient: Yes ☐   No ☒

October 24	20XX	*David W. Smith MD*
Date		Doctor's Signature
SE		David W. Smith, MD

DE 2547A Rev. 10 (9-84)

FIGURE 16-7 Medical Inquiry, Form DE 2547A. This form is mailed to the physician at any time during the life of the claim if any questions need to be answered or if the physician has failed to enter a prognosis date.

All follow-up correspondence should include the patient's name and Social Security number. The insurance billing specialist should promptly report any change of address, telephone number, or return-to-work date to the SDI office. Patients must report any income received to the SDI office because income received may affect benefits.

CONCLUSION

This chapter ends as it began—with a bit of levity. The following errors were taken from actual disability insurance application forms, completed by employees, that came across the desk of a claims adjuster.

Spelled as:	Should have been:
yellow "jonders"	yellow jaundice
"goalstones"	gallstones
"limp glands"	lymph glands
"falls teeth"	false teeth
"high pretension"	hypertension
"Pabst smear"	Pap smear
"wrecktum"	rectum

KEY POINTS

This is a brief chapter review, or summary, of the key issues presented. To further enhance your knowledge of the technical subject matter, review the key terms and key abbreviations for this chapter by locating the meaning for each in the Glossary at the end of this book, which appears in a section before the Index.

1. Disability income insurance is a type of insurance that provides periodic payments under certain conditions when the insured is unable to work because of illness, disease, or injury, not as a result of a work-related accident or condition.

2. While disabled, benefits begin after an elimination or waiting period (WP).

3. The types of disability are temporary, residual or partial, and total.

4. Disability policies may be guaranteed renewable for a specific number of years to a certain age.

5. The Social Security Administration (SSA) manages two programs that pay monthly disability benefits to people younger than age 65 who cannot work for at least 1 year because of a severe disability: Social Security Disability Insurance (SSDI) program and Supplemental Security Income (SSI) program.

6. Federal employees who have put in a certain number of years of service and who become disabled not by work-related means may be eligible for Civil Service Retirement System (CSRS) and Federal Employees Retirement System (FERS) programs.

7. Individuals on active duty fall under the Armed Services Disability program if they become disabled while serving in the military.

8. The Veterans Affairs (VA) disability program provides benefits for veterans who have suffered a service-connected disability.

9. Five states plus Puerto Rico have a State Disability Insurance (SDI) program for those who suffer a wage loss because of off-the-job illness or injury.

10. Claims for SDI must be filed within the time limits of each state's laws.

11. For disability income claims, the insured must file a proof of loss form and the attending physician must also complete a section to verify the disability.

12. For federal disability cases, the physician must submit details about the individual's disabled condition.

13. State disability claim forms must be completed by the attending physician to substantiate the claimant's condition to receive benefits.

🖥 STUDENT ASSIGNMENT

✔ Study Chapter 16.

✔ Answer the fill-in-the-blank, multiple-choice, and true/false review questions in the *Workbook* to reinforce the theory learned in this chapter and to help prepare you for a future test. Complete the assignments in the *Workbook*. These assignments will provide you with hands-on experience in working with patient histories and completing disability insurance claim forms described in this chapter.

✔ Turn to the Glossary at the end of this text for a further understanding of the key terms and key abbreviations used in this chapter.

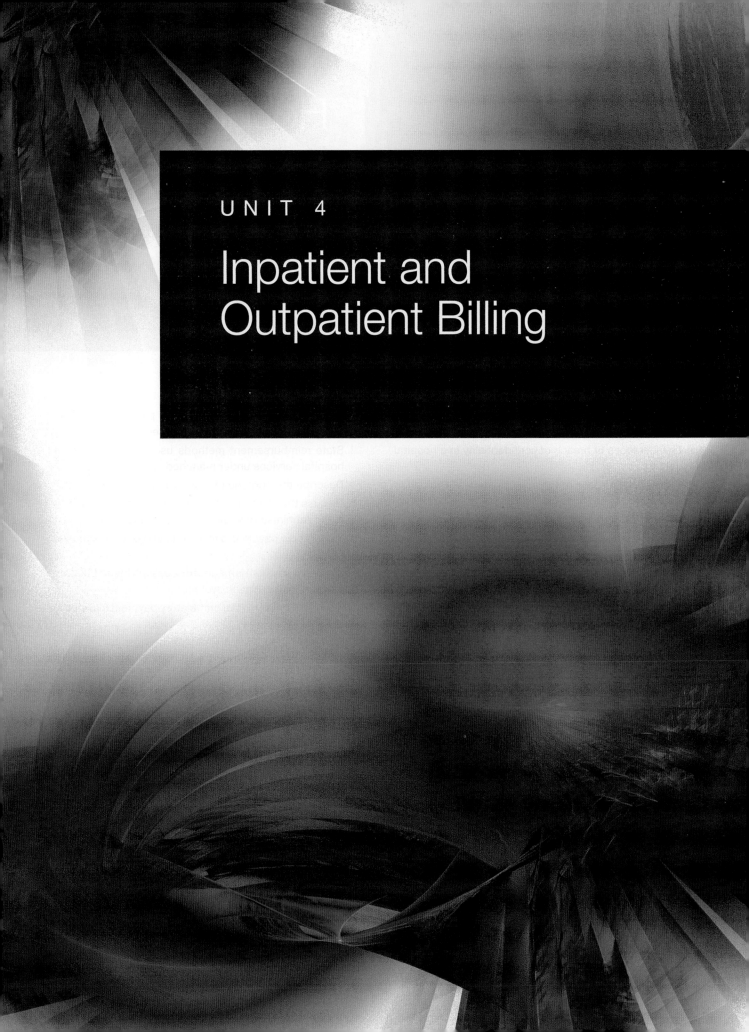

UNIT 4

Inpatient and Outpatient Billing

Hospital Billing

Payel Bhattacharya Madero

OBJECTIVES

After reading this chapter, you should be able to:

1. Name qualifications necessary to work as a hospital patient accounts representative.
2. List instances of breach of confidentiality in a hospital setting.
3. Explain the purpose of the appropriateness evaluation protocols.
4. Describe criteria used for admission screening.
5. Define and discuss the 72-hour rule.
6. Describe the quality improvement organization and its role in the hospital reimbursement system.
7. Describe the *International Classification of Diseases, Tenth Revision, Procedure Coding System* (ICD-10-PCS).
8. State the role of *International Classification of Diseases, Tenth Revision, Procedure Coding System* (ICD-10-PCS) in hospital billing.
9. Explain the basic flow of the inpatient hospital stay from billing through receipt of payment.
10. Describe the charge description master.

11. State when the CMS-1450 (UB-04) paper or electronic claim form may and may not be used.
12. State reimbursement methods used when paying for hospital services under managed care contracts.
13. Describe the purpose of diagnosis-related groups.
14. Discuss the electronic claim filing guidelines as stated in the Administrative Simplification Act of 1996.
15. Identify how payment is made on the basis of diagnosis-related groups.
16. State how payment is made on the basis of the ambulatory payment classification system.
17. Name the four types of ambulatory payment classifications.
18. Complete insurance claims in both hospital inpatient and hospital outpatient settings to minimize their rejection by insurance carriers.
19. State the general guidelines for completion of the paper CMS-1450 (UB-04) and transmission of the electronic claim form.

KEY TERMS

admission review
ambulatory payment classifications
appropriateness evaluation protocols
benefit summary sheets
capitation
case rate
charge description master

charges
clinical outliers
code sequence
complication/comorbidity
cost-based systems
cost outlier
cost outlier review
day outlier review
diagnosis-related groups

downcoding
DRG creep
DRG validation
elective surgery
grouper
inpatient
International Classification of Diseases, Ninth Revision, Clinical Modification

International Classification of Diseases, Tenth Revision, Clinical Modification
International Classification of Diseases, Tenth Revision, Procedure Coding System
Looping
major complication/comorbidity
major diagnostic categories
modifiers

outpatient
percentage of revenue
per diem
preadmission testing
principal diagnosis
procedure review
prospective payment system
Quality Improvement Organization
readmission review

reason for encounter
registered nurse
stop loss
transfer review
Uniform Bill (CMS-1450 [UB-04])
upcoding
utilization review

KEY ABBREVIATIONS

AEP	DRG	MCC	RHIA
APC	FL	MDC	RHIT
ASC	GAO	MS-DRG	RN
CC	ICD-9-CM	OPPS	TJC
CDM	ICD-10-CM	PAT	UB-04
CMHC	ICD-10-PCS	PPS	UR
CMS-1450 (UB-04)	LOS	QIO	

Service to Patients

Learn to be courteous in all interactions with co-workers and patients so that patients sense an atmosphere of high morale in the working environment. Be watchful about observing how patients and co-workers react to you and to hospital policies and procedures so that communication ends up as a positive patient encounter. Ensure that you are educated about your job duties and hospital policy; otherwise, responses to the patient may vary from employee to employee when training is not thorough. Always look and act as a professional and respond immediately to patients' questions and problems.

HEALTH INSURANCE REIMBURSEMENT

The financial relationship of the health insurer and the patient care provider is unique when compared to other business sectors in the United States. It is most important to note that the underlying factor that controls the reimbursement process is that health care providers render services and get paid afterward. The process of health care reimbursement involves collecting payment after health care services have been provided. Second, health insurance companies reserve the right to approve payment for medical services that they deem necessary for patient health. To illustrate, a patient taking herbal supplements recommended by her physician but not approved by the insurance company will have to pay out of pocket for the entire cost. Finally, health insurance companies have payment schedules for services based on the physician's work, the geographic area in which the procedure was performed, and the estimated cost of malpractice insurance.

PATIENT ACCOUNTS REPRESENTATIVE

Qualifications

A variety of jobs are available in the financial department and health information management (HIM) department, formerly known as the *medical records department*, of hospitals; therefore this chapter focuses on hospital *inpatient* and *outpatient* insurance billing and coding. Individuals who desire a position in a hospital facility business department should have knowledge and competence in the following subjects:

- *International Classification of Diseases, Ninth Revision, Clinical Modification (ICD-9-CM)* and *International Classification of Diseases,* **Tenth Revision, Clinical Modification (ICD-10-CM)** diagnostic codes
- Current Procedural Terminology (CPT), Healthcare Common Procedure Coding System (HCPCS), ICD-9-CM, and *International Classification of Diseases,*

Box 17-1	AHIMA Certifications	
Registered Health Information Technologist (RHIT)	Ensures the quality of medical records, analyzes patient data, improves patient care, and specializes in medical coding and insurance reimbursement	Medical Records Technician, Release of Information Clerk, Cancer Registrar
Registered Health Information Administrator (RHIA)	Manages patient information; administers health information systems; collects and analyzes patient data; and has a comprehensive knowledge of administrative, legal, and ethical requirements related to health care delivery	Director of Health Information Management, Facility Privacy Officer, Information Systems Implementation Manager
Certified Coding Associate (CCA)	Entry level medical coding skills across a variety of health care settings	Entry level long-term care facility coder
Certified Coding Specialist (CCS)	Mastery level coding skills across a variety of health care settings	Inpatient hospital coder

AHIMA offers a variety of different certifications for career advancement. For more information, visit www.ahima.org/certification.

Tenth Revision, Procedure Coding System (ICD-10-PCS) procedure and equipment codes
- CMS-1500 (02-12)/837P insurance claim form
- CMS-1450 (UB-04) insurance claim form
- Electronic claim submission procedure and standards
- Explanation of benefits and remittance advice documents
- Medical terminology (that is, anatomy and physiology, diseases, procedures, and treatments)
- Major health insurance programs
- Managed care plans
- Denied and delinquent claims
- Claim appeals
- Reimbursement payment posting

A hospital facility is larger than a clinic or private physician's office, so there is greater opportunity for advancement. An individual may be hired as a file clerk or insurance verifier and advance from junior to senior clerk, insurance clerk, or patient account representative. To continue professional development, patient account representatives will benefit from seeking additional credentials from the American Health Information Management Association (AHIMA) (Box 17-1). Most hospital facilities have policies that encourage career growth by promoting employees from within. To qualify for a medical coding position, previous experience is preferred. Additional qualifications are shown in Figure 17-1. See Chapter 1 for details on educational and training requirements and ethics.

Principal Responsibilities

A generic job description for a patient accounts representative in a hospital business office whose primary function is to file hospital inpatient and outpatient claims with third-party payers is shown in Figure 17-1. Prior to starting a career in health insurance reimbursement, it is important to recognize that each health insurance organization maintains individual standards for health care facilities to follow prior to releasing reimbursements. The first step to being successful as an insurance billing specialist is to gain basic knowledge of insurance programs that are managed in the geographic area. Health insurance companies publish **benefit summary sheets** that provide guidelines on medical coding expectations, reimbursement schedules, and other specific information requirements in order to complete the medical claim accurately and completely. Accurate claim processing is essential to obtain maximum reimbursement from the insurance company. Due to the lack of attention to accurate details, many hospitals hastily submit insurance claims incorrectly, receive reduced payment for services rendered, and make *adjustments* to clear the balance off of patient accounts. This practice results in a high percentage of coding inaccuracies and the loss of many dollars. To be successful in this industry, an insurance billing specialist must continually update his or her knowledge of coding and insurance program policies by attending seminars, workshops, classes, and in-house training.

ADMISSIONS PROCEDURES

Appropriateness Evaluation Protocols

The definition of *admission* from a hospital perspective is the act of accepting a patient for inpatient services related to improving the patient's quality of life through therapeutic care. To maintain a quality standard of patient care, it is important to first identify the standards of quality patient care and develop a strategy to meet these standards. Many health care organizations, such as The Joint Commission (TJC), American Hospital Association (AHA), and Centers for Medicare and Medicaid Services (CMS), provide guidance for hospitals to meet quality patient delivery goals.

Position Description

Title: Patient Accounts Representative   **Job Number: 3954**

Department: Contract Billing   Effective Date: 2/26/XX

Reports to: Patient Accounts Supervisor

Primary Function:

In a prompt and accurate manner, all hospital inpatient and outpatient health insurance claims, both initial and/or subsequent, should be filed with third-party payers. Each patient account should be followed up with the health insurance company in a timely and efficient manner to ensure maximum reimbursement for health services provided. Also responsible for ensuring patient accounts are posted with contracted reimbursements and adjustments per the terms of applicable contracts. Collection activity is needed in the collection of the outstanding balance due per the terms of applicable contracts from any responsible parties.

Principal Responsibilities

1. Processes claims within assigned responsibility in an accurate and timely manner; all insurance claim filing procedures should ensure completeness and correctness of all claims to facilitate maximum reimbursement.
    a. Investigates and assigns correct claim data according to the available health care patient data.
    b. Enters data accurately, efficiently, and consistently.
    c. Continually develops thorough knowledge of third-party payers, insurance claim requirements, UB-04 requirements by payer, electronic claims processing, and health data documentation standards for accurate coding.
2. Manages communication concerning patient accounts under HIPAA privacy and security standards via phone, mail, and other electronic media.
    a. Maintains professional correspondence standards with all clientele while facilitating thorough knowledge of confidentiality, ethical and legal billing procedures.
3. Maintains strong interdepartmental relations to ensure quality patient care.
    a. Manages all health care documentation and records in accordance with federal and state regulations.
    b. Instructs various hospital departments on effective medical records documentation to ensure maximum reimbursement.
4. Participates in mandatory education opportunities within the hospital and local health information management seminars for job and personal development.
    a. Attends workshops and seminars to ensure application of billing/coding industry changes.
    b. Takes advantage of personal development opportunities to facilitate interdepartmental relations.
5. Organizes facilitation with all hospital departments.
    a. Attends all department meetings.
    b. Contributes to improving health insurance reimbursement by communicating shifting billing/coding industry standards to varying hospital departments.

Qualifications

A background check is required for all employees who wish to work in the health care environment.

Required: High School graduate, 1 year experience in medical office setting, knowledge of basic collections and follow-up on patient accounts, and intermediate MS Office skills.

Preferred: Some college or Medical Billing School, previous hospital experience, knowledge of medical terms and billing coding, and/or advance MS Office skills.

FIGURE 17-1 Job description for patient accounts representative (hospital biller). *HIPAA,* Health Insurance Portability and Accountability Act.

APPROPRIATENESS EVALUATION PROTOCOL CRITERIA FOR ADMISSION CERTIFICATION

An admission may be certified if one of the following criteria is met:

SEVERITY OF ILLNESS (SI)
1. Sudden onset of unconsciousness or disorientation (coma or unresponsiveness).
2. Pulse rate <50 or >140.
3. Systolic blood pressure <80 or >200 mm Hg. Diastolic blood pressure <60 or >120 mm Hg.
4. Sudden onset of loss of sight or hearing.
5. History of persistent fever ≥100° F (orally) or 101° F (rectally) for more than 5 days or with white blood cell count >15,000/mm³.
6. Sudden onset of motor function loss of any body part.
7. Active, uncontrolled bleeding.
8. Electrolyte or blood gas abnormality of serum K⁺: <2.5, >6.0; serum Na⁺ <123, >156; CO_2 <20 mEq/L, >36 mEq/L (new findings).
9. Acute or progressive sensory, motor, circulatory, or respiratory embarrassment sufficient to incapacitate the patient (one of the IS criteria must also be met).
10. Electrocardiographic evidence of acute ischemia with suspicion of new myocardial infarction.
11. Wound dehiscence or evisceration.

INTENSITY OF SERVICE (IS)
12. Administration and monitoring of intravenous medications and/or fluid replacement (does not include tube feeding).
13. Surgery or procedure scheduled within 24 hours requiring general or regional anesthesia with use of equipment and facilities available only in a hospital.
14. Vital signs monitoring at least every 2 hours, including telemetry and bedside cardiac monitoring.
15. Use of chemotherapeutic agents that require continuous observation for a life-threatening toxic reaction.
16. Treatment in intensive/coronary care unit.
17. Administration of intramuscular antibiotics at least every 8 hours.
18. Intermittent or continuous respirator use at least every 8 hours.
19. Documentation on the medical record by the attending physician that the patient has been unsuccessfully treated as an outpatient *with* further documentation of how the patient is now to be treated as an inpatient.

FIGURE 17-2 Appropriateness evaluation protocol (AEP) criteria for admission certification listing severity of illness and intensity of service.

These organizations have established specific procedure guidelines that hospitals must follow to ensure quality patient care for preadmission tests, such as laboratory tests, x-rays, and electrocardiograms (ECGs). In addition, the hospital may have specific rules for observation status dictated by the AHA, the hospital administration, and the hospital medical staff. Specific criteria are used by the insurance company for admission screening. Hospitals must meet **appropriateness evaluation protocols (AEPs)** by the hospital's **utilization review (UR)** department to certify that the patient's complaints meet the hospital's guidelines to warrant admittance to the hospital. A hospital AEP for admission example is found in Figure 17-2.

From a health care reimbursement perspective, because health care services are rendered prior to receiving payment, hospitals need to evaluate each patient case to ensure future payment. The CMS has recently pushed a zero tolerance for medical errors; they will not reimburse health care practitioners for mistakes in patient care. For this reason, UR is very important to the health care reimbursement process; it is the hospital's responsibility to obtain the approved UR of the case with the insurance carrier. Therefore the UR department should review each patient case to ensure that AEPs are exceeded. The Medicare prospective payment system (PPS) requires that all patients meet at least one severity of illness (SI) or intensity of service (IS) criterion, unless otherwise indicated, to be certified for reimbursement. Within the first 24 hours, the hospital's UR department analyzes the documentation on the medical record, which must reflect how the patient meets these criteria. UR is discussed in detail later in this chapter. Figure 17-3 shows the basic flow of the inpatient admission process from the initial encounter to discharge of the patient.

Admitting Procedures for Major Insurance Programs
Preauthorization

Prior to admission to the hospital, a case manager is assigned to verify patient benefits. After an evaluation by a qualified health professional, the admitting diagnosis is provided for the case manager, who then contacts the insurance company directly for approval, or *authorization*. Without this authorization, none of the therapeutic care provided to the patient is reimbursable.

The admitting process varies according to rules set down by the patient's insurance plan and hospital rules based on guidelines from the AHA. The basic admitting procedures and preadmission authorization requirements for the major insurance programs follow.

Private Insurance (Group or Individual): It is the responsibility of the outpatient and inpatient admitting personnel to obtain complete and accurate information during initial registration of the patient. The patient must provide a current insurance card for his or her primary and secondary health care coverage. Obtain images of the front and back of all cards. Some hospital facilities employ an insurance verification clerk. He or she is responsible for contacting the insurance company (within 24 hours or on the next working day), or the insured individual's employer in workers' compensation cases, to verify the type of health insurance. The clerk also must call the insurance company to verify eligibility and benefits and determine whether prior authorization is necessary. Some facilities use the internet to obtain insurance verification from an insurance company or use a point-of-service (POS) machine. These methods are quicker and less expensive than telephone verification. Refer to Procedure 17-1 on how to perform a new patient admission and insurance verification.

Commercial Insurance and Managed Care: In today's private health care insurance industry, almost all plans have aspects of managed care.[1] There are restrictions and various policies and procedures to follow when admitting a patient who has a managed care health maintenance organization (HMO) or preferred provider organization (PPO) type of insurance. Several types of patient admissions to the hospital are recognized by managed care plans. See Chapter 11 for additional information on this subject.

Emergency Inpatient Admission: For a patient who is admitted through the emergency department (ED), the managed care program should be notified on the next working day or within 48 hours to obtain an authorization number. The plan authorizes the admission and preapproves subsequent days based on the admitting diagnosis. The case management review by the health insurance company determines the emergency status and may send written notification to the hospital and physician; the patient is also notified of his or her deductible and copayment responsibilities. ED services are billed on the CMS-1450 (UB-04) claim form, which is also known as the 837i (institutional) claim form. The admitting physician's services are billed on a CMS-1500 (02-12) insurance claim form.

Nonemergency Inpatient Admission and Elective Admission: The patient must be referred by his or her primary care physician (PCP) and obtain preliminary authorization for the length of the hospital stay prior to admission. Although the patient may have a coinsurance requirement that he or she will be responsible for after admission, the deductible is payable prior to the service. If a patient seeks health care services at a nonparticipating facility, he or she will be responsible for penalties, such as higher deductibles, higher coinsurance, and possibly no insurance coverage.

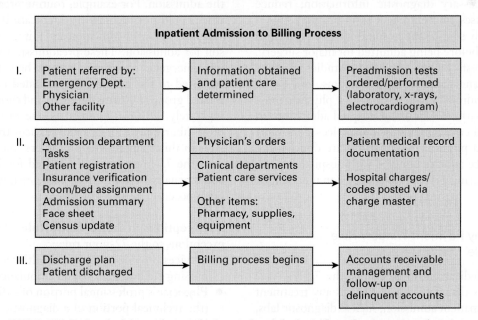

FIGURE 17-3 Referral of the patient to the hospital and the basic flow after inpatient admission. This illustration shows various services a patient might encounter during a hospital stay and ends with the patient's discharge, the billing process, and accounts receivable management.

Medicaid: Preapproval for admission is a requirement for Medicaid patients, with the exception of being admitted in an emergency. For an emergency, a certification of need for services form must accompany the insurance claim form. Many state Medicaid programs have issued specialized terminal equipment for efficient patient eligibility verification. See Chapter 13 for additional information.

Medicare: Medicare patients do not need prior approval for admission to a hospital. However, their admittance should be certified by AEPs, as previously discussed in this chapter. For patients who receive both Medicare and Medicaid or other secondary insurance benefits, Medicare is billed first. Secondary insurances are billed after Medicare has paid the claim; the claim form is processed automatically by Medicaid and many other private insurances. See Chapter 12 for detailed discussion of the Medicare program.

Tricare: As stated in Chapter 14, all admissions to a civilian hospital and ambulatory surgical facility, except for emergency cases, require precertification. The TRICARE website health care provider search can help in finding medical care when a military treatment hospital is not available. See Chapter 14 for additional information.

Workers' Compensation: Workers' compensation programs do not issue an insurance card for their insured beneficiaries. When the patient is seen on an emergency basis, an injury report must be completed and sent to the workers' compensation insurance company and the state industrial accident board before a hospital's or physician's claim may be submitted. Once the report is filed and approved, a case number is assigned by the workers' compensation insurance. Appropriate information relating to the injured patient, date of injury, insurance carrier, and employer must be obtained. Prior to admission, the insurance adjuster must authorize length of stay and all surgical procedures for an elective admission. See Chapter 15 for additional information on Worker's Compensation insurance plans.

Preadmission Testing

To obtain necessary diagnostic information, reduce inpatient expenses, and eliminate extra hospital days, a patient is usually sent to the hospital for **preadmission testing (PAT)** before being admitted for major surgery. Preadmission tests include diagnostic studies, such as routine blood and urine work, x-ray films, and ECG. For inpatient admission, a history and physical must be completed within 24 hours of hospital admission. In elective surgical cases, preadmission services (for example, history and physical examination) are done in the physician's office and are bundled with hospital services instead of appearing as separate **charges** on inpatient or outpatient bills.

Medicare 3-Day Payment Window Rule or 72-Hour Rule

When filing Medicare hospital claims, the *72-hour rule* applies. It states that if a patient receives any treatment related to the inpatient admission, such as diagnostic labs, x-rays, medical equipment, and any outpatient services within 72 hours of admission to a hospital (3-day payment window), then all such services are bundled with the inpatient service claim if these services are related to the admission. For example, routine preadmission blood work could not be billed to Medicare if it is completed within 72 hours of admission and if it is related to the reason for admission. These preadmission services, including emergency services if this is how the patient was admitted to the hospital, are included in the diagnosis-related group (DRG) assignment and should not be billed separately. DRG assignment is one of several methods of reimbursement for hospital services that are discussed later in this chapter. Medical billers that do not comply with the 72-hour rule will be cited for fraud and abuse and a penalty in the form of a fine or imprisonment may be imposed.

Exceptions to the 72-Hour Rule. The following are exceptions to the 72-hour rule:
- Services provided by home health facilities, hospices, nursing facilities (NFs), and ambulance services
- Physician's professional portion of a diagnostic service (the technical portion of a diagnostic service must be included in the inpatient bill)
- Preadmission laboratory testing when the laboratory is not contracted with the hospital

It is important to note that the 72-hour rule applies only to Medicare; therefore other health insurance companies do cover preadmission lab work, x-rays, medical equipment, and so on within 24 hours of hospital admission.

Present on Admission

Present on admission (POA) indicator codes are assigned to each diagnosis to determine whether the condition was present on admission. It can include conditions known at the time of admission, conditions present at admission but not diagnosed until later, and conditions that develop during outpatient encounters, such as ED, observation, or outpatient surgery. Medicare no longer reimburses hospitals for preventable medical errors in patient care, such as an object left in the body during surgery, catheter-associated urinary tract infection, hospital-acquired injury, and so on. The POA indicator codes are reported on the CMS 1450 (UB-04) paper or 837i claim form, Field 67. The different types of POA codes are listed in Table 17-1.

UTILIZATION REVIEW

As discussed in Chapter 11, UR is necessary to control costs in a managed care setting. UR is a formal assessment of the cost and use of components of the health care system. Each hospital should have a UR department that conducts an admission and concurrent review and prepares a discharge plan on all cases. An **admission review** is an evaluation for appropriateness and necessity of admissions. A case manager should be assigned to each patient to ensure appropriate medical care for that patient as well as a plan for his or her discharge. A concurrent review is an evaluation of health care services to determine medical necessity and appropriateness of medical care during the time services are being provided; this is done by a health care provider other than the one giving the care. This process anticipates the patient's length of stay (LOS) and concludes the expected discharge date. If the admission is found to be necessary, it is certified.

UR companies provide utilization review and case management services for self-insured employers, third-party administrators, and insurance companies. They furnish data to the person who buys their services to achieve cost savings and they generate reports on how much money has been saved.

Quality Improvement Organization Program

Quality Improvement Organizations (QIOs) work with CMS to review medical necessity, reasonableness, appropriateness, completeness, and adequacy of

Table 17-1	Present on Admission Codes
INDICATOR	**DESCRIPTION**
Y	Diagnosis was present at time of inpatient admission.
N	Diagnosis was not present at time of inpatient admission.
U	Documentation insufficient to determine if condition was present at the time of inpatient admission.
W	Clinically undetermined. Provider unable to clinically determine whether the condition was present at the time of inpatient admission.

Department of Health and Human Services: Centers for Medicare and Medicaid Services, October 2011.

inpatient hospital care for Medicare and Medicaid beneficiaries. CMS requires that all hospitals have a quality improvement program to meet accreditation standards. There is currently a national network of 53 QIOs responsible for each state and territory and the District of Columbia. QIO is governed by Titles XI and XVIII of the Social Security Act. QIOs are required to review all written quality of service complaints submitted by Medicare beneficiaries. The review addresses whether the services met professionally recognized standards of health care and may include whether the appropriate services were or were not provided in appropriate settings. The QIO's professional medical staff performs these reviews. The results of the reviews are submitted to CMS. The QIOs are responsible for the following types of review:

- Admission review for appropriateness and necessity of admissions.
- **Readmission review** on patients readmitted within 7 days with problems related to the first admission to determine whether the first discharge was premature or the second admission is medically necessary.
- **Procedure review** of diagnostic and therapeutic procedures in cases in which past abuses have been found to determine appropriateness.
- **Day outlier review** of short or unusually long length of hospital stays to determine the number of days before the day outlier threshold is reached as well as the number of days beyond the threshold. This process is done to certify necessity of admission and medical necessity of services for additional Medicare reimbursement.
- **Cost outlier review** of cases not eligible for day outlier review to determine the necessity of admission and the necessity and appropriateness of services rendered.
- **DRG validation** to find out whether the diagnostic and procedural information affecting DRG assignment is substantiated by the clinical information in the patient's chart. DRGs are discussed later in this chapter.
- **Transfer review** of cases involving a transfer to a distinct part or unit of the same hospital or other hospitals.

CODING HOSPITAL DIAGNOSES AND PROCEDURES

A health insurance claim form requires codes for the diagnosis and the procedure. Diagnosis codes come from the ICD-9-CM or ICD-10-CM code sets, depending on the health insurance medical billing requirements. Procedure codes come from the CPT; HCPCS; ICD-9-CM, Volume 3; or ICD-10-PCS. To be successful in medical coding, it is important to differentiate between the CM and PCS code sets. CM, or clinical modifications, is used for diagnosis only. PCS, or procedural coding system, is used for inpatient procedures only.

Chapter 5 provides basic information and instructions on how to use ICD-9-CM and ICD-10-CM, Volumes 1 and 2. This chapter explains the use of ICD-10-PCS. Chapter 6 gives information on CPT and HCPCS procedural codes.

As of the date of publication of this book, it has been proposed that all health care organizations need to update the current ICD-9-CM to ICD-10-CM and ICD-10-PCS by October 1, 2014. However, there may be some health insurers that will accept only ICD-9-CM, Volume 3, after the deadline; for this reason, coding procedures for both code sets are included in this chapter.

Principal Diagnosis

The **principal diagnosis** is listed as the first diagnosis on the insurance claim; this diagnosis code from the ICD-9-CM or ICD-10-CM is the reason for the patient seeking medical care. For outpatient claims, the first diagnosis is also known as the **reason for encounter**. For inpatient claims, the principal diagnosis is the reason for admission; this can also be known as the *admitting diagnosis*. For example, heart disease is the principal diagnosis if a patient initially comes in for heart transplantation. However, pneumonia is the principal diagnosis if the heart transplant patient goes home and then returns to the hospital with pneumonia. Subsequent diagnostic codes should be used for any current condition that coexists with the principal condition, complicating the treatment and management of the principal disorder. These codes are listed after the principal diagnosis. A secondary diagnosis is one that may contribute to the condition, treatment, or recovery from the condition shown as the principal diagnosis. It also may define the need for a higher level of care but is not the underlying cause. Codes for conditions that were previously treated and no longer exist should not be included. The diagnostic **code sequence** is important in billing of hospital inpatient

Example 17-1	Principal Diagnosis, Signs and Symptoms

Mr. Brown was admitted to the hospital with fever, severe abdominal pain, nausea, and vomiting.

Diagnosis:	Acute appendicitis
ICD-10-CM Dx Code:	K35.9 (acute appendicitis without generalized peritonitis)

Note: Symptoms are considered integral to the condition, so the condition should be coded.

cases because maximum reimbursement is based on the DRG system. This is explained in detail at the end of this chapter.

Rules for Coding Inpatient Diagnoses

Coding diagnoses for inpatient and outpatient cases can differ. One important difference is how uncertain diagnoses are coded. For inpatient cases, code all "rule out," "suspected," "likely," "questionable," "possible," or "still to be ruled out" as if it existed. For example, the physician documents "upper abdominal pain, rule out cholecystitis." Assign ICD-10-CM code K81.9 (cholecystitis, unspecified) for this diagnosis. This rule applies to inpatient records only.

In addition, the following rules and examples should be noted about the principal diagnosis:
- ICD-10-CM codes for signs and symptoms are not reported as principal diagnoses (Example 17-1).
- When two or more conditions meet the definition of principal diagnosis, either condition may be sequenced first unless otherwise indicated by the circumstances of admission or the therapy provided (Example 17-2).
- When a symptom is followed by a contrasting comparative diagnosis, sequence the symptom code first (Example 17-3).

Conditions that are an integral part of a documented disease process should not be coded and abnormal findings should not be coded unless the physician indicates their clinical significance.

The physician should be made aware that certain principal diagnoses are subject to 100% review by the review agency. The physician should pay special attention when using the following as principal diagnoses:
- Arteriosclerotic heart disease (ASHD)—acceptable as a diagnosis only when cardiac catheterization or open heart surgery is performed

---

Example 17-2   Two Medical Conditions

Mrs. Sanchez was admitted with acute congestive heart failure (CHF) and unstable angina. Both conditions are treated.

Diagnosis: CHF and unstable angina

ICD-10-CM Dx Code: I50.9 (congestive heart failure NOS) and I20.0 (unstable angina)

NOS, Not otherwise specified.

Note: This is the focus of many compliance reviews.

Example 17-3   Symptom as Principal Diagnosis

Miss Chan was admitted with acute epigastric abdominal pain.

Diagnosis: Epigastric abdominal pain, acute pyelonephritis versus acute gastritis

ICD-10-CM Dx Code: R10.13 (epigastric pain)
                               N10 (acute pyelonephritis)
                               K29.00 (acute gastritis without bleeding)

Note: Code symptoms first, followed by conditional diagnoses.

- Diabetes mellitus without complications
- Right or left bundle branch block
- Coronary atherosclerosis

Local hospital health information management personnel should be contacted periodically to find out whether new items have been added to this list.

CODING INPATIENT PROCEDURES

Procedural Coding Systems

The Department of Health and Human Services (DHHS) announced that final implementation of the ICD-10-CM/PCS system will occur on October 14, 2015. Currently the diagnosis and hospital procedure coding is in transition. This edition summarizes ICD-9-CM, Volume 3, and details only the ICD-10-PCS inpatient coding procedures in light of the implementation date and the publication date of this text.

The ICD-10-CM lists procedural codes used only for surgical procedures performed in the hospital. These codes can be used only on the CMS-1450

(UB-04) claim form because they represent inpatient procedures.

International Classification of Diseases, Ninth Revision, Clinical Modification, Volume 3

In ICD-9-CM, Volume 3, the code set is organized by the Tabular List and the Alphabetic Index. The Tabular List is divided into chapters that relate to operations or procedures for various body systems, with the last chapter referring to miscellaneous diagnostic, therapeutic, and prophylactic procedures. Procedure codes are two digits at the category code level, with one or two digits beyond the decimal point. The third and fourth digits differentiate unilateral or bilateral, surgical approach or technique, and condition type (for example, indirect or direct hernia). No alphabetic characters are used. All four digits must be listed when a three-digit code is followed by a fourth digit. Remember to always code to the highest level of specificity.

The Alphabetic Index is arranged by procedure (for example, incision, excision, graft, or implant) and not anatomic site. It is used to locate the procedure that is referred to as the main term. Read any notations that appear under the main term in bold type. A main term may be followed by modifiers (for example, a series of subterms in parentheses) that give differences in site or surgical technique.

International Classification of Diseases, Tenth Revision, Procedure Coding System

The coding structure in ICD-10-PCS is significantly different than that in ICD-9-CM, Volume 3. ICD-10-PCS code drafts can be downloaded for free from the CMS website.

Code Structure

The new table format of ICD-10-PCS allows for unique identification of each procedure. ICD-10-PCS codes have a seven-character alphanumeric code structure that is multi-axial, or the code set is divided by various sections and then further defined by smaller classifications. Each character contains up to 34 possible alphanumeric values. To avoid confusion with digits 0 and 1, the letters O and I are not used. The ICD-10-PCS code structure may be defined as follows:

Character:	Section	Body System	Root Operation	Body Part	Approach	Device	Qualifier
	1	2	3	4	5	6	7

Character Definitions

Character 1: Section. The Section character is the largest classification in ICD-10-PCS; the Section defines the index of the medical specialty. The most expansive section is character 0 for Medical and Surgical Procedures; for inpatient hospital billing, coders will most likely use Section 0. A list of medical specialty sections is found in Table 17-2.

Character 2: Body System. The Body System character identifies on which body system the procedure is being done. All complete ICD-10-PCS codes will have an assigned body system except the rehabilitation and mental health sections.

Character 3: Root Operation. The Root Operation character identifies the type of procedure that was performed. Root operations and their definitions can be found in Appendix C of the *Workbook*. Not all root operations can be performed on every body system. For example, the root operation fragmentation, which involves breaking solid matter in a body part into pieces, cannot be performed on the nasal sinuses; therefore a table cannot be found matching this body system with the root operation.

The tables are organized by the first three characters of the ICD-10-PCS code, which are the Section, Body System, and Root Operation. The last four characters of the ICD-10-PCS code are determined inside the table.

Character 4: Body Part. The Body Part character identifies where in the body system the procedure is done. In most cases, right and left sides of the body part are identified by different characters. The body parts are subsets of the body system; in other words, the trachea body part is not listed in the body system ear, nose, and

sinus. For accurate coding, only body parts listed in the specific table can be used; if the coder chooses body part characters that are not listed, the coding will be incorrect.

Character 5: Approach. The Approach character identifies the approach the surgeon is taking for the surgery. A list of Approach definitions can be found in Appendix D of the *Workbook*. For accurate coding, the coder must be made aware of how the surgery was performed.

Character 6: Device and Character 7: Qualifier. The Device and Qualifier characters are used to identify specific devices in use or provide information for some codes that may not be identified elsewhere. Most codes use character Z, which represents No Device or No Qualifier.

Tabular Index

The most effective way to code ICD-10-PCS is to use the Tabular Index. The Tabular Index is organized first by Section and then by Body Part. The tables are then presented by the root operation characters. This method of coding prevents coders from choosing erroneous codes; all acceptable codes are presented in the tables. For an example of an ICD-10-PCS table, see Table 17-3. Refer to Procedure 17-2 on how to use the tables in ICD-10-PCS coding.

Alphabetic Index

While ICD-10-PCS does have an Alphabetic Index, it is not advisable to rely on this index for accurate coding. The tables provide the only approved body parts, approaches, devices, and qualifiers. This information can be verified only by using the Section, Body System, and Root Operation tables in ICD-10-PCS to ensure accurate coding.

Prepare for ICD-10-PCS Coding

Due to the detail-oriented nature of the ICD-10-PCS coding set, successful coders must understand the procedures in the type of operation performed, the exact body parts, and the surgical approach. Therefore it is recommended that ICD-10-PCS coders should improve their proficiency in anatomy and physiology, medical terminology, and clinical knowledge. As a result, step-by-step procedures for locating codes in the ICD-10-PCS codebook are not detailed in text. It is recommended that a separate course on ICD-10-PCS be taken to become skillful and proficient at this task.

CODING HOSPITAL OUTPATIENT PROCEDURES

Outpatient claims are always completed on a CMS-1500 (02-12) claim form. Diagnosis codes are from the ICD-9-CM and ICD-10-CM code sets. Procedural codes are

Table 17-2	ICD-10-PCS Character 1 Section Medical Specialties
CHARACTER	**SECTION**
0	Medical and Surgical
1	Obstetrics
2	Placement
3	Administration
4	Measurement and Monitoring
5	Extracorporeal Assistance and Performance
6	Extracorporeal Therapies
7	Osteopathic
8	Other Procedures
9	Chiropractic
B	Imaging
C	Nuclear Medicine
D	Radiation Oncology
F	Physical Rehabilitation and Diagnostic Audiology
G	Mental Health
H	Substance Abuse Treatment

from the CPT and/or HCPCS code sets. ICD-9-CM, Volume 3, and ICD-10-PCS are never used for outpatient claims billing.

Healthcare Common Procedure Coding System Level I: Current Procedural Terminology

The Medicare HCPCS (pronounced "hick-picks") consists of the following two levels of coding:
- Level I: AMA CPT codes and modifiers (national codes)
- Level II: CMS-designated codes and alpha modifiers (national codes)

The CPT code set is published by the AMA and updates are published each year on January 1. Typically the CPT code set is used for procedural codes and HCPCS is used for medical equipment, medical supplies, ambulatory services, drugs, and any other auxiliary codes. Chapter 6 gives basic information and instruction on how to use the code book. Billing software must be updated with new codes to receive maximum reimbursement.

Modifiers

Modifiers are two-digit alphanumeric codes that modify or provide more detailed information on the procedure. While both CPT and HCPCS use modifiers, an experienced coder will not use CPT modifiers for HCPCS codes and vice versa. An example of a CPT modifier is AA; this modifier designates that an anesthesiologist performed the service. See Appendix A of the CPT manual or Chapter 6 of this text for a detailed explanation of CPT modifier use. Selected HCPCS/National Level II and CPT Level I modifiers that are generally approved and used for outpatient hospital billing are listed in Table 6-6 and a partial listing is shown in Table 1 of the Workbook.

MEDICAL BILLING PROCESS

The hospital takes responsibility to bill for all procedures, including inpatient and outpatient. Patients admitted to the hospital prior to surgery who need 24-hour monitored care after the procedure are considered **inpatient**. Outpatient procedures are performed on patients who are expected to return home for recovery but can also be performed in the hospital. Most hospitals have one surgical area, so all billed medical procedures occur in the same unit. Because all surgeries are completed in the hospital, ICD-10-PCS codes are used for procedure codes when billing the facility fee.

Inpatient hospital claims include charges for the surgery and aftercare in the hospital environment. Only the facility fee for the outpatient surgery is billed to the insurance company. Both inpatient and outpatient procedures should be billed on a CMS 1450 (UB-04) form.

INPATIENT MEDICAL BILLING PROCESS

The insurance billing division is often part of the hospital's business office and may be placed near the admission department, hospital cashier, or main lobby (entry and exit) of the hospital because patients need easy access. In some facilities, the financial department may be so large that it is relocated to a building at another site. The inpatient billing process involves many people and departments in the hospital. As an introduction, Figure 17-4 shows which main departments of the hospital interact as the billing process flows from beginning to end. Explanations of each hospital employee's role in this process are included in the following sections.

Table 17-3	ICD-10-PCS Table, Section 0, Body System C, Operation P		
Section	**0** Medical and Surgical		
Body System	**C** Mouth and Throat		
Operation	**P** Removal: Taking out or off a device from a body part		
BODY PART	**APPROACH**	**DEVICE**	**QUALIFIER**
A Salivary Gland	**0** Open	**0** Drainage Device	**Z** No Qualifier
	3 Percutaneous	**C** Extraluminal Device	
S Larynx	**0** Open	**0** Drainage Device	**Z** No Qualifier
	3 Percutaneous	**7** Autologous Tissue Substitute	
	7 Via Natural or Artificial Opening	**D** Intraluminal Device	
	8 Via Natural or Artificial Opening Endoscopic	**J** Synthetic Substitute	
	X External	**K** Nonautologous Tissue Substitute	
Y Mouth and Throat	**0** Open	**0** Drainage Device	**Z** No Qualifier
	3 Percutaneous	**1** Radioactive Element	
	7 Via Natural or Artificial Opening	**7** Autologous Tissue Substitute	
	8 Via Natural or Artificial Opening Endoscopic	**D** Intraluminal Device	
	X External	**J** Synthetic Substitute	
		K Nonautologous Tissue Substitute	

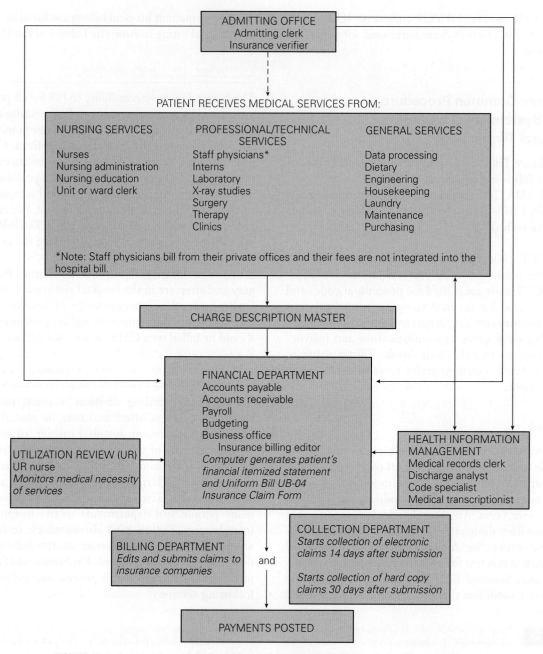

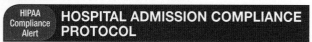

FIGURE 17-4 An overview of the basic flow of the hospital billing process for an inpatient.

Admitting Clerk

An admitting clerk registers the patient by interviewing and obtaining personal (demographic) and insurance information from the patient and admitting diagnosis or symptoms from the admitting physician or preadmission surgery data. The primary responsibility of the admitting clerk is to ensure that the collected insurance information is correct, to obtain names of family members that can make decisions on the patient's behalf, to inform the patient of their patient and privacy rights, and to collect any copayments prior to admission.

The patient is assigned a patient account number at this time; this number differs from the medical record number because a new number is assigned to each patient encounter with the same hospital while the medical record number remains the same. The patient account number is associated with all charges and payments related to the dates of the specific episode of care. Copies of the admitting face sheet are sent to the PCP or surgeon's office. Registration information, copies of all authorization and signature documents, a copy of the insurance card or cards, and a copy of the ED report if the patient is admitted through the ED are scanned in paperless facilities or assembled in a financial folder in facilities that use a traditional system and become a part of the patient's permanent medical record.

Insurance Verifier

An insurance verifier is responsible for verifying patient eligibility, obtaining authorization for admission, and confirming any copayment requirements. The insurance identifier also may telephone the patient or physician for additional data for health insurance coverage purposes. It may be necessary for additional physician's consultation reports to obtain an authorization for surgery; the insurance verifier will ensure that all documents needed are submitted to the insurance company for preauthorization of services. For workers' compensation cases, the verifier may contact the employer or insurance adjuster directly to verify coverage.

The Admission Process

Patients who are admitted for surgery will enter through the surgical prep department. During intake, the attending physician is responsible for dictating a history and physical on admission, which includes the admitting diagnosis. The attending physician and nurses enter daily notations on the patient's medical record as the patient receives medical services. A unit secretary or ward clerk inputs the physician's orders by use of a computer that electronically transmits them to other departments (for example, pharmacy, laboratory, or radiology). A handheld computer may be used in some hospitals. If supplies are used, stickers are removed from the supply item and scanned to record data. The attending physician supplies documentation for all medical and surgical reports, ending the patient's stay with a discharge summary that is sometimes known as a clinical résumé. A final progress note may be substituted for a discharge summary under specific instances—that is, when the inpatient stay does not exceed 48 hours for an uncomplicated condition. This document is transcribed by the medical transcriptionist and includes the course of treatment during the hospital stay, all diagnostic studies, consultations, admission and discharge diagnoses, operations performed, condition of patient at the time of discharge, instructions for continuing care and follow-up treatment, and time frame for postoperative office visit.

Discharge Process

Once a patient is discharged from the facility, their medical record is sent to the HIM department where a clerk will begin to assemble the patient chart. The clerk authenticates the completeness of the patient's medical record for a history and physical, other dictated reports (including procedure reports and consultations), and that all physicians' orders are signed by the attending physician. A deficiency sheet completed by the HIM clerk is placed in the paper record and the record is placed in an area where physicians can resolve the chart deficiencies. Hospitals bill for services only after the discharge summary is completed and signed by the physician. Many hospitals strive to complete charts within 3 to 4 days, and no more than 14 days, after a patient is discharged; otherwise a cash flow problem will result. Per TJC, hospital charts may be completed up to 30 days after discharge. TJC is an accrediting body for clinics, hospitals, and other federal and military facilities. It reviews the policies, patient records, credentialing procedures, and quality assurance programs of the facility.

Charge Description Master

The **charge description master (CDM)** is used to list all charges for the care provided to the patient during the encounter; some of these charges include pharmaceuticals, medical equipment, room and board, nursing care, surgical supplies, and surgical equipment. All services and items provided to the patient are coded and entered using health insurance billing software, which assists with the high volume of insurance claim filing for hospital patients.

The CDM contains the following elements:
a. *Procedure code.* CPT and HCPCS codes should correspond with the description of the procedure.
b. *Charge.* Dollar amount for each CPT and HCPCS code. The dollar amount billed is not always what is reimbursed. Reimbursement amounts depend on the patient's insurance company, managed care options, and/or private or government-sponsored insurance plan.
c. *Revenue code.* The revenue code represents a specific accommodation, ancillary service, or billing calculation related to service that is inserted in Form Locator 42 of the CMS-1450 (UB-04) claim form. This code can be either a 3-digit or a 4-digit number. Since payers vary in their revenue code preference, confirm which revenue code form is accepted by the payer. Examples are where the service was performed (0320 = Radiology); where the service may have been provided (0450 = ED);

or the total dollar amount of the services provided for a particular time frame, bill, or claim (0001 = last entry on the bill). The revenue code must be coded to the highest level of specificity. You may see a code 030X, with the "X" indicating that further breakdown is necessary to best identify the service or supply being provided. Before using a fourth digit, some revenue codes may indicate that a service should be put on a CMS-1500 (02-12) claim form instead of a CMS-1450 (UB-04) claim form. For example, durable medical equipment (DME) code 0292 must be submitted on a CMS-1500 (02-12) claim form, not on a CMS-1450 (UB-04), with the correct HCPCS and facility DME provider number. For Medicare, some revenue codes can be used only on a CMS-1500 (02-12). The facility software should be able to determine a revenue code appropriate for the same services and supplies in the outpatient and inpatient setting. A Health Insurance Portability and Accountability Act (HIPAA) compliance issue is that it would be fraudulent for a insurance billing specialist to change a revenue code so that a claim would pass edits.

The master charge list or charge description list is a computer database of what the hospital will charge for each service or supply; this list is developed by the UR department and varies from hospital to hospital. This database is unique to each hospital that accommodates the charges for items and services that may be provided to patients. The content and format of the charge master varies among facilities but the function remains the same.

For institutional facilities (for example, inpatient and outpatient departments, rural health clinics, chronic dialysis services, or adult day health care), each patient's data consisting of revenue codes, procedure codes, descriptions, charges, and medical record data are organized by the CDM and printed on a hospital paper CMS-1450 (UB-04) or stored electronically for future claim transmission.

The charge master database must be kept current and accurate to obtain proper reimbursement. It must be audited regularly; otherwise, negative impacts such as overpayment, underpayment, undercharging for services, claims rejections, fines, or penalties may result. A committee may oversee maintenance of the charge master composed of experts in coding, billing regulations, clinical procedures, and health record documentation. Because this system is automated, there is a high risk that a single coding or data mapping error could replicate and many medical claim errors could occur before being identified and corrected. *Data mapping* is a method of matching one set of data elements or individual code values to the nearest equivalents in another set, also known as *crosswalk*. Duplicate reports of CPT or HCPCS Level II codes for the same service, both by the department performing the service and by the HIM coding specialists, are common billing problems. These problems

may be prevented by regularly reviewing the charge master (sorted by CPT code number) with the coding staff so that they are aware of the codes reported via the charge master. Category III CPT codes should be reported by only one source, either the department that charges for the service or the code specialist. Category III codes are temporary codes for emergency technology, services, and procedures and are used instead of a category I unlisted code number.

In a direct data entry (DDE) system, there is usually a lag time (for example, from 1 to 4 days after patient discharge) before the bill is "dropped" by the charge master to ensure that all charges have been entered. The word "dropped" refers to the dropped time, which is the time between the discharge of the patient from the hospital and the input of the late charges to the time when the final bill is printed.

Coding Specialist

The chart is given to HIM, which is directed or managed by a registered health information administrator (RHIA) or registered health information technician (RHIT). In some situations, an RHIA or RHIT may act as a consultant to several hospitals and may not be employed by one hospital. This department is also composed of discharge analysts, coding specialists, and clerical staff. A medical record number is assigned to the patient's chart at the time of admission. This medical record number never changes (even on future admits to the same health care facility) and all records are filed under this number.

An HIM coder abstracts procedures and diagnoses from the patient's health record and assigns the appropriate codes for the services given. It is possible that the coder may use an encoder to perform this function. As discussed, an encoder is a computer software program that assigns a code to represent data. See Chapter 8 for further information.

Coding Credentials

Accuracy of coding affects the financial viability of acute care hospitals. The coder, whose job is highly analytic, should not only abstract information from the medical record and assign the correct code but also guard against the most common errors of transposing numbers and leaving off fourth and fifth digits from diagnostic codes. A majority of coders in the hospital setting have credentials and have earned a certificate or degree from an educational institute. A number of professional organizations that offer certification for coders are mentioned in Chapter 18.

Electronic Claims Submission

The Administrative Simplification provisions of HIPAA prohibited the submission of paper claims, both CMS-1500 and CMS-1450 claims, as of October 16, 2003, except under the following conditions:

- Small provider claims—the health care provider groups have limited resources and do not employ more than 25 full-time employees
- Roster billing of inoculations covered by Medicare
- Claims for payment under a Medicare-demonstrated topic that specifies claims to be submitted on paper
- Medicare secondary payer claims
- Claims submitted by Medicare beneficiaries
- Dental claims
- Claims for services or supplies furnished outside of the US by non–US providers
- Disruption in electricity or communication connections outside of a provider's control lasting more than 2 days
- Claims from providers that submit fewer than 10 claims on average during a calendar year[2]

Another element of the Administrative Simplification provisions of HIPAA is the establishment of electronic transaction data sets. As of January 1, 2012, the HIPAA X12 *Version 5010* is the new standard that regulates the transmission of specific health care transactions, which include eligibility, claim status, referrals, claims, and remittances. The upgrade to Version 5010 from Version 4010A1 will allow for ICD-10 values when they go into effect within the next few years.[3] One challenge that many insurance billing specialists face is the lack of standardization between all of the different medical billing software used in the industry. *Clearinghouses* act as an intermediary between the provider filing the claim and the insurance company accepting the claim, and vice versa. The provider submits the claim in data packets to the clearinghouse. The clearinghouse then arranges the data packets according to the required electronic transmission standards to the insurance company. The insurance company then communicates claim status to the clearinghouse, which in turn informs the provider electronically. Electronic remittance advices (ERAs) are also sent from the insurance company to the clearinghouse to the provider.

Clearinghouses will not accept paper claims on behalf of the provider and then submit Version 5010 claims to insurance companies; insurance billing specialists need to submit data packets electronically, which are then formatted into the required Version 5010.

Ensuring accurate coding is vital; therefore a systematic approach should be established when editing a claim and the same procedure should be used each time. Procedure 17-3, which shows how to edit a CMS-1450 (UB-04), may be found on the Evolve website http://evolve.elsevier.com/Fordney/handbook. This helps to train the editor to notice errors or omitted information. Insurance personnel should understand coding but in a hospital setting it is not their job to assign codes. Final code selection is done by clinical coding specialists. Reviewing form locators (FLs) 42 through 47 is the most time-consuming portion of the editing process and the area that requires experience to master. This is the area where the most errors and omissions occur. The claim form may go back to the HIM department after it is edited (where the coder verifies all codes) and to the contract department (where a contractor matches the bill with the insurance type).

Typically the insurance company will not allow all charges to be paid in full. Payments made by the insurance company are based on its fee schedule. The balance between the hospital charges and the allowable charge needs to be adjusted; this is done after the hospital has received the remittance advice. An adjustment to the account is posted, indicating the dollar amount above which the insurance carrier will not pay according to the contract. This transaction is referred to as relieving the accounts receivable on the front end and is desirable because the accounts receivable does not appear inflated.

Electronically transmit or mail all claim forms to the insurance carrier for payment and retain digital files or paper copies for the office files. Document the patient's file with the date mailed and the address to which the insurance claim was filed. The claim may be rejected or delayed if errors are not caught, leading to slow payment or nonpayment. See Chapter 7 for a list of common reasons why claims are rejected or delayed.

Clinical Documentation Improvement Specialists

Registered nurses (RNs) work as nurse clinical documentation improvement specialists and verify the doctor's orders and the medical record against each charge item on the bill. They may be onsite employees or hired offsite to come in periodically. These professionals have a background in nursing and have an interdisciplinary approach to auditing patient charts. A clean bill has no errors. An *under bill* fails to list charges that have been provided but not been billed. An *over bill* includes charges that have not been documented in the chart. A report goes to the HIM department if a coding error or omission occurs. All such accounts have coding priority. Several types of audits follow:

- *Random internal audit.* This occurs continually. Blind charts are pulled and audited to maintain quality control.
- *Audit by request.* The patient can request an audit to verify charges.
- *Defense audit.* The insurance company requests an audit. The insurance auditor may or may not (but should) meet with a hospital auditor, depending on the circumstances. Charts are pulled and audited.

LEGAL CONFIDENTIALITY ISSUES

Documents

All contents of the patient's health record are legal documents and must be kept confidential. No patient information can be disclosed or released to any individual unless a patient has signed a release authorization form. Chapter 2 contains information on confidentiality when facsimile communication is used. All confidential papers must be shredded and destroyed to prevent violations of confidentiality.

Computer Security

As you learned in Chapter 8 regarding computer security, when using a computer adhere to hospital policies with respect to the following:

- Using passwords and other encryption methods
- Policies for composition and transmission of e-mail
- Policies for use of the fax machine
- Downloading of computer data from one department to another
- Length of time that documents may be retained on computer hard drives by employees
- Procedures for deletion of confidential information
- Procedures for archiving of data
- Logging off when leaving a workstation or desk

Verbal Communication Breaches

Verbal breaches of confidentiality in a hospital setting, much like in a provider's office, can result in an insurance billing specialist being held liable and the facility being sued by a patient. A verbal breach of confidential communication is the unauthorized release of confidential information about a patient to a third party. Also, HIPAA violations carry monetary penalties and may include a jail sentence. New employees must be trained in confidentiality and asked to sign an understanding of confidentiality statement to ensure HIPAA compliance. This statement should emphasize that the employee may be subject to immediate termination in the event of a violation. Some of the following scenarios in which the patient's right to privacy has been breached in the hospital setting may be encountered by an insurance billing specialist, such as an employee overhearing co-workers discussing a patient's case, an employee who talks to family members about a patient's case, an employee who discusses a diagnosis with a co-worker, or a physician who talks on a cellphone about a patient's diagnosis.

For examples of and exercises related to medicolegal confidentiality issues, refer to Chapter 17 of the *Workbook*.

REIMBURSEMENT PROCESS

Generally, a hospital bill for inpatient care is much larger than the bill for services rendered in a physician's office. Individuals are admitted to hospitals for severe health problems and many require major surgery, resulting in considerable expense to the patient. Hospitals use and maintain highly sophisticated, expensive equipment; are located in large facilities; and employ large numbers of personnel, many of whom are state licensed and specialized. Salaries and operating costs must be recovered through patient insurance billing. However, working parents with families, elderly people, and jobless persons (even those who have insurance) have found it increasingly difficult to pay their share of the hospital bills. Consequently, accurate and timely hospital billing and good follow-up and collection techniques are in demand. In Chapter 10 you learned that a patient seeking medical care who is unable to pay for services and is ineligible for state aid should be directed to the local hospital that services recipients under the Hill-Burton Act of 1946. These hospitals obtained federal construction grants to enlarge their facilities in exchange for their provision of health care to needy patients. The DHHS will furnish the names of local hospitals that participate in this service. Patients must complete financial applications to determine eligibility before care is rendered.

Reimbursement Methods

As health insurance companies are under more pressure to reduce the cost to insure patients, more and more are converting to managed care organizations (MCOs). These organizations operate under varying contracts, policies, and guidelines, depending on individual state and federal laws. In negotiating a reimbursement contract, the managed care plan administrator tries to obtain discounted rates for participation in the plan by a hospital in exchange for an increased volume of patients. These programs use any one or a combination of various payment methods. See Chapter 11 for definitions of types of managed care plans. A brief description of some reimbursement methods follows:

- **Ambulatory payment classifications (APCs).** APC is an outpatient classification system developed by Health Systems International. This method is based on procedures rather than diagnoses. For Medicare patients, services associated with a specific procedure or visit are bundled into the APC reimbursement. More than one APC may be billed if more than one procedure is performed but discounts may be applied to any additional APCs. This topic is discussed in detail at the end of this chapter.

- *Bed leasing.* A managed care plan leases beds from a facility (for example, payment to the hospital of $300 per bed for 20 beds, regardless of whether those beds are used).

- **Capitation** or **percentage of revenue.** *Capitation* means reimbursement to the hospital on a per-member, per-month basis regardless of whether the patient is hospitalized. *Percentage of revenue* means a fixed percentage paid to the hospital to cover charges.
- **Case rate.** *Case rate* is an averaging after a flat rate (set amount paid for a service) has been given to certain categories of procedures (for example, normal vaginal delivery is $1800 and cesarean section is $2300). Utilization is expected to be 80% vaginal deliveries and 20% cesarean section; therefore the case rate is $1900 for all deliveries. Specialty procedures may also be given a case rate (for example, coronary artery bypass graft surgery or heart transplantation). *Bundled case rate* means an all-inclusive rate is paid for both institutional and professional services; for example, for coronary artery bypass graft surgery, a rate is used to pay all who provide services connected with that procedure. Bundled case rates are seen in teaching facilities in which a faculty practice plan works closely with the hospital.
- *Contract rate.* A set amount for payment to the hospital is established in the contract between the hospital and the managed care plan.
- **Diagnosis-related groups (DRGs).** A classification system called DRGs categorizes patients who are medically related with respect to diagnosis and treatment and are statistically similar in length of hospital stay. Medicare and some private hospital insurance payments are based on fixed dollar amounts determined by DRGs. DRGs are discussed in detail later in the chapter.
- *Differential by day in hospital.* The first day of the hospital stay is paid at a higher rate (for example, the first day may be paid at $1000 and each subsequent day at $500). Most hospitalizations are more expensive on the first day. This type of reimbursement method may be combined with a per diem arrangement.
- *Differential by service type.* The hospital receives a flat per-admission reimbursement for the service to which the patient is admitted. A prorated payment may be made (for example, 50% intensive care and 50% medicine) if services are mixed. Service types are defined in the contract (for example, medicine, surgery, intensive care, neonatal intensive care, psychiatry, obstetrics).
- *Fee-for-service.* The hospital is paid for each medical service provided on the basis of an established schedule of fees.
- *Fee schedule.* A comprehensive listing of charges based on procedure codes, under a fee-for-service (FFS) arrangement, or discounted FFS, states fee maximums paid by the health plan within the period of the managed care contract. Usually the fee schedule is based on CPT codes. For industrial cases, whether managed care or not, this listing may be called a *workers' compensation fee schedule.* This document is also known as a *fee maximum schedule* or *fee allowance schedule* as established by the state.
- *Flat rate.* A set amount (single charge) per hospital admission is paid by the managed care plan, regardless of the cost of the actual services the patient receives.
- **Per diem.** Per diem is a single charge for a day in the hospital regardless of actual charges or costs incurred (for example, a plan that pays $800 for each day regardless of the actual cost of service).
- *Percentage of accrued charges.* Payment calculates reimbursement on the basis of a percentage of total approved charges accrued during a hospital stay and submitted to the insurance plan.
- *Periodic interim payments (PIPs) and cash advances.* These are methods in which the plan advances cash to cover expected claims to the hospital. The fund is replenished periodically. Insurance claims may be applied to the cash advance or may be paid outside it. Generally this is done by Medicare.
- *Relative value studies or scale (RVS).* A list of procedure codes for professional services and procedures are assigned unit values that indicate the relative value of one procedure over another.
- *Resource-based relative value scale (RBRVS).* This payment system is implemented under the prospective payment system for Medicare and other government programs and provides reimbursement for outpatient services. It is based on a formula. The formula is that the relative value unit of each service must equal the sum of relative value units representing physicians' work, practice expenses, and cost of professional liability insurance.
- *Usual, customary, and reasonable (UCR).* This method is used by third-party payers to establish their fee schedules in which three fees are considered in calculating payment: (1) the usual fee is the fee typically submitted by the provider; (2) the customary fee falls within the range of usual fees charged by the provider in a geographic area; and (3) the reasonable fee meets the aforementioned criteria or is considered justifiable because of special circumstances.
- *Withhold.* In this method, part of the plan's payment to the hospital may be withheld or set aside in a bonus pool. If the hospital does not meet or exceed the criteria set, the hospital receives its bonus or withhold; other terms used are *bonus pools, capitation, risk pools,* and *withhold pools.*
- *Managed care stop-loss outliers.* **Stop loss** is a form of guarantee that may be written into a contract using one of a variety of methods. The purpose is to limit the exposure of cost to a reasonable level to prevent excessive loss. Stop loss is the least understood of reimbursement issues and can leave many thousands of dollars uncollected. There are a number of different ways in which stop loss can be applied; each contract is different. Become familiar with each contract and the stop-loss provisions in it.

The following are some methods that may be encountered:

- *Case-based stop loss.* This is the most common stop loss and can apply to the physician, on a smaller case basis, as well as to the individual hospital claim. For example, the hospital bill may run more than $1 million in cases of premature infants of extremely low birth weight. The contract may pay $2000 to $3000 per day, which may reimburse the hospital several hundred thousand dollars, but the hospital must absorb the excess. Stop-loss provisions may pay 65% of the excess over $100,000. Thus the hospital and the insurance carrier share the loss.
- *Reinsurance stop loss.* The hospital buys insurance to protect against lost revenue and receives less of a capitation fee; the amount it does not receive helps to pay for the insurance. For example, if a case has one or more claims that exceeds $100,000 in a calendar year, the plan may receive 80% of expenses in excess of $100,000 from the reinsurance company for the remainder of the year.
- *Percentage stop loss.* Some managed care contracts pay a percentage of charges when the total charge exceeds a listed contracted amount.
- *Medicare stop loss.* Medicare provides stop loss called outliers in its regulations. The day outliers for patients who remain in the hospital for long spells of illness no longer apply. Medicare provides cost outliers for those cases in which charges exceed the DRG or $30,000. DRGs are discussed at the end of this chapter.

Some reimbursement methods that are not used very much follow:

- *Charges.* In a managed care plan, charges are the dollar amounts owed to a participating provider for health care services rendered to a plan member, according to a fee schedule set by the managed care plan. This is the most expensive and least desirable type of reimbursement contract, so not many of these contracts exist.
- *Discounts in the form of sliding scale.* This is a form of discount with a limit in which the percentage amount increases, based on hospital numbers (for example, a 10% reduction in charges for 0 to 500 total bed days per year) with incremental increases in the discount up to a maximum percentage.
- *Sliding scales for discounts and per diems.* Based on total volume of business generated, this is a reimbursement method in which an interim per diem is paid for each day in the hospital. For example, a lump sum is either added to or withheld from the payment due at the end of each year to adjust for actual hospital usage. This is difficult to administer because it can be done either monthly or annually.

Hard Copy Billing

A printed paper copy of the CMS-1450 (UB-04) that is generated from the computer system is referred to as a *hard copy.* As of 2013, most health insurance companies require all claims to be submitted electronically. Some workers' compensation companies do not accept electronic insurance claims, so maintaining a practice management software program to print paper copies of the CMS-1450 (UB-04) forms is important. All secondary insurance companies and claims that require attachments also fit into this category.

Receiving Payment

Timeliness of payment may be included in a contract to encourage a hospital to join a plan (for example, an additional 4% discount for paying a clean claim within 14 days of receipt) or a hospital may demand a penalty for clean claims not processed within 30 days. Some states require this payment by law.

After receipt of payment from insurance and managed care plans, the patient is sent an explanation of benefits (EOB) that details how much the hospital was paid and the remaining patient responsibility due to a deductible, coinsurance amount, and charges for services not covered under the insurance policy. Standard bookkeeping procedures are used to post entries showing payments and adjustments. Financial management for managed care programs is discussed and shown in figures in Chapter 11 and the basic steps in the insurance claim process are illustrated in Figure 17-5.

OUTPATIENT INSURANCE CLAIMS

The term **outpatient** is used when an individual receives medical service in a section or department of the hospital and goes home the same day or receives care in a physician's office. In addition, outpatient services may occur in a clinic, imaging center, laboratory, ED, rehabilitation center, urgent care clinic, or ambulatory surgery center. If an individual has an accident, injury, or acute illness, he or she may seek the services of medical personnel in the ED of the hospital. When seen in the ED, a patient is considered an outpatient unless he or she is admitted for an overnight hospital stay. Many elective surgeries are done on an outpatient surgery basis. **Elective surgery** indicates a surgical procedure that can be scheduled in advance, is not an emergency, and is discretionary on the part of the physician and patient. Elective procedures are those that are deferrable, which means that the patient will not experience serious consequences if the operation is postponed or there is failure to undergo the operation. Some insurance policies require a second opinion for elective surgery. The insurance company may not pay if the patient does not seek a second opinion and chooses to undergo surgery. See Chapter 12 for elective surgery and the Medicare program. Patients may receive certain types of therapy and diagnostic testing services on an outpatient basis.

Hospital Professional Services

Although physicians make daily hospital visits to their patients, perform surgeries, discharge patients from the hospital, and are called to the hospital to provide consultations and ED treatment, their professional services are submitted on the CMS-1500 (02-12) insurance claim form by the physician and not by the hospital billing department. Only services provided by the hospital should be submitted by the hospital unless the hospital is billing for physicians who are on the hospital payroll. Such hospital services include the following:

● ED facility fee (supplies)
● Laboratory (technical component)
● Radiology (technical component)
● Physical and occupational therapy facility fee

Personnel who work in these departments (for example, ED physician, pathologist, radiologist, and physical therapist) might be employees of the hospital. The hospital submits bills for professional services in that situation and these charges are submitted on a CMS-1500 (02-12) form. The professional charges are billed independently if the physician is not an employee.

Using the hospital for surgical or medical consultations that could be done in a specialist's office should be avoided unless the patient physically requires admission.

This necessity should be documented. If a patient is admitted for consultation only, the entire payment for hospital admission will be denied, as will any physician fees involved.

BILLING PROBLEMS

A patient has the right to request, examine, and question a detailed statement, as mentioned in the Patient's Bill of Rights, a nationally recognized code of conduct published by the AHA. A bill should never show unexplained codes or items without descriptions. A brief hospital stay may translate into hundreds of individual charges. If the bill lumps charges together under broad categories, such as pharmacy, surgical supplies, and radiology, and the patient requests an itemized invoice, it should be provided at no cost to the patient. In fact, consumer advocates and policies governing the Medicare program encourage consumers to scrutinize their hospital bills for mistakes. The hospital may receive a call or letter from the patient asking for an explanation of the charges if they seem exorbitant. Sometimes, hospital billing personnel, a hospital patient representative or advocate, the attending physician, and his or her staff may be able to explain a confusing charge to the patient's satisfaction.

Medicare, Medicaid, and some insurance companies have begun to stop reimbursing hospitals for never events.

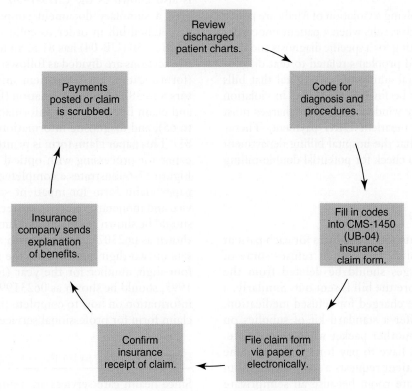

FIGURE 17-5 The life cycle of an insurance claim.

Never events are surgical procedures that are performed on the wrong side, wrong site, wrong body part, or wrong person (for example, an object left inside a patient during surgery, use of the wrong blood type during a transfusion, or infection from a urinary catheter). Some hospitals do not charge for never events whereas other facilities may charge for certain ones.

Common billing errors are as follows:
- Incorrect name; use of maiden name instead of married name
- Wrong subscriber; patient's name listed in error
- Covered days versus noncovered days

Duplicate Statements

Duplicate billing, which may confuse the patient, can occur when a patient receives inpatient and outpatient preadmission tests or services. Perhaps a test was canceled and rescheduled and a charge is shown for the canceled test or perhaps several physicians consulted on a case and each ordered the same test or therapy. Possibly a technician took the incorrect amount of blood or produced an unclear radiograph, submitted a charge for the service performed in error as well as for the correct service, and thereby generated two charges for one test. These examples are hospital personnel errors.

Double Billing

Another example involving a violation of Medicare policy is double billing, which results when a patient undergoes routine outpatient testing for a specific diagnosis and then develops unanticipated problems related to that diagnosis that require hospital admission. A hospital that bills for such services may be fined because it is in violation of the Medicare 3-day window rule. Such charges must be bundled into the inpatient DRG payment. Therefore it is imperative that the hospital billing department develop procedures to check for potential double-billing problems.

Phantom Charges

Physicians order admission procedures for each patient who enters the hospital. If a patient refuses some of these tests, the charges should be deleted from the financial records before the bill is sent out. Similarly, a patient should not be charged for refused medication. The hospital may offer a standard kit of supplies on admission or a new-mother packet when appropriate. A patient should not have to pay for supplies that he or she refuses. If a patient requests a semiprivate room but is sent to a private room because all semiprivate rooms are occupied, the patient should not be billed

at the higher rate. Phantom charges may appear if a scheduled test is canceled by a physician or the patient is released early, making it imperative to check the dates and times of admission and discharge. Charges that should appear on a patient's itemized statement may be missing because the charges were transferred to the wrong patient's bill. This requires a review of the patient's medical records. A charge should be deleted from the bill when it cannot be accounted for by a review of the patient's medical record or by talking to the attending physician.

HOSPITAL BILLING CLAIM FORM

Uniform Bill Claim Form

The **Uniform Bill (CMS-1450 [UB-04])** claim form is used by institutional facilities (for example, acute care facilities, dialysis centers, inpatient skilled nursing facilities, or rehabilitation centers) to report fees related to surgery only; the CMS-1500 form is used to report all professional and technical services.

In 1982, the UB-82 claim form was developed for hospital claims and printed in green ink. A revision was issued in 1992, which became known as the Uniform Bill (UB-92). Because it was determined that an update of this form was necessary, a new form called the *UB-04 claim form* made its appearance in 2007. The Uniform Bill (UB-04) paper or electronic claim form is also known as the *CMS-1450*. This form is considered a summary document supported by an itemized or detailed bill in order to collect the facility fee. The CMS-1450 (UB-04) has 81 form locators (fields) and its five sections are divided as follows: provider information (form locators 1 to 7), patient information (form locators 8 to 38), billing information (form locators 39 to 49 and claim line 23), payer information (form locators 50 to 65), and diagnostic information (form locators 66 to 81). This paper claim form is printed in red ink on white paper for processing with optical scanning equipment. Figure 17-6 illustrates a completed CMS-1450 (UB-04) paper claim form for inpatient services. Dates of service and monetary values are entered (for example, $200 should be shown as 200 00, and June 23, 2007, should be shown as 062307). Dates of birth are entered using two sets of two-digit numbers for the month and day and a four-digit number for the year (for example, June 23, 1995, should be shown as 06231995). See Chapter 7 for information on how to complete the CMS-1500 (02-12) claim form for professional services.

PREDETERMINING PAYMENT

Since health care services are reimbursed after they are rendered, it can be challenging to forecast future income.

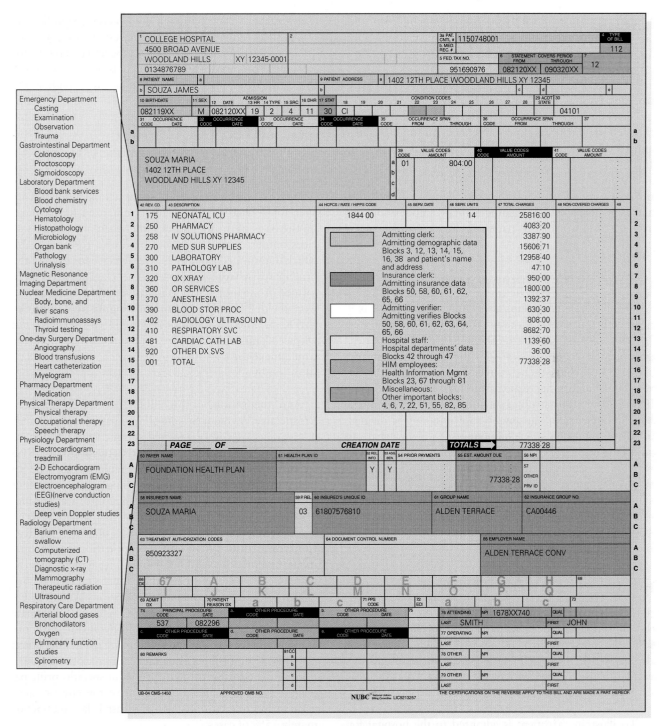

FIGURE 17-6 Scannable Uniform Bill (CMS-1450 [UB-04]) insurance paper claim form completed for an inpatient showing hospital departments that input data for hospital services. *Colored blocks* indicate data obtained by various hospital personnel. Job titles and the exact data each person obtains may vary from facility to facility. Form locator guidelines vary and may not always follow the visual guide presented here.

In the past, physicians would be reimbursed by **cost-based systems,** in which insurance companies would make payments based on the amount charged. There were some discrepancies when using cost-based systems for reimbursement.

1. The amount charged would vary from physician to physician, even though the same service was rendered.
2. The amount charged would not take into account variables such as where the physician practiced, malpractice insurance rates, and the amount of work.

3. There was no uniformity of reimbursements, so insurance companies could not forecast costs relating to the medical procedure.

To solve these discrepancies, Medicare created the **prospective payment system (PPS).** This system took into account the work that went into the medical service, the geographic area, and malpractice insurance rates and developed a standards rate per medical procedure. In time, Medicaid, TRICARE, and other private insurance companies developed similar PPSs to standardize the costs of delivering health care. PPSs take a statistical analysis and base their reimbursement amounts on the average care provided to patients who are assigned specific diagnoses.

DIAGNOSIS-RELATED GROUPS

A diagnosis-related group, also known as a DRG, is a prospective payment structure on which hospital fee reimbursements are based. The DRG groups diseases, possible related diseases, and medical treatment into a single code, which then produces a relative weight for reimbursement. The relative weight is then multiplied by the hospital's base unit rate and equals the amount to be reimbursed. The hospital's base unit rate is divided into labor and nonlabor components; the labor share is adjusted by the wage index, dependent on the state in which the hospital operates. The thought process behind this concept is that patients who present with similar symptoms will use similar hospital resources through their patient care encounter, and have similar length of stay, and therefore would incur the same costs and should be reimbursed the same.

History

The concept of DRGs was developed by Professors John D. Thompson and Robert B. Fetter at Yale University and tested in New Jersey from 1977 to 1979. The goal was to develop a scheme of patient classification for utilization review that combined patient diagnosis, related medical care required, and hospital costs in one relative value.

To illustrate, a patient is admitted to the hospital for appendicitis. Routine care for appendicitis includes laparoscopic surgery to remove the appendix and a 1-night stay in the hospital. The relative weight reflects the costs to care for the routine patient with this diagnosis. Hospital case managers are responsible for submitting the patient's diagnosis to their insurance company's utilization review, which then preauthorizes the patient for hospital admission.

The purpose of a DRG-based two-tiered system used for Medicare reimbursement was to hold down rising health care costs. Therefore Medicare reimbursement as a whole was expected to and did decrease significantly under the original DRG payment system. In 2008, the system was renamed Medicare Severity Diagnosis-Related Group (MS-DRG), which is a more complex three-tiered system. Extensive changes were made to the program and this system is designed to increase reimbursement for sicker patients.

The Medicare Severity Diagnosis-Related Group (MS-DRG) System

The DRG system changed hospital reimbursement from a fee-for-service system to a lump sum, fixed-fee payment on the basis of the diagnoses rather than on time or services rendered. The fees were fixed by a research team, which determined a national "average" fee for each of the principal discharge diagnoses. The classifications were formed from more than 10,000 ICD-9-CM codes that were divided into 25 basic **major diagnostic categories (MDCs).** The classifications for ICD-10-CM have not yet been published but it was announced that Medicare would make the transition to the new coding system classification by October 1, 2015.

As of the printing of this edition, Medicare's Inpatient Prospective Payment System (IPPS) has 745 MS-DRGs. These diagnoses were assigned specific values commensurate with severity of illness whereas the original DRGs were assigned values based on geographic areas, types of hospitals, depreciation values, teaching status, and other specific criteria. MS-DRGs are split into a maximum of three payment tiers on the basis of patient severity as determined by the presence of a **major complication/comorbidity (MCC),** a **complication/comorbidity (CC),** or no CC. The amount of payment may be increased by documenting in the patient's medical record any comorbid conditions or complications. When referring to DRGs, the abbreviation CC is used to indicate such complications or comorbidities (and not the more common interpretation, chief complaint, found in patient charting). Comorbidity is defined as a preexisting condition that, because of its effect on the specific principal diagnosis, will require more intensive therapy or cause an increase in length of stay by at least 1 day in approximately 75% of cases.

To obtain MS-DRG information, go to the *Federal Register*'s website each October 1 for the update.

Hospital facilities contract with Medicare to supply acute inpatient care and agree to accept a predetermined amount of reimbursement based on the diagnoses and procedures related to the patient during his or her inpatient hospital stay. The diagnoses stated on the discharge summary and the procedures performed during the stay are the basis for payment. Each diagnosis and procedure is grouped into MS-DRGs that contain similar amounts and types of hospital resources. Using a software program called a **grouper,** this information is keyed in and the program calculates and assigns the MS-DRG payment group. These MS-DRGs are weighted to reflect the average costs for inpatient care. **Looping** is the grouper process of searching all listed diagnoses for the presence of any comorbid condition or complication or searching all procedures for operating room procedures or more specific procedures.

When the ICD-10 is implemented, a reimbursement crosswalk that identifies ICD-9 and corresponding ICD-10 codes and MS-DRGs should be used. If an ICD-10 code combines the descriptions of two separate ICD-9 codes, the ICD-10 code replaces the more commonly used ICD-9 code. In some cases, several general ICD-9 codes in a "cluster" may be replaced with one specific ICD-10 code.

A case that cannot be assigned to an appropriate DRG because of an atypical situation is called a **cost outlier.** Outliers are unique cases in which costs incurred require higher reimbursements. These cases require extensive documentation as to why the case should be processed as an outlier. These atypical situations are as follows:
1. **Clinical outliers:**
   a. Unique combinations of diagnoses and surgeries causing high costs
   b. Very rare conditions
2. Long length of stay due to an MCC or CC
3. Low-volume DRGs
4. Inliers (hospital case falls below the mean average or expected length of stay)
5. Death
6. Patient leaving against medical advice
7. Admitted and discharged on the same day

The current federal plan for outliers is the full DRG rate plus an additional payment for the services provided. An unethical practice, **DRG creep,** is to code a patient's DRG category for a more severe diagnosis than indicated by the patient's condition. This is also called **upcoding.**

In hospital billing, **downcoding** can also erroneously occur when sequencing several diagnoses (for example, listing a normal pregnancy as the primary diagnosis for payment and complications in the secondary position when the patient remained in the hospital for an extended number of days). Additional examples are discussed in Chapter 6.

If a patient is discharged with two or more conditions and the physician fails to indicate the "most resource-intensive" or "most specific" diagnosis as the principal diagnosis, the DRG assessment will be incorrect, resulting in decreased reimbursement to the health care facility (Examples 17-4 and 17-5). It is the responsibility of the

---

Example 17-4   Comorbid Condition and Complication

A patient has had congestive heart failure (CHF) for several years and is admitted with an admitting diagnosis of chest pain and principal diagnosis of anterior wall myocardial infarction (MI). While hospitalized, the patient experiences atrial fibrillation.

ICD-10-CM

Principal diagnosis:	I21.09 acute transmural myocardial infarction of anterior wall
Comorbid condition (CC):	I50.9 congestive heart failure NOS
Complication:	I48.0 atrial fibrillation

NOS, Not otherwise specified.

Example 17-5   Comorbid Condition and Complication

A patient has had chronic obstructive pulmonary disease (COPD) for the past 6 months and is admitted with an admitting diagnosis of chest pain and a principal diagnosis of anterior wall myocardial infarction (MI). While hospitalized, the patient experiences respiratory failure.

ICD-10-CM

Principal diagnosis:	I21.09 acute transmural myocardial infarction of anterior wall
Comorbid condition:	J44.9 chronic obstructive pulmonary disease, unspecified
Complication:	J96.9 respiratory failure, unspecified

---

attending physician to certify the sequencing of the principal diagnosis and other diagnoses on the basis of his or her best judgment.

Both examples warrant additional payment because of comorbid conditions and complications.

Diagnosis-Related Groups and the Physician's Office

Even though DRGs affect Medicare hospital payments, the individual in a physician's office who communicates the admitting diagnosis to the hospital can greatly affect the DRG assignment. Remember the following points:
1. Give all of the diagnoses authorized by the physician, if there are more than one, when calling the hospital to admit a patient so that the hospital personnel can use their expertise in listing the primary and secondary diagnoses.

2. Ask the physician to review the treatment or procedure in question when a hospital representative calls about a test, length of stay, or treatments ordered by the attending physician. The hospital needs this information to justify a higher-than-average bill to Medicare.

3. Get to know hospital personnel on a first-name basis so that you can call on these hospital experts when the physician or patients have DRG-related questions.

OUTPATIENT CLASSIFICATION

In late 2000, under the requirements of the Balanced Budget Act of 1997, the CMS implemented a PPS for Medicare beneficiaries. This was a move from a cost-based reimbursement system to a line-item billing system for ambulatory surgery centers and hospital outpatient services. The CMS has categorized outpatient services into an ambulatory payment classification system. Some Medicaid programs and private payers have embraced this system because of the escalation of outpatient costs.

Ambulatory Payment Classification (APC) System

Ambulatory surgery categories (ASCs) were adopted for 1-day surgery cases that were derived from the surgery section of the CPT. ASCs used disease and procedural coding classification systems to supply the input to the grouper to assign ASCs.

Recently the General Accounting Office (GAO) ordered Congress to begin conversion of surgical, radiologic, and other diagnostic services to an ambulatory payment classification (APC) system effective August 1, 2000, which replaced ASCs. The more than 500 APCs are continually being modified (added to) and deleted. Because of this constant state of change, APC information is updated and released twice a year in the *Federal Register*.

APCs are applied to the following:

- Ambulatory surgical procedures
- Chemotherapy
- Clinic visits
- Diagnostic services and diagnostic tests
- ED visits
- Implants
- Outpatient services furnished to patients in nursing facilities that are not packaged into nursing facility consolidated billing (services commonly furnished by hospital outpatient departments that nursing facilities are not able to provide [computed tomography, magnetic resonance imaging, or ambulatory surgery])
- Partial hospitalization services for community mental health centers (CMHCs)
- Preventive services (colorectal cancer screening)

- Radiology, including radiation therapy
- Services for patients who have exhausted Medicare Part A benefits
- Services to hospice patients for treatment of a nonterminal illness
- Surgical pathology

Hospital Outpatient Prospective Payment System

The development process for APCs is similar to that used for DRGs; however, the procedure code, not the diagnosis code, is the primary axis of classification. The reimbursement methodology is based on median costs of services and facility cost to determine charge ratios in addition to copayment amounts. There is also an adjustment for area wage differences, which is based on the hospital wage index currently used for inpatient services. This hospital Outpatient Prospective Payment System (OPPS) may be updated annually, not periodically. An APC group may have a number of services or items packaged within it so that separate payment cannot be obtained.

Ambulatory Payment Classification Status

Categories of services have payment status indicators consisting of alpha code letters or symbols. They are the following:

Category	Payment Status Indicator
A	Durable medical equipment (DME), prosthetics, and orthotics
A	Physical, occupational, and speech therapy
A	Ambulance
A	Erythropoietin (EPO) for patients with end-stage renal disease (ESRD)
A	Clinical diagnostic laboratory services
A	Physician services for patients with ESRD
A	Screening mammography
C	Inpatient procedures
E	Noncovered items and services
F	Acquisition of corneal tissue
G	Drug/biologic pass-through payment
H	Device pass-through payment
K	Non–pass-through drug/biologic
N	Incidental services, packaged into APC rate
P	Partial hospitalization
S	Significant procedure, not discounted when multiple
T	Significant procedure, multiple procedure reduction applies
V	Visit to clinic or ED
X	Ancillary service

Partial hospitalization refers to a distinct and organized intensive psychiatric outpatient day treatment program designed to provide patients with profound and disabling mental health conditions with an individual, coordinated, comprehensive, and multidisciplinary treatment program.

Types of Ambulatory Payment Classifications

The four types of APCs are as follows:

1. **Surgical Procedure APCs.** These are surgical procedures for which payment is allowed under the PPS (for example, cataract removal, endoscopies, biopsies). Surgical APCs are assigned on the basis of CPT codes.
2. **Significant Procedure APCs.** These consist of nonsurgical procedures that are the main reason for the visit and account for the majority of the time and services used during the visit (for example, psychotherapy, computed tomography and magnetic resonance imaging, radiation therapy, chemotherapy administration, partial hospitalization). Significant procedure APCs are selected on the basis of CPT codes.
3. **Medical APCs.** These include encounters with a health care professional for evaluation and management services. The medical APC is determined by site of service (clinic or ED), level of the evaluation and management service (CPT code), and diagnosis from 1 of 20 diagnostic categories (ICD-10-CM code).
4. **Ancillary APCs.** These involve diagnostic tests or treatments not considered to be significant procedure APCs (for example, plain x-ray film, ECGs, or cardiac rehabilitation). Ancillary APCs are assigned on the basis of CPT codes.

It is possible that multiple APCs can be used when billing for a visit. Use of CPT modifiers for hospital outpatient visits affects APC payments; therefore it is important to accurately apply correct modifiers when applicable.

Most hospitals use a type of encoder program in which the CPT code is input and an APC group code number is assigned. For example, if CPT code number 99282 is input for a low-level ED visit, the encoder assigns APC Group 610. Use of an unbundling reference book may be helpful in assigning a CPT code; it is preferable to use the code that will generate the highest APC payment.

The data that hospitals submit during the first years of implementation of the APC system are vitally important to the revision of weights and other adjustments that affect payment in future years. The APC data that appear on the CMS-1450 (UB-04) paper claim form are shown in Figure 17-7.

DATES OF
SERVICE

REVENUE
CODES

HCPCS/CPT
CODES

Note: When multiple
procedures are
performed, the codes
should be sequenced in
proper order and match
the diagnoses listed in
Blocks 80 and 81.

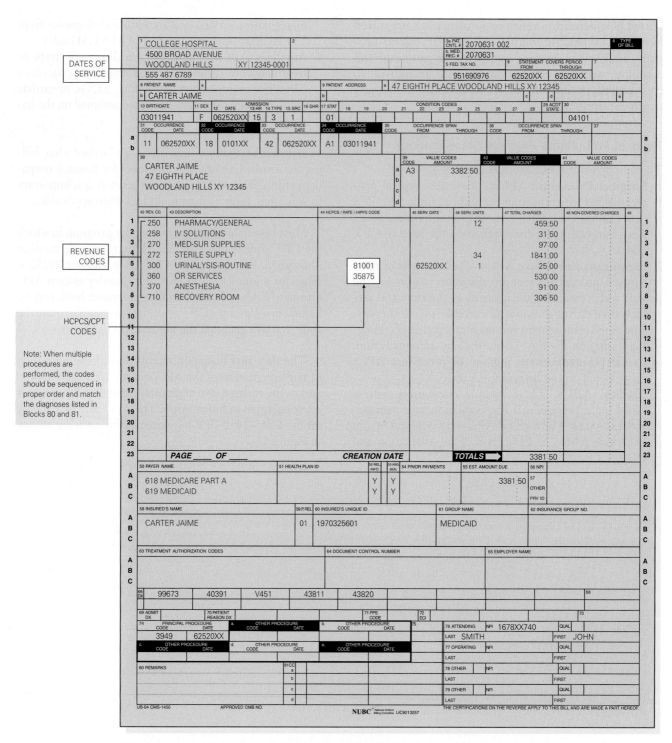

FIGURE 17-7 Scannable Uniform Bill (CMS-1450 [UB-04]) insurance paper claim form showing placement of ambulatory payment classification (APC) data for an outpatient for submission to insurance company.

PROCEDURE 17-1

New Patient Admission and Insurance Verification

1. Interview the patient and obtain complete and accurate information during initial registration. If this is an emergency inpatient admission, the managed care program should be notified on the next working day or within 48 hours to obtain an authorization number.
2. Write down the information from the employee at the physician's office who has telephoned for admittance of the patient.
3. Make photocopies of the front and back of all insurance cards.
4. Contact the insurance company or the insured individual's employer to verify the type of health insurance or telephone the insurance company to verify eligibility and benefits and determine whether prior authorization is necessary.
5. Obtain an approved signed treatment authorization request for elective admissions for a Medicaid or TRICARE patient.
6. Collect any copayment or deductible.
7. Obtain information about the injured patient, industrial accident, insurance carrier, and employer for a patient injured on the job.
8. Get an authorization for admission, length of stay, and all surgical procedures for an elective admission of a patient injured on the job from the workers' compensation insurance adjuster.
9. Ask the patient to read and sign the necessary hospital admitting documents (for example, Notice of Privacy document, surgical consent form, and financial agreement).

PROCEDURE 17-2

ICD-10-PCS Table Coding

The basic steps in coding for an endoscopic esophagostomy from ICD-10-PCS are as follows:

1. Locate the needed table from the index. Each table represents a three-character code for the Section, Body System, and Root Operation. In the case of coding for an esophagostomy, the correct table should be 0DB (see Table 17-4).
2. The next character is the body part. An esophagostomy is performed on the esophagus, so character 4 will be 5.
3. The next character is the approach. The information about the approach used can be found in the procedure report. Definitions of the approach can be found in the *Workbook*, Appendix D. Since the example surgery states endoscopic, the approach character will be 8.
4. The next character is device. The table contains only one character for device, so the device character will be Z.
5. The final character is qualifier. Because the purpose of the surgery is not defined as diagnostic, the qualifier character will be Z.
6. The complete seven-digit ICD-10-PCS code for the endoscopic esophagostomy is 0DB58ZZ.

For further ICD-10-PCS exercises, refer to Chapter 17 of the *Workbook*.

Table 17-4	ICD-10-PCS Table, Section 0, System D, Operation B

Section	**0** Medical and surgical
Body system	**D** Gastrointestinal system
Operation	**B** Excision: Cutting out or off, without replacement, a portion of a body part

BODY PART	APPROACH	DEVICE	QUALIFIER
1 Esophagus, upper			
2 Esophagus, middle			
3 Esophagus, lower			
4 Esophagogastric junction			
5 Esophagus			
7 Stomach, pylorus			
8 Small intestine			
9 Duodenum			
A Jejunum	**0** Open		
B Ileum	**3** Percutaneous		
C Ileocecal valve	**4** Percutaneous endoscopic	**Z** No device	**X** Diagnostic
E Large intestine	**7** Via natural or artificial opening		**Z** No qualifier
F Large intestine, right	**8** Via natural or artificial opening endoscopic		
G Large intestine, left			

KEY POINTS

This is a brief chapter review, or summary, of the key issues presented. To further enhance your knowledge of the technical subject matter, review the key terms and key abbreviations for this chapter by locating the meaning for each in the Glossary at the end of this book, which appears in a section before the Index.

1. A primary job function of a patient service representative is to promptly file hospital inpatient and outpatient claims with third-party payers, following up in a timely and efficient manner, to ensure that maximum reimbursement is received for services provided.

2. Under HIPAA, patients' financial and medical records, verbal communications, and computer security in a hospital must be confidential.

3. A patient is considered an inpatient on admission to the hospital for an overnight stay for medical services.

4. To obtain necessary diagnostic information, reduce inpatient expenses, and eliminate extra hospital days, a patient is usually sent to the hospital for preadmission testing (PAT).

5. Medicare policy that states if a patient receives diagnostic tests and hospital outpatient services within 72 hours of admission to a hospital, all such tests and services are combined (bundled) with inpatient services only if services are related to the admission.

6. The CMS administers the Quality Improvement Organization (QIO) program, which is responsible for the following types of reviews: admissions, readmissions, procedures, day outliers, cost outliers, diagnosis-related group (DRG) validations, and transfers.

7. For coding and billing outpatient claims, CPT and HCPCS codes are used for procedures and ICD-10-CM for diagnosis.

8. For coding and billing inpatient claims, ICD-10-CM is used for diagnoses and ICD-10-PCS is used for procedures. In 2014, ICD-10-PCS will replace Volume 3 of ICD-9-CM.

9. The principal diagnosis is the condition that is assigned a code representing the diagnosis established after study that is chiefly responsible for the admission of the patient to the hospital.

10. The diagnostic code sequence is important in billing of hospital inpatient cases because maximum payment is based on the DRG system.

11. After an admitting clerk registers and admits a patient, an insurance verifier must confirm the insurance coverage.

12. All hospital services are coded with an internal code and link various hospital departments via a computer system called a charge description master (CDM). It contains the charges for items and services provided to each patient.

13. The UB-04 claim form, also known as CMS-1450 (02/12), is the institutional uniform claim form developed by the National Uniform Billing Committee for hospital inpatient and outpatient billing and payment transactions.

14. Managed health care programs operate under varying contracts, policies, and guidelines and use any one or a combination of various payment methods to reimburse hospital facilities for their services.

15. After receiving payment from insurance and managed care plans, the patient is sent a net bill that lists any owed deductible, coinsurance amount, and charges for services not covered under the insurance policy.

16. When an individual receives medical service in a section or department of the hospital and goes home on the same day, he or she is classified as an outpatient.

17. A patient classification system that categorizes patients who are medically related with respect to principal diagnosis, presence of a surgical procedure, age, presence or absence of significant complications, and treatment and who are statistically similar in length of hospital stay is referred to as a DRG. Medicare hospital insurance payments are based on relative value units multiplied by the hospital's base unit rate for a principal diagnosis as listed in MS-DRGs.

18. A method developed by the CMS for outpatient hospital reimbursement based on procedures that have similar clinical characteristics and similar costs rather than on diagnoses is known as the ambulatory payment classification (APC) system.

💻 STUDENT ASSIGNMENT

✔ Study Chapter 17.
✔ Answer the fill-in-the-blank, multiple-choice, true/false, and mix and match review questions and assignments in the *Workbook* to reinforce the theory learned in this chapter and to help you prepare for a future test.

✔ Complete the assignments in the *Workbook* and Evolve to gain hands-on experience in analyzing and editing information from computer-generated CMS-1450 (UB-04) claim forms for inpatient and outpatient hospital billing. One of the assignments will assist you in further enhancing your diagnostic coding skills in relation to DRGs. These problems point out the value of coding properly in terms of proper diagnostic sequence, indicating the variance in payment.

✔ Turn to the Glossary at the end of this text for a further understanding of the key terms and key abbreviations used in this chapter.

References

1. Claxton G: *How Private Insurance Works: A Primer*. Retrieved from http://www.kff.org/insurance/upload/How-Private-Insurance-Works-A-Primer-Report.pdf, 2012.
2. Centers for Medicare and Medicaid Services: *Administrative Simplification Compliance Act Self Assessment*. Retrieved from http://www.cms.gov/Medicare/Billing/ElectronicBillingEDITrans/ASCASelfAssessment.html, 2012.
3. Blue Cross Blue Shield of Massachusetts: *HIPAA Version 5010 Frequently Asked Questions*. Retrieved from https://www.bluecrossma.com/staticcontent/HIPPA_V5010_FAQ.pdf, 2012.

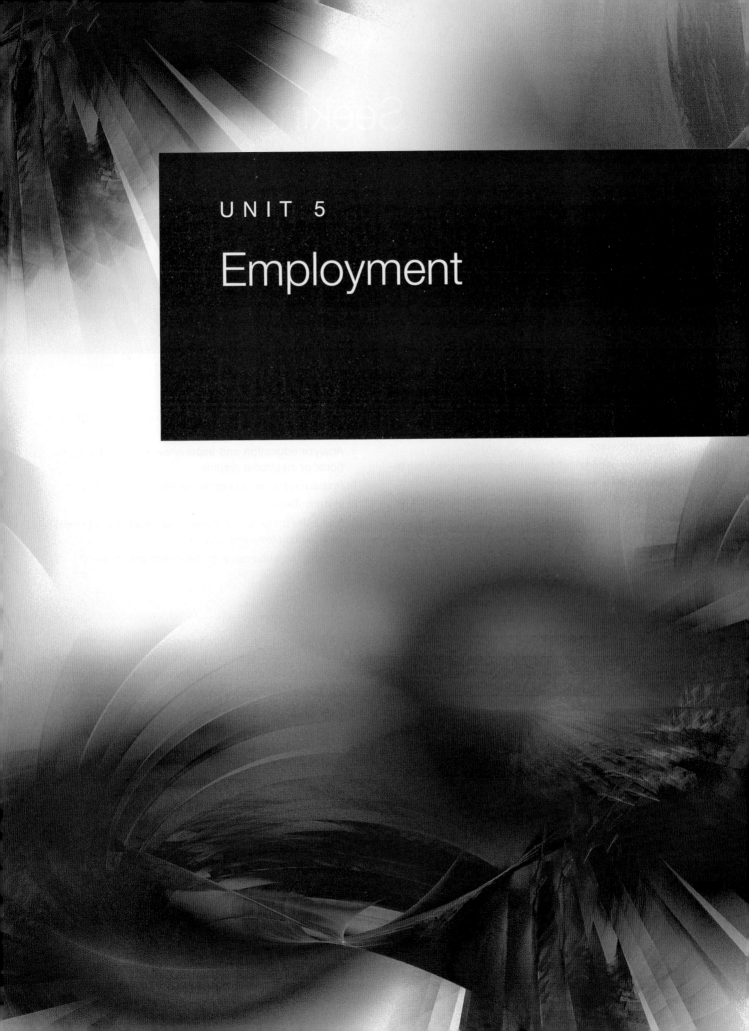

UNIT 5

Employment

CHAPTER 18

Seeking a Job and Attaining Professional Advancement

Marilyn Takahashi Fordney

OBJECTIVES

After reading this chapter, you should be able to:

1. Prepare to find a position as an insurance billing specialist, claims assistance professional, or electronic claims processor.
2. State types of certification and registration available to insurance billers and coders.
3. State and discuss various actions to take to search for a job.
4. Search online for employment opportunities and discuss job fairs.
5. List guidelines for completing an electronic job application form.
6. Compose a letter of introduction to accompany the résumé.
7. Analyze education and experience to prepare a traditional or electronic résumé.
8. Prepare responses to common interview questions.
9. Identify illegal interview questions.
10. Name the items to assemble for an electronic portfolio and discuss follow-up letters.
11. Explore the business aspects of self-employment.

KEY TERMS

application form
blind mailing
business associate agreement
certification
Certified Coding Specialist
Certified Coding
 Specialist–Physician
Certified Medical Assistant
Certified Medical Billing Specialist
Certified Professional Coder

chronologic résumé
claims assistance professional
combination résumé
continuing education
cover letter
employment agencies
functional résumé
immigrant
interview
mentor

National Certified Insurance and
 Coding Specialist
networking
portfolio
Registered Medical Assistant
Registered Medical Coder
registration
résumé
self-employment
service contract

KEY ABBREVIATIONS

AAPC	CCAP	CECP	CMRS
AHIMA	CCS	CMA	CPC
CAP	CCS-P	CMBS	CPC-A

CPC-H	HRS	RMA
ECP	NCICS	RMC
EEOC	PAHCOM	USCIS

Service to Patients

An insurance billing specialist has other service-oriented positions, such as collection manager, claims assistant professional for elderly patients, and insurance counselor, that focus on attention to patient needs. Whatever you decide to specialize in as far as a career related to insurance billing and coding is concerned, remember that the most important aspect of your job is patient care.

EMPLOYMENT OPPORTUNITIES

Insurance Billing Specialist

Employment opportunities are available throughout the United States (US) for insurance billing specialists who attain coding skills, knowledge of insurance programs, and expertise in completing insurance claims accurately. In addition to the skills necessary for performance on the job, ask yourself the following questions to determine whether you need to sharpen your job-seeking techniques:

- Are you motivated and interested in finding a job?
- Can you communicate effectively in an interview?
- Do you enjoy good health?
- Are you mature?
- Do you have good grooming and manners?

The increase in the knowledge necessary and volume of paperwork associated with insurance claims, medical record keeping, and state and government agencies means a corresponding increase in the need for an insurance billing specialist. Because an individual can choose a number of different types of positions, this chapter provides information on each.

You can work in one of two ways: either employed by someone or self-employed after a number of years of experience (Figure 18-1). The following are some of the choices in this career field:

- Insurance billing specialist
- Electronic claims processor (ECP)
- Medicare or Medicaid billing specialist
- Claims assistance professional (CAP)
- Coding specialist (freelance or employed)
- Physician Coding Specialist (PCS)

Some hospital facilities and physicians prefer credentialed coders or insurance billers and advertise for the following:

- **Certified Medical Billing Specialist (CMBS)**
- Certified Medical Reimbursement Specialist (CMRS)
- **Certified Professional Coder (CPC)**
- Certified Professional Coder–Apprentice (CPC-A)
- Certified Professional Coder–Hospital (CPC-H)
- **Certified Coding Specialist (CCS)**
- **Certified Coding Specialist–Physician (CCS-P)**
- Certified Electronic Claims Processor (CECP)
- Certified Claims Assistance Professional (CCAP)
- Facility Coding Specialist (FCS)
- Health Care Reimbursement Specialist (HRS)
- **National Certified Insurance and Coding Specialist (NCICS)**
- **Registered Medical Coder (RMC)**

Becoming certified is certainly an essential goal if one seeks career advancement and the steps to accomplish this, as well as certification in other careers allied to this one, are detailed at the end of this chapter.

Claims Assistance Professional

Contact local hospitals to determine whether they have patients who require insurance help if you want to establish yourself as a self-employed **claims assistance professional (CAP)** (in addition to some of the aforementioned positions). You can also call on small employers to determine

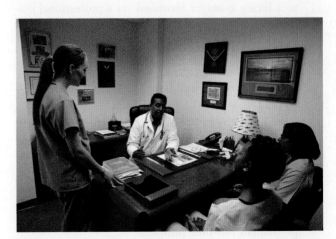

FIGURE 18-1 Staff conference discussing applicants for potential interviews.

whether they need assistance explaining their health insurance policies or enhancing insurance benefits.

JOB SEARCH

You can seek employment in several ways. You may wish to be employed by a physician, hospital, medical facility, insurance company, or managed care organization (MCO). You may choose to be self-employed if you have had a number of years of experience or you may even choose some type of combination situation. The following lists suggested actions to take to search for a job:

1. Explore the internet using a smartphone, tablet, or computer. Visit websites of professional billing and coding organizations. Review the advertisements placed on Craigslist. Make it easy to be found, such as being on LinkedIn, ExecuNet, or other professional networking sites. Upload your résumé to as many databases as possible. Search names of professional offices and hospitals near your location to contact.

2. Join a professional organization, as mentioned later in this chapter, to network with others in the same career field and to hear about job openings (Figure 18-2). Put a notice about your availability in the chapter newsletter.

3. Attend meetings and workshops in this career field to keep up to date and network with others.

4. Contact the school placement personnel, complete the necessary paperwork, and leave a résumé on file if you have just completed a course at a community college or trade school. Always prepare two types of résumés: one for posting via computer technology and one to give to an employer in person. A résumé for humans might use the words "career successes" and "accomplishments" but a computer scanner might see "work experience."

5. Spread the word to those who work in medical settings and those who might hear of openings in medical facilities, such as classmates, instructors, school counselors, relatives, and friends. If you are introducing yourself to a hiring manager identified via a professional colleague, type the colleague's name in the e-mail subject line (for example, "John Doe referred me") so that the manager is less likely to delete your e-mail.

6. Contact pharmaceutical representatives who visit physicians' offices and hospitals for employment information or leads.

7. Visit public and private **employment agencies,** including temporary and temporary-to-permanent agencies. Before signing with an agency, ask whether the employer or applicant pays the agency fee.

8. Inquire at state and federal government offices and their employment agencies.

9. Look for part-time employment that might lead to a permanent full-time position.

10. Check bulletin boards in personnel offices of hospitals and clinics frequently for posted job offerings.

11. Go to your local medical society to determine whether it has a provision for supplying job leads.

12. Send a blind mailing of the résumé, including a cover letter, to possible prospects. A **blind mailing** means to send information to employers whom you do not know personally and who have not advertised for a job opening. This may result in a positive response with either a request to complete an application form or an invitation for an interview.

13. Visit your city's chamber of commerce and ask for some of their publications that contain membership directories, names of major professional employers in specific areas, and brochures describing regional facts.

14. Subscribe to an online principal newspaper of the city where employment is desired. Read help wanted advertisements in the classified section, especially in the Sunday newspaper. Positions of interest might be listed as insurance billing specialist, reimbursement manager, insurance claims manager, insurance coordinator, insurance biller, coding/reimbursement specialist, reimbursement coordinator, coder/abstracter, electronic claims processor, and so on. Do not be discouraged by specific requirements in an advertisement; apply anyway. Send or transmit an e-mail with your résumé and a cover letter the next day. Some employers give priority to candidates who respond within the first 3 or 4 days after a job announcement because they believe it is an indication that someone is truly interested in the position. Many jobs are not advertised and there could be an opening available for which you qualify.

15. E-mail or telephone job hotlines of large medical clinics in your area.

16. Visit job locations unannounced (referred to as "cold calling").

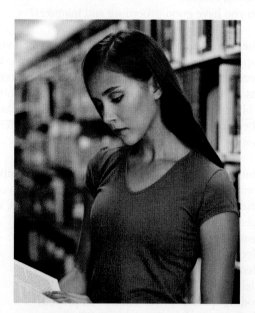

FIGURE 18-2 Student scanning a professional journal for job leads.

Online Job Search

Because of vast communication available via the internet, newspaper and magazine classified advertisements may become resources of the past. An individual with a mobile device, tablet, or computer can access online services. Many websites on the internet incorporate text, sound, graphics, animation, and video. It is possible to locate potential employers who are offering jobs to health care workers at their websites by using various search engines. At some sites you can find detailed descriptions of posted positions and locate opportunity postings by location or employer. You may be able to find and respond to a specific job of interest by delivering an online résumé, attaching a cover letter, and updating your posting as often as needed. Some websites allow you to receive e-mailed job alerts. Employers may use automated résumé scanning to sort e-mailed résumés for key words. Use standard typefaces and font sizes between 10 to 14 points. Keep text lines under 74 characters and use boldface for section headings. You must have a 95% to 100% key word match for the position; therefore sprinkle your résumé and cover letter with the verbiage used in the job advertisement. Key words can be entered at the end of the document. To make them unnoticeable, select the words and make the font color white; they will not appear when printed or viewed on the monitor but the electronic scan will see them when sorting.

You can gain internet access in several ways (computer, mobile device, or tablet). Your school may allow you to access the internet on campus. Many libraries have computers with free internet service. If you have a mobile device, tablet, or computer, you may wish to subscribe to either a commercial online service with internet access or an internet service in your locale (Figure 18-3).

Internet

Once online, go to a web index to locate a search engine, such as Yahoo (www.yahoo.com) or Google (www.google.com), that lists different options to explore. Helpful websites are www.jobsearch.about.com and www.indeed.com.com/jobs that features templates and examples. One valuable resource is Career Magazine (www.careermag.com), which lets you browse through hundreds of national job openings in a variety of fields. Check out America's Job Bank, which has job postings that you can browse according to field, location, and career type. MedSearch America is a health employment service that posts jobs for hospitals, MCOs, and pharmaceutical companies. MedSearch, Monster Board, and Online Career Center combined to form Monster.com. Job seekers can send their résumés via e-mail for free online posting by going to www.monster.com and www.indeed.com.

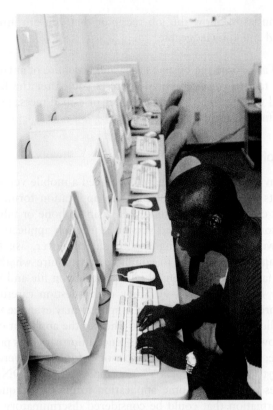

FIGURE 18-3 Student doing an online job search.

If you subscribe monthly to a commercial online service, you can network by posting a notice on a bulletin board with your résumé or a note stating that you are looking for a particular type of position in a given locale.

Job Fairs

Annual community events feature job fairs at community colleges and technical trade schools. Some job fairs are sponsored by professional associations. Job recruiters set up booths with information about their companies and available positions; however, they do not have much time to spend with each job seeker. Thus it is wise to go prepared and practice a 30-second introduction before attending. This introduction should consist of a quick overview of your career goals, experience, skills, training, education, and personal strengths. Be sure to explain what you can offer the employer. These are usually day-long events and you may want to investigate a number of participating employers' booths.

Go prepared by dressing professionally and carrying a binder or folder with plenty of copies of your résumé to give to the company representatives you meet. Résumés should be neat, clean, and not folded, wrinkled, or coffee stained. Take a pen, pencil, and notepad to obtain information. Research the employers attending so that you know which ones you will visit. Keep a positive attitude and approach each employer with confidence and enthusiasm. Show the job recruiter that you are interested and knowledgeable.

Take home the business card and brochure of anyone you talk to who genuinely interests you. After the fair, send that person a follow-up letter or e-mail message to reaffirm your interest.

Application

A savvy employer may have developed a mobile version of its job website to complete an application form. In that case, access the internet via a smartphone or tablet to complete a simplified version of the job application. However, when visiting a potential employer, ask for an **application form** to complete and inquire whether the facility keeps potential job applicants on file and for how long (Figure 18-4). Study each question carefully before answering because the employer may evaluate the application itself to determine whether the applicant can follow instructions. Furnish as much information as possible; if a question does not apply or cannot be answered, insert "no," "none," "NA" (not applicable), or "DNA" (does not apply). Some application forms may request information that could be considered discriminatory. If this situation occurs, use your best judgment on whether to insert or omit an answer. When visiting a potential employer for an application form, be sure you have prepared in advance for an interview in case an opportunity arises on that first visit.

Follow these guidelines when completing an application form:

1. Read the whole application form because some instructions may appear on the last page or last line.
2. Read the fine print and instructions: "Please print," "Put last name first," or "Complete in your own handwriting." This indicates an ability to follow directions or instructions.
3. Print if your handwriting is poor and abbreviate only when there is lack of space.
4. Complete the application in black ink unless pencil is specified.
5. Refer to data from a portfolio, sample application form, or résumé that has been checked for accuracy; use this information to copy onto each new application form. Be neat.
6. List correct dates of previous employment so they will be accurate if the employer seeks verification. If a question is presented asking the reason for leaving a position, insert "to be discussed during the interview."
7. Name specific skills such as procedural coding, diagnostic coding, knowledge of insurance programs, ability to complete and/or transmit the CMS-1500 (02-12) claim form, typing or keyboarding (number

of words per minute), fluency in a second language, knowledge of medical terminology, and knowledge and use of computer software.
8. When a question is asked about salary amount, write in "negotiable" or "flexible" and then discuss this during the interview.
9. Sign the application after completion.
10. Reread the entire form, word for word, to find any errors of omission or commission. This avoids having to apologize during an interview for a mistake.

Letter of Introduction

Individuals spend days perfecting a résumé but throw together an e-mail message, letter of introduction, or **cover letter** in minutes. This is a mistake. The main goal of the cover letter is to get the employer to take notice of the potential employee and résumé so that an interview appointment can be made. A cover letter may be in the form of an e-mail message, so make sure the subject line is clean and specific to the job you want (for example, bilingual health insurance specialist seeks billing position). Messages or letters should be typed, addressed to a specific person, and customized to each potential employer. If the advertisement gives a telephone number, call and ask for the name of the person doing the interviewing so that the message or letter can include that person's name. When the name is unknown, use "Dear Sir or Madam," "To Whom It May Concern," or a less formal "Hello" or "Good Morning." If a medical practice has a website, go to the website to learn if you need to follow guidelines for submitting résumés and if attachments to e-mails are acceptable.

Do not repeat everything in the résumé in your letter of introduction. Begin with an attention grabber and get right to the point so that the employer knows what you want and why. The message or letter should explain how your qualifications and skills would benefit the employer. Use key words that appear in the "position wanted" advertisement. Employers use applicant tracking systems (ATSs) to find and screen candidates, so include skill-oriented key words to boost your chance of being discovered. End the message or letter by requesting an interview and be sure to attach or enclose a résumé. Always include telephone numbers (home and cell) and the time of day when you are available.

Reread the message or letter to check for typos and errors in grammar, punctuation, and spelling. Avoid the use of "I" in the sentence structure (Figure 18-5). E-mail the message to a friend and ask him or her to check the content and style.

APPLICATION FOR POSITION / Medical or Dental Office

(In answering questions, use extra blank sheet if necessary)

AN EQUAL OPPORTUNITY EMPLOYER

No employee, applicant, or candidate for promotion, training or other advantage shall be discriminated against (or given preference) because of race, color, religion, sex, age, physical handicap, veteran status, or national origin.

PLEASE READ CAREFULLY AND WRITE OR PRINT ANSWERS TO ALL QUESTIONS. DO NOT TYPE.

Date of application *7-2-20XX*

A. PERSONAL INFORMATION

Name - Last	First	Middle	Home Tel. (555) *439-4800*	E-mail (optional) *valasquezj@gmail.com*
Valasquez	*Jennifer*	*M*	Bus. Tel. ( )	Cell Phone (optional) *555-301-2612*

Present address: Street *1234 Martin Street* (Apt.#) City *Woodland Hills* State *XY* Zip *12345*

Person to notify in case of emergency or accident - name: *Elena Sanchez*

Address: *20 South M Street Woodland Hills, XY 12345* Telephone: *555-261-0707*

B. EMPLOYMENT INFORMATION

Position desired: *insurance biller* **X** Full-time Part-time Either Date available for employment: *7-6-20XX* Wage/salary expectations: *negotiable*

List hrs./days you prefer to work: *M-F 8-5 PM* List any hrs./days you are not available: (Except for times required for religious practices or observances) Can you work overtime, if necessary? **X** Yes No

Are you employed now?: Yes **X** No If so, may we inquire of your present employer? No Yes, if yes: Name of employer: Phone number: ( )

Have you applied for a position with this office before? **X** No Yes If Yes, when?: Month and year _____ Location _____

Are you able to perform the essential functions of the job for which you are applying? .... **X** Yes No

If no, describe the functions that cannot be performed. _____

Have you ever been convicted of a criminal offense (felony or serious misdemeanor)? *(Convictions for marijuana-related offenses that are more than two years old need not be listed.)* Yes No

If yes, state nature of the crime(s), when and where convicted and disposition of the case. _____

(Note: We comply with the ADA and consider reasonable accommodation measures that may be necessary for eligible applicants/employees to perform essential functions. Hire may be subject to passing a medical examination, and to skill and agility tests.)

(Note: No applicant will be denied employment solely on the grounds of conviction of a criminal offense. The nature of the offense, the date of the offense, the surrounding circumstances and the relevance of the offense to the position(s) applied for may, however, be considered.)

Referred by/or where did you learn of this job? *Read advertisement in newspaper*

Can you, upon employment, submit verification of your legal right to work in the United States? **X** Yes No

Submit proof that you meet legal age requirement for employment? **X** Yes No

Language(s) applicant speaks or writes (if use of a language other than English is relevant to the job for which the applicant is applying: *Spanish*

C. EDUCATION HISTORY

	Name and address of schools attended (include current)	Number of months/ years attended	Highest grade/ level completed	Diploma/degree(s) obtained/areas of study
High school	*ABC High School, Woodland Hills, XY*	*2000-2004*	*12*	*Diploma*
College	*Vocational-Tech School, Woodland Hills, XY*	*2005*		Degree/major *Certificate*
Post graduate	*Montana State Univ., Woodland Hills, XY*	*2005-2007*		Degree/major *24 credits*
Business/trade/technical				Course/diploma/license/ certificate
Other				Course/diploma/license/ certificate

Specific training, skills, education, or experiences which will assist you in the job for which you have applied. *See resume*

Membership/professional or civic organizations (excluding those that disclose race, color, religion or national origin) *Amer. Acad. of Professional Coders*

Future educational plans *Continuing education—preparing for certification in coding*

Military - did you serve in the armed forces? **X** No Yes, if yes, branch? _____
Training relevant to position for which you are applying:

D. SPECIAL SKILLS (Check below the kinds of work you have done)

Front Office		Back Office	
X Accounts receivable	**X** Filing	Blood counts	Phlebotomy
Bookkeeping	**X** Medical terminology	Dental assistant	Urinalysis
X Collections	Medical transcription	Dental hygienist	X-ray
X Data entry	Receptionist	Injections	Other:
X Electronic/medical billing	Other:	Nursing/assisting	Other:

Other kinds of tasks performed or skills that may be applicable to position:

Office equipment/machines used: *computer, calculator, printer*

Computer programs used: *Word, Excel*

Keyboarding/ typing speed *65 wpm*

FIGURE 18-4 Application for Position / Medical or Dental Office form. *(Courtesy Bibbero Systems, Inc., Petaluma, Calif. Telephone: [800] 242-2376; fax: [800] 242-9330; website: www.bibbero.com.)*

Continued

E. EMPLOYMENT RECORD ☐ INFORMATION SUPPLIED ON ATTACHED RÉSUMÉ

LIST MOST RECENT EMPLOYMENT FIRST (Full or Part-Time)   May we contact your previous employer(s) for a reference? ☒ Yes ☐ No

| 1) Employer/Company name | Type of business: |
| St. John's Outpatient Clinic | Hospital outpatient medical clinic |

| Address   Street   City   State   Zip code | Worked performed. Be specific: |
| 24 Center St.   Woodland Hills, XY   12345 | |

| Phone number |
| (555) 782-0155 |

Your position	Dates Mo. Yr. Mo. Yr.
Insurance billing specialist	From 6	07 To 6	09
Supervisor's name	Hourly rate/salary
Candice Johnson	Starting $12/hr Final $15/hr
Reason for leaving   Professional advancement

| 2) Employer/Company name | Type of business: |
| Eastern Airlines | Airline transportation |

| Address   Street   City   State   Zip code | Worked performed. Be specific: |
| Orlando FL | |

| Phone number |
| (555) 350-7000 |

Your position	Dates Mo. Yr. Mo. Yr.
Receptionist	From 1	99 To 1	2000
Supervisor's name	Hourly rate/salary
Gary Stevens	Starting $9/hr Final $11.50/hr
Reason for leaving   Career change

| 3) Employer/Company name | Type of business: |

| Address   Street   City   State   Zip code | Worked performed. Be specific: |

| Phone number ( ) |

Your position	Dates Mo. Yr. Mo. Yr.
	From To
Supervisor's name	Hourly rate/salary
	Starting Final
Reason for leaving

F. REFERENCES — List below two persons NOT related to you who have knowledge of your work performance within the last three years.

(1) _____ Furnished upon request _____
 Name   Address   Telephone number   (☐ Work ☐ Home)   Occupation   Years acquainted
(2) _____
 Name   Address   Telephone number   (☐ Work ☐ Home)   Occupation   Years acquainted

Please feel free to add any information which you feel will help us consider you for employment

DO NOT ANSWER ANY QUESTIONS IN THIS SECTION UNLESS THE BOXES ARE CHECKED - If the employer has checked the box next to the question, the information requested is needed for a legally permissible reason, including, without limitation, national security considerations, a legitimate occupational qualification or business necessity. The Civil Rights Act of 1964 prohibits discrimination in employment because of race, color, religion, sex or national origin. Federal law also prohibits discrimination based on age, citizenship and disability. The laws of most States also prohibit some or all of the above types of discrimination as well as some additional types such as discrimination based upon ancestry, marital status and sexual preference.

	Provide dates you attended school:	Elementary From To		☐	Number of dependents, including yourself	
☐	High School From To	College From To		☐	Are you a Vietnam veteran?	☐ Yes ☐ No
	Other (give name and dates)			☐	Sex ☐ Male ☐ Female	
☐	Marital status ☐ Single ☐ Engaged ☐ Married ☐ Separated ☐ Divorced ☐ Widowed	☐ Date of marriage		☐	Are you a U.S. citizen?	☐ Yes ☐ No
☐	What was your previous address?			☐	How long at previous address?____ years	
☐	State names of relatives and friends working for us, other that your spouse.			☐	How long at present address?____ years	
☐	Have you ever been bonded? ☐ Yes ☐ No If "Yes," with what employers?			☐	Are you over 18 years of age? If not, employment is subject to verification of age.	☐ Yes ☐ No

READ THE FOLLOWING CAREFULLY, THEN SIGN AND DATE THE APPLICATION

The information provided in this Application for Employment is true, correct, and complete. If employed, any misstatement or omission of fact on this application may result in my dismissal. I understand that acceptance of an offer of employment does not create a contractual obligation upon the employer to continue to employ me in the future. If you decide to engage an investigative consumer reporting agency to report on my credit and personal history I authorize you to do so. If a report is obtained you must provide, at my request, the name of the agency so I may obtain from them the nature and substance of the information contained in the report.

If requested, I hereby agree to submit to binding arbitration all disputes and claims arising out of the submission of this application. I further agree, in the event that I am hired by the company, that all disputes that cannot be resolved by informal internal resolution which might arise out of my employment with the company, whether during or after that employment, will be submitted to binding arbitration. I agree that such arbitration shall be conducted under the rules of the American Arbitration Association. This application contains the entire agreement between the parties with regard to dispute resolution, and there are no other agreements as to dispute resolution, either oral or written.

Date: 7-2-20XX _____   Signature: _____ Jennifer M. Valasquez _____

FIGURE 18-4, cont'd

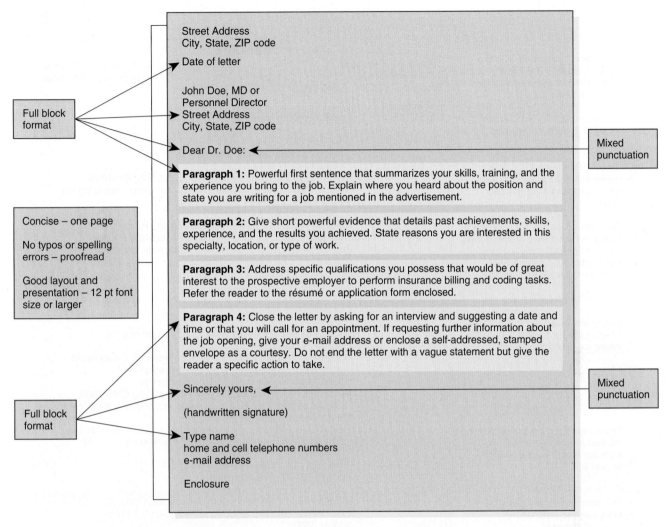

FIGURE 18-5 Suggested content for a letter of introduction to accompany a résumé. Typed in full-block style with mixed punctuation.

Résumé

The current trends is to use social media, such as Twitter and LinkedIn, which have quickly become job boards as well as places to hunt for candidates and research applicants. However, this presents the problem of trying to write a 140-character résumé—a single tweet summarizing one's experience and unique attributes. Because we are in a transitional period, the old style of résumé will continue to be mentioned.

A traditional **résumé** is a data sheet designed to sell job qualifications to prospective employers. A résumé that highlights information related to the position the applicant is trying to obtain should be created and therefore résumés will differ for each job. There are several formats from which to choose:

● A **chronologic résumé** gives recent experiences first, with dates and descriptive data for each job.

● A **functional résumé** states the qualifications or skills that an individual is able to perform.

● A **combination résumé** summarizes the applicant's job skills as well as educational and employment history. The combination style is the best choice for an insurance billing specialist (Figure 18-6).

A results-oriented résumé focuses on results, not characteristics. It helps prospective employers reduce the risks that are associated with hiring because it shows what the job seeker has accomplished and his or her attitude toward work.

The ideal length for a résumé is one page. It can be typed on an 8½- × 14-inch page and reduced to letter size. The résumé should be keyed or typed, not handwritten, on high-quality, wrinkle-free bond off-white or white paper. It should be single spaced internally with double

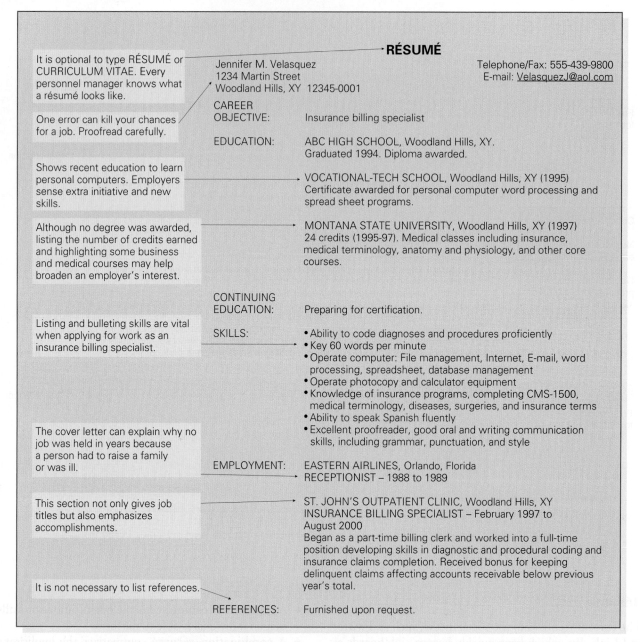

It is optional to type RÉSUMÉ or CURRICULUM VITAE. Every personnel manager knows what a résumé looks like.

One error can kill your chances for a job. Proofread carefully.

Shows recent education to learn personal computers. Employers sense extra initiative and new skills.

Although no degree was awarded, listing the number of credits earned and highlighting some business and medical courses may help broaden an employer's interest.

Listing and bulleting skills are vital when applying for work as an insurance billing specialist.

The cover letter can explain why no job was held in years because a person had to raise a family or was ill.

This section not only gives job titles but also emphasizes accomplishments.

It is not necessary to list references.

RÉSUMÉ

Jennifer M. Velasquez
1234 Martin Street
Woodland Hills, XY 12345-0001

Telephone/Fax: 555-439-9800
E-mail: VelasquezJ@aol.com

CAREER OBJECTIVE: Insurance billing specialist

EDUCATION: ABC HIGH SCHOOL, Woodland Hills, XY.
Graduated 1994. Diploma awarded.

VOCATIONAL-TECH SCHOOL, Woodland Hills, XY (1995)
Certificate awarded for personal computer word processing and spread sheet programs.

MONTANA STATE UNIVERSITY, Woodland Hills, XY (1997)
24 credits (1995-97). Medical classes including insurance, medical terminology, anatomy and physiology, and other core courses.

CONTINUING EDUCATION: Preparing for certification.

SKILLS:
• Ability to code diagnoses and procedures proficiently
• Key 60 words per minute
• Operate computer: File management, Internet, E-mail, word processing, spreadsheet, database management
• Operate photocopy and calculator equipment
• Knowledge of insurance programs, completing CMS-1500, medical terminology, diseases, surgeries, and insurance terms
• Ability to speak Spanish fluently
• Excellent proofreader, good oral and writing communication skills, including grammar, punctuation, and style

EMPLOYMENT: EASTERN AIRLINES, Orlando, Florida
RECEPTIONIST – 1988 to 1989

ST. JOHN'S OUTPATIENT CLINIC, Woodland Hills, XY
INSURANCE BILLING SPECIALIST – February 1997 to August 2000
Began as a part-time billing clerk and worked into a full-time position developing skills in diagnostic and procedural coding and insurance claims completion. Received bonus for keeping delinquent claims affecting accounts receivable below previous year's total.

REFERENCES: Furnished upon request.

FIGURE 18-6 Example of a combination résumé stressing education and skills. Personal data may be excluded as a result of the Civil Rights Act of 1964, enforced by the Equal Employment Opportunity Commission (EEOC).

spacing between main headings and balanced spacing for all four margins. Laser-printed résumés give a professional appearance. You might want to have a longer (two-page maximum) résumé on hand to offer during an interview.

Under the Civil Rights Act of 1964, enforced by the Equal Employment Opportunity Commission (EEOC), information about height, weight, birth date, marital status, Social Security number, and physical condition may be omitted. Additional items to omit are salary requirements, reason for leaving jobs, date of résumé preparation, date available to begin work, references,

and vague references to time gaps. Questions about these items might be asked during an interview. If you were laid off and have a gap between jobs, get involved in volunteer projects or consulting opportunities, even if you work for free. This allows you to use your skills and can then be described on your résumé. Hobbies and outside interests that relate to the profession might be included. Membership or leadership positions held in professional organizations related to the medical field might be mentioned. A photograph is not necessary but might be included if it will be of value to the interviewer for recall purposes.

The format may include the following:

- *Title.* Résumé, Personal Data Sheet, Biographic Sketch, or Curriculum Vitae.
- *Heading.* At the beginning of the résumé, list your name, phone number, and e-mail address. Mailing addresses are being phased out, so simply noting your city and state is acceptable. A Quick Response (QR) code using an online résumé maker to point recruiters to a digital version of the résumé might include a video, social media profile, or online portfolio containing work samples.
- *Summary.* This may be a statement as to why the employer should be interested in you. Use action words as shown in Figure 18-6 and avoid the personal pronoun.
- *Education.* Name high school, college, any business school attended, and **continuing education** classes, city and state, degree, and date received. List in reverse chronologic order. Grade average and awards or scholastic honors may be included.
- *Professional experience.* Name all employers in reverse chronologic order with addresses, telephone numbers, and dates of employment. Include summer, full-time, part-time, and temporary jobs as well as externship and volunteer work. Detail achievements, not duties (for example, "possess strong communication, service to patients, and organizational skills" or "consistently surpassed collection goals by 10% or more each year").
- *Skills.* List keyboarding words per minute, computer equipment operated, experience in medical practice management software programs, accurate procedure and diagnostic coding including knowledge of modifiers, expertise in insurance claims completion and submission, knowledge of medical terminology and insurance terminology, bookkeeping (posting charges, payments, and adjustments to accounts receivable journal), experience in preparing appeals for denied claims, resubmittal of delinquent claims, ability to explain insurance programs and plans (for example, benefits, requirements, and submission of claims), ability to abstract information from patients' medical and financial records, and ability to review insurance payments from explanation of benefits (EOB) documents. If you are fluent in another language, provide this information. Telephone and reception skills also might be mentioned. Skills might be placed near the top of the résumé where they will catch a résumé screener's eye.
- *References.* Type in the phrase "Furnished on request." Prepare approximately five references on a separate sheet and be sure to contact the persons referenced before an interview.
- *Final details.* It is acceptable to e-mail or fax a résumé to an employer who advertises a job opening but gives no guidelines on how to submit the résumé. It is

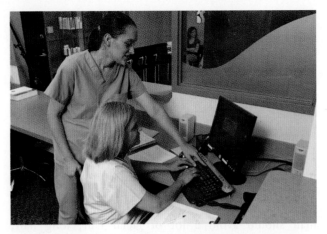

FIGURE 18-7 Insurance billing student at an externship site.

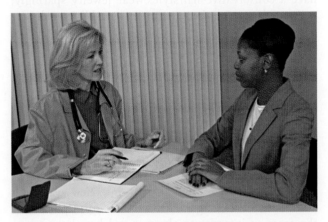

FIGURE 18-8 Student being interviewed for an insurance billing position.

wise to use every advantage possible in a competitive employment market in which time is of the essence (Figure 18-7).

Proofread the résumé carefully for spelling, punctuation, grammar, and typographic errors. Ask a friend or professional individual with excellent English skills to read and critique it. Remember that the résumé is only a foot in the door and not what is going to land that job for you—you are!

Interview

After looking for a potential employer, preparing a résumé, and completing an application, the final step in landing a job is the face-to-face interview. An **interview** is a formal consultation with questions by an employer to evaluate the qualifications of a prospective job applicant (Figure 18-8).

Make the best impression possible on the prospective employer as soon as you walk through the door. It is a well-known fact that the first 30 seconds makes either a positive or negative impression. Hiring depends on positive qualities. Concentrate on good grooming and a fresh, relaxed appearance. Display a warm, positive, and interested attitude. When speaking, employers want job candidates who are well spoken and articulate. Use proper grammar, avoid using slang, slow down your speaking, and maintain eye contact.

A female applicant should wear a clean skirt, dress, or tailored suit and nylon stockings with low-heeled pumps. A male applicant should wear a clean dark suit or sport coat, conservative necktie, white shirt, plain slacks, plain socks, and well-shined shoes. A man should avoid a lot of facial hair, long hair, earrings, and heavy aftershave lotion. A woman should have a conservative hairstyle; wear jewelry sparingly; and avoid heavy makeup, a low-cut neckline, a sleeveless dress, strong perfume, and dark or bright nail polish.

Do not answer a cellphone or send a text during the interview. Do not smoke or chew gum. Use a proper deodorant. Eliminate nervous habits. It has been found that when applicants have similar skills and education, the decision to hire has been based on physical appearance at the interview.

Figure 18-9 is an example of an interview evaluation and reference investigation form. This form points out the areas an interviewer observes and how impressions are rated.

Research before the interview to know whether the salary (when offered) is acceptable. If you want to ask questions about benefits, do not appear to be overly interested in them.

If possible, choose a good time for the interview and arrive promptly. It has been found that late Monday and Friday afternoons between 4:00 and 5:00 PM are not good times for interviews because Mondays are usually catch-up, heavily-scheduled days and Fridays are getaway days. Research has proved that the likelihood of hiring the last person interviewed for a position is greater than that of hiring those interviewed first. Carry something in your hand (for example, portfolio with notepad, résumé, and other documents) so that you are not showing nervousness or anxiety, which might detract and be detrimental during the interview.

Role-playing is a good method to use to prepare for an interview. Give a friend a list of questions to ask you and then try to answer the questions spontaneously without stumbling. Videotape or audiotape the session, if possible, to see or hear what the employer will experience.

Questions an interviewer might ask about personal life (marital status), family planning, pregnancy, provision for child care, religious preference, club memberships, height, weight, dependents, age (birth date), ethnic background, maiden name, native language, physical or psychiatric problems, spouse's employment and earnings, credit rating, and home and automobile ownership are illegal and do not have to be answered. (It is not considered discriminatory if an employer wants to know whether an applicant smokes.) Three suggestions for handling an illegal question follow:
1. Answer the question and ignore the fact that you know it is illegal.
2. Answer with, "I think the question is not relevant to the requirements of this position."
3. Refuse to answer and contact the nearest EEOC office.

Shake the interviewer's hand at the conclusion of the meeting (Figure 18-10). Ask how long it will be before a job offer or denial is forthcoming and then leave with a "thank you." If the job is offered at the interview and you are not sure about accepting, ask, "How soon do you need to know?" This will allow time to think and compare job offers before making a commitment.

Portfolio

Prepare in advance for the interview by organizing a web **portfolio.** This may give you a leg up in the job market. Scan in letters of recommendation (from former employers, teachers, family physician, professional friends, or community leaders), school diplomas or degrees, transcripts, certificates, names and addresses of references, a résumé, timed typing test certified by an instructor, some neatly typed insurance claim forms with evidence of coding skills, and any other items related to prior education and work experience. When completing an online job application, insert a link to your web-based portfolio.

Immigrant

Any employee that has immigrant status must have an Employment Eligibility Verification Form I-9 on file with his or her employer. As discussed in Chapter 12, an **immigrant** is an individual who is not a citizen or national of the United States but belongs to another country or people (also referred to as an *alien* or *foreigner*). Form I-9 can be obtained by calling the Department of Homeland Security, US Citizenship and Immigration Services (USCIS) at (800) 870-3676 or by downloading the form directly from the USCIS website (www.uscis.gov). Within 3 days of being hired,

		SUMMARY OF EVALUATION	

INTERVIEW EVALUATION AND REFERENCE INVESTIGATION FORM

	THIS IS ☐ 1ST INTERVIEW ☐ 2ND INTERVIEW ☐ 3RD INTERVIEW	POINTS FROM (21 CATEGORIES) APPLICATION AND INTERVIEW (FRONT)	
		POINTS FROM REFERENCES (1 TO 3 CATEGORIES FROM BACK)	

NAME OF APPLICANT:	DATE	**TOTAL POINTS =** (Front and Back)	
ADDRESS:	PHONE	**OVERALL IMPRESSION:** Divide total points by number of categories rated (24 maximum categories).	

RATING: EXCELLENT – 3 POINTS
GOOD – 2 POINTS
FAIR – 1 POINT
POOR – 0 POINTS

POSITION APPLIED FOR:

FROM APPLICATION FOR POSITION, GAUGE APPLICANT IN FOLLOWING AREAS	EXC	GOOD	FAIR	POOR
1. NECESSARY SKILLS FOR THIS POSITION?				
2. SUITABLE ADVANCEMENT HISTORY?				
3. AN EMPLOYMENT HISTORY THAT POINTS TOWARD DEPENDABILITY?				
4. STABILITY (REMAINED IN ONE PLACE OF RESIDENCE AND ONE JOB FOR A REASONABLE LENGTH OF TIME)?				
5. THE PROPER EDUCATIONAL BACKGROUND TO FILL THE POSITION?				
6. SALARY REQUIREMENT COMMENSURATE WITH POSITION?				
7. LEGIBLE HANDWRITING?				
8. LIMITATION ON WORKING HOURS?				

(left margin vertical text: APPLICATION SECTION REFERENCE)

FROM THE PERSONAL INTERVIEW – (SHOULD BE SPECIFIC QUALITIES – OBJECTIVE)				
9. SUFFICIENT CAPABILITY TO HANDLE ANY SITUATION THAT MAY ARISE WHEN ALONE IN OFFICE?				
10. AN APPROPRIATE ATTITUDE TOWARD WORK?				
11. APPROPRIATE DICTION, GRAMMAR, ARTICULATION?				
12. POISE?				
13. SELF CONFIDENCE (NOT OVER-CONFIDENCE)?				
14. TACT?				
15. SUFFICIENT MATURITY FOR JOB?				
16. AN ABILITY TO EXPRESS ONESELF WELL?				
17. AN INITIATIVE OR INTEREST IN LEARNING?				
18. ABILITY TO WORK WITH OTHERS IN OFFICE?				
19. APPROPRIATE APPEARANCE (NEAT, CLEAN; SUITABLE TO BUSINESS)				
20. ENERGY, VITALITY, AND PERCEIVED ABILITY TO HANDLE PRESSURE OF POSITION?				
21. EAGERNESS TO OBTAIN THE POSITION IN QUESTION?				
NOTES:	COLUMNAR TOTALS			
	TOTAL POINTS THIS PAGE			

DIRECTIONS FOR USE OF FORM:

1. Look over your ratings. A zero score on any one VITAL question should automatically eliminate applicant. Add up the total rating points and enter in the SUMMARY OF EVALUATION BLOCK in the upper right-hand corner of this page.
2. After finishing all interviews, choose the "best bets" and check their references using the reverse side of this form.
3. Enter, as above, the results of your reference check and then your overall impression (E – Excellent, G – Good, F – Fair, P – Poor).

ORDER # 72-120 ● BIBBERO SYSTEMS, INC. ● PETALUMA, CA. ● (REV.07/03)
TO REORDER CALL TOLL FREE: (800) BIBBERO (800-242-2376) OR FAX (800) 242-9330   MFG IN U.S.A.
(PLEASE TURN OVER)

FIGURE 18-9 Example of an interview evaluation and reference investigation form. *(Courtesy Bibbero Systems, Inc., Petaluma, Calif. Telephone: [800] 242-2376; fax: [800] 242-9330; website: www.bibbero.com.)*

Continued

NOTES:

RATING: 0 - POOR,   1 - FAIR,   2 - GOOD,   3 - EXCELLENT

REFERENCE INVESTIGATION	

1.

OFFICE CONTACTED	PHONE: ( ) DATE
PERSON CONTACTED	TITLE OR POSITION:
HOW LONG HAVE YOU KNOWN THIS PERSON?	TITLE/POSITION THIS PERSON HELD?
BETWEEN WHAT DATES WAS THIS PERSON EMPLOYED BY YOU?	FROM TO
RESPONSIBILITIES?	SATISFACTORILY COMPLETED?
WAS THIS PERSON CONSISTENTLY COOPERATIVE?	WHAT WERE SHORTCOMINGS?
DID THIS PERSON GET ALONG WELL WITH OTHERS?	
WAS THIS PERSON TRUSTWORTHY/DEPENDABLE?	ATTENDANCE RECORD:
REASON FOR LEAVING?	SALARY LEVEL:
WOULD YOU REHIRE THIS PERSON?	
NOTES:	
	RATING:

2.

OFFICE CONTACTED	PHONE: ( ) DATE
PERSON CONTACTED	TITLE OR POSITION:
HOW LONG HAVE YOU KNOWN THIS PERSON?	TITLE/POSITION THIS PERSON HELD?
BETWEEN WHAT DATES WAS THIS PERSON EMPLOYED BY YOU?	
RESPONSIBILITIES?	
WAS THIS PERSON CONSISTENTLY COOPERATIVE?	
DID THIS PERSON GET ALONG WELL WITH OTHERS?	
WAS THIS PERSON TRUSTWORTHY/DEPENDABLE?	ATTENDANCE RECORD:
REASON FOR LEAVING?	SALARY LEVEL:
WOULD YOU REHIRE THIS PERSON?	
NOTES:	
	RATING:

3.

OFFICE CONTACTED	PHONE: ( ) DATE
PERSON CONTACTED	TITLE OR POSITION:
HOW LONG HAVE YOU KNOWN THIS PERSON?	TITLE/POSITION THIS PERSON HELD?
BETWEEN WHAT DATES WAS THIS PERSON EMPLOYED BY YOU?	
RESPONSIBILITIES?	
WAS THIS PERSON CONSISTENTLY COOPERATIVE?	
DID THIS PERSON GET ALONG WELL WITH OTHERS?	
WAS THIS PERSON TRUSTWORTHY/DEPENDABLE?	ATTENDANCE RECORD:
REASON FOR LEAVING?	SALARY LEVEL:
WOULD YOU REHIRE THIS PERSON?	
NOTES:	
	RATING:

INTERVIEWER _____ DATE:_____ | TOTAL POINTS THIS PAGE: |

FIGURE 18-9, cont'd

an employee must show one of the following: a naturalization certification (citizen papers), an alien registration receipt card, a temporary resident receipt card, or an employment authorization card. One of these items should be available in the event that it is requested by the prospective employer during the interview.

Follow-Up Letter

Write a follow-up letter or send an e-mail message within 24 hours of the interview. Thank the person for the interview and restate your interest in the position (Figure 18-11).

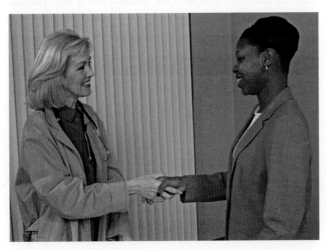

FIGURE 18-10 Job applicant concluding an interview with an office manager.

This keeps your name before the potential employer. Telephone to express continued interest in the position if no response is heard within the time frame given.

SELF-EMPLOYMENT

Setting Up an Office

When an individual wants to be his or her own boss **(self-employment),** it is usually wise to become educated and have some experience in the chosen career before undertaking this task. Having a positive and effective rapport with the public, as well as a strong background in insurance, is desirable for the individual who wants to work independently as an insurance billing specialist. Outpatient hospital and physician billing experience in several specialties is important if you choose to focus on outpatient billing and coding services. If you specialize in hospital services billing and coding, experience is necessary, especially because it is not common for a hospital to outsource these services to a small billing company. If coding services are to be part of the billing company's offerings, the coding professional should be certified by a reputable professional organization, such as the American Academy of Professional Coders (AAPC) or American Health Information Management Association (AHIMA).

Street Address
City, State, ZIP code
Date of letter

John Doe, MD or
Personnel Director
Street Address
City, State, ZIP code

Dear Dr. Doe:

Thank you for spending your valuable time yesterday to interview me for the insurance billing specialist position in your clinic.

I hope that you will allow me the opportunity to prove my abilities as I feel that I am able to perform the work with expertise. Meeting your staff was most enjoyable, and it would certainly be pleasurable working with them as a team.

I am looking forward to hearing from you in the near future.

Sincerely yours,

(handwritten signature)

Type name

FIGURE 18-11 Example of a thank-you letter sent after an interview.

HIPAA Compliance Alert — SECURITY POLICIES WHEN WORKING FROM HOME

The Health Insurance Portability and Accountability Act (HIPAA) security rules indicate that working from home requires the same security policies and practices as when working in the office. However, no specific policies are given. It is up to each covered entity to establish these documents on the basis of its security risk assessment. Security measures should address the technical setup. For example, a typical security policy might stipulate that the telecommuter use a dedicated computer with a virtual private network solution, antivirus software, and firewall if the computer is connected to the internet and the office. Management of work papers and disks and the computer work environment (protected from family and visitors) also may be indicated. Additionally, privacy compliance policies apply at home just as they do when working in an office.

One must have something to offer clients when marketing and selling one's services and skills. This knowledge and expertise can be gained only with years of experience and persistence. Full-time commitment, hard work, dedication, and many long hours to obtain clients are encountered when beginning a business. Be cautious when purchasing billing service software and obtain a complete picture of what hardware is necessary, how the program works, and the benefits it offers to your clients.

If you work a while before striking out independently, you will make contacts on the job that may help to build clientele. Networking is extremely important and may open up many opportunities when starting and growing a successful business. Many times it is who the individual knows that may get a foot in the potential client's door.

An insurance billing specialist can work as an independent contractor to have flexible hours, work from home, and reduce a medical practice's overhead. Some communities prohibit residents from telecommuting or operating a home-based business, although most allow it with restrictions. Working at home requires self-discipline and one must develop a schedule and stick to it. Good time management is essential. It takes additional hours to advertise, obtain clients, bill, and perform bookkeeping tasks. Box 18-1 is a checklist of tasks that must be done to establish a new business.

Planning Your Business

Every successful business endeavor begins with a smart business plan. This is a road map that can guide your business from start-up to continuous success. A business plan addresses facts and figures pertinent to your business and financial abilities and assesses your objectives and goals. Visit www.entrepreneur.com/howto/bizplan/ for a complete guide on writing a business plan.

Professional Mailing Address

No doubt you will receive mail, so it is important to establish a professional address. It is always wise to rent a post office box. Doing this creates a business-oriented mailing address, helps to maintain confidentiality in mailings you receive about clients and patient accounts, and protects you from unwanted visitors to your home. Visit the website of the Internal Revenue Service (IRS) at www.irs.gov/Businesses/Small-Businesses-&-Self-Employed for self-employed and small business resources.

Finances to Consider
Taxes

You must decide on what form of business entity you will be (that is, sole proprietor, partnership, or corporation). It is advisable to seek the services of a lawyer, accountant, or both before legally establishing a business and making appropriate selection of the tax options involved. Set up detailed financial records from the beginning, even if an accountant is to be hired. Obtain simplified bookkeeping software for use on the computer. Expert advice is essential and helps to develop a successful business; a business could fail without it.

Establishing a business in a home may result in some deductions, so obtain all of the information you can from your accountant and the IRS regarding important laws concerning small business and self-employment taxes. Keep receipts and complete records of income and expenses because these are extremely important for IRS purposes.

Check stubs, copies of hours worked, and identifying data on clients must be retained for the period of time stipulated by the IRS. The following is a record retention schedule:

- Bank statements and canceled checks: 7 years
- Expired contracts: 7 years
- Financial statements: permanently
- General correspondence: 1 to 5 years
- Payroll records and summaries: 7 years
- Income tax returns: permanently
- Worksheets and supporting documents: 7 years

Keep a record of business travel expenses and document mileage. Travel log books are available at stationery stores.

Box 18-1 New Business Checklist

The following is a checklist to help you in starting a new home business. This is not a complete list of items to consider nor the exact order to accomplish them in; however, important points are covered in this list.

- Define your services and construct a business plan. Make sure you forecast for success. Will this business be viable? Can you accomplish the services you will promise to carry out? Can you financially afford this endeavor?
- Research whether you need to obtain a business license from the business license section of your city hall. Regulations vary in each city licensing office. You might have to obtain a home occupation permit from the planning department and have it signed by your landlord if you are renting. The city may have guidelines on hours of business, pedestrian and vehicular activity, noise, and so on in residential areas. Determine whether your county has rules on operating a small business from home.
- Consider a name for your business. File a fictitious business name (doing business as [DBA]) at the county clerk's office by obtaining the proper form for completion. If you use your given name, you do not have to file a fictitious business name.
- Decide what address to use. You may want to obtain a post office box number instead of using your home address. This will help with a professional mailing address as well as protect you from unexpected visitors to your home.
- Consult with an accountant for advice on the tax structure of your company (for example, sole proprietor, corporation). Learn about what expenses are deductible. Depending on how you set up your business, some possible tax breaks are depreciation of office equipment; declaring a room of your home as an office; subscriptions to professional publications; dues to professional associations; expenses associated with your automobile; telephone, photocopying, and office supplies (for example, stationery, books, photocopy and fax paper); promotion and advertising (for example, postage, meals with business associates, website development and fees); and any expenses pertaining to meetings, conventions, workshops, or seminars (for example, registration fees, lodging, meals, transportation, parking). Visit www.irs.gov to learn more about how taxes can affect your business.
- Obtain the insurance that you need: health insurance, disability insurance, life insurance, liability insurance, workers'

compensation (if you have employees), and so on. Insurance called "release of information insurance" or "errors and omissions insurance" with a "hold harmless" clause is available to protect you against loss of material. Consider a retirement plan, such as an individual retirement account or a Keogh plan.

- Obtain a separate telephone number and possibly a fax number to separate "home" from "business." However, you might consider using your existing telephone number and switching to a business listing. Having a business listing allows you to be listed in the Yellow Pages of your telephone directory. Remember that advertising can be expensive, so be sure that this falls within your budget.
- Create a website advertising your services, incorporating a video clip and web-based portfolio with other visuals as well as links to LinkedIn, Facebook, and Twitter.
- Open a bank account. Many banks offer small business accounts with nominal monthly fees. For example, you can open an account "Jane Doe DBA 123 Claims Service."
- Create a professional image through business cards, stationery, and invoice billing forms. You can find resources on the internet or in software programs to print your own.
- Stay current in the industry with up-to-date reference books. Begin to assemble a library to include a good medical dictionary, procedural and diagnostic code books, compliance handbooks, trade journals, and so on.
- Start a contact database and begin to advertise your business using some of the following methods: visiting offices, mailing flyers, advertising in trade journals or your local newspaper, sending announcements, putting up signs (be sure to get permission), and sending personalized letters to prospects (hospitals, clinics, and physician's offices).
- If you have opened an office at a location outside of your home, make sure you have reviewed a proper lease before signing it and consider the finances needed for items such as utility deposits (that is, water, gas, and electricity). Rent, renovation, and janitorial or trash services must also be considered.
- Some contracts include a statement on confidentiality assuring the contracting facility that all patient data are handled in a confidential manner.

Start-Up Expenses

Money is necessary for equipment, computer software, overhead, taxes, stationery, preprinted statements and forms, and a myriad other expenses. It is vital to have sufficient funds to run the business for a period of 1 year or more. It is imperative that this be accrued before vacating a full-time job. This will help to eliminate a lot of fear and anxiety over not having enough business clients. A common reason for business failure is running out of the money necessary to keep the business going. It may take a year or more to begin seeing a profit, so one must be patient. This is where the business plan becomes a useful resource!

If an individual has had no business management experience, courses may be taken to gain knowledge and instill confidence in these areas before beginning a business. Attend workshops and lectures on starting a business that are offered by financial institutions, universities, community colleges, or private institutions.

Bank Account

Open a bank account that is separate from your own personal checking account. This smart approach saves a lot of time in the future when it comes to sorting out expenses and working on taxes. Also, think about the professional image that a business check will convey. Most banks have small business account services, including those for the self-employed. Shop around and visit several banks, if you do not already have a preference, and compare monthly fees and transaction capabilities.

Business Name, Plan, and License

Some towns or counties require a business license to operate a business. This may include working from your home office. Check with your local offices to determine whether an application or fee is required. This is the time to choose an appropriate business name and get applicable town and county licenses.

A business name should be easy to remember and explain what your company does. For example, ABC's #1 Medical Billing Service tells potential clients that the company works with health care related to billing and insurance claims.

A successful business must start with a smart business plan. This guides and helps your small business with financial and business strategies. It would be wise to meet with an accountant, an attorney, or a business consultant to help get your company started in the right direction.

For more information about business planning, visit the US Small Business Association (SBA) website at www.sba.gov.

Insurance

It is sometimes required that business owners protect income and property from unexpected loss. The following are types of insurance to investigate:

- Professional liability/errors and omissions protects you and your company from claims if your client holds you responsible for errors or the failure to perform as promised in your service contract. Coverage can include legal costs and may pay for resulting judgments against you.
- Business interruption insurance and property insurance in case of fire, theft, or disaster protects your assets and may help you in the recovery of data.
- Disability insurance if one becomes unable to work because of illness or injury can include yourself and/or an employee.
- Health and life insurance covers health care for you and/or employee(s) as well as life insurance.

Business Associate under the Health Insurance Portability and Accountability Act

The Health Insurance Portability and Accountability Act (HIPAA) rules apply to most billing companies as a business associate when a relationship is formed with one or more health care providers for whom you perform billing services.

Business associate: (Sect: 160.103)

A person (or organization) who,

(i) On behalf of such covered entity performs, or assists in the performance of a function or activity involving the use or disclosure of individually identifiable health information, including claims processing or administration, data analysis, processing or administration, utilization review, quality assurance, billing, benefit management, practice management, and repricing;

or

(ii) Provides, other than in the capacity of a member of the workforce of such covered entity, legal, actuarial, accounting, consulting, data aggregation, management, administrative, accreditation, or financial services, where the provision of the service involves the disclosure of individually identifiable health information from such covered entity or arrangement, or from another business associate of such covered entity or arrangement, to the person.[1]

Therefore if your billing company gets personal health information from a covered entity to perform a function or activity on behalf of that covered entity, your relationship is likely that of a business associate and your responsibilities must be defined with a business associate agreement.

The Business Associate Agreement

The **business associate agreement** must give "satisfactory assurances" to the covered entity on whose behalf the business associate performs services and must include, according to HIPAA rules, the following terms as set forth in the regulation:

- Business Associate agrees to not use or disclose protected health information (PHI) other than as permitted or required by the Agreement or as required by law.
- Business Associate agrees to use appropriate safeguards to prevent use or disclosure of the PHI other than as provided for by this Agreement.
- Business Associate agrees to mitigate, to the extent practicable, any harmful effect that is known to Business Associate of a use or disclosure of PHI by Business Associate in violation of the requirements of this Agreement. (This provision may be included if it is appropriate for the Covered Entity to pass on its duty to mitigate damages to a Business Associate.)
- Business Associate agrees to report to Covered Entity any use or disclosure of the PHI not provided for by this Agreement of which it becomes aware.
- Business Associate agrees to ensure that any agent including a subcontractor, to whom it provides PHI received from, or created or received by Business Associate on behalf of, Covered Entity agrees to the same restrictions and conditions that apply through this Agreement to Business Associate with respect to such information.
- Business Associate agrees to provide access, at the request of Covered Entity, and in the time and manner

[insert negotiated terms], to PHI in a Designated Record Set, to Covered Entity or, as directed by Covered Entity, to an Individual in order to meet the requirements under 45 CFR § 164.524. (Not necessary if business associate does not have PHI in a designated record set.)

● Business Associate agrees to make any amendment(s) to PHI in a Designated Record Set that the Covered Entity directs or agrees to pursuant to 45 CFR § 164.526 at the request of Covered Entity or an Individual, and in the time and manner [insert negotiated terms]. (Not necessary if business associate does not have PHI in a designated record set.)

● Business Associate agrees to make internal practices, books, and records, including policies and procedures and PHI, relating to the use and disclosure of PHI received from, or created or received by Business Associate on behalf of, Covered Entity available [to the Covered Entity, or] to the Secretary, in a time and manner [insert negotiated terms] or designated by the Secretary, for purposes of the Secretary determining Covered Entity's compliance with the Privacy Rule.

● Business Associate agrees to document such disclosures of PHI and information related to such disclosures as would be required for Covered Entity to respond to a request by an Individual for an accounting of disclosures of PHI in accordance with 45 CFR § 164.528.

● Business Associate agrees to provide to Covered Entity or an Individual, in time and manner [insert negotiated terms], information collected in accordance with Section [insert section number in contract where provision (i) appears] of this Agreement, to permit Covered Entity to respond to a request by an Individual for an accounting of disclosures of PHI in accordance with 45 CFR § 164.528.[2]

Service Contract

The service contract is a separate document from the business associate agreement. The **service contract** is a necessary document that defines the duties and obligations of each party involved in the business relationship. Contracts or agreements should be made in writing, signed, and notarized. For example, a contract should define the following:

● Who is responsible for the coding (the physician or the billing service)?
● What will be the routine for claim submission?
● Is there a per-claim processing fee or is there a flat monthly fee?
● Who is responsible for follow-up on collection procedures (telephone calls or letters)?
● Who pays for rebilling, photocopying of records, mailing fees, and clearinghouse charges? Is this included in a flat monthly service fee?

● Under whose name will bills be sent to patients (the physician or the billing service)?
● Will the billing service telephone number appear on the statement or will a toll-free or local number be used?
● How will the telephone be answered?
● What are the charges for coding consultation services?
● What are the coverage arrangements for absence or illness?
● How will information be protected and handled between the client and billing company?

If there is any change in the terms of the agreements, write an addendum to the original agreement and have both parties sign to acknowledge the change. Be sure that all agreements and contracts have proper effective and termination dates. Remember that renegotiation is possible when the contract expires.

> **HIPAA Compliance Alert**
> ### CONFIDENTIALITY STATEMENT
> Some contracts may include a statement on confidentiality assuring the contracting facility that all patient data will be handled in a confidential manner.

Pricing Your Services

Define your services and work out a structured fee schedule, making sure to review state laws regarding percentage billing. (Percentage billing is illegal in some states.) It is imperative that you get legal advice when creating contracts and agreements.

A variety of methods are used to price services, such as a percentage of reimbursement or an annual, hourly, or per-claim fee. Deciding on which method depends on the type of client being served and the work to be done. For example, a CAP may bill in 15-minute increments. Contact other billing and insurance services, preferably outside the area, to learn what they are charging because in-area competitors may be reluctant to divulge that information.

Security and Equipment

The most important consideration when starting your business is privacy and security of the health information and business documents that you will handle and be responsible for. Review the security suggestions outlined in Chapter 8.

An initial equipment checklist may include the following:
● Computer
● Laser or ink jet printer

- Paper
- Current billing and coding manuals and books
- Desk supplies such as stapler, paper clips, and self-adhesive notes
- Locking file cabinets
- Fax machine

Also consider using separate computer backup protection (for example, a surge protector with battery power) to guard against faulty wiring or power failure. This gives you more than 10 minutes to back up your current project and then shut down. These are available at office stores for about $100.

Shop smart. Research upcoming sales and lease programs, rebates, upgrade trade-ins, and service plans.

Research the various medical billing software programs and ask for demonstration software before purchasing. Also look for a reputable clearinghouse. Compare functionality, customer service, technical support, and prices.

Marketing, Advertising, Promotion, and Public Relations

Marketing refers to how a business is presented or advertised to promote sales. Marketing strategies vary, depending on the section of the public that is targeted. When promoting a medical billing service, develop a well-organized marketing plan and follow basic guidelines to reach a specific target audience.

Ways to market a business and the reasons for marketing strategies are presented in Table 18-1.

At this point, you should be ready to start marketing your business. If you are creative, you can design your own business cards and have them printed. A classic white card with black print conveys professionalism. You can also find matching stationery sets and create flyers, brochures, newsletters, surveys, and so on. Obtain financial data to help convince clients that the service you are offering is better and can do more for their businesses than what they presently have. Save them time and money! Stress being honest, reliable, committed, efficient, and professional and offer them something they cannot do for themselves.

Put yourself in front of office managers and health care providers to advertise your services. Consider visiting the health care offices in your area and be sure to follow up with visits and calls. Be careful with offices that have a sign stating "No Soliciting." If you see this sign, respect it and jot down the address to mail

Table 18-1	Business Marketing and Strategies
STRATEGY	**REASON**
Obtain professionally printed stationery and business cards.	Enhances professional image.
Pass out business cards at professional meetings.	Advertises availability and services. Helps with networking.
Develop a business name and logo for the company.	Enables potential clients to identify that you are in business.
Ensure accuracy of all printed materials.	When items are not professionally assembled or proofread to eliminate typographical errors, a potential client receives a doubtful or negative image of the company.
Develop a professional flyer and distribute it to medical facilities and physicians' offices.	Introduces company name, advertises services, and describes benefits.
Follow up with a personal visit or telephone call.	A friendly voice and professional image offer personal services and let potential clients know that you are available and interested.
Advertise in the journal or newsletter of the county medical society and state medical association.	Potential clients read such publications and advertisements of this nature lend to your credibility.
Place an ad in the newspaper or on cable television.	Circulates business within the county.
Sign up for an ad on Google or put an ad in the local Yellow Pages.	Solicits a wider range of prospective clients.
Join a local chamber of commerce to network with members and network using social media, such as LinkedIn.	Networking and advertising can be the best public relations tool.
Network via computer using the internet's discussion and career boards, such as America Online and Yahoo.	Offers a wide range of contacts.
Promote your business with a professionally developed website.	Search engines will help find you. Websites deliver immediate, detailed information about your company.
Check with established businesses to determine whether they are overloaded with work, the owner needs a vacation, or they need help with a temporary situation because of illness.	Present your services as a help, not a threat to current office staff.

them literature instead. Also, note that solicitation by fax is illegal according to the Federal Communications Commission:

Enacted by Congress in 1991, the Telephone Consumer Protection Act (TCPA) restricts the use of the telephone and facsimile machine to deliver unsolicited advertisements. Under the TCPA, one may not send an unsolicited advertisement to a fax machine. In addition, those sending fax messages or transmitting artificial or prerecorded voice messages are subject to certain identification requirements.

Marketing can be tough and intimidating. Networking with other colleagues and professionals and persistence will pay off.

Documentation

Besides keeping documentation received from your client, keep written records of the number of hours worked, the quantity of work done each day, and the corrections applied to the work by officials in the contracting facility or hospital. Retain any written coding guideline from the contracting facility or hospital.

Professional Associations, Certification, and Registration

More exacting professional requirements have evolved because of specialization in the allied health careers. Certification and registration are two ways of exhibiting professional standards (Table 18-2). **Certification** is a statement issued by a board or association verifying that a person meets professional standards. **Registration** may be accomplished in two ways: as an entry in an official registry or record that lists names of persons in an occupation who have satisfied specific requirements or by attaining a certain level of education and paying a registration fee. In the latter method, if registration is required, an unregistered person may be prevented from working in a career for which he or she is otherwise qualified.

Membership in professional organizations helps in keeping up to date. Most of these associations have student, as well as active and associate, membership categories. You can inquire whether there is a local chapter or state organization affiliated with the national association. Benefits of belonging to a professional organization, in addition to certification and recertification, include problem solving, continuing education, and employment opportunities. Local meetings can keep you knowledgeable by providing guest speakers on topics of current interest. The newsletters and journals published by these organizations keep you abreast of current trends either as a subscriber or as a benefit when becoming a member.

Mentor and Business Incubator Services

A valuable vehicle for career development is to find a mentor in the business. A **mentor** is a guide or teacher who offers advice, criticism, wisdom, guidance, and perspective to an inexperienced but promising protégé to help reach a life goal. Decide what kind of help you want (for example, technical, general feedback, or managerial) and then look for a mentor whose background, values, and style are similar to yours. Be willing to face criticism with a positive attitude and express gratitude when excellence is praised.

Another way to develop a business and obtain management assistance is to seek the services of a business incubator. A *business incubator* is an environment that grows and nurtures small businesses through their early years of existence by offering an array of business assistance services, shared resources, and networking. An incubator facility can be an actual building that has several small business tenants. It is run by managers and staff who offer business advice and referral services to tenants and many additional services, such as high-speed internet; conference rooms; secretarial, mail, and courier service; fax; copier; printer; TV, DVD, and VCR; break room; and free parking.

Networking

Another avenue to pursue for career development is networking. **Networking** is the exchange of information or services among individuals, groups, or institutions and making use of professional contacts. To do this, join as many organizations as possible because it can be difficult to keep abreast of ongoing changes in the insurance industry when you are self-employed. Many of the professional organizations publish monthly newsletters or quarterly journals, offer certification, and plan national conventions, state conferences, and regional meetings.

CAPs should attend local meetings for Medicare recipients. Join local volunteer service organizations and the chamber of commerce to network with others. Contact the Leads Club at (800) 783-3761 or the National Association for Female Executives at (800) 927-6233 for potential client leads and networking.

Reassess and Continue with Success

Once your billing service is under way, you will find it necessary to routinely assess the overall health of the business. Review your business plans and make sure you are following the guidelines. Make changes where applicable and revise your strategies and goals. Running your own successful business is challenging and highly rewarding both emotionally and financially. Good luck!

Table 18-2 Certification and Registration

CERTIFICATION TITLE (ABBREVIATION)	DESCRIPTION TO OBTAIN CERTIFICATION OR REGISTRATION	PROFESSIONAL ASSOCIATION MAILING ADDRESS	TELEPHONE NUMBER	WEBSITE	E-MAIL ADDRESS
• Advanced Coding Specialist (ACS) • Specialty Coding Professional (SCP) • Certified Compliance Professional–Physician (CCP-P)	2 to 3 years of experience and working knowledge of coding in the specialty	Board of Medical Specialty Coding 9737 Washington Blvd. Suite 200 Gaithersburg, MD 20878	(800) 897-4509	www.advanced medicalcoding .com	info@medical specialty coding.com
Certified Billing and Coding Specialist (CBCS)	Graduate of health care training program or 1 or more year(s) of full-time job experience; exam or home study certification program	National Healthcare Association 11161 Overbrook Road Leawood, KS 66211	(800) 499-9092	www.nhanow.com	info@nhanow .com
Certified Bookkeeper (CB)	Self-study program and employment experience; pass 3 tests	American Institute of Professional Bookkeepers 6001 Montrose Road Suite 500 Rockville, MD 20852	(800) 622-0121	www.aipb.org	info@aipb.org
• Certified Coding Associate (CCA) • Certified Coding Specialist (CCS) • Certified Coding Specialist–Physician (CCS-P) • Certified in Healthcare Privacy and Security (CHPS)	Self-study program; pass certification examination	American Health Information Management Association (AHIMA) 233 N. Michigan Ave. 21st Floor Chicago, IL 60601-5809	(800) 335-5535	www.ahima.org	info@ahima.org
• Certified Cardiology Coding Specialist (CCCS) • Certified ENT Coding Specialist (CENTCS) • Certified Family Practice Coding Specialist (CFPCS) • Certified Gastroenterology Coding Specialist (CGCS) • Certified General Surgery Coding Specialist (CGSCS) • Certified Internal Medicine Coding Specialist (CIMCS) • Certified Nephrology Coding Specialist (CNCS) • Certified OB/GYN Coding Specialist (COBGCS) • Certified Orthopedics Coding Specialist (COCS) • Certified Pediatrics Coding Specialist (CPEDCS) • Certified Podiatry Coding Specialist (CPODCS) • Certified Pulmonary Medicine Coding Specialist (CPMCS) • Certified Urology Coding Specialist (CUCS) • Certified Multi-Specialty Coding Specialist (CMSCS)	Active member of Professional Association of Healthcare Coding Specialists, employed as a coder with 2 years experience, 6 college credit course hours in coding	Professional Association of Healthcare Coding Specialists (PAHCS) 218 E. Bearss Ave. #354 Tampa, FL 33613	(888) 708-4707	www.pahcs.org	info@pahcs.org

Certification	Requirements	Organization	Phone	Website	Email
Certified Healthcare Financial Professional (CHFP)	60 hours of college or university and complete core exam and one specialty exam within 2-year period	Healthcare Financial Management Association (HFMA) 3 Westbrook Corporate Center Suite 600 Westchester, IL 60154-5700	(800) 252-4362	www.hfma.org	webmaster@FinancialProfessionalhfma.com
Claims assistant professional (CAP)	No formal certification process	Alliance of Claims Assistance Professionals (ACAP) 9600 Escarpment Suite 745-65 Austin, TX 78749	(888) 394-5163	www.claims.org	capinfo@claims.org
Certified Healthcare Billing and Management Executive (CHBME)	Complete comprehensive program; pass proficiency test	Healthcare Billing and Management Association (HMBA) 1540 South Coast Highway Suite 203 Laguna Beach, CA 92651	(877) 640-4262	www.hbma.com	info@hbma.com
Certified in Healthcare Compliance (CHC)	Have work experience, continuing education, and pass examination	Health Care Compliance Association 6500 Barrie Road Suite 250 Minneapolis, MN 55435	(888) 580-8373	www.hcca-info.org	info@hcca-info.org
Certified Health Data Analyst (CHDA)	Eligibility requirements and pass examination; pass CHPS examinations	American Health Information Management Association (AHIMA) 233 N. Michigan Ave. 21st Floor Chicago, IL 60601-5809	(800) 335-5535	www.ahima.org	info@ahima.com
• Certified Information Systems Security Professional (CISSP) • Systems Security Certified Practitioner (SSCP)	Pass examination and submit endorsement form	International Information Systems Security Certifications Consortium, Inc. 1964 Gallows Road Suite 210 Vienna, VA 22182	(866) 462-4777	www.isc2.org	isc2@asestores.com
Certified Medical Assistant (CMA)	Graduate from accredited medical assisting program; apply to take national certifying examination	American Association of Medical Assistants (AAMA) 20 North Wacker Drive Suite 1575 Chicago, IL 60606	(800) 228-2262	www.aama-ntl.org	Visit website

Continued

Table 18-2 Certification and Registration—cont'd

CERTIFICATION TITLE (ABBREVIATION)	DESCRIPTION TO OBTAIN CERTIFICATION OR REGISTRATION	PROFESSIONAL ASSOCIATION MAILING ADDRESS	TELEPHONE NUMBER	WEBSITE	E-MAIL ADDRESS
Certified Medical Billing Specialist (CMBS)	Complete 6 courses and provide evaluation of billing performance by supervisor	Medical Association of Billers (MAB) 2620 Regatta Dr. Suite 102 Las Vegas, NV 89128	(702) 240-8519	www.physicianswebsites.com	medassocb@aol.com
Certified Medical Manager (CMM)	Examination for supervisors or managers of small-group and solo practices	Professional Association of Health Care Office Management (PAHCOM) 1576 Bella Cruz Dr. Suite 360 Lady Lake, FL 32159	(800) 451-9311	www.pahcom.com	pahcom@pahcom.com
Certified Medical Practice Executive (CMPE) • Nominee first level • Certification second level • Fellow third level	• First level—Eligible group managers join; membership/nominee • Second level—Complete 6- to 7-hour examination • Third level—Mentoring project of thesis	Medical Group Management Association (MGMA), American College of Medical Practice Executives (affiliate) 104 Inverness Terrace East Englewood, CO 80112-5306	(877) 275-6462	www.mgma.com	acmpe@mgma.com
Certified Medical Coder (CMC) • Certified Medical Insurance Specialist (CMIS) • Certified Medical Compliance Officer (CMCO)	Self-study program and successfully pass exam	Practice Management Institute 9501 Console Drive Suite 100 San Antonio, TX 78229-2033	(800) 259-5562	www.pmimd.com	info@pmimd.com
Certified Medical Reimbursement Specialist (CMRS)	Self-study program; successfully pass 18 sections of examination	American Medical Billing Association (AMBA) 2465 E. Main Davis, OK 73030	(580) 369-2700	www.ambanet.net/cmrs.htm	larry@brightok.net
Certified Medical Transcriptionist (CMT)	Self-study program and successfully pass written and practical examinations offered by Medical Transcription Certification Commission (MTCC)	Association for Healthcare Documentation Integrity (AHDI) 4230 Kiernan Avenue Suite 130 Modesto, CA 95356	(800) 982-2182	www.ahdionline.org	ahdi@ahdionline.org
Certified Patient Account Technician (CPAT) • Certified Clinic Account Technician (CCAT) • Certified Clinic Account Manager (CCAM)	Complete self-study course; pass standard examination administered twice yearly	American Association of Healthcare Administrative Management (AAHAM) National Certification Examination Program 11240 Waples Mill Road Suite 200 Fairfax, VA 22030	(703) 281-4043	www.aaham.org	moayad@aaham.org

Certification	Requirements	Organization/Address	Phone	Website	Email
• Certified Professional Coder (CPC) • Certified Professional Coder–Apprentice (CPC-A) • Certified Professional Coder–Hospital (CPC-H)	Independent study program; examination approximately 5 hours (CPC) and 8 hours (CPC-H) in length	American Academy of Professional Coders (AAPC) 2480 South 3850 West Suite B Salt Lake City, UT 84120	(800) 626-CODE	www.aapc.com	info@aapc.com
• Facility Coding Specialist (FCS) • Physician Coding Specialist (PCS)		American College of Medical Coding Specialists (ACMCS) 1540 South Coast Highway Suite 203 Laguna Beach, CA 92651	(800) 946-9402	www.acmcs.org	info@acmcs.org
Healthcare Reimbursement Specialist (HRS)	Successfully complete open-book examination	National Electronic Billers Alliance (NEBA) 2226-A Westborough Blvd. #504 South San Francisco, CA 94080	(650) 359-4419	www.nebazone.com	mmedical@aol.com
National Certified Insurance and Coding Specialist (NCICS)	Graduate from an insurance program; sit for certification examination given by independent testing agency at many school sites across the nation	National Center for Competency Testing 7007 College Blvd. Suite 385 Overland Park, KS 66211	(800) 875-4404	www.ncctinc.com	staff@ncctinc.com
Registered Medical Assistant (RMA)	Sit for certification exam	American Medical Technologists (AMT) 10700 West Higgins Road Suite 150 Rosemont, IL 60018	(800) 275-1268	www.amt1.com	amtmail@aol.com
Utilization Review Accreditation Commission (URAC) Accredited Consultant	Application	Utilization Review Accreditation Commission (URAC) 1220 L Street, NW Suite 400 Washington, DC 20005	(202) 216-9010	www.urac.org	ita@urac.org
	Examination, work experience, and continuing education	Health Care Compliance Association 6500 Barrie Road Suite 250 Minneapolis, MN 55435	(888) 580-8373	www.hcca-info.org	info@hcca-info.org
	Pass examination and submit endorsement form	International Information Systems Security Certifications Consortium, Inc. 1964 Gallows Road Suite 210 Vienna, VA 22182	(866) 462-4777	www.isc2.org	isc2@asestores.com

PROCEDURE 18-1

Creating an Electronic Résumé

Once a medical position has been identified, a résumé may be e-mailed or a hard copy may be faxed. The basic steps for creating a résumé are as follows:

1. Compose a résumé using computer software with accurate spelling features and be sure to keep it simple. Each line should be no more than 65 characters in length.

2. Discard traditional résumé-writing techniques, such as focusing on action verbs. Instead, think of descriptive key words, such as *medical biller, education, work experience, skills, knowledge,* and *abilities.* To catch a résumé screener's eye, you might insert a section about skills at the top of the résumé.

3. Avoid the use of decorative graphics and complex typefaces, bulleted lists, complicated page formatting, symbols, underlining, and italics. These features may not appear the same on an employer's computer online.

4. Consider inserting a Quick Response (QR) code when using an online résumé maker to direct recruiters to a digital version of your résumé. This might include a video, social media profile, or online portfolio that could contain work samples or audio files.

5. When applying for an entry-level position, use only one page. However, if you are experienced, electronic résumés may be three to four pages. Save your résumé using a file name such as medical biller, medical coding specialist, or insurance biller because in some tracking systems this may help get you past the filters instead of using "myrésumé."

6. Proofread the résumé and save the electronic résumé in a job search file.

7. Study the potential employer's online guides presenting special procedures for sending e-mail and files.

8. Use the word processing software's "copy and paste" feature and enter the information in an e-mail or, if you save it as an electronic file, it can be transmitted as an attachment to an e-mail message.

9. Do not post a letter of introduction when posting a résumé to a bulletin board. Upload the résumé to post online using the file transfer feature.

10. After you send a résumé electronically, mail a hard copy and call the hiring manager directly to follow up. Be assertive.

PROCEDURE 18-2

Compose, Format, Key, Proofread, and Print a Cover Letter

1. Assemble materials: computer, printer, letterhead paper, envelopes, attachments, thesaurus, English dictionary, medical dictionary, and pen or pencil.

2. Obtain recipient's name, address, and title and choose letterhead style (modified or full block format with mixed punctuation). Refer to Figure 18-5.

3. Turn computer on and select the word processing software program (that is, Microsoft Word). Open a blank document.

4. Key the date line beginning three lines below letterhead and format in the location for the chosen style.

5. Double space down and insert the recipient's title, name, and address. If necessary, double space down for an attention line.

6. Double space down and key the salutation. Use open or mixed punctuation.

7. Double space down and key the reference line (Re or Subject) in the location for chosen letter style.

8. Double space down and key the body (content) of the letter in single-spaced format. Paragraphs should match the chosen format. Always double space down between paragraphs. Save your file every 15 minutes.

9. Proofread the letter on screen for typos, spelling, grammar, and auto-correction errors.

10. If a second page is needed, key that page with a heading (name, page number, and date) in vertical or horizontal format.

11. Key a complimentary close, making sure it is in the location for the chosen style.

12. Drop four spaces down and key the sender's name and title with credentials as shown on the letterhead.

13. When keyboarding a letter for an individual, double space down and insert the sender's and typist's reference initials in lowercase letters, separating the two sets of initials with a colon or slash (for example, HWN:mtf). This step is eliminated when typing your own cover letter.

14. If enclosures or attachments accompany the letter, single or double space down to insert "CC" for copy or "Enc" for enclosures or attachments.

15. If necessary to insert a postscript, double space down to insert "P.S."

16. Save the file to the hard drive before printing a hard copy and proofread the letter, making final corrections.

17. Print two copies, one to be sent and one to be retained in the files.

18. Prepare an envelope. If the letter is to be sent registered or certified, insert mailing instructions on the envelope.

19. Sign the letter, fold it, and insert it with enclosures into the envelope for mailing.

Bonding (10): An insurance contract by which, in return for a stated fee, a bonding agency guarantees payment of a certain sum to an employer in the event of a financial loss to the employer by the act of a specified employee or by some contingency over which the employer has no control.

Breach (2): Breaking or violation of a law or agreement.

Breach of confidential communication (2): Breach means "breaking or violation of a law or agreement." In the context of the medical office, it means the unauthorized release of information about the patient.

Buffing (11): A physician's justifying the transference of sick, high-cost patients to other physicians in a managed care plan.

Bundled codes (6): To group more than one component (service or procedure) into one Current Procedural Terminology (CPT) code.

Business associate (2): A person who, on behalf of the covered entity, performs or assists in the performance of a function or activity involving the use or disclosure of individually identifiable health information, including claims processing or administration, data analysis, process or administration, utilization review, quality assurance, billing, benefit management, practice management, and repricing.

Business associate agreement (8, 18): Contract between the provider and a clearinghouse that submits the electronic claims on behalf of the provider.

By report (BR) (15): A report must be submitted with the claim when the notation "BR" follows the procedure code description. This term is sometimes seen in workers' compensation fee schedules.

Cable modem (8): A modem used to connect a computer to a cable television system that offers online services.

Cancelable (3): A renewal provision in an insurance agreement that grants the insurer the right to cancel the policy at any time and for any reason.

Capitation (11, 17): A system of payment used by managed care plans in which physicians and hospitals are paid a fixed per capita amount for each patient enrolled over a stated period of time, regardless of the type and number of services provided; reimbursement to the hospital on a per-member/per-month basis to cover costs for the members of the plan. Capitation can also mean a set amount to be paid per claim.

Carcinoma in situ (5): Cancer confined to the site of origin without invasion of neighboring tissues.

Carve outs (11): Medical services not included within the capitation rate as benefits of a managed care contract and that may be contracted for separately.

Case rate (17): An averaging after a flat rate is given to certain categories of procedures.

Cash flow (1, 10): In a medical practice, the amount of actual cash generated and available for use by the medical practice within a given period of time.

Catastrophic cap (14): The maximum dollar amount that a member has to pay under TRICARE or CHAMPVA in any fiscal year or enrollment period for covered medical bills.

Catchment area (14): In the TRICARE program, an area, defined by zip codes, that is approximately 40 miles in radius surrounding each United States military treatment facility.

Categorically needy (13): Aged, blind, or disabled individuals or families and children who meet financial eligibility requirements for Aid to Families with Dependent Children (AFDC), Supplemental Security Income (SSI), or an optional state supplement.

Centers for Medicare and Medicaid Services (CMS) (12): Formerly known as the Health Care Financing Administration (HCFA), CMS divides responsibilities among three divisions: the Center for Medicare Management, the Center for Beneficiary Choices, and the Center for Medicaid and State Operations.

Certification (18): A statement issued by a board or association verifying that a person meets professional standards.

Certified Coding Specialist (CCS) (18): A title received by a person after appropriate training and by passing a certification examination administered by the American Health Information Management Association (AHIMA) for hospital-based coding.

Certified Coding Specialist–Physician (CCS-P) (18): A title received by a person after appropriate training and by passing a certification examination administered by the American Health Information Management Association (AHIMA) for physician-based coding.

Certified Medical Assistant (CMA) (18): A title received by a person after appropriate training and by passing a certification examination administered by the American Association of Medical Assistants (AAMA).

Certified Medical Billing Specialist (CMBS) (18): A title received by a person after appropriate training and by passing a certification examination administered by either the American Association of Medical Billers (AAMB) in Los Angeles or the Medical Association of Billers (MAB) in Las Vegas.

Certified Professional Coder (CPC) (18): A title received by a person after appropriate training and the passing of a certification examination administered by the American Academy of Professional Coders (AAPC).

CHAMPVA (3, 14): See Veterans Health Administration.

Charge description master (CDM) (17): A computer program that is linked to various hospital departments and includes procedure codes, procedure descriptions, service descriptions, fees, and revenue codes; also known as charge master or procedure code dictionary.

Charges (17): The dollar amount a hospital bills an outlier case on the basis of the itemized bill.

Chief complaint (CC) (4, 5): A patient's statement describing symptoms, problems, or conditions as the reason for seeking health care services from a physician.

Chronic (4): A medical condition persisting over a long period of time.

Chronologic résumé (18): A data sheet that outlines experience and education by dates.

Churning (11): When physicians see a high volume of patients—more than medically necessary—to increase revenue. May be seen in fee-for-service or managed care environments.

Civil Monetary Penalty (CMP) (2): Federal statute that imposes fines and sanctions to combat health care fraud and abuse and is imposed on individuals or health care facilities that do not comply with the Centers for Medicare and Medicaid Services (CMS) regulations.

Civil Service Retirement System (CSRS) (16): A program for federal employees hired before 1984.

Civilian Health and Medical Program of the Department of Veterans Affairs (CHAMPVA) (3, 14): See Veterans Health Administration.

Claim (3): A bill sent to an insurance carrier requesting payment for services rendered; also known as encounter record.

Claim attachments (8): Documents that contain information, hard copy or electronic, related to a completed insurance claim that assists in validating the medical necessity or explains the medical service or procedure for payment (for example, operative report, discharge summary, invoice).

Claims assistance professional (CAP) (1, 18): A practitioner who works for the consumer and helps patients to organize, complete, file, and negotiate health insurance claims of all types to obtain maximum benefits as well as tells patients what checks to write to providers to eliminate overpayment.

Claims examiner (15): In industrial cases, a representative of the insurer who authorizes treatment and investigates, evaluates, and negotiates the patient's insurance claim and acts for the company in the settlement of claims; also known as claims adjuster, claims representative, and claims administrator.

Claims-review type of foundation (11): A type of foundation that provides peer review by physicians to the numerous fiscal agents or carriers involved in its area.

Clean claim (7): A completed insurance claim form submitted within the program time limit that contains all necessary information without deficiencies so that it can be processed and paid promptly.

Clearinghouse (2, 8): An independent organization that receives insurance claims from the physician's office, performs software edits, and redistributes the claims electronically to various insurance carriers.

Clinical outliers (17): Cases that cannot adequately be assigned to an appropriate diagnosis-related group (DRG), owing to unique combinations of diagnoses and surgeries, rare conditions, or other unique clinical reasons. Such cases are grouped together into clinical outlier DRGs and therefore are considered outliers.

Cloned note (4): 1. Entry in a patient's medical record worded exactly like or similar to the previous entries. 2. Medical documentation that is worded exactly the same from patient to patient. Cloned notes are considered a misrepresentation of the medical necessity requirements for insurance coverage of medical services and can trigger audits.

Closed panel program (11): A form of health maintenance organization (HMO) that limits the patient's choice of personal physicians to only those doctors practicing in the HMO group practice within the geographic location or facility. A physician must meet narrow criteria to join a closed panel.

Clustering (2): Reporting one level of service for all patient visits, regardless of the patient's presenting problem or the amount of work or time spent with the patient.

Code of Medical Ethics (10): A code of medical ethics written by Thomas Percival in 1803.

Code sequence (17): The correct order of diagnostic codes (1, 2, 3, 4) when submitting an insurance claim that affects maximum reimbursement. Other factors affecting maximum reimbursement are accurate diagnostic code selection and linking the proper service or procedures provided to the patient.

Code set (8): Any set of codes with their descriptions used to encode data elements, such as tables of terms, medical concepts, medical diagnostic codes, or medical procedure codes.

Coinsurance (3, 13): 1. A cost-sharing requirement under a health insurance policy providing that the insured will assume a percentage of the costs for covered services. 2. For Medicare, after application of the yearly cash deductible, the portion of the reasonable charges (20%) for which the beneficiary is responsible. 3. In the Medicaid Qualified Medicare Beneficiary (MQMB) program, the amount of payment that is above the rate that Medicare pays for medical services. The state assumes responsibility for payment of this amount.

Collateral (10): Any possession, such as an automobile, furniture, stocks, or bonds, that secures or guarantees the discharge of an obligation.

Collection ratio (10): The relationship between the amount of money owed and the amount of money collected in reference to the doctor's accounts receivable.

Combination code (5): A code from one section of the procedural code book combined with a code from another section that is used to completely describe a

Ergonomic (15): Science and technology that seek to fit the anatomic and physical needs of the worker to the workplace.

Essential modifiers (5): In ICD-10-CM, subterms that are indented two spaces to the right under main terms. They are referred to as essential modifiers because their presence changes the diagnostic code assignment.

Established patient (4): An individual who has received professional services within the past 3 years from the physician or another physician of the same specialty who belongs to the same group practice.

Estate administrator (10): One who takes possession of the assets of a decedent, pays the expenses of administration and the claims of creditors, and disposes of the balance of an estate in accordance with the statutes governing the distribution of decedent's estates.

Estate executor (10): One who takes possession of the assets of a decedent, pays the expenses of administration and the claims of creditors, and disposes of the balance of an estate in accordance with the decedent's will.

Ethics (1): Standards of conduct generally accepted as a moral guide for behavior by which an insurance billing or coding specialist may determine the appropriateness of his or her conduct in a relationship with patients, the physician, co-workers, the government, and insurance companies.

Etiology (5): The cause of disease; the study of the cause of a disease.

Etiquette (1): Customs, rules of conduct, courtesy, and manners of the medical profession.

Exchanges (3): Organized marketplace where uninsured individuals and small-business owners can find health insurance coverage and select from all of the qualified health plans available in their area. Also referred to as *Health Benefit Exchanges.*

Excludes 1 (5): Word with number that is one of the conventions used in the diagnostic code book titled *International Classification of Diseases,* Tenth Revision, Clinical Modification (ICD-10-CM). This indicates that the code excluded should never be used at the same time as the code above the Excludes 1 note. An Excludes 1 is when two conditions cannot occur together (for example, congenital form versus acquired form of a condition). A note instructs the reader to go to another code for the excluded condition. This convention does not appear in the former ICD-9-CM code books.

Excludes 2 (5): Word with number that is one of the conventions used in the diagnostic code book titled *International Classification of Diseases,* Tenth Revision, Clinical Modification (ICD-10-CM). This note represents "Not included here" and indicates that the condition excluded is not part of the condition represented by the code but a patient may have both conditions at the same time. When an Excludes 2 note

appears under a code, it is acceptable to use both the code and the excluded code together. This convention does not appear in the former ICD-9-CM code books.

Exclusion(s) (3, 16): Provisions written into the insurance contract denying coverage or limiting the scope of coverage.

Exclusive provider organization (EPO) (3, 11): A type of managed health care plan that combines features of health maintenance organizations (HMOs) and preferred provider organizations (PPOs). It is referred to as "exclusive" because it is offered to large employers who agree not to contract with any other plan. EPOs are regulated under state health insurance laws.

Expanded problem focused (EPF) (4): A phrase used to describe a level of history or physical examination.

Explanation of benefits (EOB) (9): A document detailing services billed and describing payment determinations; also known in Medicare, Medicaid, and some other programs as a remittance advice (RA). In the TRICARE program, it is called a summary payment voucher.

Explanation of Medicare benefits (EOMB) (8): See Remittance advice (RA).

Expressed contract (3): A verbal or written agreement.

Extended (3): To carry forward the balance of an individual financial accounting record.

External audit (4): A review done after claims have been submitted (retrospective review) of medical and financial records by an insurance company or Medicare representative to investigate suspected fraud or abusive billing practices.

External causes of morbidity (5): Classification of codes used for external causes of injury rather than disease. The code description refers to the circumstances that caused an injury rather than the nature of the injury. The codes are also used in coding adverse reactions to medications.

Extraterritorial (15): State laws effective outside the state by either specific provision or court decision. In workers' compensation cases, benefits under the state law that apply to a compensable injury of an employee hired in one state but injured outside that state.

Facility billing (1): Charging for services done in hospitals, acute care hospitals, skilled nursing or long-term care facilities, rehabilitation centers, or ambulatory surgical centers.

Facility provider number (7): A facility's (hospital, laboratory, radiology office, or nursing facility) provider number to be used by the facility to bill for services, or by the performing physician to report services done at that location.

Family history (FH) (4): A review of medical events in the patient's family, including diseases that may be hereditary or place the patient at risk.

Federal Employees' Compensation Act (FECA) (15): An Act instituted in 1908 providing benefits for on-the-job injuries to all federal employees.

Federal Employees Retirement System (FERS) (16): A program for federal employees hired after 1984 or those hired before 1984 who switched from Civil Service Retirement System (CSRS) to FERS.

Fee-for-service (FFS) (11): A method of payment in which the patient pays the physician for each professional service performed from an established schedule of fees.

Fee schedule (6, 10, 15): A list of charges or established allowances for specific medical services and procedures. See also Relative value studies (RVS).

Financial accounting record (3, 10): An individual record indicating charges, payments, adjustments, and balances owed for services rendered; also known as a ledger.

Fiscal agent (13): An organization under contract to the state to process claims for a state Medicaid program; insurance carrier handling claims from physicians and other suppliers of service for Medicare Part B; also referred to as Medicare administrative contractor (MAC), formerly fiscal intermediary.

Formal referral (11): An authorization request (telephone, fax, or completed form) required by the managed care organization contract to determine medical necessity and grant permission before services are rendered or procedures performed.

Formulary (12): List of drugs that a health insurance plan covers as a benefit.

Foundation for medical care (FMC) (3, 11): An organization of physicians sponsored by a state or local medical association concerned with the development and delivery of medical services and the cost of health care.

Fraud (2): An intentional misrepresentation of the facts to deceive or mislead another.

Functional résumé (18): A data sheet that highlights qualifications and skills.

Future purchase option (16): See Cost-of-living adjustment.

Garnishment (10): A court order attaching a debtor's property or wages to pay off a debt.

Gatekeeper (11): In the managed care system, this is the physician who controls patient access to specialists and diagnostic testing services.

Global surgery policy (6): A Medicare policy relating to surgical procedures in which preoperative and postoperative visits (24 hours before [major] and day of [minor]), usual intraoperative services, and complications not requiring additional trips to the operating room are included in one fee.

Group National Provider Identifier (group NPI) (7): A number assigned to a group of physicians submitting insurance claims under the group name and reporting income under one name.

Grouper (17): The computer software program that assigns diagnosis-related groups (DRGs) of discharged patients using the following information: patient's age, sex, principal diagnosis, complications/comorbid conditions, principal procedure, and discharge status.

Guaranteed renewable (3, 16): A clause in an insurance policy that means the insurance company must renew the policy as long as premium payments are made. However, the premium may be increased when it is renewed. These policies may have age limits of 60, 65, or 70 years or may be renewable for life.

Guarantor (3): An individual who promises to pay the medical bill by signing a form agreeing to pay or who accepts treatment, which constitutes an expressed promise.

Health benefits advisor (HBA) (14): An individual at military hospitals or clinics who is there to help TRICARE beneficiaries obtain medical care through the military and through TRICARE.

Health care finder (HCF) (14): Health care professionals, generally registered nurses, who are located at TRICARE service centers (TSCs) to act as a liaison between military and civilian providers, verify eligibility, determine availability of services, coordinate care, facilitate the transfer of records, and perform first level medical review. HCFs help TRICARE beneficiaries and providers with preauthorization of medical services.

Health Care Fraud Prevention and Enforcement Action Team (HEAT) (2): Group created in 2009 by the Department of Justice and the Department of Health and Human Services to build and strengthen programs to combat Medicare and Medicaid fraud and to crack down on fraud perpetrators.

Health care provider (2): A provider of medical or health services and any other person or organization who furnishes bills or is paid for health care in the normal course of business.

Health insurance (3): A contract between the policyholder or member and insurance carrier or government program to reimburse the policyholder or member for all or a portion of the cost of medical care rendered by health care professionals; generic term applying to lost income arising from illness or injury; also known as accident and health insurance or disability income insurance.

Health Insurance Claim Form (CMS-1500 [02-12]) (7): Known as CMS-1500. A universal insurance claim form developed and approved by the American Medical Association (AMA) Council on Medical Service and the Centers for Medicare and Medicaid Services (CMS). It is used by physicians and other professionals to bill outpatient services and supplies to TRICARE, Medicare, and some Medicaid programs as well as some private insurance carriers and managed care plans.

Health maintenance organization (HMO) (3, 11): The oldest of all prepaid health plans. A comprehensive health care financing and delivery organization that provides a wide range of health care services with an emphasis on preventive medicine to enrollees within a geographic area through a panel of providers. Primary care physician "gatekeepers" are usually reimbursed via capitation. In general, enrollees do not receive coverage for the services from providers who are not in the HMO network, except for emergency services.

Health record (4): Written or graphic information documenting facts and events during the rendering of patient care. Also known as medical record.

Healthcare Common Procedure Coding System (HCPCS) (6): The Centers for Medicare and Medicaid Services' (CMS's) Common Procedure Coding System. A three-tier national uniform coding system developed by the CMS, formerly Health Care Financing Administration (HCFA), used for reporting physician or supplier services and procedures under the Medicare program. Level I codes are national Current Procedural Terminology (CPT) codes. Level II codes are HCPCS national codes used to report items not covered under CPT. Level III codes are HCPCS regional or local codes used to identify new procedures or items for which there is no national code. Pronounced "hick-picks."

Hearing (16): The second level of the appeal process for an individual applying for Social Security Disability Insurance (SSDI) or Supplemental Security Income (SSI). This is a hearing before an administrative law judge who had no part in the initial or reconsideration disability determination.

High complexity (HC) (4): A phrase used to describe a type of medical decision making when a patient is seen for an evaluation and management (E/M) service.

High risk (3): A high chance of loss.

HIPAA Omnibus Rule (2): Regulation that became effective in 2013 under the Health Insurance Portability and Accountability Act (HIPAA) that modified privacy and security rules for covered entities and their business associates.

HIPAA Transaction and Code Set (TCS) rule (8): This regulation under the Health Insurance Portability and Accountability Act (HIPAA) defines the standardized methods for transmitting electronic health information. The TCS process includes any set of HIPAA-approved codes with their descriptions used to encode data elements, such as tables of terms, medical concepts, medical diagnostic codes, or medical procedure codes. TCS regulations were implemented to streamline electronic data interchange.

History of present illness (HPI) (4): A chronologic description of the development of the patient's present illness from the first sign or symptom or from the previous encounter to the present.

Hospice (12): A public agency or private organization primarily engaged in providing pain relief, symptom management, and supportive services to terminally ill patients and their families in their own homes or in a homelike center.

Hospital insurance (12): A program providing basic protection against the costs of hospital and related after-hospital services for individuals eligible under the Medicare program. Known as Medicare Part A.

Immigrant (18): An individual belonging to another country or people; a foreigner. Referred to as an immigrant when a person from another country comes to settle.

Implied contract (3): A contract between physician and patient not manifested by direct words but implied or deduced from the circumstance, general language, or conduct of the patient.

In-area (11): Within the geographic boundaries defined by a health maintenance organization (HMO) as the area in which it will provide medical services to its members.

Incomplete claim (7): Any Medicare claim missing necessary information; such claims are identified to the provider so that they may be resubmitted.

Indemnity (3): Benefits paid to an insured while disabled; also known as reimbursement.

Indemnity Health Insurance (3): Traditional or fee-for-service health insurance plan that allows patients maximum flexibility and choice of provider for a fixed monthly premium. Medical services are paid at a percentage of covered benefits after an annual deductible is paid. Providers are paid each time a service is rendered on a fee-for-service basis. Also referred to as indemnity benefits plan.

Independent (or individual) practice association (IPA) (3, 11): A type of health maintenance organization (HMO) in which a program administrator contracts with a number of physicians who agree to provide treatment to subscribers in their own offices. Physicians are not employees of the managed care organization (MCO) and are not paid salaries. They receive reimbursement on a capitation or fee-for-service basis; also referred to as a medical capitation plan.

Individually identifiable health information (IIHI) (2): Any part of an individual's health information, including demographic information (for example, address, date of birth) collected from the individual, that is created or received by a covered entity.

Injury (15): In a workers' compensation policy, this term signifies any trauma or damage to a body part or disease sustained, arising out of, and in the course of employment, including injury to artificial members and medical braces of all types.

Inpatient (17): A term used when a patient is admitted to the hospital for overnight stay.

Inquiry (9): See Tracer.

In situ (5): A description applied to a malignant growth confined to the site of origin without invasion of neighboring tissues.

Insurance adjuster (15): An individual at the workers' compensation insurance carrier overseeing an industrial case, authorizing diagnostic testing and medical treatment, and communicating with the provider of medical care.

Insurance balance billing (10): A statement sent to the patient after his or her insurance company has paid its portion of the claim.

Insurance billing specialist (1): A practitioner who carries out claims completion, coding, and billing responsibilities and may or may not perform managerial and supervisory functions; also known as an insurance claims processor, reimbursement specialist, medical billing representative, or senior billing representative.

Insurance poster (9): Individual working for a medical practice or hospital that inserts payments received, adjustments (credits or write-offs), and denials from insurance companies, patients, and governmental agencies into patient financial accounts. Also known as insurance payment poster, payment coordinator, payment representative, or reimbursement coordinator.

Insurance posting (9): Process of applying payments and adjustments (credits or write-offs) to patient financial accounts.

Insured (3): An individual or organization protected in case of loss under the terms of an insurance policy.

Intelligent character recognition (ICR) (7): Same as Optical character recognition.

Intermediate care facility (ICF) (12): Institution furnishing health-related care and services to individuals who do not require the degree of care provided by acute care hospitals or nursing facilities.

Internal review (4): The process of going over financial documents before and after billing to insurance carriers to determine documentation deficiencies or errors.

International Classification of Diseases, Ninth Revision, Clinical Modification (ICD-9-CM) (5, 17): A diagnostic code book that uses a system for classifying diseases and operations to assist collection of uniform and comparable health information. A code system to replace this is ICD-10, which is being modified for use in the United States.

International Classification of Diseases, Tenth Revision, Clinical Modification (ICD-10-CM) (5, 17): A diagnostic code book that uses a system for classifying diseases and operations to assist collection of uniform and comparable health information. It has been modified, was implemented on October 1, 2013, and replaces ICD-9-CM Volumes 1 and 2 when submitting insurance claims for billing hospital and physician office medical services.

International Classification of Diseases, Tenth Revision, Procedure Coding System (ICD-10-PCS) (5, 17): Procedural code system developed by 3M Health Information Systems (HIS) under contract with the Centers for Medicare and Medicaid Services (CMS). When implemented on October 1, 2014, it replaced ICD-9-CM Volume 3 for hospital inpatient procedure reporting in the United States.

Interview (18): Meeting an individual face to face for evaluating and questioning a job applicant.

Intoxication (5): A diagnostic coding term that relates to an adverse effect rather than a poisoning when drugs, such as digitalis, steroid agents, and so on, are involved.

Invalid claim (7): Any Medicare claim that contains complete, necessary information but is illogical or incorrect (for example, listing an incorrect provider number for a referring physician). Invalid claims are identified to the provider and may be resubmitted.

Itemized statement (10): A detailed summary of all transactions of a patient's account: dates of service, detailed charges, payments (copayments and deductibles), date on which the insurance claim was submitted, adjustments, and account balance.

Late effect (5): An inactive residual effect or condition produced after the acute phase of an illness or injury has ended.

Ledger card (3, 10): See Financial accounting record.

Legible (4): Pertaining to a health record, data that is easily recognizable by individuals outside of a medical practice who are unfamiliar with the particular handwriting.

Lien (10, 15): A claim on the property of another as security for a debt. In litigation cases, it is a legal promise to satisfy a debt owed by the patient to the physician out of any proceeds received on the case.

Limiting charge (12): A percentage limit on fees, specified by legislation, that nonparticipating physicians may bill Medicare beneficiaries above the fee schedule amount.

List service (listserv) (1): An online computer service run from a website where questions may be posted by subscribers.

Long-term disability insurance (16): A provision to pay benefits to a covered disabled person to age 65.

Looping (17): The automated grouper (computer software program that assigns diagnosis-related groups [DRGs]) process of searching all listed diagnoses for the presence of any comorbid condition or complication or of searching all procedures for operating room procedures or other specific procedures.

Lost claim (9): An insurance claim that cannot be located after sending it to an insurer.

Low complexity (LC) (4): Phrase used to describe a type of medical decision making when a patient is seen for an evaluation and management (E/M) service.

Major complication/comorbidity (MCC) (17): Main underlying condition or other condition that arises or exists along with the condition for which the patient is receiving treatment. Used in diagnostic-related group (DRG) reimbursement.

Major diagnostic category (MDC) (17): A broad classification of diagnoses. There are 83 coding system–oriented MDCs in the original diagnosis-related groups (DRGs) and 23 body system–oriented MDCs in the revised set of DRGs.

Major medical (3): A health insurance policy designed to offset heavy medical expenses resulting from catastrophic or prolonged illness or injury.

Malignant tumor (5): An abnormal growth that has the properties of invasion and metastasis (for example, transfer of diseases from one organ to another). The word "carcinoma" refers to a cancerous or malignant tumor.

Managed care organization (MCO) (11): A generic term applied to a managed care plan. May apply to exclusive provider organization (EPO), health maintenance organization (HMO), preferred provider organization (PPO), integrated delivery system, or other different managed care arrangement. MCOs are usually prepaid group plans and physicians are typically paid by the capitation method.

Mandated benefit (3): Health service (treatment or procedure) required by state and/or federal law that may be given to a patient for a specific health condition. This health service may be delivered by certain types of health care providers for some categories of dependents, such as children placed for adoption. Also referred to as mandated services.

Manual billing (10): Processing statements by hand; may involve typing statements or photocopying the patient's financial accounting record and placing it in a window envelope, which then becomes the statement.

Maternal and Child Health Program (MCHP) (3, 13): A state service organization to assist children younger than 21 years of age who have conditions leading to health problems.

Medicaid (3, 13): A federally aided, state-operated, and state-administered program that provides medical benefits for certain low-income persons in need of health and medical care. California's Medicaid program is known as Medi-Cal.

Medi-Cal (13): California's version of the nationwide program known as Medicaid. See Medicaid.

Medical billing representative (1): See Insurance billing specialist.

Medical decision making (MDM) (4): Health care management process done after performing a history and physical examination on a patient that results in a plan of treatment. It is based on establishing one or more diagnoses and/or selecting a management or treatment option, amount of data or complexity of data reviewed, and complications and/or morbidity or mortality.

Medical necessity (4, 5, 9, 12): The performance of services and procedures that are consistent with the diagnosis in accordance with standards of good medical practice, performed at the proper level, and provided in the most appropriate setting. Medical necessity must be established (via diagnostic or other information presented on the individual claim under consideration) before the carrier may make payment.

Medical report (4): A permanent, legal document (letter or report format) that formally states the consequences of the patient's examination or treatment. See also Health record.

Medical service order (15): An authorization given to the physician, either written or verbal, to treat the injured or ill employee.

Medically needy (MN) (13): Persons in need of financial assistance or whose income and resources will not allow them to pay for the costs of medical care; also called medically indigent in some states.

Medically (or psychologically) necessary (3, 14): Medical or psychological services considered appropriate care and generally accepted by qualified professionals to be reasonable and adequate for the diagnosis and treatment of illness, injury, pregnancy, and mental disorders or that are reasonable and adequate for well-baby care.

Medicare (3, 12): A nationwide health insurance program for people age 65 years of age and older and certain disabled or blind persons regardless of income, administered by Centers for Medicare and Medicaid Services (CMS). Local Social Security offices take applications and supply information about the program.

Medicare administrative contractor (MAC) (12): Insurance carrier that receives and processes claims from physicians and other suppliers of service for Medicare Part B; formerly referred to as fiscal intermediary, Medicare carrier, fiscal agent, Medicare Part B carrier, or contractor.

Medicare/Medicaid (Medi-Medi) (3, 12): Refers to an individual who receives medical or disability benefits from both Medicare and Medicaid programs; sometimes referred to as a Medi-Medi case or a crossover.

Medicare Part A (12): Hospital benefits of a nationwide health insurance program for persons age 65 years of age and older and certain disabled individuals regardless of income, administered by Centers for Medicare and Medicaid Services (CMS). Local Social Security offices take applications and supply information about the program.

Medicare Part B (12): Medical insurance of a nationwide health insurance program for persons age 65 years of age and older and certain disabled individuals regardless of income, administered by Centers for Medicare and Medicaid Services (CMS). Local Social Security offices take applications and supply information about the program.

Medicare Part C (12): Medicare Plus (+) Choice plans offer a number of health care options in addition to those available under Medicare Part A and Part B. Plans may include health maintenance organizations (HMOs), fee-for-service plans, provider-sponsored organizations, religious fraternal benefit societies (RFBSs), and Medicare medical savings accounts.

Medicare Part D (12): Stand-alone prescription drug plan, presented by insurance and other private companies that offer drug coverage that meets the standards established by Medicare. Other names for these plans are Part D private prescription drug plans (PDPs) or Medicare Advantage prescription drug plans (MA-PDs).

Medicare secondary payer (MSP) (12): The primary insurance plan of a Medicare beneficiary that must pay for any medical care or services first before Medicare is sent a claim.

Medicare Summary Notice (MSN) (12): A document received by the patient explaining amount charged, Medicare approved, deductible, and coinsurance for medical services rendered.

Medigap (MG) (12): A specialized supplemental insurance policy devised for the Medicare beneficiary that covers the deductible and copayment amounts typically not covered under the main Medicare policy written by a nongovernmental third-party payer. Also known as Medifill.

Member (3): Person covered under an insurance program's contract, including (1) the subscriber or contract holder who is the person named on the membership identification card and (2) in the case of (a) two-person coverage, (b) one adult–one child coverage, or (c) family coverage, the eligible family dependents enrolled under the subscriber's contract.

Mentor (18): Guide or teacher who offers advice, criticism, wisdom, guidance, and perspective to an inexperienced but promising protégé to help reach a life goal.

Metastasis (5): Process in which tumor cells spread and transfer from one organ to another site.

Military Treatment Facility (MTF) (14): All uniformed service hospitals or health clinics; also known as military hospitals or uniformed service hospitals.

Mitigation (2): For a breach of privacy under the Health Insurance Portability and Accountability Act (HIPAA), this means to alleviate the severity, reduce, or make mild any harmful effects of such violation.

Moderate complexity (MC) (4): A phrase used to describe a type of medical decision making when a patient is seen for an evaluation and management (E/M) service.

Modifier (6, 17): In Current Procedural Terminology (CPT) coding, a two-digit add-on number placed after the usual procedure code number to indicate a procedure or service has been altered by specific circumstances. The two-digit modifier may be separated by a hyphen. In HCPCS Level II coding, one-digit or two-digit add-on alpha characters, placed after the usual procedure code number (Example G-1).

Example G-1

27372-51

Multipurpose billing form (3): See Encounter form.

Multiskilled health practitioner (MSHP) (1): An individual cross-trained to provide more than one function, often in more than one discipline. These combined functions can be found in a broad spectrum of health-related jobs ranging in complexity, including both clinical and administrative functions. The additional skills added to the original health care worker's job may be of a higher, lower, or parallel level. The terms *multiskilled, multicompetent,* and *cross-trained* can be used interchangeably.

National alphanumeric codes (12): Alphanumeric codes developed by the Health Care Financing Administration (HCFA). See Healthcare Common Procedure Coding System (HCPCS).

National Certified Insurance and Coding Specialist (NCICS) (18): An insurance and coding certification that is awarded by an independent testing agency, the National Center for Competency Testing (NCCT).

National Provider Identifier (NPI) (7): A Medicare lifetime 10-digit number issued to providers. When adopted, it will be recognized by Medicaid, Medicare, TRICARE, and CHAMPVA programs and eventually may be used by private insurance carriers.

National Standard Format (NSF) (8): The name of the standardization of data to reduce paper and have more accurate information and efficient organization.

Neoplasm (5): Benign or malignant tumor.

Netback (10): Evaluating a collection agency's performance by taking the amount of monies collected and subtracting the agency's fees.

Networking (18): Exchanging information or services among individuals, groups, or institutions and making use of professional contacts.

Never event (6): Incident related to a wrong surgical device, patient protection, care management, environment, or criminal occurrence that results in injury or death due to error in health care management or failure to follow standard care or institutional practices or policies. Also referred to as serious reportable event.

New patient (NP) (4): An individual who has not received any professional services from the physician or another physician of the same specialty who belongs to the same group practice within the past 3 years.

No charge (NC) (10): Waiving the entire fee owed for professional care.

Noncancelable clause or policy (3, 16): An insurance policy clause that means the insurance company cannot increase premium rates and must renew the policy until the insured reaches the age stated in the contract. Some disability income policies have noncancelable terms.

Nondisability (ND) claim (15): A claim for an on-the-job injury that requires medical care but does not result in loss of working time or income.

Nonessential modifiers (5): In ICD-10-CM, modifiers that provide additional description and are enclosed in parentheses. They are referred to as nonessential modifiers because their presence or absence does not affect the diagnostic code assigned.

Nonexempt assets (10): One's total property (in bankruptcy cases) not falling in the exemption category, including money, automobile equity, and property, more than a specified amount, depending on the state in which the person lives.

Nonparticipating (nonpar) physician or provider (3, 12, 14): 1. A provider who does not have a signed agreement with Medicare and has an option about assignment. The physician may not accept assignment for all services or has the option of accepting assignment for some services and collecting from the patient for other services performed at the same time and place. 2. A provider who decides not to accept the determined allowable charge from an insurance plan as the full fee for care. Payment goes directly to the patient in this case and the patient is usually responsible for paying the bill in full.

Non-physician practitioner (NPP) (4): Health care provider who meets state licensing requirements to provide specific medical services. Medicare allows payment for services furnished by NPPs, including but not limited to advance registered nurse practitioners (ARNPs), certified registered nurse practitioners, clinical nurse specialists (CNSs), licensed clinical social workers (LCSWs), physician assistants (PAs), nurse midwives, physical therapists, speech therapists, and audiologists. Also referred to as midlevel practitioner, midlevel provider, or physician extender.

Nonprivileged information (2): Information consisting of ordinary facts unrelated to the treatment of the patient. The patient's authorization is not required to disclose the data unless the record is in a specialty hospital or in a special service unit of a general hospital, such as the psychiatric unit.

Not elsewhere classifiable (NEC) (5): This term is used in the ICD-9-CM diagnostic coding system when the code lacks the information necessary to code the term in a more specific category.

Not otherwise specified (NOS) (5): Unspecified. Used in ICD-9-CM numeric code system for coding diagnoses.

Notice of Privacy Practices (NPP) (2): Under the Health Insurance Portability and Accountability Act (HIPAA), a document given to the patient at the first visit or at enrollment explaining the individual's rights and the physician's legal duties in regard to protected health information (PHI).

Nursing facility (NF) (12): A specially qualified facility that has the staff and equipment to provide skilled nursing care and related services that are medically necessary to a patient's recovery; formerly known as a skilled nursing facility (SNF).

Occupational illness (or disease) (15): An abnormal condition or disorder caused by environmental factors associated with employment. It may be caused by inhalation, absorption, ingestion, or direct contact.

Occupational Safety and Health Administration (OSHA) (15): A federal agency that regulates and investigates safety and health standards in work locations.

Official Coding Guidelines for Coding and Reporting (5): Set of rules developed to accompany and complement the official conventions and instructions provided within the ICD-10-CM coding manual. The guidelines include definitions, standards, rules, general coding guidelines, and 21 chapter-specific guidelines. Adherence to the guidelines when assigning an ICD-10-CM diagnosis code is required under the Health Insurance Portability and Accountability Act (HIPAA) and has been adopted for all health care settings.

Optical character recognition (OCR) (7): A device that can read typed characters at very high speed and convert them to digitized files that can be saved on disk. Also known as intelligent character recognition (ICR).

Optionally renewable (3): An insurance policy renewal provision in which the insurer has the right to refuse to renew the policy on a date and may add coverage limitations or increase premium rates.

Ordering physician (4): The physician ordering non-physician services for a patient (for example, diagnostic laboratory tests, pharmaceutical services, or durable medical equipment [DME]) when an insurance claim is submitted by a non-physician supplier of services. The ordering physician also may be the treating or performing physician.

Other health insurance (OHI) (14): Health care coverage for TRICARE beneficiaries through an employer, an association, or a private insurer. A student in the family may have a health care plan through school.

Outpatient (17): A patient who receives services in a health care facility, such as a physician's office, clinic, urgent care center, emergency department, or ambulatory surgical center, and goes home the same day.

Overpayment (9): Money paid over and above the amount due by the insurer or patient.

Paper claim (7): An insurance claim submitted on paper, including those optically scanned and converted to an electronic form by the insurance carrier.

Partial disability (16): A disability from an illness or injury that prevents an insured person from performing one or more of the functions of his or her regular job.

Participating (par) physician or provider (3, 11, 12, 14): 1. A physician who contracts with a health maintenance organization (HMO) or other insurance company to provide services. 2. A physician who has agreed to accept a plan's payments for services to subscribers (for example, some Blue plans). Eighty percent of practicing American physicians are participating physicians. 3. A physician who agrees to accept payment from Medicare (80% of approved charges) plus payment from the patient (20% of approved charges) after the $100 deductible has been met. 4. One who accepts TRICARE assignment. Payment goes directly to the provider. The patient must still pay the cost-share outpatient deductible and the cost of care not covered by TRICARE. See Assignment.

Partnership program (14): A program that allows TRICARE-eligible individuals to receive inpatient or outpatient treatment from civilian providers of care in a military hospital or from uniformed services providers of care in civilian facilities.

Password (8): A combination of letters and numbers that each individual is assigned to access computer data.

Past history (PH) (4): A patient's past experiences with illnesses, operations, injuries, and treatments.

Patient registration form (3) A questionnaire designed to collect demographic data and essential facts about medical insurance coverage for each patient seen for professional services; also called patient information form.

Peer review (9): The review of a patient's case by one or more physicians using federal guidelines to evaluate another physician regarding the quality and efficiency of medical care. This is done to discover overuse or misuse of a plan's benefits.

Pending claim (7): An insurance claim held in suspense because of review or other reason. These claims may be cleared for payment or denied.

Per capita (11): See Capitation.

Percentage of revenue (17): The fixed percentage of the collected premium rate that is paid to the hospital to cover services.

Per diem (17): A single charge for a day in the hospital regardless of any actual charges or costs incurred.

Permanent and stationary (P and S) (15): A phrase used when a workers' compensation patient's condition has become stabilized and no improvement is expected. It is only after this declaration that a case can be rated for a compromise and release.

Permanent disability (PD) (15): An illness or injury (impairment of the normal use of a body part) expected to continue for the lifetime of the injured worker that prevents the person from performing the functions of his or her regular occupation, therefore impairing his or her earning capacity.

Personal insurance (3): An insurance plan issued to an individual (or his or her dependents); also known as individual contract.

Petition (15): A formal written request commonly used to indicate an appeal; also means any request for relief other than an application.

Phantom billing (2): Billing for services not performed.

Physical examination (PE or PX) (4): Objective inspection or testing of organ systems or body areas of a patient by a physician.

Physically clean claim (7): Insurance claims with no staples or highlighted areas. The bar code area has not been deformed.

Physician provider group (PPG) (11): A physician-owned business that has the flexibility to deal with all forms of contract medicine and still offer its own packages to business groups, unions, and the general public.

Physician Quality Reporting Initiative (PQRI) (12): Voluntary pay-for-reporting program for providers who successfully report quality information related to services provided to patients under Medicare Part B between July 1 and December 31, 2007.

Physician's fee profile (5): A compilation of each physician's charges and the payments made to him or her over a given period for each specific professional service rendered to a patient.

Placeholder (5): Last or seventh character that composes an ICD-10-CM diagnostic code indicated by an "X" that is used to allow space for future code expansion or to meet the requirement of coding to the highest level of specificity.

Point-of-service (POS) option (14): Individuals under the TRICARE program can choose to get TRICARE-covered nonemergency services outside the prime network of providers without a referral from the primary care manager and without authorization from a health care finder.

Point-of-service (POS) plan (3, 11): A managed care plan in which members are given a choice as to how to receive services, whether through a health maintenance organization (HMO), preferred provider organization (PPO), or fee-for-service plan. The decision is made at the time the service is necessary (for example, "at the point of service"); sometimes referred to as open-ended HMOs, swing-out HMOs, self-referral options, or multiple option plans.

Poisoning (5): A condition resulting from an overdose of drugs or chemical substances or from the wrong drug or agent given or taken in error.

Portfolio (18): A compilation of items that represents a job applicant's skills.

Posted (3): To record or transfer financial entries, debit or credit, to an account (for example, daysheet, financial account record [ledger], bank deposit slip, check register, journal).

Preadmission testing (PAT) (17): Treatment, tests, and procedures done 48 to 72 hours before admission of a patient to the hospital. This is done to eliminate extra hospital days.

Preauthorization (3, 14): A requirement of some health insurance plans to obtain permission for a service or procedure before it is done and to see whether the insurance program agrees that it is medically necessary.

Precertification (3): A procedure done to determine whether treatment (surgery, tests, or hospitalization) is covered under a patient's health insurance policy.

Predetermination (3): A financial inquiry done before treatment to determine the maximum dollar amount the insurance company will pay for surgery, consultations, postoperative care, and so forth.

Preexisting conditions (3): Illnesses or injuries acquired by the patient before enrollment in an insurance plan. In some insurance plans, preexisting conditions are excluded from coverage temporarily or permanently or may disqualify membership in the plan.

Preferred provider organization (PPO) (3, 11): A type of health benefit program in which enrollees receive the highest level of benefits when they obtain services from a physician, hospital, or other health care provider designated by their program as a "preferred provider." Enrollees may receive substantial, although reduced, benefits when they obtain care from a provider of their own choosing who is not designated as a "preferred provider" by their program.

Premium (3, 12): The cost of insurance coverage paid annually, semiannually, or monthly to keep the policy in force. In the Medicare program, the monthly fee that enrollees pay for Medicare Part B medical insurance. This fee is updated annually to reflect changes in program costs.

Prepaid group practice model (11): A plan under which specified health services are rendered by participating physicians to an enrolled group of persons, with fixed periodic payments made in advance, by or on behalf of each person or family. If a health insurance carrier is involved, it contracts to pay in advance for the full range of health services to which the insured is entitled under the terms of the health insurance contract. Such a plan is one form of a health maintenance organization (HMO).

Prepayment audit (4): Review of a submitted claim by an insurance carrier that is pended with a request to the physician to submit a copy of the patient's medical record to support the claim before payment is generated. The insurance carrier reviews the record to determine payment or nonpayment of the claim. Sometimes referred to as prospective audit.

Primary care manager (PCM) (14): A physician who is responsible for coordinating and managing all of the TRICARE beneficiary's health care unless there is an emergency.

Primary care physician (PCP) (4, 11): A physician (for example, family practitioner, general practitioner, pediatrician, obstetrician/gynecologist, general internist) who oversees the care of patients in a managed health care plan (HMO or PPO) and refers patients to specialists (for example, cardiologists, oncologists, surgeons) for services as needed. Also known as a gatekeeper.

Primary diagnosis (5): Initial identification of the condition or chief complaint for which the patient is treated for outpatient medical care.

Principal diagnosis (5, 17): A condition established after study that is chiefly responsible for the admission of the patient to the hospital.

Prior approval (PA) (13): The evaluation of a provider request for a specific service to determine the medical necessity and appropriateness of the care requested for a patient. Also called prior authorization in some states.

Privacy (2): The condition of being secluded from the presence or view of others.

Privacy officer, privacy official (PO) (2): An individual designated to help the provider remain in compliance by setting policies and procedures and by training and managing the staff regarding Health Insurance Portability and Accountability Act (HIPAA) and patient rights; usually the contact person for questions and complaints.

Privileged information (2): Data related to the treatment and progress of the patient that can be released only when written authorization of the patient or guardian is obtained.

Problem focused (PF) (4): A phrase used to describe a type of medical decision making when a patient is seen for an evaluation and management (E/M) service.

Procedure code numbers (6): Five-digit numeric codes that describe each service the physician renders to a patient.

Procedure review (17): A review of diagnostic and therapeutic procedures to determine appropriateness.

Professional billing (1): Charging for services performed by physicians or non-physician practitioners (NPPs).

Professional component (PC) (6): The portion of a test or procedure (containing both a professional and a technical component) that the physician performs (for example, interpreting an electrocardiogram [ECG], reading an x-ray, making an observation and determination using a microscope).

Professional courtesy (10): A discount or exemption from charges given to certain people at the discretion of the physician rendering the service. It is rarely used in current medicine.

Prospective audit (4): See Prepayment audit.

Prospective payment system (PPS) (12, 17): A method of payment for Medicare hospital insurance based on diagnosis-related groups (DRGs) (a fixed dollar amount for a principal diagnosis).

Prospective review (4): The process of going over financial documents before billing is submitted to the insurance company to determine documentation deficiencies and errors.

Protected health information (PHI) (2): Any data that identify an individual and describe his or her health status, age, sex, ethnicity, or other demographic characteristics, whether or not that information is stored or transmitted electronically.

Psychotherapy notes (2): Notes recorded in any medium by a health care provider who is a mental health professional documenting or analyzing the contents of conversation during a private counseling session or a group, joint, or family counseling session and that are separate from the rest of the individual's medical record.

Quality assurance program (14): A plan that continually assesses the effectiveness of inpatient and outpatient care in the TRICARE and CHAMPVA programs.

Quality Improvement Organization (QIO) (12, 17): A program that replaces the peer review organization program and is designed to monitor and improve the usage and quality of care for Medicare beneficiaries.

Qui tam action (2, 12): An action to recover a penalty brought on by an informer in a situation in which one portion of the recovery goes to the informer and the other portion goes to the state or government.

Readmission review (17): A review of patients readmitted to a hospital within 7 days with problems related to the first admission, to determine whether the first discharge was premature or the second admission is medically necessary.

Real time (8): Online interactive communication between two computer systems allowing instant transfer of information.

Reason for the encounter (17): First diagnosis stated or listed for an outpatient insurance claim.

Reasonable fee (6, 12): A charge is considered reasonable if it is deemed acceptable after peer review even though it does not meet the customary or prevailing criteria. This includes unusual circumstances or complications requiring additional time, skill, or experience in connection with a particular service or procedure. In Medicare, the amount on which payment is based for participating physicians.

Rebill (resubmit) (9): To send another request for payment for an overdue bill to either the insurance company or the patient.

Recipient (13): A person certified by the local welfare department to receive the benefits of Medicaid under one of the specific aid categories; an individual certified to receive Medicare benefits.

Reconsideration (16): The first level of appeal process for an individual applying for Social Security Disability Insurance (SSDI) or Supplemental Security Income (SSI). It is a complete review of the claim by a medical or psychological consultant or disability examiner team who did not take part in the original disability determination.

Recovery Audit Contractor (RAC) Initiative (12): Proposal of legislation that originally created a demonstration program that became permanently implemented when Congress enacted the Tax Relief and Health Care Act (TRHCA) of 2006. This extended the RAC program

to all 50 states by 2010. Its goals are to identify Medicare underpayments and overpayments and recover overpayments using automated review and complex review. An automated review is done electronically without human review and complex review is done using human review of the medical record.

Referral (4): The transfer of the total or specific care of a patient from one physician to another. In managed care, a request for authorization for a specific service.

Referring physician (4): A physician who sends the patient for testing or treatment noted on the insurance claim when it is submitted by the physician performing the service.

Regional contractor (14): For TRICARE and CHAMPVA, the insurance company that handles the claims for care received within a particular state or country. Also known as claims processor and formerly known as fiscal agent, fiscal carrier, or fiscal intermediary. For Medicare, see Medicare administrative contractor (MAC).

Regional office (RO) (16): A Social Security state office.

Registered Medical Assistant (RMA) (18): A title earned by completing appropriate training and passing a registry examination administered by the American Medical Technologists (AMT).

Registered Medical Coder (RMC) (18): A registered title awarded after completion of coursework given by the Medical Management Institute (MMI) with recertification requirements.

Registered nurse (RN) (17): Individual who has graduated from a course of study at a state-approved school of nursing, passed the National Council Licensure Examination (NCLEX-RN), and been licensed by appropriate state authority. Registered nurses are the most highly educated of nurses with the widest scope of responsibility, including, at least potentially, all aspects of nursing care. RNs work in a variety of settings (for example, hospital facilities, medical offices and clinics, public health departments, schools).

Registration (18): Entry in an official registry or record that lists names of persons in an occupation who have satisfied specific requirements or by attaining a certain level of education and paying a registration fee.

Reimbursement (9,10): Repayment; the term used when insurance payment is pending.

Reimbursement specialist (1): See Insurance billing specialist.

Rejected claim (7, 9): An insurance claim submitted to an insurance carrier that is discarded by the system because of a technical error (omission or erroneous information) or because it does not follow Medicare instructions. It is returned to the provider for correction or change so that it may be processed properly for payment.

Relative value studies or scale (RVS) (6): A list of procedure codes for professional services and procedures that are assigned unit values that indicate the relative value of one procedure over another.

Relative value unit (RVU) (6, 12): A monetary value assigned to each service on the basis of the amount of physician work, practice expenses, and cost of professional liability insurance. These three RVUs are then adjusted according to geographic area and used in a formula to determine Medicare fees.

Remittance advice (RA) (9, 12): A document detailing services billed and describing payment determination issued to providers of the Medicare or Medicaid program; also known in some programs as an explanation of benefits (EOB).

Resident physician (4): A physician who has finished medical school and is performing one or more years of training in a specialty area on the job at a hospital (medical center).

Residual benefits (16): A term used in disability income insurance for disability that is not work related. It is the payment of partial benefits when the insured is not totally disabled.

Residual disability (16): A disability from an illness or injury that prevents an insured person from performing one or more of the functions of his or her regular job. This is sometimes referred to as partial disability. See also Partial disability.

Resource-based relative value scale (RBRVS) (6, 12): A system that ranks physician services by units and provides a formula to determine a Medicare fee schedule.

Respite care (12): A short-term hospice inpatient stay for a terminally ill patient to give temporary relief to the person who regularly assists with home care of a patient.

Respondeat superior (1): "Let the master answer." Refers to a physician's liability in certain cases for the wrongful acts of his of her assistant(s) or employee(s).

Résumé (18): A summary of education, skills, and work experience, usually in outline form.

Retrospective review (4): The process of going over financial documents after billing an insurance carrier to determine documentation deficiencies and errors.

Review (9): To look over a claim to assess how much payment should be made.

Review of systems (ROS) (4): An inventory of body systems obtained through a series of questions used to identify signs or symptoms that the patient might be experiencing or has experienced.

Running balance (3): An amount owed on a credit transaction; also known as outstanding or unpaid balance.

Secondary diagnosis (5): A reason subsequent to the primary diagnosis for an office or hospital encounter that may contribute to the condition or define the need for a higher level of care but is not the underlying cause. There may be more than one secondary diagnosis.

Second-injury fund (15): See Subsequent-injury fund (SIF).

Secured debt (10): A debt (an amount owed) in which a debtor pledges certain property (collateral), in a written security agreement, to the repayment of the debt.

Security officer (2): A person who protects the computer and networking systems within the practice and implements protocols, such as password assignment, backup procedures, firewalls, virus protection, and contingency planning for emergencies.

Security Rule (2): Health Insurance Portability and Accountability Act (HIPAA) regulations related to the security of electronic protected health information (ePHI) that, along with regulations related to electronic transactions and code sets, privacy, and enforcement, compose the Administrative Simplification provisions.

Self-Directed Health Plan (SDHP) (3): See Consumer Directed Health Plan (CDHP).

Self-employment (18): Working for oneself, with direct control over work, services, and fees.

Self-referral (11): A patient in a managed care plan that refers himself or herself to a specialist. The patient may be required to inform the primary care physician (PCP).

Senior billing representative (1): See Insurance billing specialist.

Sequelae (5, 15): Diseased conditions after and usually resulting from a previous disease.

Service area (11): The geographic area defined by a health maintenance organization (HMO) as the locale in which it will provide health care services to its members directly through its own resources or arrangements with other providers in the area.

Service benefit program (14): A program (for example, TRICARE) that provides benefits without a contract guaranteeing the indemnification of an insured party against a specific loss; there are no premiums. TRICARE Standard is considered a service benefit program.

Service-connected injury (14): Injury incurred by a service member while on active duty or incurred during reserve duty with a military unit.

Service contract (18): A document that enumerates the obligations of a billing service and a medical practice stating the responsible party for each specific duty and task.

Service retiree (14): An individual who is retired from a career in the armed forces; also known as a military retiree.

Share of cost (13): The amount the patient must pay each month before he or she can be eligible for Medicaid; also known as liability or spend down.

Short-term disability insurance (16): A provision to pay benefits to a covered disabled person as long as he or she remains disabled, up to a specified period not exceeding 2 years.

Skip (10): A debtor who has moved and neglected to give a forwarding address (that is, skipped town).

Social history (SH) (4): An age-appropriate review of a patient's past and current activities (for example, smoking, diet intake, alcohol use).

Social Security Administration (SSA) (16): Administers Social Security Disability Insurance (SSDI) and Supplemental Security Income (SSI) programs for disabled persons.

Social Security Disability Insurance (SSDI) program (16): A federal entitlement program for long-term disability under Title II of the Social Security Act. It provides monthly benefits to workers and those self-employed who meet certain conditions.

Social Security number (SSN) (7): An individual's tax identification number issued by the federal government.

Sponsor (14): For the TRICARE program, the service person (active duty, retired, or deceased) whose relationship makes the patient (dependent) eligible for TRICARE.

Staff model (11): The type of health maintenance organization (HMO) in which the health plan hires physicians directly and pays them a salary.

Standard transactions (8): The electronic files in which medical data are compiled to produce a specific format.

State Children's Health Insurance Program (SCHIP) (3, 13): A state child health program that operates with federal grant support under Title V of the Social Security Act. In some states this program may be known as Maternal and Child Health Program (MCHP) or Children's Special Health Care Services (CSHCS).

State Disability Insurance (SDI) (3, 16): See Unemployment Compensation Disability.

State license number (7): A number issued to a physician who has passed the state medical examination indicating his or her right to practice medicine in the state where issued.

State preemption (2): A complex technical issue not within the scope of the health care provider's role; refers to instances when state law takes precedence over federal law.

Statute of limitations (10): A time limit established for filing lawsuits; may vary from state to state.

Stop loss (11, 17): An agreement between a managed care company and a reinsurer in which absorption of prepaid patient expenses is limited; or limiting losses on an individual expensive hospital claim or professional services claim; form of reinsurance by which the managed care program limits the losses of an individual expensive hospital claim.

Straightforward (SF) (4): Phrase used to describe a type of medical decision making when a patient is seen for an evaluation and management (E/M) service.

Subpoena (4): "Under penalty." A writ that commands a witness to appear at a trial or other proceeding and give testimony.

Subpoena duces tecum (4): "In his possession." A subpoena that requires the appearance of a witness with his or her records. Sometimes the judge permits the mailing of records and it is not necessary for the physician to appear in court.

Sub rosa films (15): Videotapes made without the knowledge of the subject; used to investigate suspicious claims in workers' compensation cases.

Subscriber (3): The contract holder covered by an insurance program or managed care plan who either has coverage through his or her place of employment or has purchased coverage directly from the plan or affiliate. This term is used primarily in Blue Cross and Blue Shield plans.

Subsequent-injury fund (SIF) (15): A special fund that assumes all or part of the liability for benefits provided to a worker because of the combined effect of a work-related impairment and a preexisting condition; also known as second-injury fund.

Summary payment voucher (14): The document that the fiscal agent sends to the provider or beneficiary, showing the service or supplies received, allowable charges, amount billed, amount TRICARE paid, how much deductible has been paid, and the patient's cost-share.

Supplemental benefits (16): Disability insurance provisions that allow benefits to the insured to increase the monthly indemnity or receive a percentage of the policy premiums if an individual keeps a policy in force for 5 or 10 years or does not file any claims.

Supplemental Security Income (SSI) (12, 13, 16): A program of income support for low-income aged, blind, and disabled persons established by Title XVI of the Social Security Act.

Surgical package (6): Surgical procedure code numbers include the operation; local infiltration, digital block, or topical anesthesia; and normal, uncomplicated postoperative care. This is referred to as a package and one fee covers the whole package.

Suspended claim (9): An insurance claim that is processed by the insurance carrier but held in an indeterminate (pending) state about payment because of an error or the need for additional information.

Suspense (9): The pending indeterminate state of an insurance claim because of an error or the need for more information.

Syndrome (5): Another name for a symptom complex (a set of complex signs, symptoms, or other manifestations resulting from a common cause or appearing in combination, presenting a distinct clinical picture of a disease or inherited abnormality).

T-1 (8): A T-carrier channel that can transmit voice or data channels quickly.

Taxonomy codes (8): Numeric and alpha provider specialty codes that are assigned and classify each health care provider when transmitting electronic insurance claims.

Teaching physician (4): A physician who is responsible for training and supervising medical students, interns, or residents and who takes them to the bedsides of patients in a teaching hospital to review course and treatment.

Technical component (6): Portion of a test or procedure (containing both a technical and a professional component) that pertains to the use of the equipment and the operator who performs it (for example, electrocardiogram [ECG] machine and technician, radiography machine and technician, microscope and technician).

Temporary disability (TD) (15, 16): The recovery period after a work-related injury during which the employee is unable to work and the condition has not stabilized; a schedule of benefits payable for the temporary disability.

Temporary disability insurance (TDI) (16): See Unemployment Compensation Disability (UCD).

Tertiary care (11): Services requested by a specialist from another specialist (for example, neurosurgeons, thoracic surgeons, intensive care units).

The Joint Commission (TJC) (17): Formerly Joint Commission on Accreditation of Healthcare Organizations (JCAHO). Established in 1951 as Joint Commission on Accreditation of Hospitals (JCAH). It is a nonprofit accrediting body for clinics, hospitals, and other federal and military facilities. TJC reviews the policies, patient records, credentialing procedures, and quality assurance programs of the facility. When TJC awards official approval, it means the quality and high standards of the facility have been met after its scrutiny. This is the goal of every facility that goes through the process about every 3 years.

Third-party liability (15): Third-party liability exists if an entity is liable to pay the medical cost for injury, disease, or disability of a person hurt during the performance of his or her occupation and the injury is caused by an entity not connected with the employer.

Third-party subrogation (15): The legal process by which an insurance company seeks from a third party, who has caused a loss, recovery of the amount paid to the policyholder.

Total disability (16): A term that varies in meaning from one disability insurance policy to another. For example, a liberal definition might read: "The insured must be unable to perform the major duties of his or her specific occupation."

Total, permanent service-connected disability (14): A total, permanent disability incurred by a service member while on active duty.

Tracer (9): An inquiry made to an insurance company to locate the status of an insurance claim (for example, claim in review, claim never received).

Trading partner (8): See Business associate.

Trading partner agreement (8): See Business associate agreement.

Transaction (2): The transmission of information between two parties to carry out financial or administrative activities related to health care.

Transfer review (17): Review of transfers to different areas of the same hospital that are exempted from prospective payment.

Treating, or performing, physician (4): A provider who renders a service to a patient.

TRICARE (3): A three-option managed health care program offered to spouses and dependents of service personnel with uniform benefits and fees implemented nationwide by the federal government.

TRICARE Extra (14): A preferred provider organization (PPO)–type of TRICARE option in which the individual does not have to enroll or pay an annual fee. On a visit-by-visit basis, the individual may seek care from an authorized network provider and receive a discount on services and reduced cost-share (copayment).

TRICARE for Life (TFL) (14): A health care program that offers additional TRICARE benefits as a supplementary payer to Medicare for uniformed service retirees, their spouses, and survivors age 65 years of age or older.

TRICARE Prime (14): A voluntary health maintenance organization (HMO)–type option for TRICARE beneficiaries.

TRICARE service center (TSC) (14): An office staffed by TRICARE Health Care Finders and beneficiary service representatives.

Turfing (11): Transferring the sickest high-cost patients to other physicians so that the provider appears as a "low-utilizer" in a managed care setting.

Unbundling (6): The practice of using numerous Current Procedural Terminology (CPT) codes to identify procedures normally covered by a single code; also known as itemizing, fragmented billing, exploding, or a la carte medicine; billing under Medicare Part B for non-physician services to hospital inpatients furnished to the hospital by an outside supplier or another provider. Under the new law, unbundling is prohibited and all non-physician services provided in an inpatient setting will be paid as hospital services.

Uncertain behavior (5): Phrase used to describe certain types of neoplasms or lesions when future cell response cannot be predicted.

Unemployment Compensation Disability (UCD) (3, 16): Insurance that covers off-the-job injury or sickness and is paid for by deductions from a person's paycheck. This program is administered by a state agency and is sometimes also known as State Disability Insurance (SDI) or temporary disability insurance (TDI).

Uninterruptible power supply (UPS) (8): Electrical equipment that provide instantaneous emergency power to computers, data centers, and telecommunications equipment when the main power fails so there is no data loss or business disruption.

Unsecured debt (10): Any debt (amount owed) that is not secured or backed by any form of collateral.

Upcoding (6, 17): Deliberate manipulation of Current Procedural Terminology (CPT) codes for increased payment.

Urgent care (14): Medically necessary treatment that is required for illness or injury that would result in further disability or death if not treated immediately.

Use (2): The sharing, employment, application, utilization, examination, or analysis of individually identifiable health information (IIHI) within an organization that holds such information.

Usual, customary, and reasonable (UCR) (3, 6): A method used by insurance companies to establish their fee schedules in which three fees are considered in calculating payment: (1) the usual fee is the fee typically submitted by the physician, (2) the customary fee falls within the range of usual fees charged by providers of similar training in a geographic area, and (3) the reasonable fee meets the aforementioned criteria or is considered justifiable because of special circumstances. UCR uses the conversion factor method of establishing maximums, the method of reimbursement used under Medicaid by which state Medicaid programs set reimbursement rates using the Medicare method or a fee schedule, whichever is lower.

Utilization review (UR) (11, 17): A process, based on established criteria, of reviewing and controlling the medical necessity for services and providers' use of medical care resources. Reviews are carried out by allied health personnel at predetermined times during the hospital stay to assess the need for the full facilities of an acute care hospital. In managed care systems, such as a health maintenance organization (HMO), reviews are done to establish medical necessity, thus curbing costs. Also called utilization or management control.

Verbal referral (11): A primary care physician (PCP) informs the patient and telephones to the referring physician that the patient is being referred for an appointment.

Veteran (14): Any person who has served in the armed forces of the United States, especially in time of war; is no longer in the service; and has received an honorable discharge.

Veterans Affairs (VA) disability program (16): A program for honorably discharged veterans who file claim for a service-connected disability.

Veterans Affairs (VA) Outpatient Clinic (3): A facility where medical and dental services are rendered to a veteran who has a service-related disability.

Veterans Affairs (VA) outpatient clinic card (16): An identification card belonging to a retired member of the armed forces that is shown when receiving medical or dental services for service-related disabilities from a clinic.

Veterans Health Administration (CHAMPVA) (3, 14): Formerly known as Civilian Health and Medical Program of the Department of Veterans Affairs. A program for veterans with total, permanent, service-connected disabilities or surviving spouses and dependents of veterans who died of service-connected disabilities.

Volume performance standard (VPS) (12): The desired growth rate for spending on Medicare Part B physician services, set each year by Congress.

Voluntary disability insurance (16): A majority of employees of an employer voluntarily consent to be covered by an insured or self-insured disability insurance plan instead of a state plan.

Waiting period (WP) (15, 16): For disability insurance, the initial period of time when a disabled individual is not eligible to receive benefits even though unable to work; for workers' compensation, the days that must elapse before workers' compensation weekly benefits become payable. Also known as elimination period.

Waiver of premium (16): A disability insurance policy provision that an employee does not have to pay any premiums while disabled.

Whistleblowers (12): Informants who report physicians suspected of defrauding the federal government.

Withhold (11): A portion of the monthly capitation payment to physicians retained by the health maintenance organization (HMO) until the end of the year to create an incentive for efficient care. If the physician exceeds utilization norms, he or she will not receive it.

Work hardening (15): An individualized program of therapy using simulated or real job duties to build up strength and improve the worker's endurance so he or she can work up to 8 hours per day. Sometimes work site modifications are instituted to get the employee back to gainful employment.

Workers' Compensation Appeals Board (WCAB) (15): The board that handles workers' compensation liens and appeals.

Workers' compensation insurance (3, 15): A contract that insures a person against on-the-job injury or illness. The employer pays the premium for his or her employees.

Write-off (10): Assets or debts that have been determined to be uncollectable and are therefore adjusted off the accounting books as a loss.

Z codes (5): A classification of ICD-10-CM coding used to describe environmental events, circumstances, and conditions as the external cause of injury, poisoning, and other adverse effects. Z codes are also used in coding adverse reactions to medications.

zeroization (4): Method to dispose of confidential or sensitive information by writing repeated sequences of ones and zeros over the data.

Key Abbreviations

Chapter number(s) is (are) shown in parentheses after each term.

AAMA (American Association of Medical Assistants) (1)

AAMB (American Association of Medical Billers) (3)

AAPC (American Academy of Professional Coders) (3, 18)

ABC (alternative billing code) (6)

ABN (Advance Beneficiary Notice of Noncoverage) (12)

ACA (American Collectors Association) (1)

ADSM (active duty service member) (3, 14)

AEP (appropriateness evaluation protocol) (17)

AHA (American Hospital Association) (5, 6)

AHIMA (American Health Information Management Association) (1, 5, 18)

AIDS (acquired immunodeficiency syndrome) (16)

ALJ (administrative law judge) (9)

AMA (American Medical Association) (1)

AME (agreed medical evaluator) (15)

ANSI (American National Standards Institute) (8)

APC (ambulatory payment classification) (17)

A/R (accounts receivable) (3, 10)

ARRA (American Recovery and Reinvestment Act) (2, 4)

ASC (ambulatory surgery category) (17)

ASC X12 (Accredited Standards Committee X12) (8)

ASCA (Administrative Simplification Compliance Act) (7)

ASET (Administrative Simplification Enforcement Tool) (8)

ASHD (arteriosclerotic heart disease) (1)

ASP (application service provider) (8)

ATM (automatic teller machine) (8, 10)

BR (by report) (15)

C (comprehensive [level of history or examination]) (4)

C and R (compromise and release) (15)

CAC (computer-assisted coding) (5)

CAP (claims assistance professional) (1, 12, 18)

CC (chief complaint) (4, 5)

CC (complication/comorbidity) (17)

CCAP (Certified Claims Assistance Professional) (18)

CCI (Correct Coding Initiative) (12)

CCS (Certified Coding Specialist) (18)

CCS-P (Certified Coding Specialist–Physician) (18)

CCU (coronary care unit) (4)

CD (compact disk) (2)

CDHP (Consumer Directed Health Plan) (3)

CDM (charge description master) (17)

CDT (Current Dental Terminology) (7, 8)

CE (consultative examiner) (16)

CECP (Certified Electronic Claims Processor) (18)

CERT (Comprehensive Error Rate Testing) (2)

CF (conversion factor) (6)

CHAMPVA (Civilian Health and Medical Program of the Department of Veterans Affairs) (3, 14)

CLIA (Clinical Laboratory Improvement Amendments) (2, 12)

CM (Clinical Modification) (5)

CMA (Certified Medical Assistant) (18)

CMBS (Certified Medical Billing Specialist) (18)

CMHC (community mental health center) (17)

CMP (Civil Monetary Penalty) (2)

CMP (competitive medical plan) (3)

CMRS (Certified Medical Reimbursement Specialist) (18)

CMS (Centers for Medicare and Medicaid Services) (2, 9, 10, 12)

CMS-1450 (UB-04) (Centers for Medicare and Medicaid Services; Uniform Bill) (17)

CMS-1500 (02-12) (Centers for Medicare and Medicaid Services Health Insurance Claim Form) (7)

COB (coordination of benefits) (3)

COBRA (Consolidated Omnibus Budget Reconciliation Act) (3, 12)

copay (copayment) (11)

CPC (Certified Professional Coder) (18)

CPC-A (Certified Professional Coder–Apprentice) (18)

CPC-H (Certified Professional Coder–Hospital) (18)

CPT (Current Procedural Terminology) (5, 6)

CSRS (Civil Service Retirement System) (16)

D (detailed [level of history or examination]) (4)

DAB (departmental appeal board) (9)

DC (doctor of chiropractic) (12)

DCG (diagnostic cost group) (12)

DDE (direct data entry) (8)

DDS (Disability Determination Services) (16)

DEERS (Defense Enrollment Eligibility Reporting System) (14)

DEFRA (Deficit Reduction Act) (12, 13)

DHHS (Department of Health and Human Services) (2, 8)

DM (diabetes mellitus) (5)
DME (durable medical equipment) (6, 7, 12)
DNA (does not apply) (7)
DoD (Department of Defense) (3)
DOJ (Department of Justice) (2)
DOS (date of service) (3)
DRG (diagnosis-related group) (17)
DSL (digital subscriber line) (8)
dx or Dx (diagnosis) (4)
EBP (employee benefit plan) (11)
ECG (electrocardiogram) (6)
e-check (electronic check) (10)
ECP (electronic claims processor) (18)
ED or ER (emergency department or emergency room) (4, 6)
EDI (electronic data interchange) (8)
EEOC (Equal Employment Opportunity Commission) (18)
EFT (electronic funds transfer) (8)
EGHP (employee group health plan) (12)
EHR (electronic health record) (4, 8)
EIN (employer identification number) (7)
E/M (evaluation and management) (4, 6)
e-mail (electronic mail) (1)
EMC (electronic medical claim) (8)
EMG (emergency) (7)
EMR (electronic medical record) (4)
EMTALA (Emergency Medical Treatment and Active Labor Act) (6)
EOB (explanation of benefits) (6, 9)
EOMB (explanation of Medicare benefits) (8)
EPF (expanded problem focused [level of history or examination]) (4)
ePHI (electronic protected health information) (2, 8)
EPO (exclusive provider organization) (3, 11)
EPSDT (Early and Periodic Screening, Diagnosis, and Treatment) (7, 13)
ERA (electronic remittance advice) (8, 12)
ERISA (Employee Retirement Income Security Act) (9, 10, 11, 15)
ESRD (end-stage renal disease) (12)
FACT (Fair and Accurate Credit Transactions) (10)
FBI (Federal Bureau of Investigation) (2)
FCA (False Claims Act) (2)
FCBA (Fair Credit Billing Act) (10)
FCRA (Fair Credit Reporting Act) (10)
FDCPA (Fair Debt Collection Practices Act) (10)
FDIC (Federal Deposit Insurance Corporation) (2)
FECA (Federal Employees' Compensation Act) (15)
FEHBA (Federal Employee Health Benefit Act) (10)
FERA (Federal Enforcement and Recovery Act of 2009) (2)
FERS (Federal Employees Retirement System) (16)
FH (family history) (4)
FL (form locators) (17)
FMC (foundation for medical care) (3, 11)

FPL (federal poverty level) (13)
FSA (flexible spending account) (3)
FTC (Federal Trade Commission) (6, 9, 10)
FTM (full-time manager) (14)
FTP (file transfer protocol) (2)
GAF (geographic adjustment factor) (6)
GAO (General Accounting Office) (17)
GED (general equivalency diploma) (1)
GEM (general equivalence mapping) (5)
GPCIs (geographic practice cost indices) (6, 12)
HAC (Health Administration Center) (14)
HBA (health benefits advisor) (14)
HBMA (Healthcare Billing and Management Association) (3)
HC (high complexity [medical decision making]) (4)
HCERA (Health Care and Education Reconciliation Act) (3)
HCF (health care finder) (14)
HCFAC (Health Care Fraud and Abuse Control [program]) (2)
HCPCS (Healthcare Common Procedure Coding System) (6)
HDHP (high-deductible health plan) (3)
HEAT (Health Care Fraud Prevention and Enforcement Action Team) (2)
HEDIS (Health Plan Employer Data Information Set) (11)
HFMA (Healthcare Financial Management Association) (3)
HHS (Department of Health and Human Services) (2, 8)
HIM (health information management) (4)
HIPAA (Health Insurance Portability and Accountability Act) (1, 2, 9)
HITECH (Health Information Technology for Economic and Clinical Health [Act]) (2)
HIV (human immunodeficiency virus) (4, 16)
HMO (health maintenance organization) (3, 9, 10, 11)
HO (hearing officer) (9)
HPI (history of present illness) (4)
HPID (health plan identifier) (8)
HRA (health reimbursement account) (3)
HRS (Health Care Reimbursement Specialist) (18)
HSA (health savings account) (3)
IAIABC (International Association of Industrial Accident Boards and Commissions) (15)
ICD-9-CM (*International Classification of Diseases*, Ninth Revision, Clinical Modifications) (5, 17)
ICD-10-CM (*International Classification of Diseases*, Tenth Revision, Clinical Modifications) (5, 17)
ICD-10-PCS (*International Classification of Diseases*, Tenth Revision, Procedure Coding System) (5, 17)
ICD-11 (*International Classification of Diseases*, Eleventh Revision) (5)
ICF (intermediate care facility) (12)

ICR (intelligent character recognition or image copy recognition) (7)

ICU (intensive care unit) (4, 12)

IIHI (individually identifiable health information) (2)

IME (independent medical evaluator) (15)

IPA (independent [or individual] practice association) (3, 11)

IRS (Internal Revenue Service) (8)

LC (low complexity [medical decision making]) (4)

LCD (local coverage determination) (12)

LGHP (large group health plan) (12)

LHWCA (Longshore and Harbor Workers' Compensation Act) (15)

listserv (list service) (1)

LLQ (left lower quadrant) (4)

LMP (last menstrual period) (7)

LOS (length of stay) (17)

LUQ (left upper quadrant) (4)

MAAC (maximum allowable actual charge) (12)

MAB (Medical Association of Billers) (3)

MAC (Medicare administrative contractor) (8, 12)

MC (moderate complexity [medical decision making]) (4)

MCC (major complication/comorbidity) (17)

MCHP (Maternal and Child Health Program) (3, 13)

MCO (managed care organization) (11)

MDC (major diagnostic category) (17)

MDM (medical decision making) (4)

Medi-Medi (Medicare/Medicaid) (3, 12)

MG (Medigap) (12)

MGMA (Medical Group Management Association) (3)

MHS (Military Health System) (14)

MIP (Medicare Integrity Program) (2)

MMA (Medicare Prescription Drug, Improvement, and Modernization Act) (12)

MN (medically needy) (13)

MQMB (Medicaid Qualified Medicare Beneficiary) (13)

MRI (magnetic resonance imaging) (5)

MSA (medical savings account) (3, 12)

MS-DRG (Medicare Severity Diagnosis-Related Group) (17)

MSDS (material safety data sheet) (15)

MSHP (multiskilled health practitioner) (1)

MSN (Medicare Summary Notice) (12)

MSO (management services organization) (1)

MSP (Medicare secondary payer) (7, 12)

MTF (Military Treatment Facility) (14)

MTS (Medicare Transaction System) (8)

MU (meaningful use) (4)

NA or N/A (not applicable) (7, 10)

NAS (Nonavailability Statement) (14)

NC (no charge) (10)

NCCI (National Correct Coding Initiative) (6)

NCD (national coverage determination) (12)

NCHS (National Center for Health Statistics) (5)

NCICS (National Certified Insurance and Coding Specialist) (18)

NCQA (National Committee for Quality Assurance) (11)

ND (nondisability [claim]) (15)

NDC (National Drug Code) (8)

NEC (not elsewhere classifiable) (5)

NEMB (Notice of Exclusions from Medicare Benefits) (12)

NF (nursing facility) (12)

nonpar (nonparticipating [provider or physician]) (3, 12, 14)

NOS (not otherwise specified) (5)

NP (new patient) (4)

NPI (National Provider Identifier) (7, 9)

NPP (non-physician practitioner) (1, 4)

NPP (Notice of Privacy Practices) (2, 3)

NSF (nonsufficient funds or not sufficient funds) (10)

NSF (National Standard Format) (8)

NUCC (National Uniform Claim Committee) (7)

OASDI (Old Age, Survivors, and Disability Insurance) (12)

OBRA (Omnibus Budget Reconciliation Act) (12, 13)

OCNA (Other Carrier Name and Address) (12)

OCR (Office of Civil Rights) (2)

OHI (other health insurance) (14)

OIG (Office of the Inspector General) (2, 12)

OOY (over-one-year [claims]) (13)

OPPS (Outpatient Prospective Payment System) (17)

OR (operating room) (12)

ORT (Operation Restore Trust) (2)

OSHA (Occupational Safety and Health Administration) (2, 15)

PA (prior approval) (13)

P&P (policies and procedures) (2)

P and S (permanent and stationary) (15)

PAHCOM (Professional Association of Health Care Office Management) (3, 18)

par (participating [physician or provider]) (3, 12, 14)

PAT (preadmission testing) (17)

PAYRID (payer identification) (12)

PC (professional component) (6)

PCM (primary care manager) (14)

PCP (primary care physician) (4, 11)

PD (permanent disability) (15)

PE or PX (physical examination) (4)

PF (problem focused [level of history or examination]) (4)

PFFS (private fee-for-service [plan]) (12)

PFSH (past, family, or social history) (4)

PH (past history) (4)

PHI (protected health information) (2, 18)

PIN (provider identification number) (12)

PMS (practice management software or practice management system) (3, 8)

PO (privacy officer or privacy official) (2)

PO (postoperative) (4)
POR (problem-oriented record [system]) (4)
POS (place-of-service) (3, 4, 8, 9)
POS (point-of-service) (3, 11, 13, 14)
PPACA (Patient Protection and Affordable Care Act) (3)
PPG (physician provider group) (11)
PPO (preferred provider organization) (3, 11)
PPS (prospective payment system) (12)
PQRI (Physician Quality Reporting Initiative) (12)
PSO (provider-sponsored organization) (12)
QI (Qualifying Individuals [program]) (13)
QIO (Quality Improvement Organization) (11, 12, 17)
QISMC (Quality Improvement System for Managed Care) (11)
QMB (qualified Medicare beneficiary) (13)
QME (qualified medical evaluator) (15)
RA (remittance advice) (9, 12, 13)
RAC (Recovery Audit Contractor) (2, 12)
RBRVS (resource-based relative value scale) (6, 12)
RCU (respiratory care unit) (4)
RFBS (religious fraternal benefit society) (12)
RHIA (registered health information administrator) (17)
RHIT (registered health information technician) (17)
RLQ (right lower quadrant) (4)
RMA (Registered Medical Assistant) (18)
RMC (Registered Medical Coder) (18)
RN (registered nurse) (17)
RO (regional office) (16)
R/O (rule out) (4)
ROA (received on account) (3)
ROM (range-of-motion) (15)
ROS (review of systems) (4)
RUQ (right upper quadrant) (4)
RVS (relative value studies or scale) (6)
RVU (relative value unit) (6, 12)
SCHIP (State Children's Health Insurance Program) (3, 13)
SDHP (Self-Directed Health Plan) (3)
SDI (State Disability Insurance) (3, 16)
SDP (Self-Disclosure Protocol) (2)
SF (straightforward [medical decision making]) (4)
SH (social history) (4)
SHCP (Supplemental Health Care Program) (14)

SHOP (Small Business Health Options Program) (3)
SIF (subsequent-injury fund) (15)
SLMB (Specified Low-Income Medicare Beneficiary) (13)
SOAP (subjective objective assessment plan) (4)
SOF (signature on file) (3, 7, 12)
SOR (source-oriented record [system]) (4)
SSA (Social Security Administration) (16)
SSDI (Social Security Disability Insurance) (16)
SSI (Supplemental Security Income) (12, 13, 16)
SSN (Social Security number) (7)
TANF (Temporary Assistance to Needy Families) (13)
TC (technical component) (6)
TCS (Transaction and Code Set [rule]) (8)
TD (temporary disability) (15)
TDI (temporary disability insurance) (16)
TEFRA (Tax Equity and Fiscal Responsibility Act) (12, 13)
TFL (TRICARE for Life) (14)
TILA (Truth in Lending Act) (10)
TJC (The Joint Commission) (17)
TMA (TRICARE Management Activity) (14)
TPO (treatment, payment, or health care operations) (2)
TPR (TRICARE Prime Remote) (14)
TPRADFM (TRICARE Prime Remote for Active Duty Family Members) (14)
TSC (TRICARE service center) (14)
UB-04 (Uniform Bill–04) (17)
UCD (Unemployment Compensation Disability) (3, 16)
UCR (usual, customary, and reasonable) (6)
UPS (uninterruptible power supply) (8)
UR (utilization review) (11, 17)
USCIS (US Citizenship and Immigration Services) (18)
USFHP (Uniformed Services Family Health Plan) (14)
VA (Veterans Affairs) (3, 14, 16)
VPS (volume performance standard) (12)
W2 (wage and tax statement) (10)
WCAB (Workers' Compensation Appeals Board) (15)
WHO (World Health Organization) (5)
WNL (within normal limits) (4)
WP (waiting period) (15)
ZPIC (Zone Program Integrity Contractor) (2)

Index

Page numbers followed by *b*, *t*, and *f* indicate boxes, tables, and figures, respectively.